Cornelis J.P. Thijn

Radiology of the Hand

A Diagnostic Synopsis of Many General Diseases

Foreword by Louis A. Gilula

With 787 Figures

Springer-Verlag
Berlin Heidelberg NewYork Tokyo

Professor Dr. CORNELIS J.P. THIJN

Department of Radiology
State University Hospital
Groningen (Netherlands)

Radiographs prepared by
HARRY VAN DER ZWAAG

The cover design shows Fig. 1 on p. 34

ISBN 3-540-15345-4 Springer-Verlag Berlin Heidelberg New York Tokyo
ISBN 0-387-15345-4 Springer-Verlag New York Heidelberg Berlin Tokyo

Library of Congress Cataloging in Publication Data. Thijn, Cornelis Jacob Pieter, 1933- Radiology of the hand. Includes bibliographies and index. 1. Hand–Radiology. 2. Hand–Diseases–Diagnosis. 3. Diagnosis, Radioscopic. I. Title. [DNLM: 1. Handradiology. WE 830 T439r] RC951.T474 1985 617'.575'0757 85-10011
ISBN 0-387-15345-4 (U.S.)

Reproduction of figures: Gustav Dreher GmbH, Stuttgart.

Typesetting, printing, and bookbinding: Universitätsdruckerei H. Stürtz AG, Würzburg.
2121/3130-543210

Foreword

The continual growth of radiologic information makes it increasingly difficult for the practitioner to maintain current clinical knowledge. Radiologic textbooks containing much material for the practicing clinician are often impossible to review thoroughly. Such radiographic texts describing the hand as a window to the understanding of systemic disease are available, but there has been an absence of books which present an easily assimilated synopsis of this material.

Professor Thijn has elegantly presented all the major and many minor features of diseases and conditions that affect the skeleton, using hand roentgenograms as a window. He has also included numerous illustrations of key associated roentgenographic manifestations elsewhere in the body. His organized presentation of each entity, including introductory remarks, radiographic findings in the hand and other sites, differential diagnosis, and key references, forms a structure through which an appropriate evaluation of a clinical case may be made.

The concise synopsis of each disease entity, well illustrated by superb roentgenograms, provides an excellent structure for both the student first learning about such conditions and the practitioner researching an explanation for particular roentgenographic findings.

Professor Thijn has attempted, and I believe has succeeded admirably, to provide a source from which a student or practitioner of radiology may readily arrive at a differential diagnosis of an observed radiographic feature.

LOUIS A. GILULA, M.D.

Professor of Radiology
CoDirector, Musculoskeletal Section
Mallinckrodt Institute of Radiology
Washington University School of Medicine
St. Louis Missouri USA

Acknowledgments

Although the majority of the radiographs depicted are in the possession of the University Hospital of Groningen, a number of other colleagues have made important contributions for which I am most grateful. Material was drawn from the carefully documented radiological collections of Dr. G. Goedhard of the De Wever Hospital in Heerlen and Dr. M. Meradji of the Sophia Children's Hospital in Rotterdam.

The portion of the text dealing with bone tumors was written in close collaboration with Prof. Dr. J.D. Mulder and Dr. H.M.J.A. Kroon of the Netherlands Committee on Bone Tumours. The majority of the illustrations of these tumors are from the files of this committee.

I would like to thank my daughter Karin for her enormous help in typing the manuscript.

The following colleagues and radiological departments were helpful in the composition of this book, either by giving permission to use radiographs or by providing advice:

Dr. G.P.A. Smit	Department of Pediatrics, University Hospital, Groningen, Holland
Dr. C.R. Staalman	Emma Children's Hospital, Amsterdam, Holland
Dr. H.E. Schütte	St. Elisabeth's Hospital, Haarlem, Holland
Prof. Dr. H. Doorenbos	Department of Endocrinology, University Hospital, Groningen, Holland
Dr. R.L.F. Nienhuis	Department of Rheumatology, University Hospital, Groningen, Holland
Dr. A.A. Wouda	Department of Medicine, University Hospital, Groningen, Holland
Dr. A. Jonkers	Refaja Hospital, Stadskanaal, Holland
Prof. Dr. B. van Linge	Department of Orthopedics, University Hospital, Rotterdam, Holland
Dr. J.T. Wilmink	Department of Radiodiagnosis, University Hospital, Groningen, Holland
R.N. Laurini	Department of Pathology, University Hospital, Groningen, Holland
Dr. R. Dorsay	Kaiser Institute, San Francisco, USA
Dr. H. Loose	Freeman Hospital Newcastle, Great Britain
Dr. D.J. Sieniewicz	Bayview-Eglinton Radiology Department Toronto, Canada

Department of Radiodiagnosis, University Hospital, Rotterdam, Holland
Department of Radiodiagnosis, University Hospital, Nijmegen, Holland
Department of Anthropogenetics, University Hospital, Groningen, Holland

C.J.P. THIJN

Contents

1 Osteochondrodysplasias

1.1 Growth Defects of Tubular Bones and/or Spine

1.1.1 Thanatophoric Dysplasia

The most obvious clinical features of this sporadically occurring disorder are shortened limbs, a normal-sized trunk, a narrow thorax, a large head with a prominent forehead, and a protuberant abdomen. The affected infants are still-born or die of respiratory failure within hours or days after birth.

Radiographic Findings [1–3]

Hand

Very short tubular bones (especially first metacarpal)
Cupped and flared metaphyses
Bowing of tubular bones

Other Sites

Thorax: small short ribs
cupped anterior rib ends
small scapulae
Spine: platyspondylisis
relatively normal vertebral arches
wide intervertebral disc spaces
Pelvis: narrow sacroiliac notches
abnormal iliac bones
flat acetabula
short pubic bones
Long tubular bones: bowing (telephone-receiver configuration)
cupped metaphyses
flared metaphyses
Skull: prominent forehead
shortened skull base
Abdomen: bulging

Differential Diagnosis

Achondrogenesis [3–5]
Homozygous achondroplasia [3]
Torrance type short-limbed platyspondylic dwarfism [6]

References

1 Kaufman RL, Rimoin DL, Mc Alister WH, Kissane IM (1970) Thanatophoric dwarfism. Am J Dis Child 120:53–60
2 Saldino RM (1971) Lethal short-limbed dwarfism: achondrogenesis and thanatophoric dwarfism. AJR 112:185–189
3 Langer LO, Spranger JW, Greinacher I, Herdman RC (1969) Thanatophoric dwarfism. A condition confused with achondrogenesis and homozygous achondroplasia. Radiology 92:285–294
4 Kozlowski K, Masel J, Kunze D (1978) Neonatal death dwarfism. Fortschr Geb Röntgenstr Nuklearmed Ergänzungsband 129:626–633
5 Beluffi G (1977) Achondrogenesis, Type I. Fortschr Geb Röntgenstr Nuklearmed Ergänzungsband 127:341–344
6 Kaibara M, Yokoyama K, Nakano H (1983) Torrance type of lethal neonatal short-limbed platyspondylic dwarfism. Skeletal Radiol 10:17–19

a b

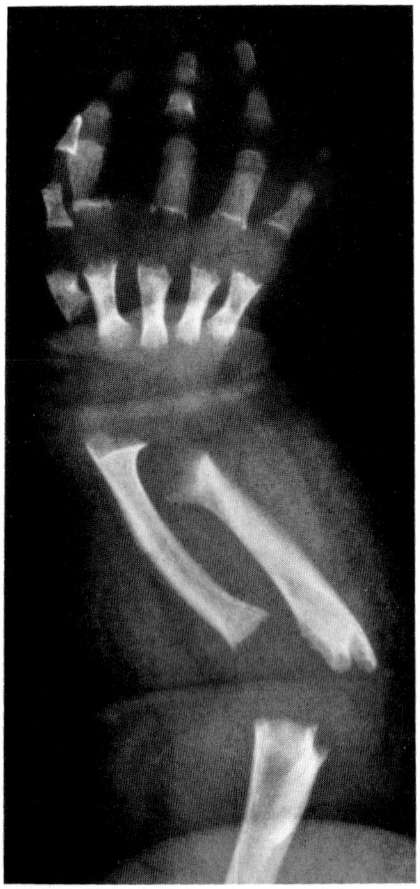

1

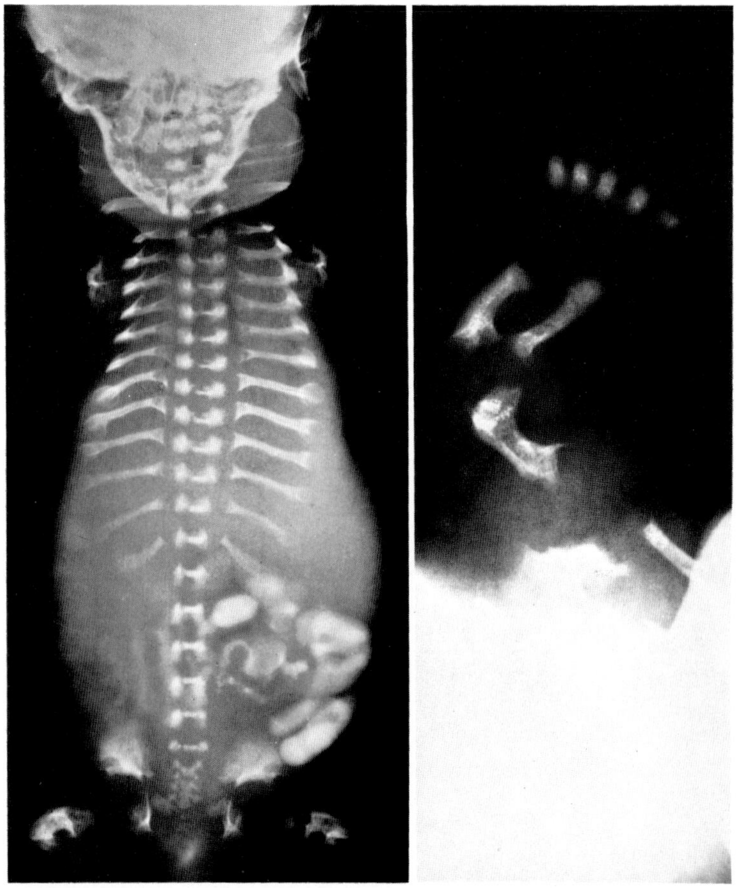

2

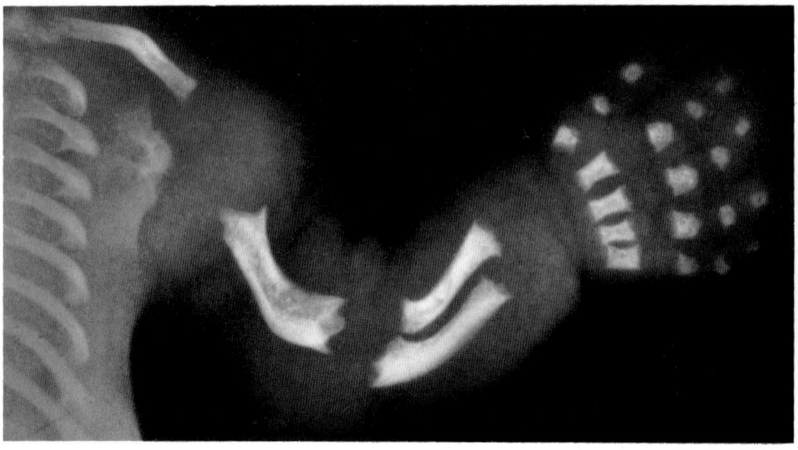

a

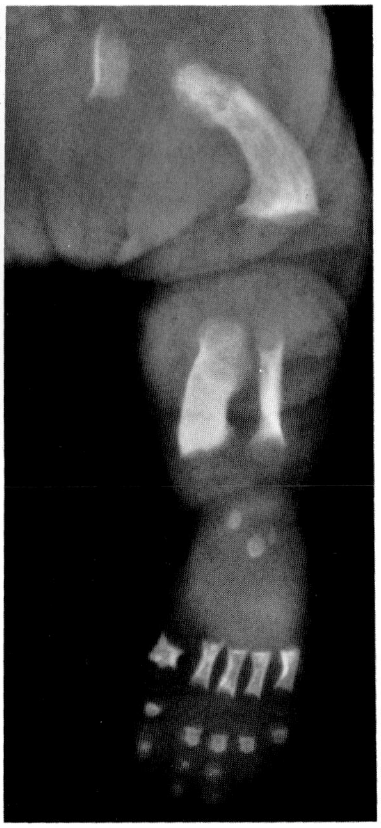

3 b

Fig. 1. Thanatophoric dysplasia. Still-born baby with shortened tubular bones, cupping and flaring of the metaphyses

Fig. 2a, b. Thanatophoric dysplasia. Still-born baby with typical abnormalities of tubular bones (telephone-receiver configuration), vertebral bodies, ribs, scapulae, and pelvic bones. **a** Head and trunk; **b** leg

Fig. 3a, b. Thanatophoric dysplasia. Characteristic deformation of the long tubular bones and very short tubular bones in the hand (**a**) and foot (**b**)

1.1.2 Chondrodysplasia Punctata

Synonyms: dysplasia epiphysealis punctata, stippled epiphyses, chondrodystrophia calcificans congenita

According to the International Nomenclature of Constitutional Diseases of Bone [1], chondrodysplasia punctata can be subdivided into an autosomal recessive rhizomelic type, an autosomal dominant type (Conradi-Hünermann), and a number of other types. In the rhizomelic and Conradi-Hünermann types, facies and skin changes are present; the intellect is normal in the latter. Severe shortening of the humerus and femur is a hallmark in the rhizomelic type. When the diagnosis has not been made in early childhood, it can be difficult to classify the abnormalities at an older age [2]. Patients with the rhizomelic type usually die before the age of 1 year. The prognosis of the Conradi-Hünermann patients is better, and survival into adult life is not uncommon [3–5, 7, 8].

Radiographic Findings [3–7]

	Rhizomelic type	Conradi-Hünermann type
Hand/foot		
Stippled densities in carpals and tarsals	+	+
Long tubular bones		
Symmetric shortening of humerus and femur	severe	absent or mild
Stippled densities	+	+
Splayed metaphyses	+	+
Spine		
Stippled densities (para) vertebral	±	+
Deformity of vertebral bodies	+ (coronal clefts)	+
Later on: platyspondylisis	–	+
Skull		
Flat facies, hypertelorism, low nasal bridge	+	+
Larynx/trachea		
Stippled densities	infrequently	frequently

Differential Diagnosis

Multiple epiphyseal dysplasia (Sect. 1.1.11)
Hypothyroidism (Sect. 7.2.1)
Spondyloepiphyseal dysplasia
Zellweger syndrome (cerebrohepatorenal syndrome)
Warfarin embryopathy

References

1 Special Report (1978) International nomenclature of constitutional diseases of bone. AJR 131:352–354
2 Kozlowski K (1980) Chondrodysplasia punctata in a nine year old girl presenting as "unclassified multiple malformation syndrome". Pediatr Radiol 9:236–238
3 Spranger JW, Bidder U, Voelz C (1970) Chondrodysplasia punctata (chondrodystrophia calcificans). Typ Conradi-Hünermann. Fortschr Geb Röntgenstr Nuklearmed Ergänzungsband 113:717–727
4 Spranger JW, Bidder U, Voelz C (1971) Chondrodysplasia punctata (chondrodystrophia calcificans) II. Der rhizomele Typ. Fortschr Geb Röntgenstr Nuklearmed Ergänzungsband 114:327–335
5 Cremin BJ, Beighton P (1978) Bone dysplasias of infancy. A radiological atlas. Springer, Berlin Heidelberg New York
6 Kaufmann HJ, Mahbouri S, Spackman TJ, Capitano MA, Kirkpatrick J (1976) Tracheal stenosis as a complication of chondrodysplasia punctata. Ann Radiol (Paris) 19:203–210
7 Sheffield LJ, Danks DM, Mayne V, Hutchinson AL (1976) Chondrodysplasia punctata – 23 cases of a mild and relatively common variety. J Pediatr 89:916–922
8 Hack WWM, Derksen-Samson JF, Grimberg RThTh, Harten JJ van der (1984) Chondrodysplasia punctata congenita: een genetisch heterogeen ziektebeeld. Tijdschr Kindergeneeskd 52:16–23

Fig. 2a–c. Same patient as ▷ Fig. 1. **a** Stippled densities in the larynx and trachea. **b** Stippled densities in the carpal bones and in the epiphyses of the radius, ulna, and humerus. **c** Characteristic pattern of densities in the pelvic bones and the proximal ends of the femora

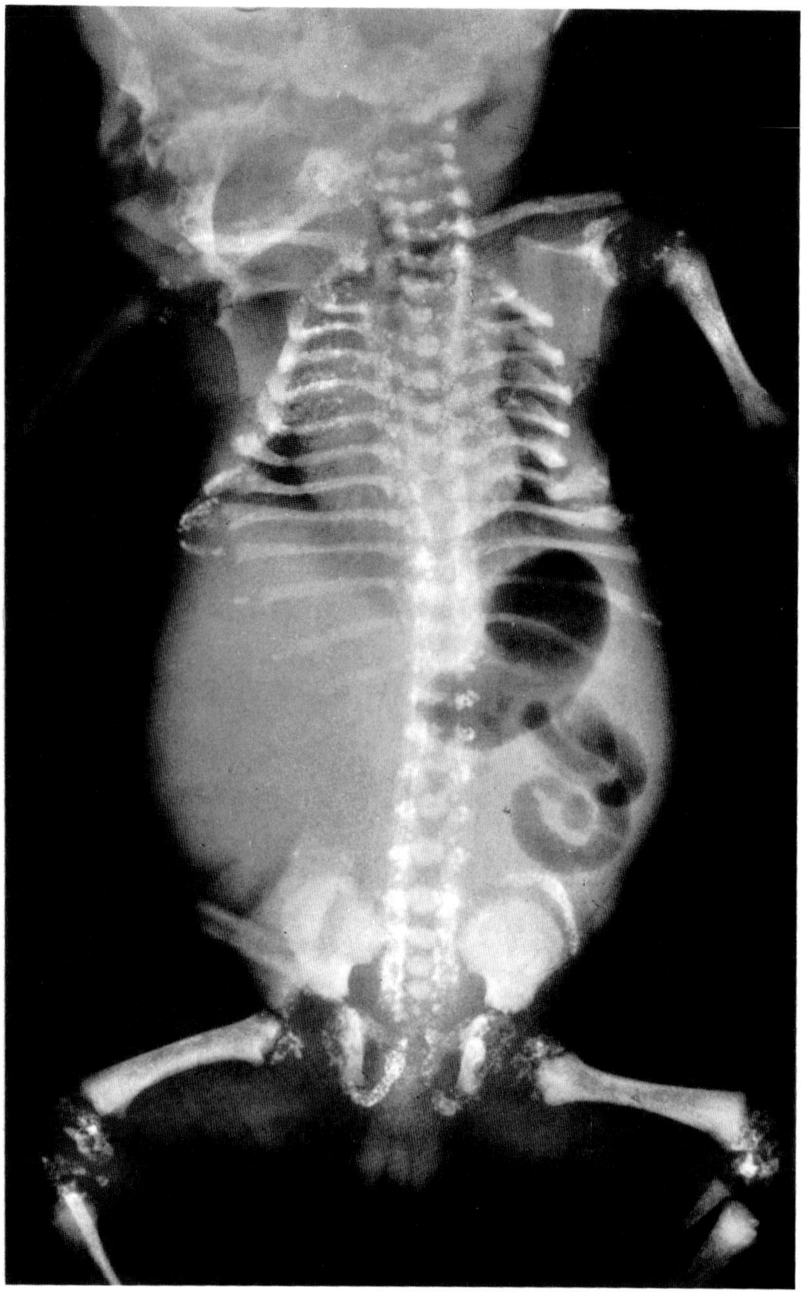

Fig. 1. Chondrodysplasia punctata (Conradi-Hünermann type). Newborn baby with numerous stippled densities along the vertebral column, at the rib ends, and in the epiphyses of the long tubular bones

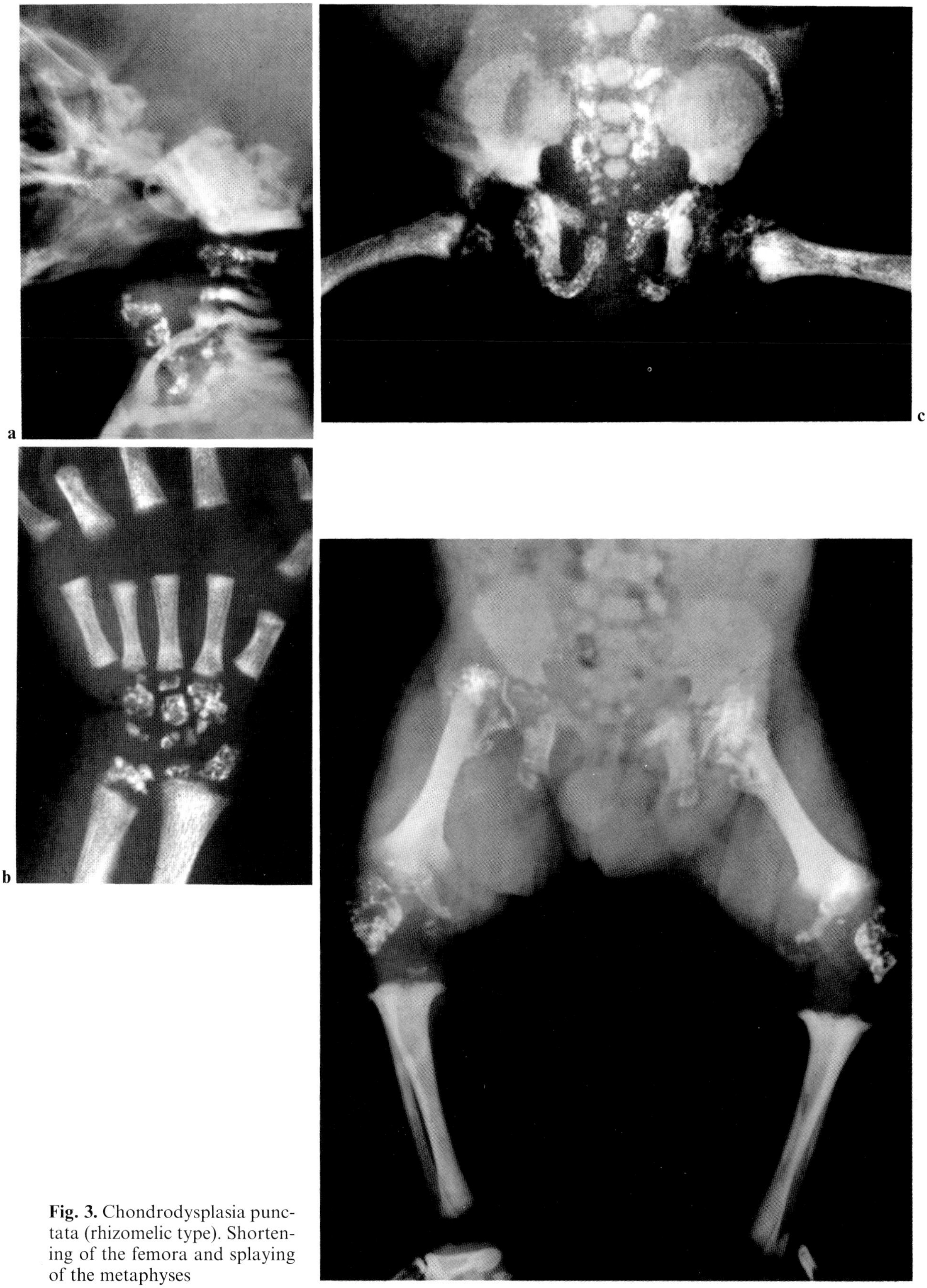

Fig. 3. Chondrodysplasia punctata (rhizomelic type). Shortening of the femora and splaying of the metaphyses

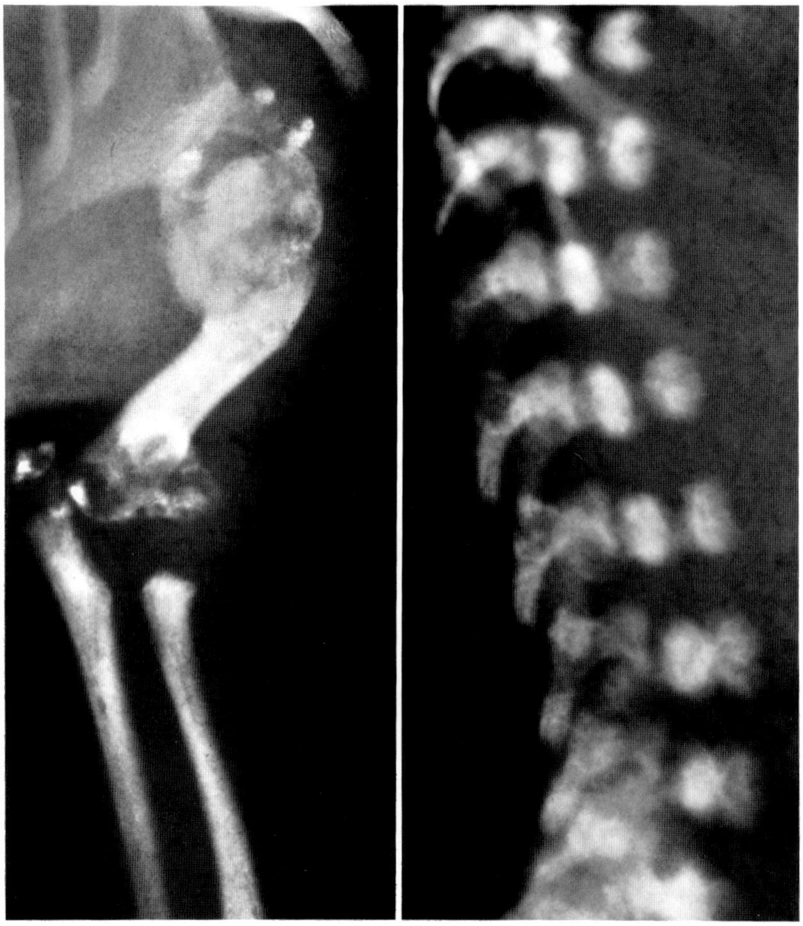

Fig. 4a, b. Same patient as Fig. 3. **a** Severe shortening of the humerus with splaying of the metaphyses. **b** The coronal clefts in the lumbar vertebrae and the absence of paravertebral stippled densities are typical features in the rhizomelic type of chondrodysplasia punctata

1.1.3 Achondroplasia and Hypochondroplasia

Patients with achondroplasia characteristically present with short stature, shortening of the limbs, skull changes (bulging forehead, large cranium, depressed nasal bridge), and vertebral changes (including narrowing of the interpeduncular distances). The intelligence is normal and the inheritance is of the autosomal dominant type. Most of the cases are heterozygous, and new gene mutations occur frequently (80%). Homozygous achondroplasia is rare and results in early death.
The etiology is based on a biochemical defect related to abnormalities in chondrocyte proliferation and formation of a fully developed hypertrophic zone [1]. Because of this impaired endochondral ossification, bulbous masses of cartilage are formed at the ends of the long tubular bones.

Hypochondroplasia is an autosomal dominant disorder and presents less severe radiographic findings than achondroplasia. The hands in patients with hypochondroplasia may be radiographically normal or only slightly abnormal [2].

Radiographic Findings [3–7]

Hand
Trident-shaped
Short tubular bones, particularly second to fourth metacarpals and proximal phalanges
Cupping of epiphyses
Irregular metaphyses

Other Sites
Long tubular bones: shortening and thickening
irregular epiphyses
metaphyseal irregularity and flaring
curving of tubular bones

Pelvis: horizontal sacrum
underdeveloped iliac wings
small pelvic cavity
narrow sacroiliac notches
flat acetabular roof

Lumbar spine: progressive caudal narrowing of interpeduncular distances
anterior "beaking"
lordosis
posterior scalloping of vertebral bodies
some platyspondylisis
increased height of intervertebral discs
spinal stenosis

Skull: bulging forehead
depressed nasal bridge
small base
small foramen magnum
basilar impression

Comparative findings in achondroplasia and hypochondroplasia (after WALKER et al. [2])

	Achondroplasia 48 patients	Hypochondroplasia 24 patients
Hand		
Short metacarpals	+(50%)	normal
Long tubular bones		
Long fibula	+(100%)	+(75%)
Genu varum	+(15%)	+(8%)
Abnormal femoral metaphysis	+	–
Limb shortening	+	±
Pelvis: square ilia	+	±(or normal)
Spine		
Lumbar lordosis	+	±
Narrowing of interpeduncular distances L1–4 (normally 0%)	+(69%)	+(17%)
Equal interpeduncular distances L1–4 (normally 59%)	+(31%)	+(83%)
Thoracolumbar kyphosis	+(50%)	–
Skull abnormalities	+	±

Differential Diagnosis

Mucopolysaccharidosis (Sect. 6.1.1)
Pseudoachondroplasia

References

1 Pedrini-Mille A, Pedrini V (1982) Proteoglycans and glucosaminoglycans of human achondroplastic cartilage. J Bone Joint Surg [Am] 64a:39–46
2 Walker BA, Murdoch JL, Mc Kusick VA, Langer LO, Beals RK (1971) Hypochondroplasia. Am J Dis Child 122:95–104
3 Wynne-Davies R, Walsh WK, Gormley J (1981) Achondroplasia and hypochondroplasia. Clinical variation and spinal stenosis. J Bone Joint Surg [Br] 63b:508–515
4 Silverman FN (1973) Achondroplasia. Progr Pediatr Radiol 4:94–124
5 Cremin BJ, Beighton P (1978) Bone dysplasias of infancy. Springer, Berlin Heidelberg New York
6 Langer LO Jr, Baumann PA, Gorlin RJ (1967) Achondroplasia. AJR 100:12–26
7 Poznanski AK (1984) The hand in radiologic diagnosis. Saunders, Philadelphia

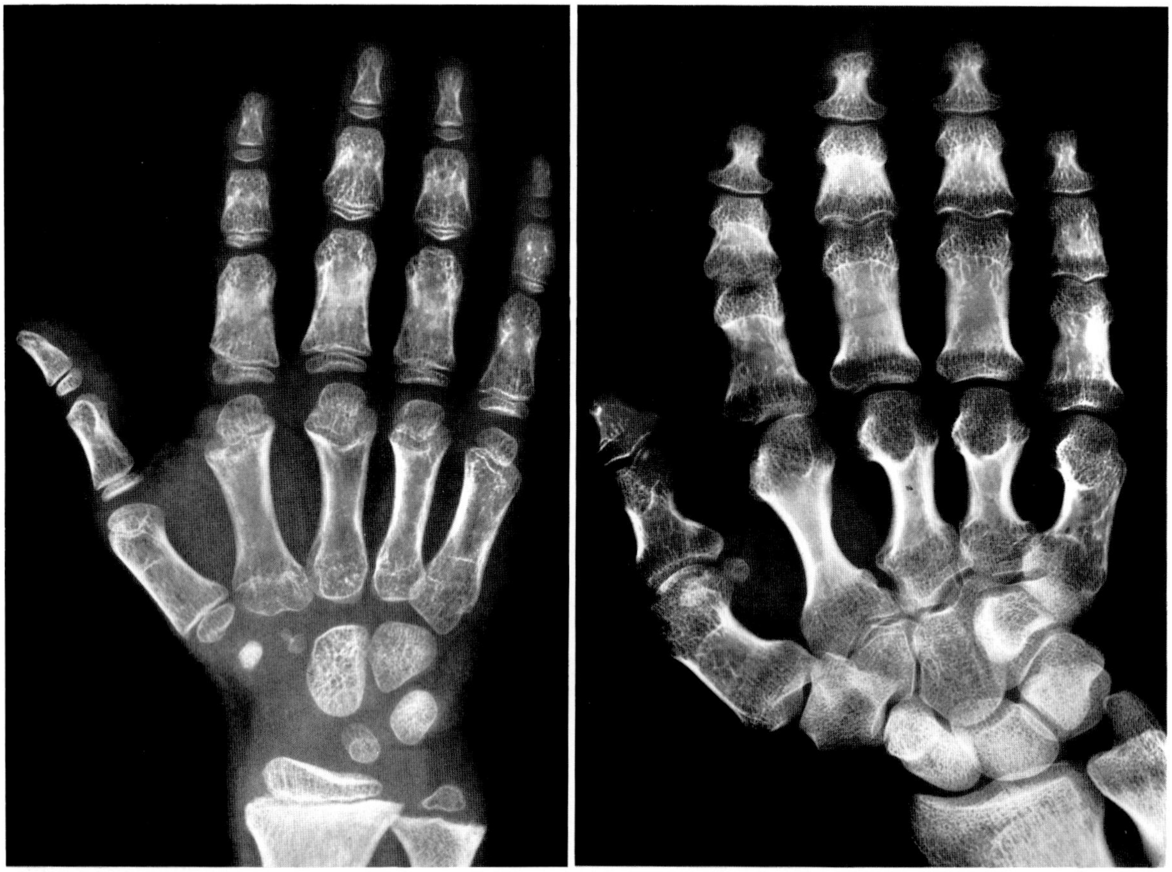

1a b

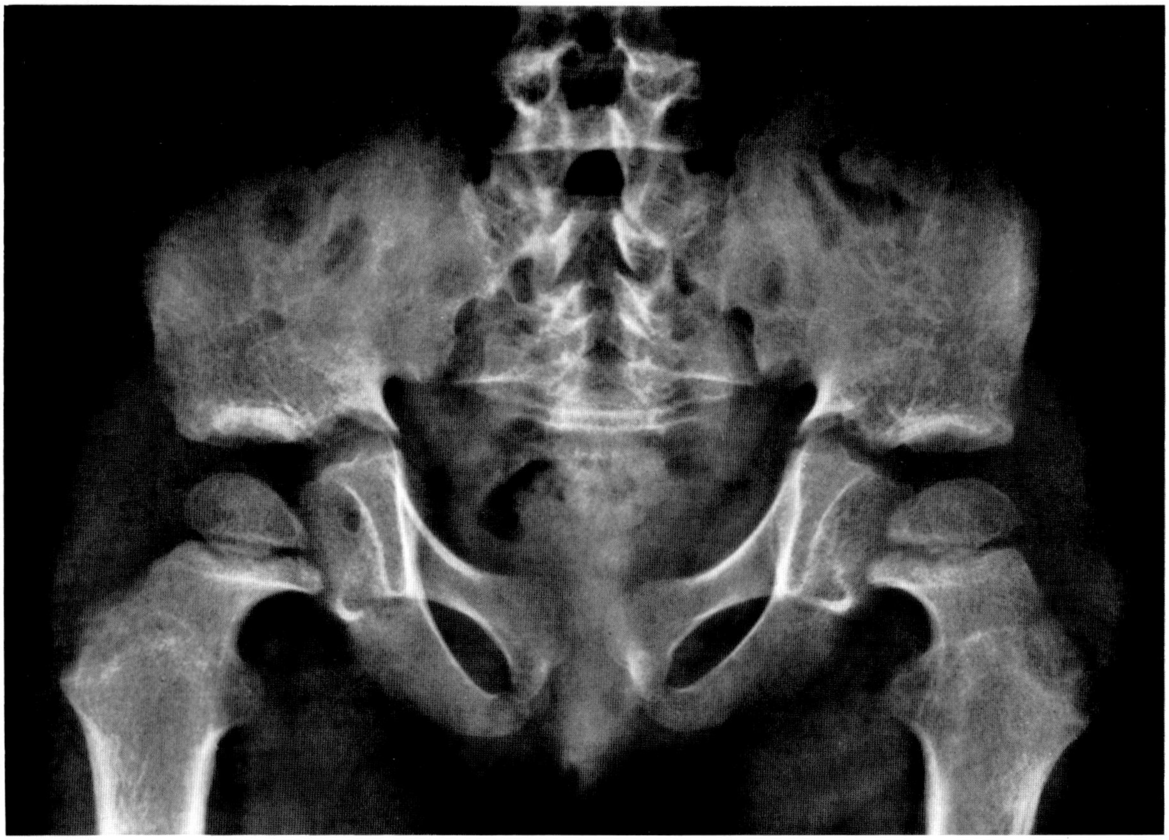

2

Fig. 3. Same patient as Fig. 2. Lumbar spine: Scalloping of posterior surfaces of vertebral bodies and slight thoracolumbar kyphosis

Fig. 4. Same patient as Fig. 2. Right lower limb: The metaphyses are all abnormally splayed. The fibula is long and some curving of the long tubular bones is present

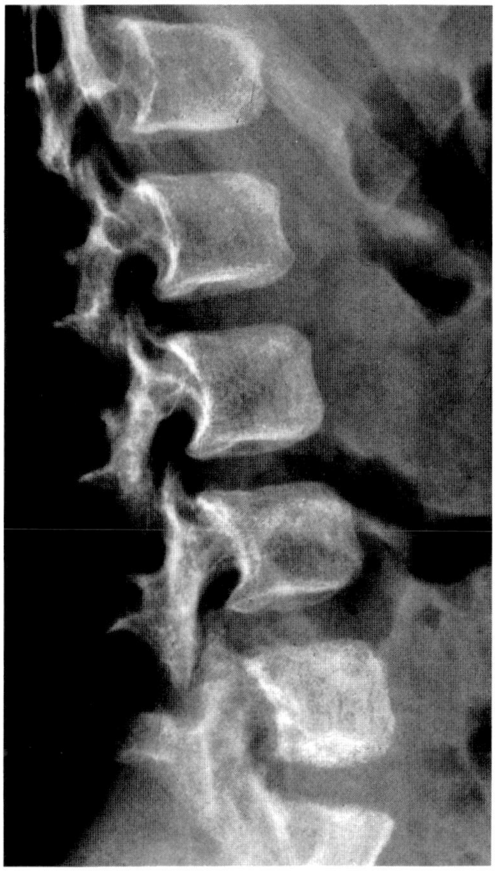

3

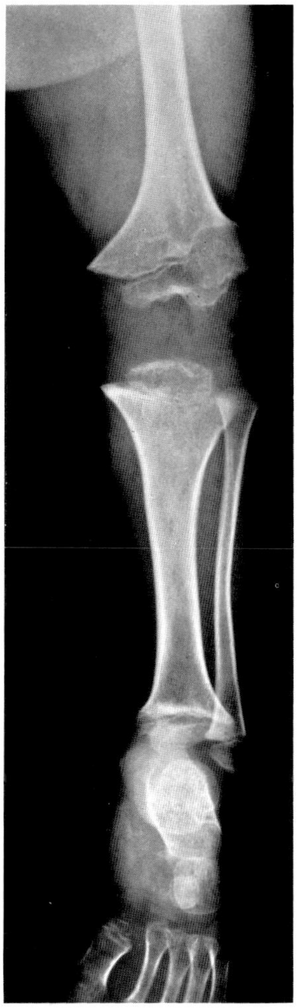

4

◁ **Fig. 1a, b.** Achondroplasia. **a** In an 8-year-old girl: Shortening of metacarpals and phalanges, irregular metaphyses of radius and ulna, most phalanges widened. **b** In a 19-year-old man: Uniform and severe shortening and widening of metacarpals and phalanges

Fig. 2. Achondroplasia in a 5-year-old girl. Narrowing of interpeduncular distances, small pelvic cavity, and narrow sacroiliac notches. Flat acetabular roofs and irregularities of femoral metaphyses

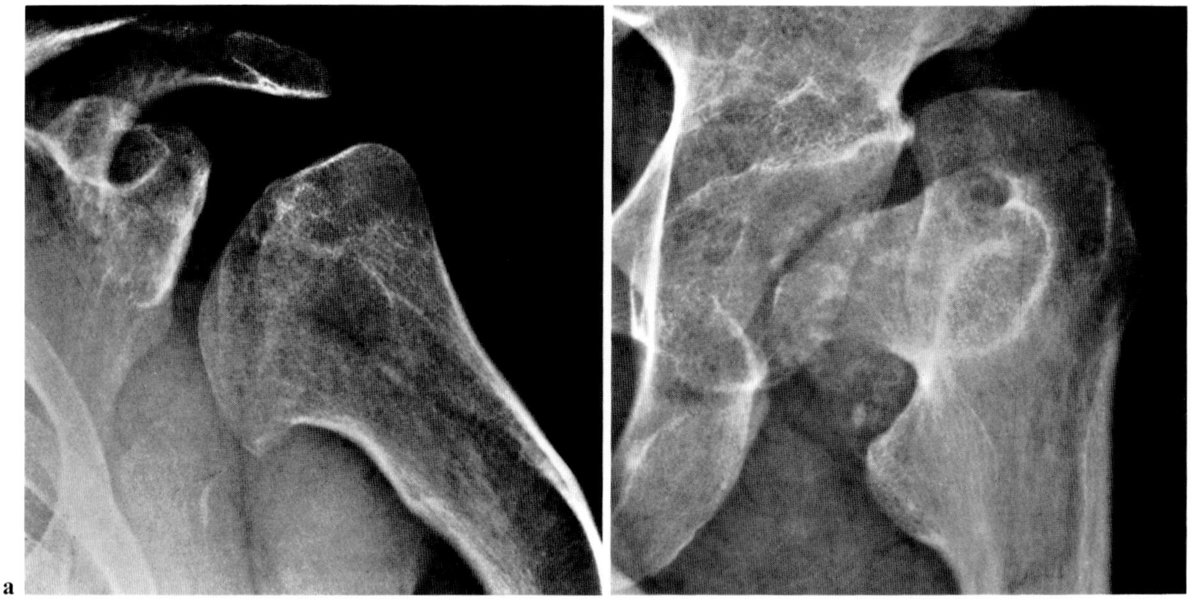

Fig. 5a, b. Achondroplasia in an adult male. **a** Shoulder: Small and irregular glenoid cavity with plump humeral head and some curving of shaft. **b** Hip: Small and deformed femoral head with coxa vara deformity

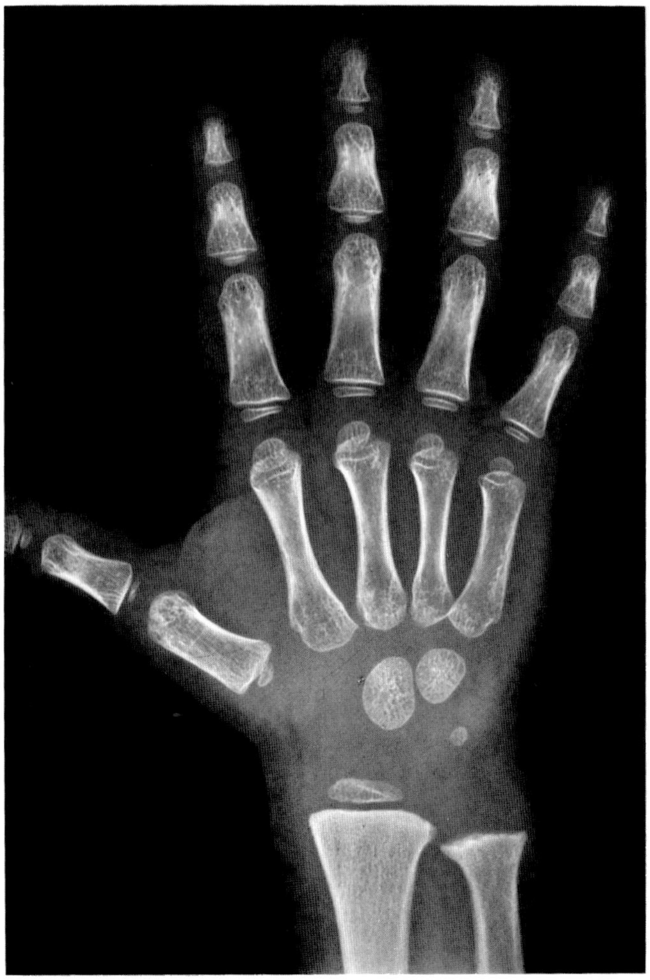

Fig. 6. Hypochondroplasia in a 4-year-old boy. Short stature, deep lumbar lordosis, and shortening of limbs. The lengths of the phalanges and metacarpals are normal, as is the relation of the lengths of the phalanges to the lengths of the metacarpals. The interpeduncular distances L1–4 in this patient are all the same (21 mm)

1.1.4 Diastrophic Dysplasia

This autosomal recessive form of dwarfism is characterized by severe shortening of the limbs, club feet, typical deformities of the hands, inflammation of the pinnae of the ears, restricted mobility of joints and progressive scoliosis. The intelligence is normal. There are flexion contractures and progressive dislocation of major joints. Hypermobile (hitchhiker) thumbs are present, although the other fingers tend to show restricted mobility of the interphalangeal joints. Survival into later adult life is possible [1].

Radiographic Findings [2–4]

Hand

Short and wide tubular bones
Very small, round, oval, or triangular first metacarpal
Abducted and proximally positioned thumb
Abnormal ossification of epiphyses and wide metaphyses
Wide distal end of radius
Bizarrely formed carpals
Precocious appearance of carpals
Supernumerary carpals (distal row)
Increased carpal angle
Symphalangism
Ulnar deviation of hand
Stub thumb

Other Sites

Long tubular bones: short and broad with widened metaphyses
retarded ossification and flattening of epiphyseal centers
coxa vara
cone-shaped epiphysis at distal femur
flat humeral heads
wide proximal end of ulna
dislocation of one or more large joints (hips, elbows)
Foot: clubfoot
short first metatarsal
Skull: micrognathia
cleft palate
Spine: hypoplasia of odontoid
subluxation C1–2
hypoplasia of bodies of cervical vertebrae (kyphosis)
irregular deformities of vertebral bodies
diminished interpeduncular distances
progressive scoliosis
Trachea: tracheomalacia

Differential Diagnosis

Arthrogryposis multiplex congenita (Sect. 7.1.1)
Achondroplasia (Sect. 1.1.3)

References

1 Hollister DW, Lachman RS (1976) Diastrophic dwarfism. Clin Orthop 114:61–66
2 Stover CN, Hayes JT, Holt JF (1963) Diastrophic dwarfism. AJR 89:914–922
3 Langer LO (1965) Diastrophic dwarfism in early infancy. AJR 93:399–402
4 Saule H (1975) Diastrophic dwarfism. Radiology 15:50–54

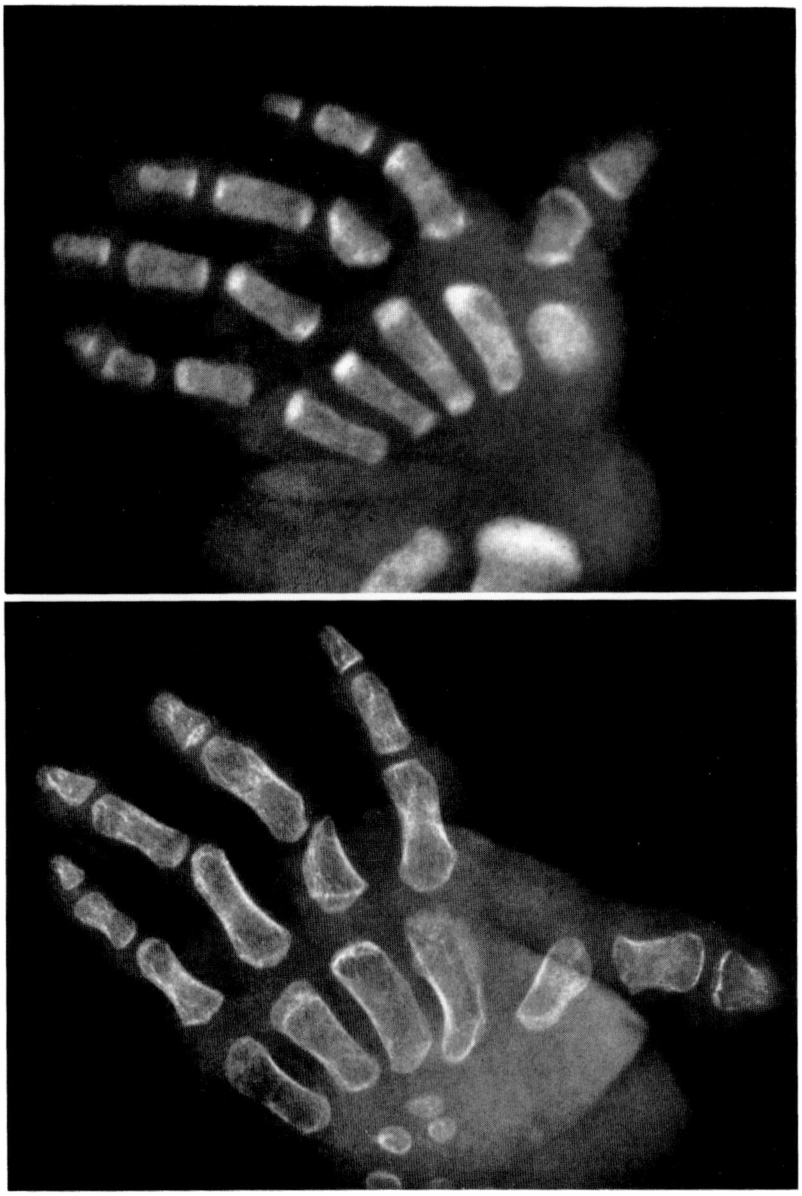

a

b

Fig. 1 a, b. Diastrophic dysplasia. **a** Abnormally formed metacarpals and phalanges with ulnar deviation. **b** At 1 year of age: Characteristic hitch-hiker thumb and precocious appearance of carpals. Probably supernumerary carpal bones

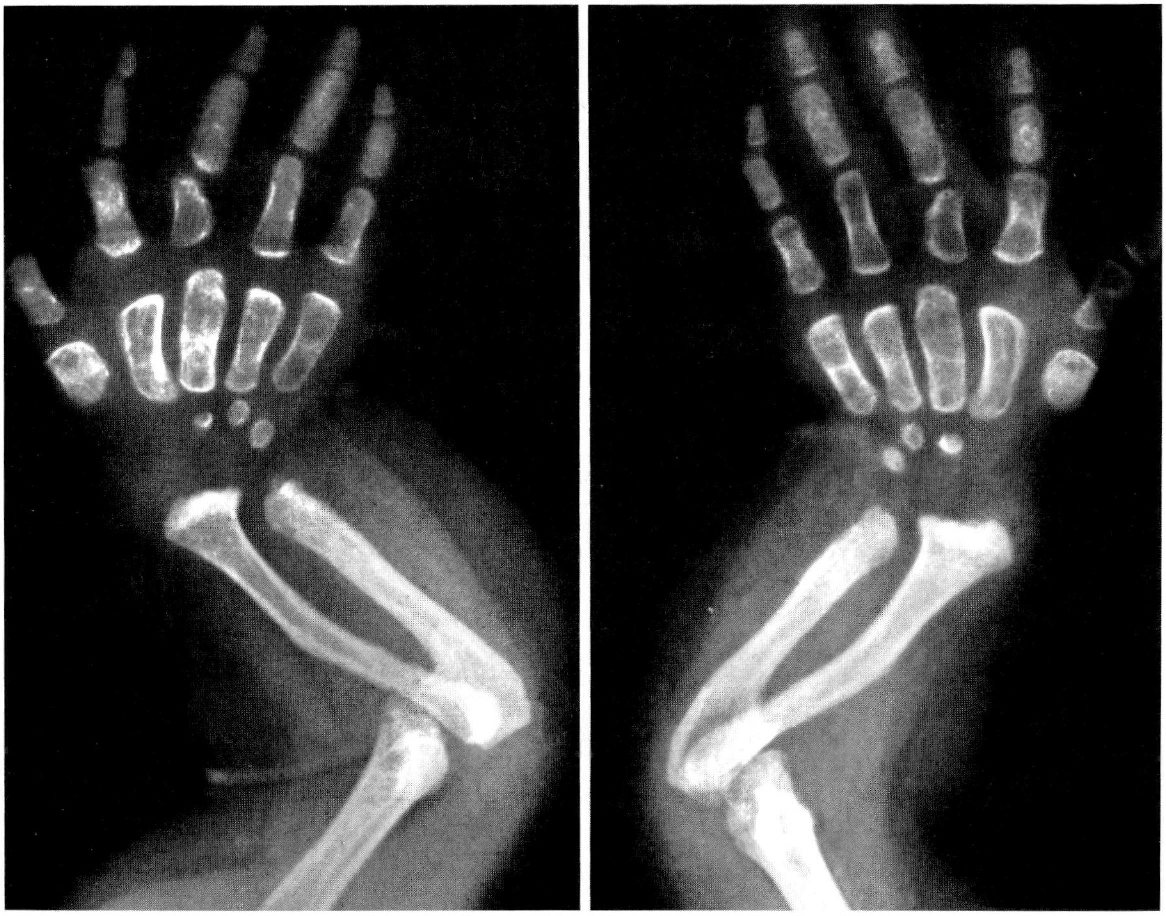

Fig. 2. Same patient as Fig. 1. Both arms at 6 months of age: Dislocation of elbows and shortened radius and ulna. The distal end of the radius is wide, carpal ossification is precocious, and the tubular bones of the hand are all abnormally shortened and widened

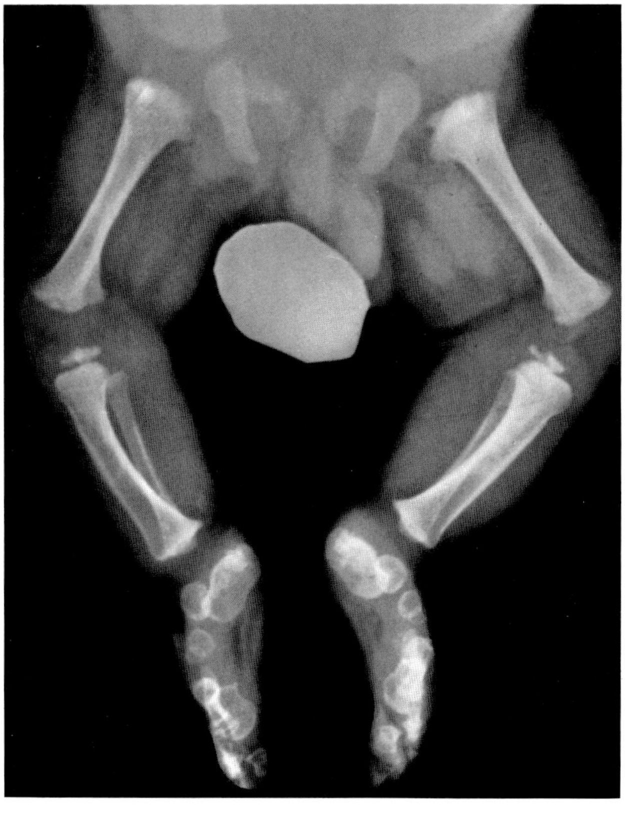

Fig. 3. Same patient as Fig. 1. Both legs at 6 months of age: Short and broad femora and tibiae, wide metaphyseal areas, and retarded ossification of flattened epiphyses

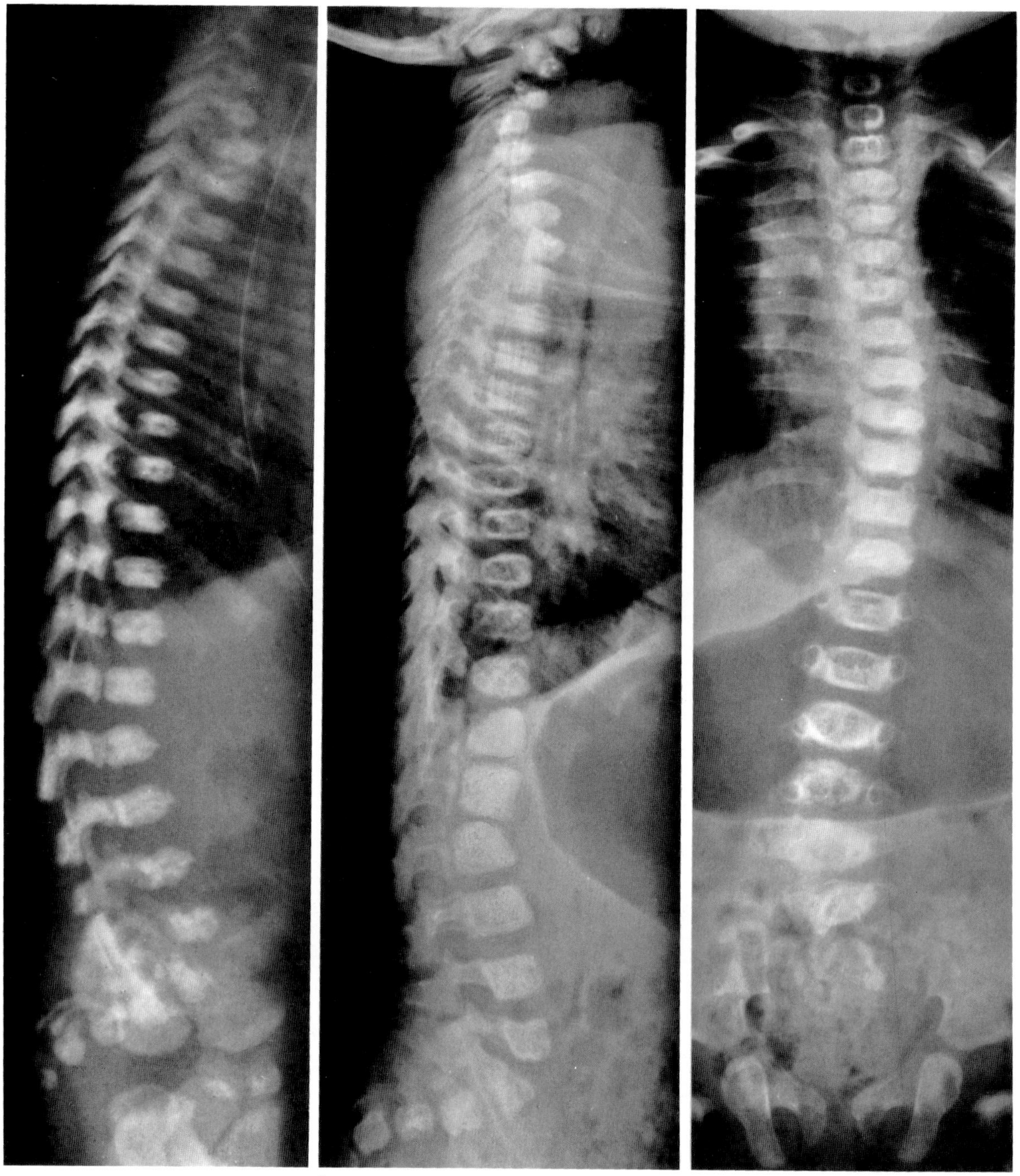

a b c

Fig. 4a–c. Diastrophic dysplasia. **a** At birth: slight kyphosis in lumbar spine. **b**, **c** At 6 months of age: Hypoplasia of vertebral bodies in cervical spine with kyphosis. Kyphotic angle in lumbar spine and progressive scoliosis. Abnormally curved sacrum

1.1.5 Metatropic Dysplasia

Metatropic dysplasia is a rare and probably autosomal recessive disorder characterized by relatively short limbs, a relatively long trunk, and a narrow thorax. With increasing age, a transformation takes place into a form of dwarfism with a relatively short trunk and relatively long extremities. Other clinical features are rapidly progressive kyphoscoliosis and limited movement of the major joints.
In some cases of metatropic dysplasia a tail-like appendage in the coccygeal area may be encountered.

Radiographic Findings [1–5]
Hand
Short tubular bones
Metaphyseal flaring
Hourglass appearance (especially of proximal phalanges)
Delayed skeletal maturation
Irregular carpal bones
Hyperextensible finger joints

Other Sites
Long tubular bones: shortening
delayed ossification of epiphyses
metaphyseal flaring and exaggerated constriction in midportions of shafts; newborn: dumbbell configuration; older: battle-ax configuration (abnormalities of metaphyses tend to regress)
Thorax: narrow and small
short ribs with wide anterior ends
prominent sternum
Spine: delayed ossification of vertebral bodies
platyspondylisis (especially in thoracic spine)
widening of intervertebral discs
kyphoscoliosis (may be present at birth)

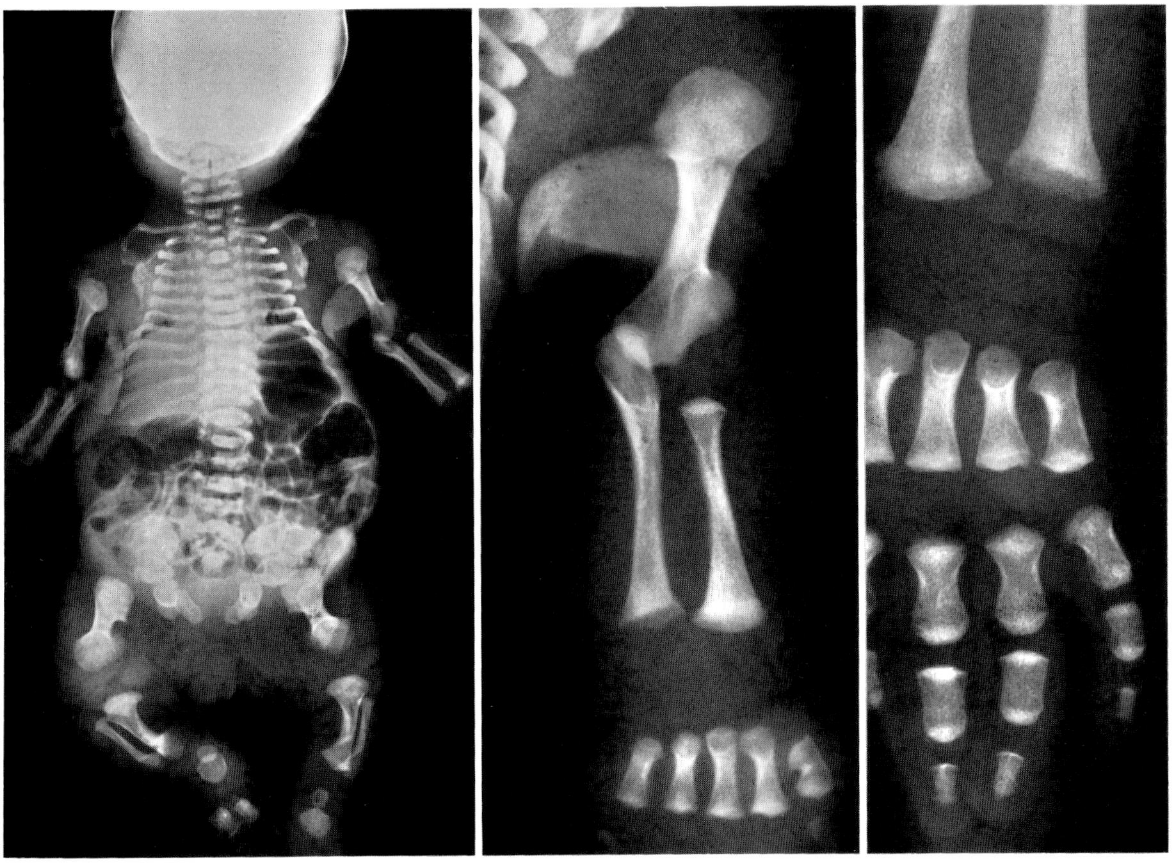

a b, c

Fig. 1 a–c. Metatropic dysplasia in a newborn child. **a** Flared metaphyses of long tubular bones and dumbbell configuration. Vertebral bodies flat, thorax small and narrow. Widening of anterior rib ends. **b** Dumbbell configuration of long tubular bones. **c** Biconcave deformities of short tubular bones, especially proximal phalanges (hourglass deformities). Peculiar indentation of first metacarpal

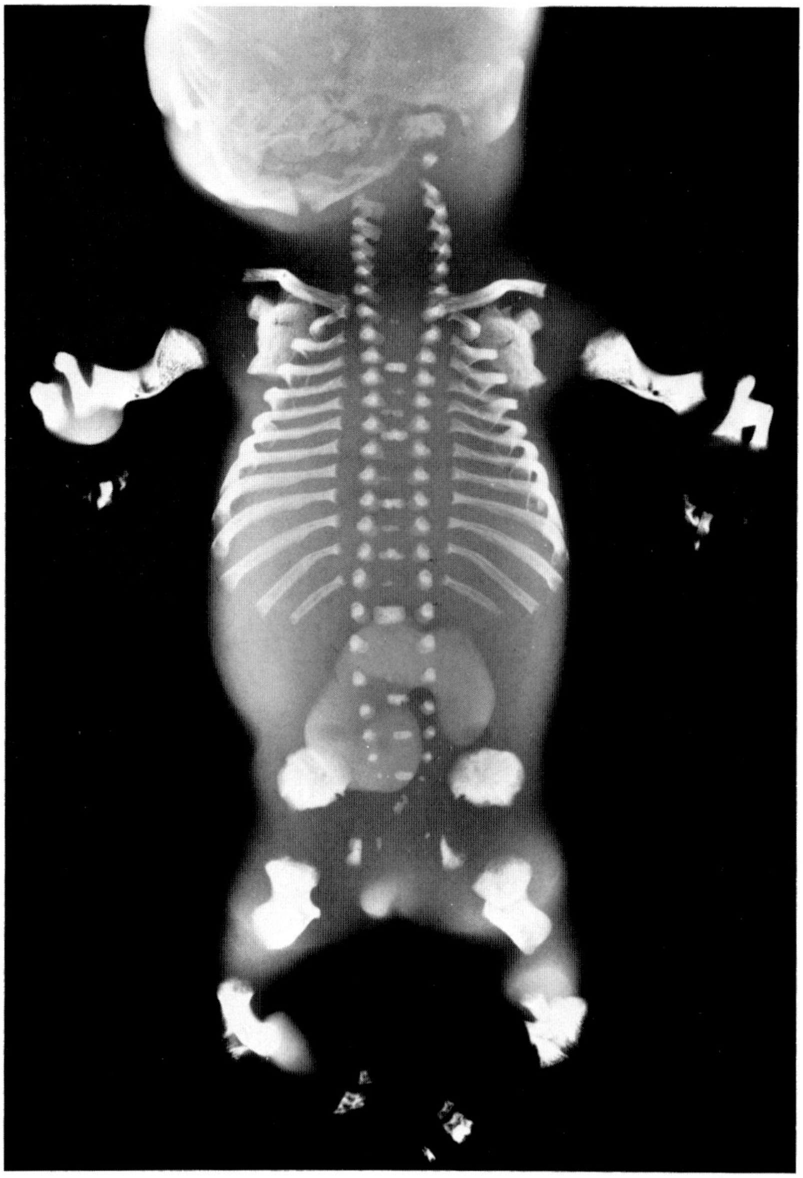

Fig. 2. Metatropic dysplasia in an 18-week fetus. Very thin or even absent ossification centers of vertebral bodies, short, dumbbell-shaped long tubular bones

occasional progressive narrowing of interpeduncular distances

Skull: cleft palate

Pelvis: iliac wings small and flared
acetabular roof flat and irregular
small sacroiliac notches

Differential Diagnosis

Achondroplasia (Sect. 1.1.3)
Diastrophic dysplasia (Sect. 1.1.4)
Metaphyseal chondrodysplasia (Sect. 1.1.10)
Mucopolysaccharidosis (Sect. 6.1.1)
Weissenbacher-Zweymuller syndrome [4]
Kniest's syndrome [6]

References

1 Silverman FN (1968) A differential diagnosis of achondroplasia. Radiol Clin North Am 6:223–237
2 Spranger J (1967) Der metatropische Zwergwuchs. Radiologe 7:385–387
3 Cremin BJ, Beighton P (1978) Bone dysplasias in infancy. Springer, Berlin Heidelberg New York
4 Rimoin DL, Siggers DC, Lachman RS, Silberberg R (1976) Metatropic dwarfism, the Kniest syndrome and pseudoachondroplastic dysplasias. Clin Orthop 114:70–82
5 Poznanski AK (1984) The hand in radiologic diagnosis. Saunders, Philadelphia
6 Haller JO, Berdon WE, Robinow M, Slovis TL, Baker DH, Johnson GF (1975) The Weissenbacher-Zweymuller syndrome of micrognathia and rhizomelic chondrodysplasia at birth with subfrequent normal growth. AJR 125:936–943

1.1.6 Chondroectodermal Dysplasia

Synonym: Ellis-van Creveld syndrome

The clinical features of this autosomal recessive disorder are mild short-limbed dwarfism, dysplastic nails, sparse hair, impaired dentition, polydactyly of the hands, genital malformation, and congenital heart anomalies (60%–75%). The cause seems to be deficient development in the ectodermal and mesenchymal tissues of the primitive limb bud. Only a small proportion of the victims survive into adult life [1–4].

Radiographic Findings [2–4]

Hand

Postaxial polydactyly (well-developed digit)
Fusion of fifth and sixth metacarpals
Short tubular bones, especially distal and middle phalanges
Hypoplastic and thin distal phalanges
Cone-shaped epiphyses
Supernumerary carpals (especially between hamate and capitate)
Carpal fusion (hamate and capitate)

Other Sites

Thorax: shortened ribs with broad anterior ends
congenital heart disease (60%–75%)
Long tubular bones: short and heavy
enlarged proximal end of ulna
enlarged distal end of radius
dislocation of radial head
wide proximal end of tibia with hypoplasia of lateral tibial plateau (genu valgum, knock-knee)
bowing of femur and humerus
Pelvis: flared and hypoplastic iliac wings (trident-shaped acetabula)
small sacroiliac notches

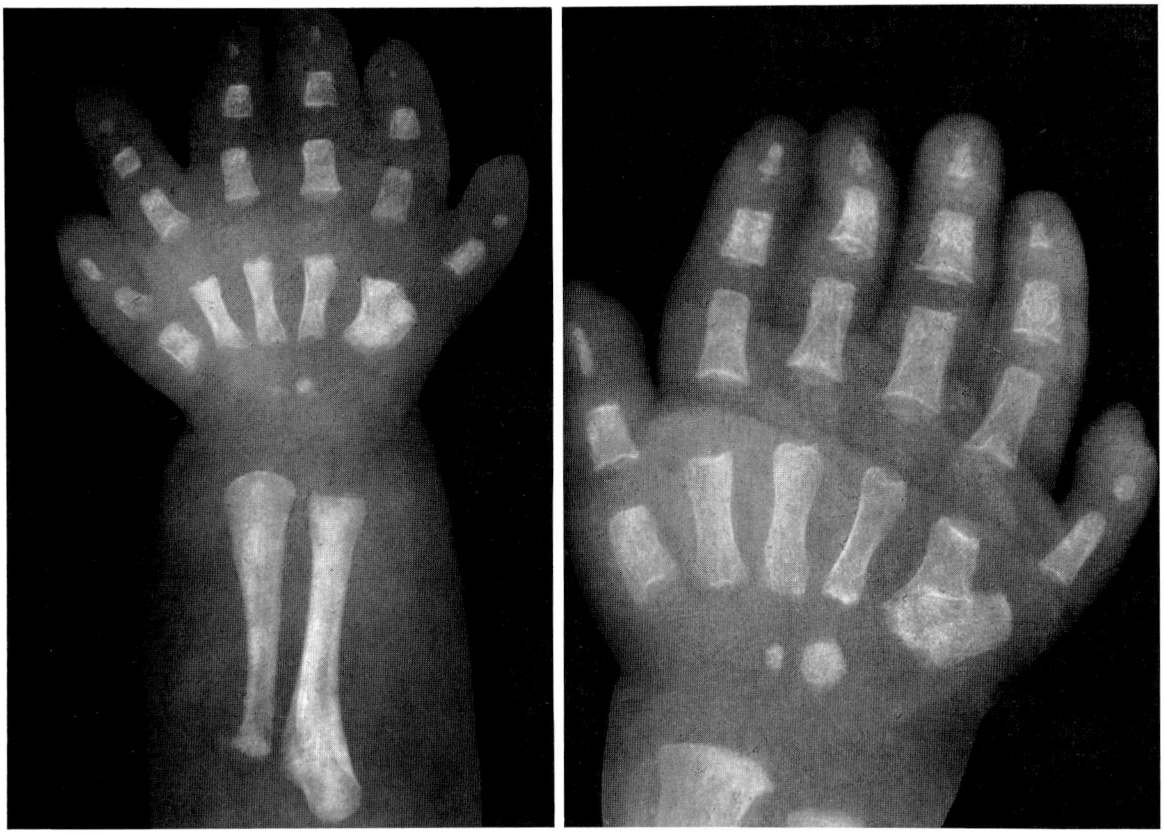

a b

Fig. 1a, b. Chondroectodermal dysplasia. **a** Fusion of fifth and sixth metacarpals and postaxial polydactyly. Hypoplasia of tubular bones, especially distal phalanges. Broad and coned distal end of radius and proximal end of ulna. **b** Postaxial polydactyly with characteristic fusion of fifth and sixth metacarpals. Several cone-shaped epiphyses and small, thin distal phalanges

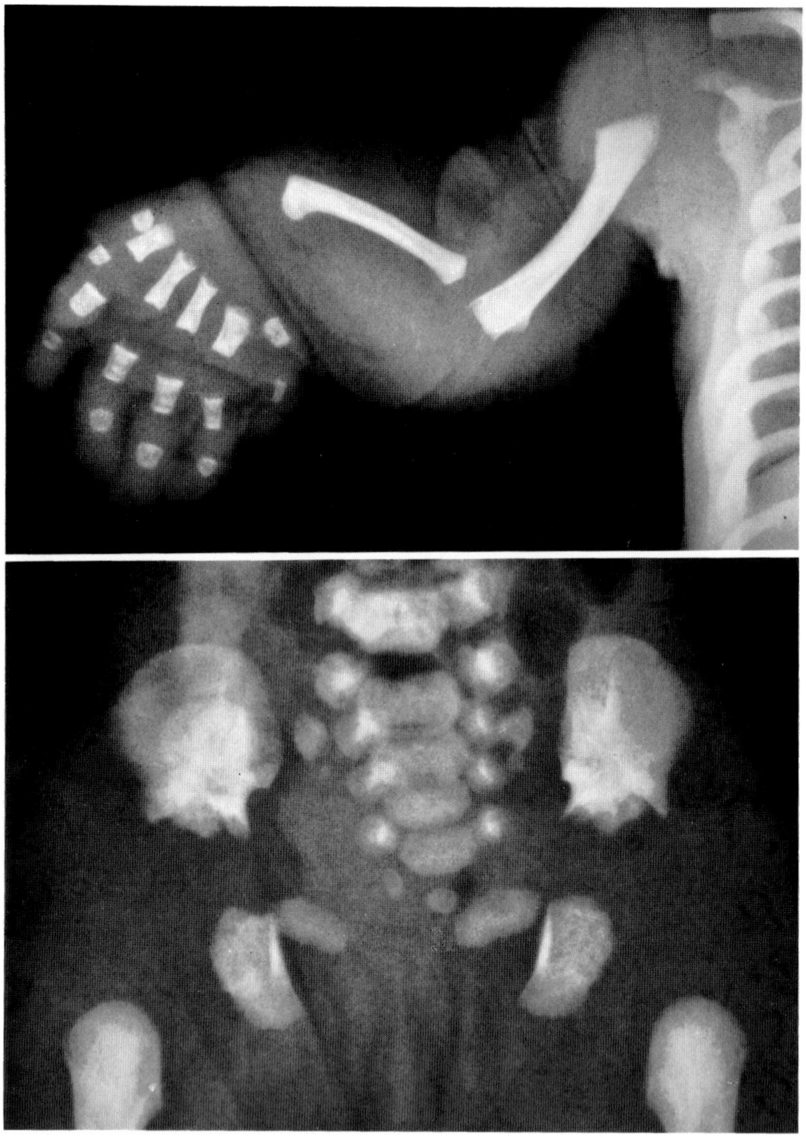

b

Fig. 2 a, b. Chondroectodermal dysplasia in a newborn boy. **a** Aplasia of ulna and postaxial polydactyly, short tubular bones, distal phalanges not yet ossified. **b** Broad iliac wings and irregular acetabula with central spurs (trident-shaped)

Foot: polydactyly
symmetatarsalism
Miscellaneous: dysplastic teeth
occasional renal abnormalities and/or hydrocephalus

Differential Diagnosis

Asphyxiating thoracic dysplasia (Sect. 1.1.7)

References

1 Ellis RWB, van Creveld S (1940) A syndrome characterized by ectodermal dysplasia, polydactyly, chondrodysplasia and congenital morbus cordis. Arch Dis Child 15:65–84
2 Ellis RWB, Andrew JD (1962) Chondroectodermal dysplasia. J Bone Joint Surg [Br] 44b:626–630
3 Bützler HO, Henscher L, Mennicken U, Franz Chr, Hiller HJ (1973) Die Röntgendiagnose der Skelettveränderungen des Ellis-van Creveld-Syndromes im Wachstumsalter. Fortschr Geb Röntgenstr Nuklearmed Ergänzungsband 118:537–552
4 Caffey J (1953) Chondroectodermal dysplasia (Ellis-van Creveld disease). Report of three cases. AJR 68:875–886

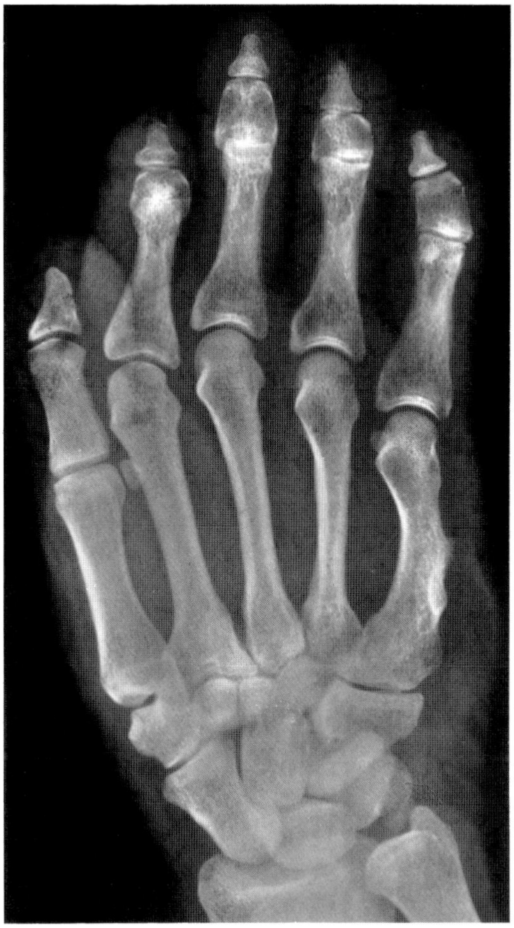

Fig. 3. Chondroectodermal dysplasia in a 49-year-old man. Previous surgery for postaxial polydactyly. Shortening of middle and distal phalanges, accessory carpal between hamate and capitate, hypoplasia of fingernails

Fig. 4a, b. Same patient as Fig. 3. **a** Wide proximal end of tibia and some hypoplasia of lateral part of tibial plateau. **b** Protrusion of femoral condyles into deformed tibial plateau

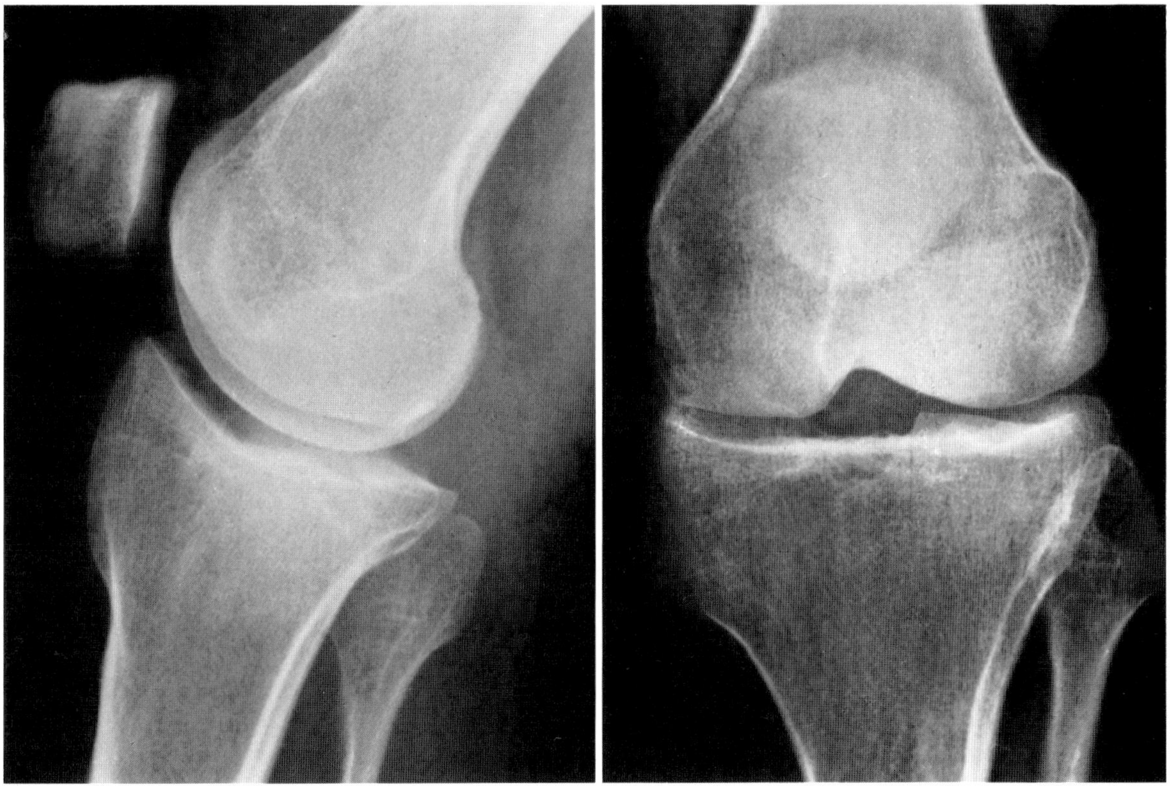

a **b**

1.1.7 Asphyxiating Thoracic Dysplasia

Synonyms: thoracic-pelvic-phalangeal dystrophy, Jeune's syndrome

Asphyxiating thoracic dysplasia is thought to be an autosomal recessive disorder. At birth the thorax is narrow and immobile with short and horizontal ribs. This causes primarily abdominal respiratory motion. In a number of patients, asphyxia and pneumonia are the reasons for early death. With increasing age, the thorax enlarges and severe pulmonary complications occur less frequently [1–5].

Radiographic Findings [1–5]

Hand
Cone-shaped epiphyses
Metaphyseal irregularities
Brachydactyly
Polydactyly (20%)

Other Sites
Thorax: bell-shaped
short horizontally placed ribs with bulbous anterior ends
inverted clavicles
incomplete ossification of sternum
Pelvis: horizontal acetabular roof, trident-shaped with central spur
short iliac wings
Long tubular bones: occasionally some shortening

Differential Diagnosis

Disorders with cone-shaped epiphyses (Sect. 2.2.9)
Disorders with brachydactyly (Sect. 2.2.11)
Disorders with polydactyly (Sect. 2.2.13)
Chondroectodermal dysplasia (Sect. 1.1.6)

References

1 Cremin BJ, Beighton P (1978) Bone dysplasias of infancy. Springer, Berlin Heidelberg New York
2 Langer LO (1968) Thoracic-pelvic-phalangeal dystrophy. Asphyxiating thoracic dystrophy of the newborn, infantile thoracic dystrophy. Radiology 91:447–456
3 Kozlowski K, Masel J (1976) Asphyxiating thoracic dystrophy without respiratory distress. Pediatr Radiol 5:30–33
4 Jequier JC, Favreau-Ethier M, Gregoire H (1973) Asphyxiating thoracic dysplasia. In: Kaufman HJ (ed) Intrinsic diseases of bone. Karger, Basel (Progress in pediatric radiology, vol 4)
5 Kozlowski K, Masel J, Morrish L, Kunze D (1978) Neonatal death dwarfism. Fortschr Geb Röntgenstr Geb Nuklearmed Ergänzungsband 129:626–633

Fig. 1a, b. Asphyxiating thoracic dysplasia. **a** In a 7-day-old girl: Cone-shaped epiphyses in proximal phalanges. **b** In a 4-year-old boy: Cone-shaped epiphyses in all phalanges and shortened tubular bones ▷

Fig. 2. Same patient as Fig. 1b. Asphyxiating thoracic dysplasia. Narrow thorax with short and horizontal ribs, cupped anterior rib ends ▷

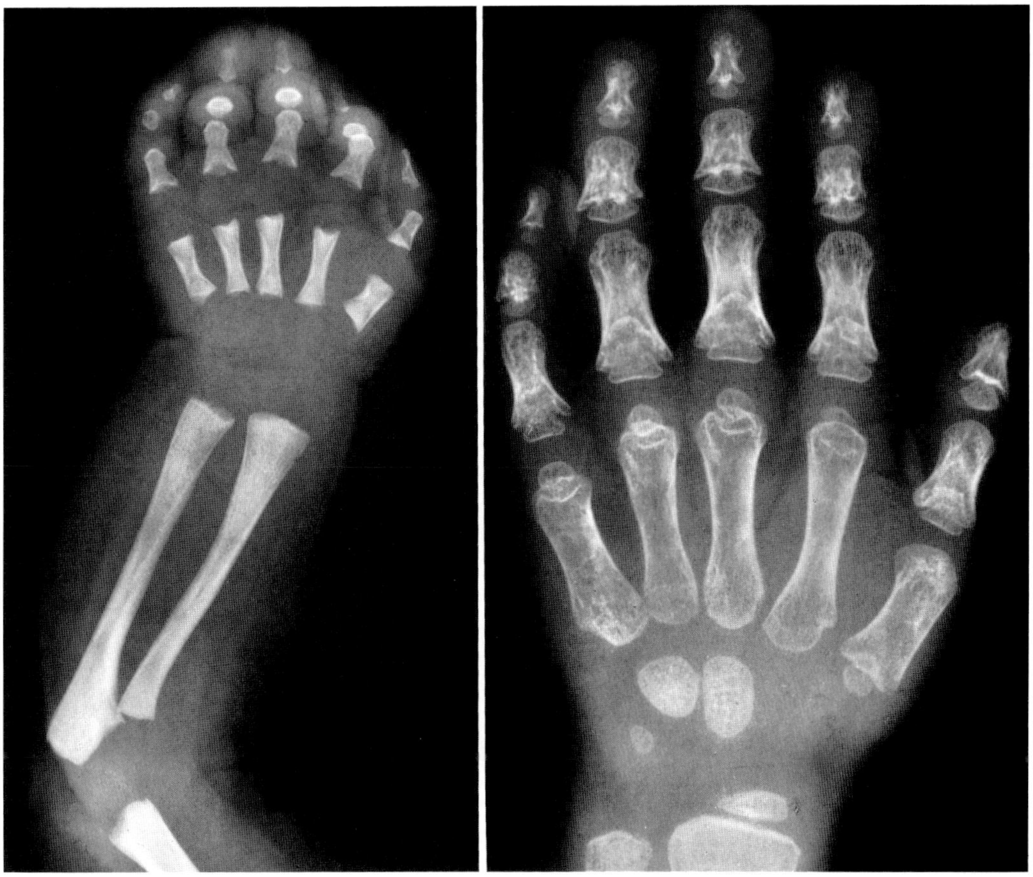

1a b

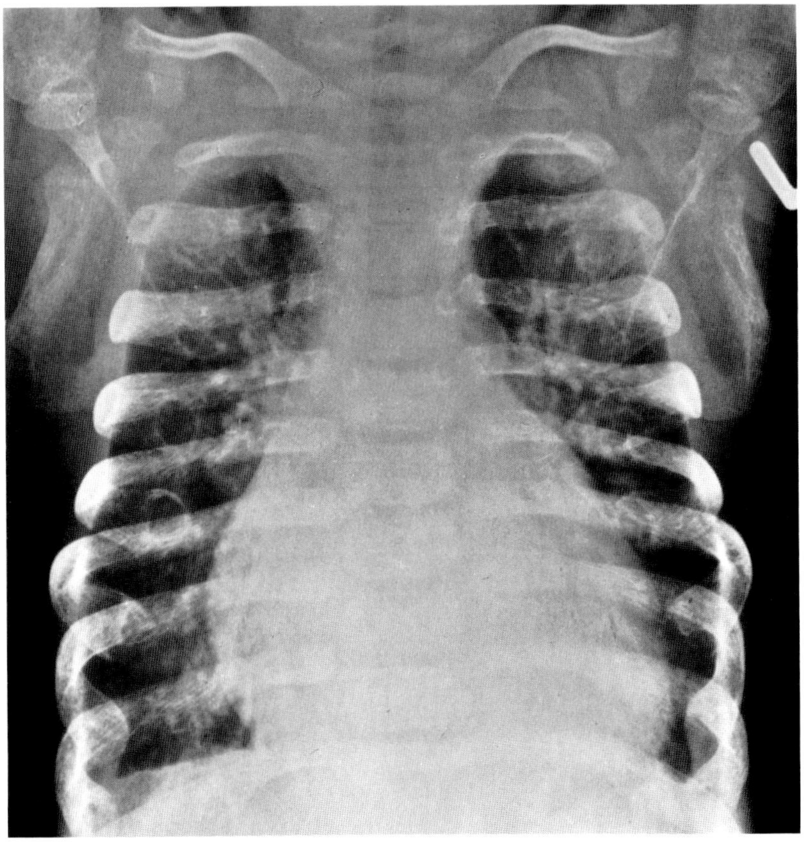

2

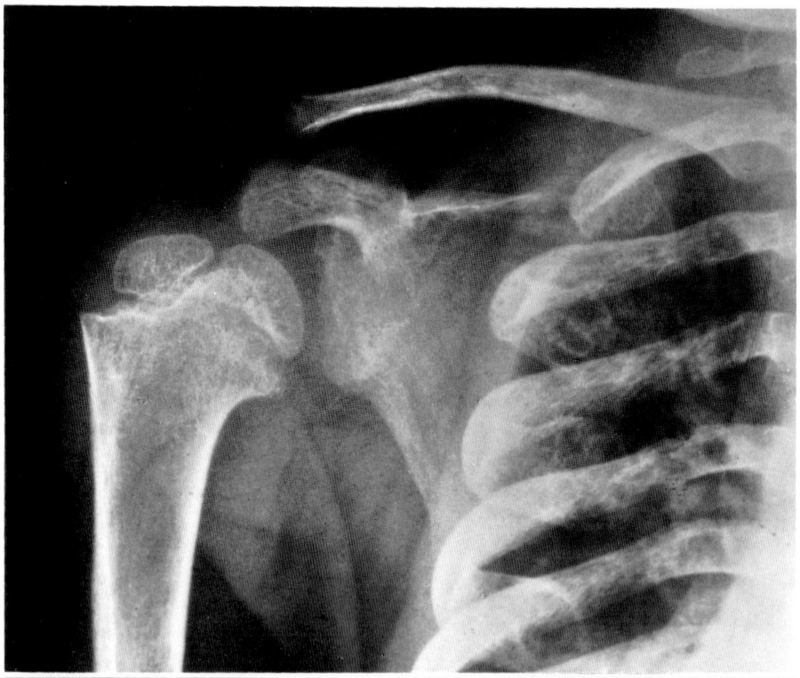

a

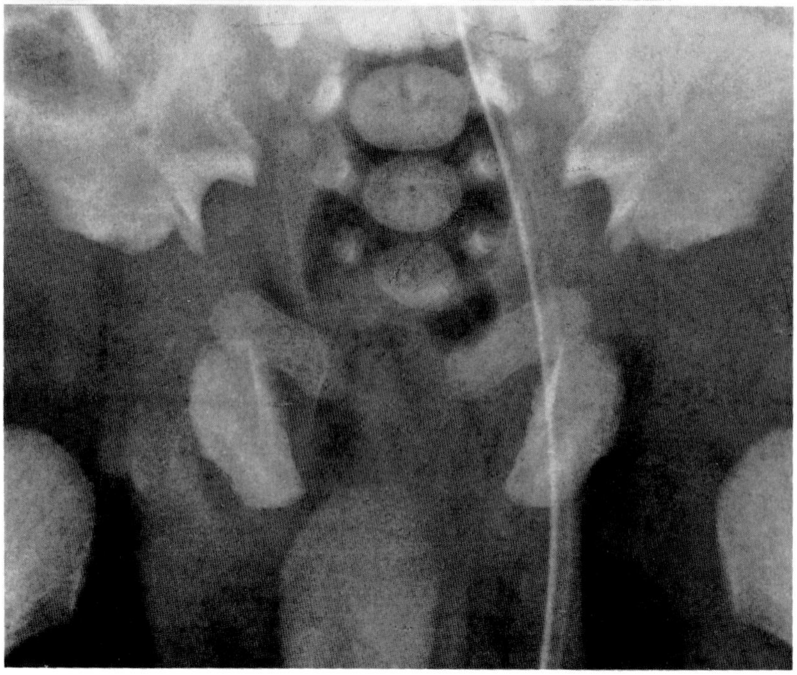

b

Fig. 3a, b. Asphyxiating thoracic dysplasia. **a** Same patient as Fig. 1b: Inversion of clavicle, broad and cupped rib ends. **b** Same patient as Fig. 1a: Peculiarly shaped acetabula with reduction of acetabular angles, medial spurs

1.1.8 Cleidocranial Dysplasia

Cleidocranial dysplasia is an autosomal dominant condition with considerable variation in expression. Hypoplasia or even aplasia (10%) of the clavicles permits abnormal mobility of the shoulders and arms. The adult height is subnormal, and the head usually shows a prominent forehead, persistence of the anterior fontanelle, and abnormal dentition [1, 2]. Additional findings are a narrow pelvis, narrow hypermobile joints, and short nails.

Radiographic Findings [1–3]

Hand

Supernumerary epiphyses (especially second and fifth metacarpals)
Thickened epiphyses of distal phalanges
Cone-shaped epiphyses
Hypoplasia of phalanges (especially distal phalanges)
Pointed tufts
Delayed skeletal maturation

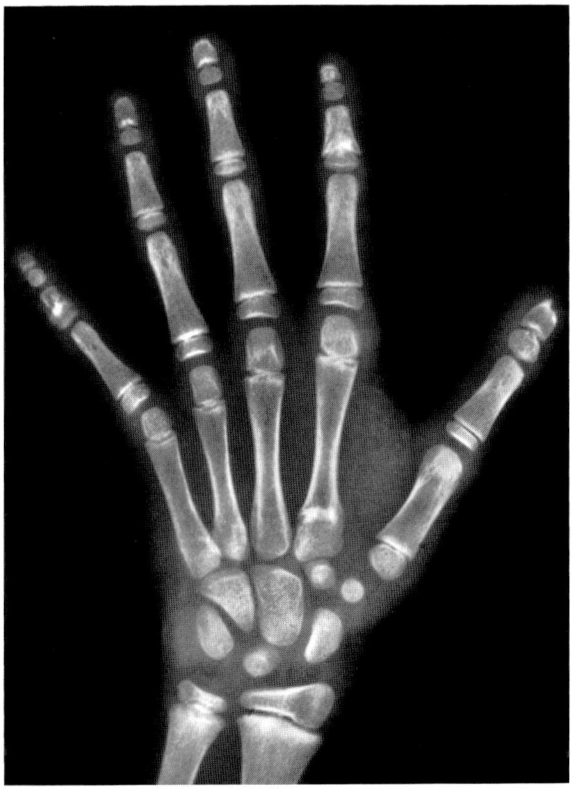

1

Fig. 1. Cleidocranial dysplasia. Thickened epiphyses of distal phalanges, cone-shaped epiphyses and shortening of middle phalanges at second and fifth fingers, pseudoepiphysis at proximal end of second metacarpal, hypoplastic distal phalanges with irregular tufts

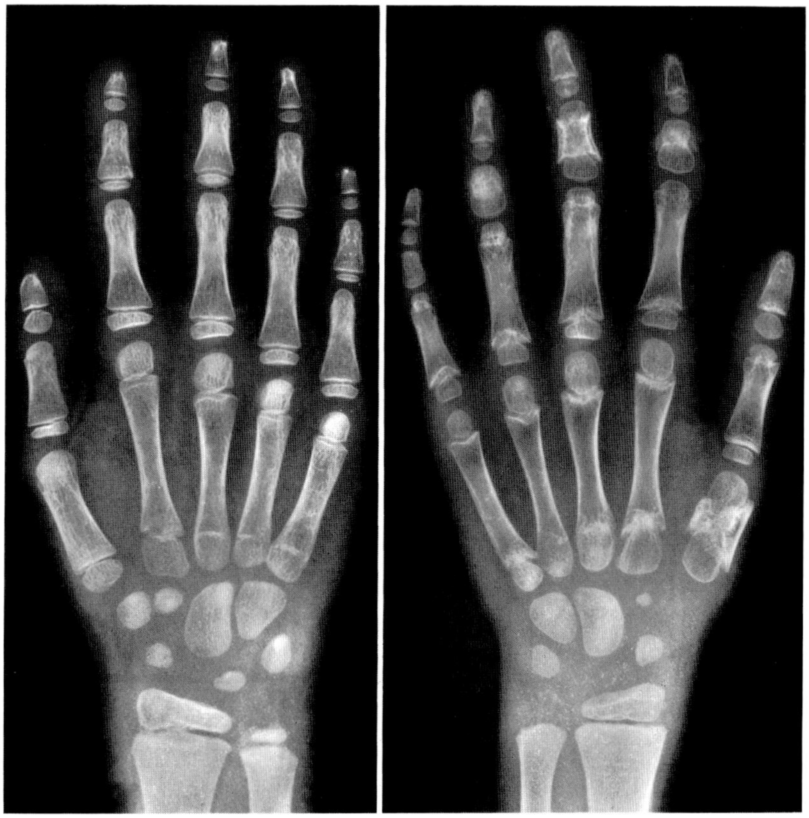

2a **b**

Fig. 2a, b. Cleidocranial dysplasia. **a** In a 7-year-old boy: Thickened epiphyses of distal phalanges, extra epiphysis at proximal end of second metacarpal, pseudoepiphyses in other metacarpals, hypoplastic distal phalanges with irregular and eroded tufts. **b** In an 11-year-old boy: Delayed skeletal maturation, multiple cone-shaped and bracket-shaped epiphyses, short middle phalanges, supernumerary cone-shaped epiphyses at proximal ends of metacarpals a

b

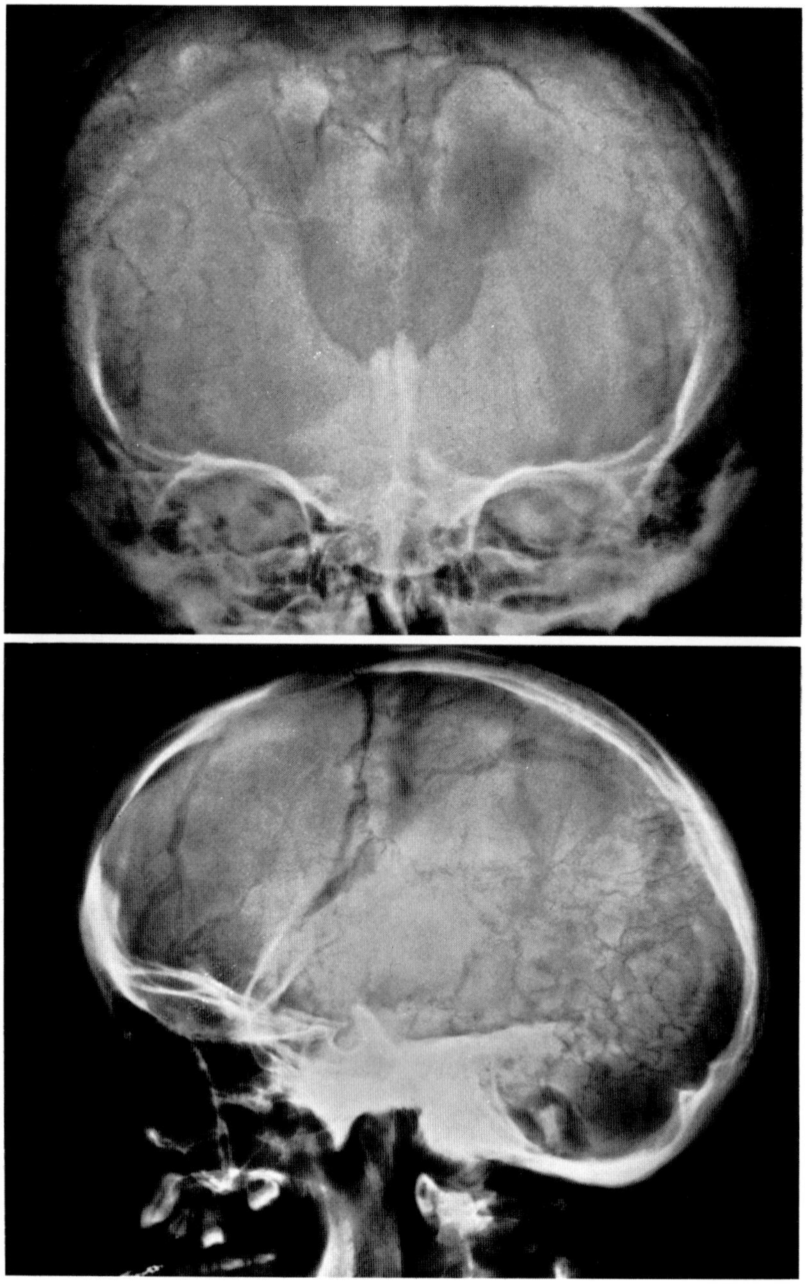

Fig. 3a, b. Cleidocranial dysplasia in a 20-year-old woman. **a** Open anterior fontanelle. **b** Wormian bones

Occasional enlarged second metacarpal and/or acro-osteolysis

Other Sites

Skull: persistence of anterior fontanelle
poor ossification
wormian bones
abnormal dentition
hypertelorism

Clavicles: hypoplasia or aplasia (10%)

Pelvis: poor ossification of pubic bones resulting in wide gap at symphysis

Spine: neural arch defects
hemivertebrae
spondylolisthesis

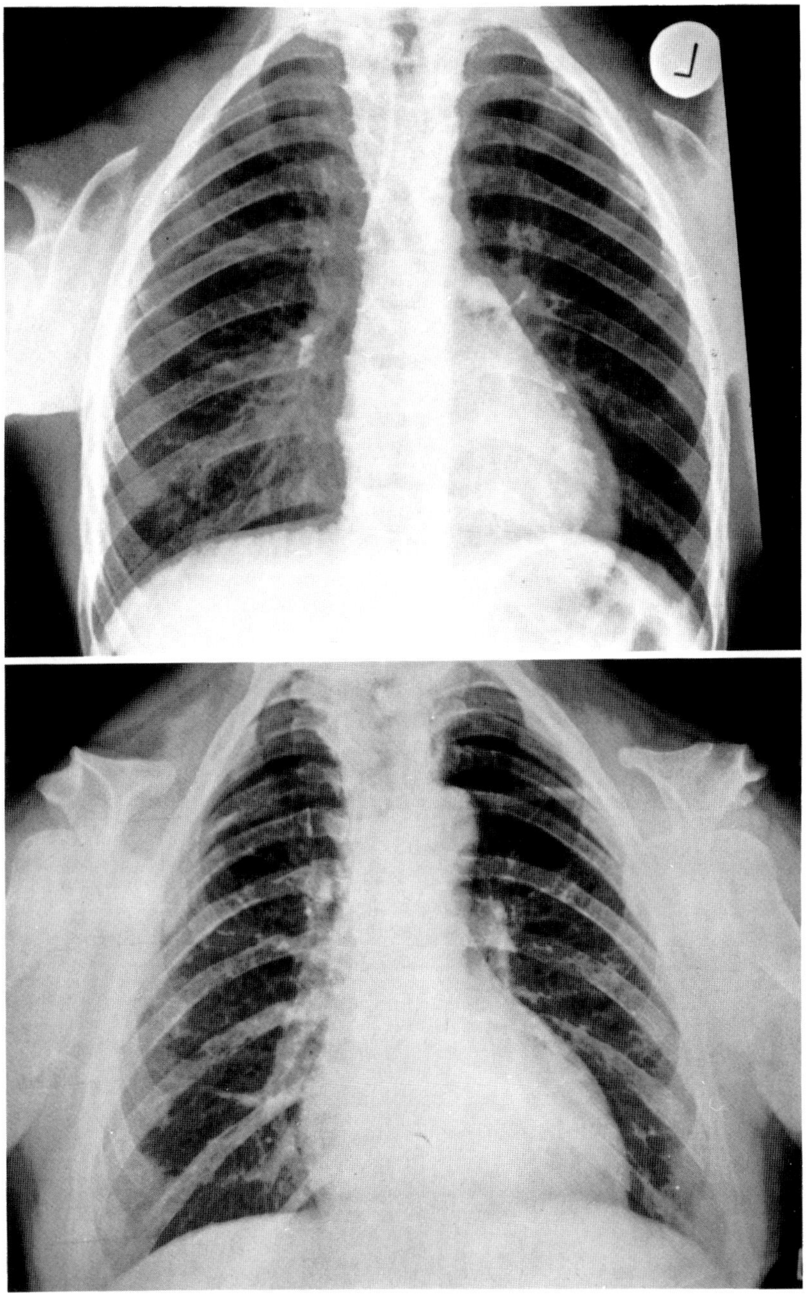

a

b

Fig. 4a, b. Cleidocranial dysplasia. **a** Aplasia of right clavicle, hypoplasia of left clavicle. **b** Hypoplasia of both clavicles

Differential Diagnosis

Brachydactyly (Sect. 2.2.11)
Cone-shaped epiphyses (Sect. 2.2.9)
Wormian bones
- osteogenesis imperfecta (Sect. 1.2.1)
- pyknodysostosis (Sect. 1.2.3)
- pachydermoperiostosis (Sect. 1.2.8)
- Hadju-Cheney syndrome (Sect. 3.1.1)
- hypothyroidism (Sect. 7.2.1)

References

1 Jarvis JL, Keats TE (1974) Cleidocranial dysostosis. A review of 40 new cases. AJR 121:5–16
2 Keats TE (1967) Cleidocranial dysostosis. Some atypical roentgen manifestations. AJR 100:71–79
3 Eventov I, Reider-Grosswasser I, Weiss S, Legun C, Schorr S (1979) Cleidocranial dysplasia. A family study. Clin Radiol 30:323–328

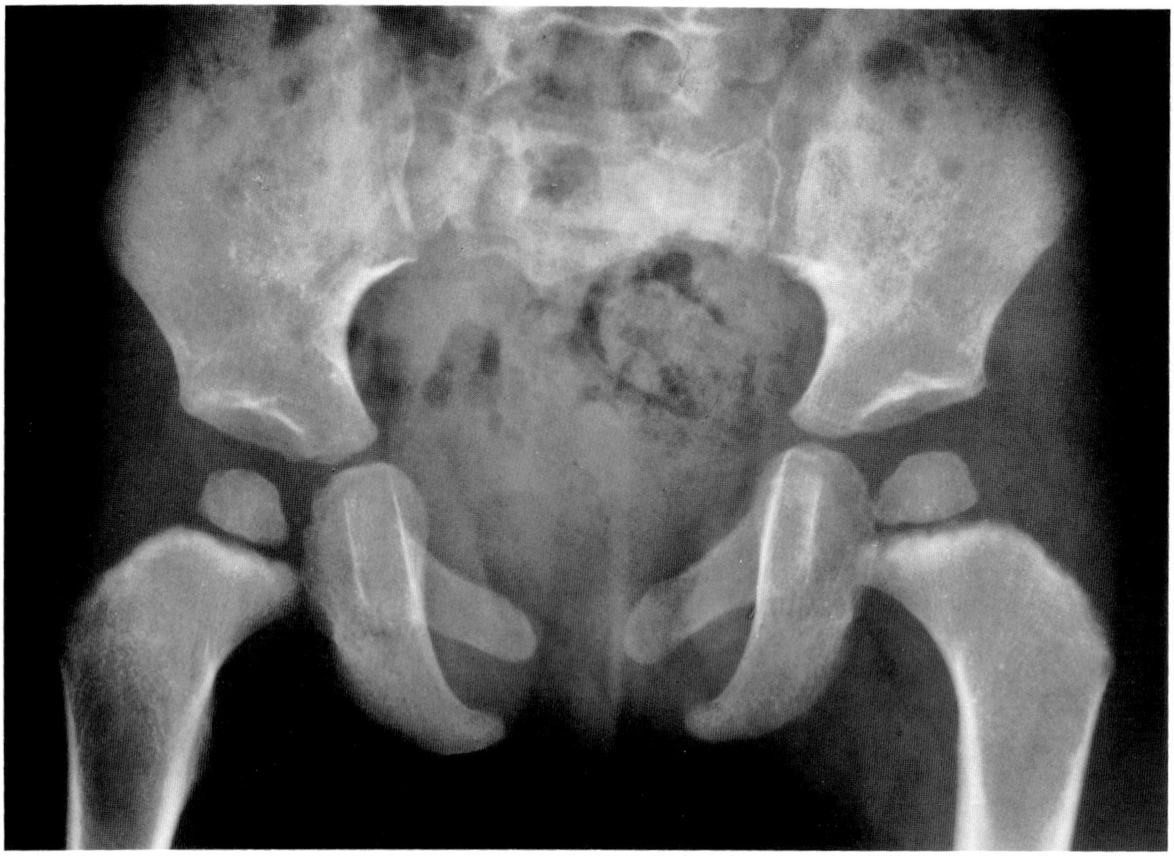

Fig. 5. Cleidocranial dysplasia in a 4-year-old boy. Wide gap at symphysis

1.1.9 Larsen's Syndrome

This autosomal dominant or recessive syndrome is characterized by a flattened facies, prominent forehead, depression of the nasal bridge, cleft palate, and widely spaced eyes [1, 2]. Multiple congenital dislocations of the large joints, infantile respiratory distress from tracheomalacia, and deformities of the fingers and toes are also encountered.

The pathogenesis of this disorder is not entirely clear, but is probably caused by generalized mesenchymal disturbance. In early childhood, knee, hip and elbow dislocations are the most important features. With increasing age, dysplastic alterations appear at the small tubular bones.

Radiographic Findings [1–6]

Hand

Supernumerary carpals
Brachytelephalangy
Brachymetacarpia
Polydactyly
Syndactyly

Other Sites

Foot: supernumerary tarsals
  double ossification center in calcaneus
Larynx: tracheomalacia
Major joints: dislocation
Spine: hypoplastic cervical vertebrae
  abnormal segmentation, especially of cervical spine
  separate processi transversus of lumbar spine
  fusion of vertebral arches
Skull: facial abnormalities
  hydrocephalus

Differential Diagnosis

Diastrophic dysplasia (Sect. 1.1.4)
Marfan's syndrome (Sect. 5.2)
Arthrogryposis multiplex congenita (Sect. 7.1.1)

Otopalatodigital syndrome [7]
Ehlers-Danlos syndrome
Congenital laxity

References

1 Larsen LJ, Schottsteadt ER, Bost FC (1950) Multiple congenital dislocations associated with characteristic facial abnormality. J Pediatr 37:574–581
2 Silverman FN (1972) Larsen's syndrome: congenital dislocation of the knees and other joints. Distinctive facies and frequently cleft palate. Ann Radiol (Paris) 15:297–328
3 Steel HH, Kohl EJ (1972) Multiple congenital dislocations associated with other skeletal anomalies (Larsen's syndrome) in three siblings. J Bone Joint Surg [Am] 54a:75–82
4 Habermann ET, Sterling A, Dennis RI (1976) Larsen's syndrome: a heritable disorder. J Bone Joint Surg [Am] 58a:558–561
5 Galanski M, Statz A (1978) Radiologic findings in Larsen's syndrome. Fortschr Geb Röntgenstr Nuklearmed Ergänzungsband 128:534–537
6 Giedion A (1981) Osteochondrodysplasien. In: Schinz HR (1981) Lehrbuch der Röntgendiagnostik, vol II, 2. Thieme, Stuttgart
7 Poznanski AK, Macpherson RI, Gorlin RJ, Garn SM, Nagy JM, Gall JC Jr, Stern AM, Dijkman DJ (1973) The hand in the oto-palato-digital syndrome. Ann Radiol [Paris] 16:203–209

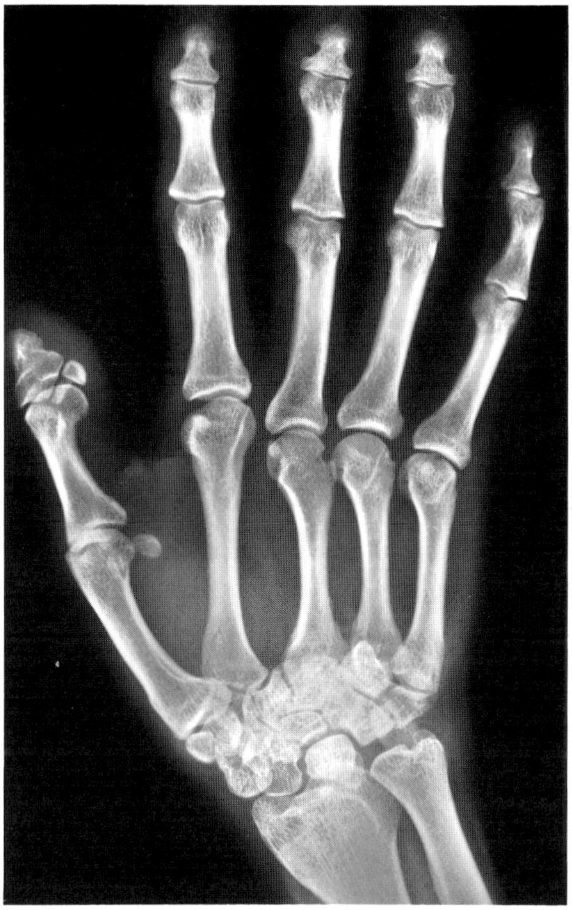

1

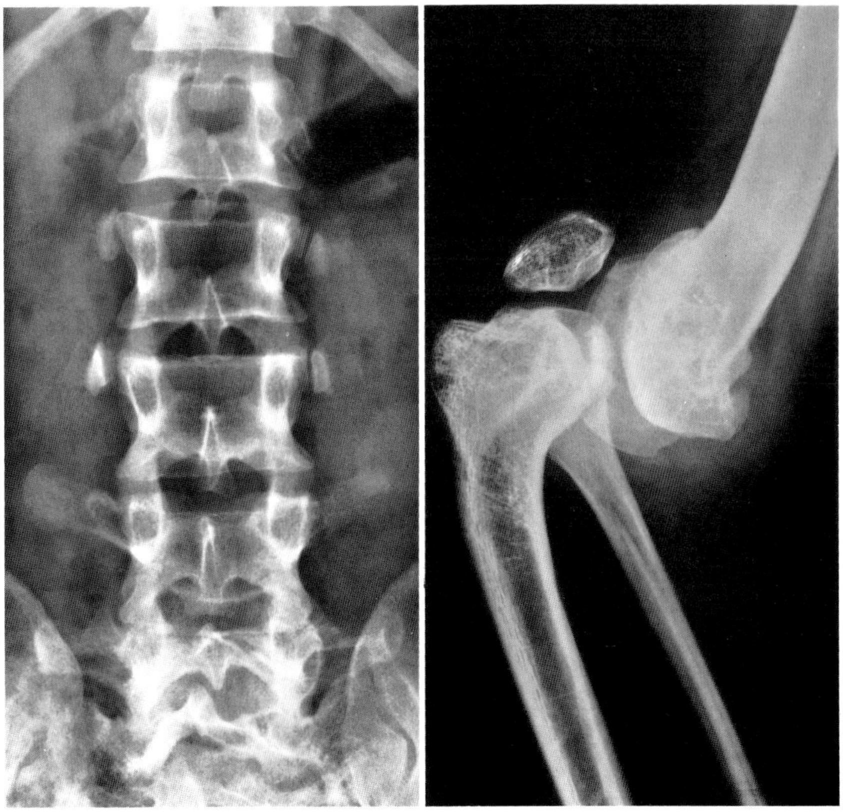

a b 2

Fig. 1. Larsen's syndrome in a 31-year-old man. Supernumerary carpals, significant shortening of third and fourth metacarpals and most distal phalanges

Fig. 2a, b. Same patient as Fig. 1. **a** Processi transversus of L2 and L3 not fused with vertebral bodies. **b** Dislocation of knee

1.1.10 Metaphyseal Chondrodysplasia

According to the International Nomenclature of Constitutional Diseases of Bone [1], four types of metaphyseal chondrodysplasia have been classified: the Jansen type [2], the Schmid type [3], the McKusick type ('cartilage-hair hypoplasia') [4–6] and the Schwachman type (with exocrine pancreatic insufficiency and cyclic neutropenia) [7–10]. The Jansen type is autosomal dominant, the Schmid type is autosomal dominant, the McKusick type is autosomal recessive, and the Schwachman type is autosomal recessive.

Radiologically, the differential diagnosis between the types is rather difficult. The Jansen type presents the most severe abnormalities, and diagnosis of it is usually easy. On the basis of hand radiographs, accurate diagnosis of the other three entities can often not be made [9, 10].

Radiographic Findings [2–5, 7, 9, 10]

Hand

Metaphyses of radius and ulna:
- widening
- cupping
- high degree of mineralization
- bizarre ossification (JANSEN)

Growth plate of radius and ulna widened
Cone-shaped epiphyses (McKUSICK)
Delayed skeletal maturation (JANSEN, McKUSICK, SCHWACHMAN)
Short and slender distal phalanges (McKUSICK)
Irregular carpals (JANSEN, McKUSICK)
Increased carpal angle (JANSEN)

Other Sites

Long tubular bones: shortening and bowing coxa vara
Thorax: widened anterior rib ends
Skull: hypertelorism
Spine: lumbar lordosis

Differential Diagnosis

Rickets (Sect. 6.2)
Other acquired metaphyseal abnormalities (Fig. 4)

References

1 Special report (1978) International nomenclature of constitutional diseases of bone. AJR 131:352–354
2 Holt JF, Poznanski AK (1973) Metaphyseal chondrodysplasia – type Jansen. Sem Roentgenol 8:166–167
3 Deut CE, Normand ECS (1964) Metaphyseal dysostosis. Type Schmid. Arch Dis Child 39:444–449
4 Wiedemann HR, Spranger J, Kosenow W (1967) Knorpel-Haar-Hypoplasie. Arch. Kinderheilkd 176:74–85
5 Ray HC, Dorst JP (1973) Cartilage-hair hypoplasia. In: Kaufman HJ (ed) Intrinsic diseases of bone. Karger, Basel (Progress in pediatric radiology, vol 4)
6 Beals RK (1968) Cartilage-hair hypoplasia. J Bone Joint Surg [Am] 50^a:1245–1248
7 Taybi H, Mitchell AD, Friedman GD (1969) Metaphyseal dysostosis and the associated syndrome of pancreatic insufficiency and blood disorders. Radiology 93:563–571
8 Schwachman H, Diamond LK, Oski FA, Khaw KT (1964) The syndrome of pancreatic insufficiency and bone marrow dysfunction. J Pediatr 65:645–663
9 Sutcliffe J, Stanley P (1973) Metaphyseal chondrodysplasias. In: Kaufmann HJ (ed) Intrinsic diseases of bone. Karger, Basel, pp 250–269 (Progress in pediatric radiology, vol 4)
10 McLennan TW, Steinbach HL (1974) Schwachman's syndrome: the broad spectrum of bony abnormalities. Radiology 112:167–173

Differentiation between the four types of metaphyseal chondrodysplasia on the basis of hand radiographs

	JANSEN	SCHMID	McKUSICK	SCHWACHMAN
Radius and ulna				
Wide growth plate	+ +	+		±
Irregular metaphysis	+ bulging	+ mild	+ significant	+
Shortening of tubular bones	+ severe	+ mild	+ significant	± mild
Short slender distal phalanges			+	
Irregular carpals	+		±	
Delayed skeletal maturation	+	+ mild	+ severe	+
Increased carpal angle	+		+	±

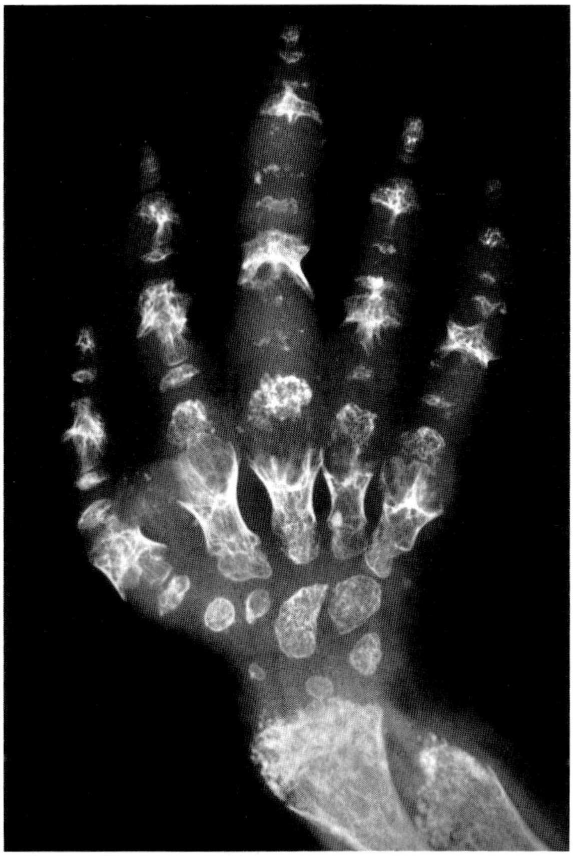

Fig. 1. Metaphyseal chondrodysplasia (Jansen type) in a 5-year-old girl. Severe metaphyseal abnormalities with cupping and lucencies, widened epiphyseal plates, and irregular carpals

Fig. 2a, b. Metaphyseal chondrodysplasia (Schmid type). **a** In a 2-year-old boy: Cupped and flared ulnar metaphysis, metaphysis of radius also abnormal, increased bone density adjacent to these metaphyses. Some delay in skeletal maturation. **b** In a 5-year-old girl: Somewhat irregular radial and ulnar metaphyses with sclerotic margins. Epiphysis in distal phalanx of thumb cone-shaped, demarcation of several phalangeal metaphyses slightly irregular. Delayed skeletal maturation
▽

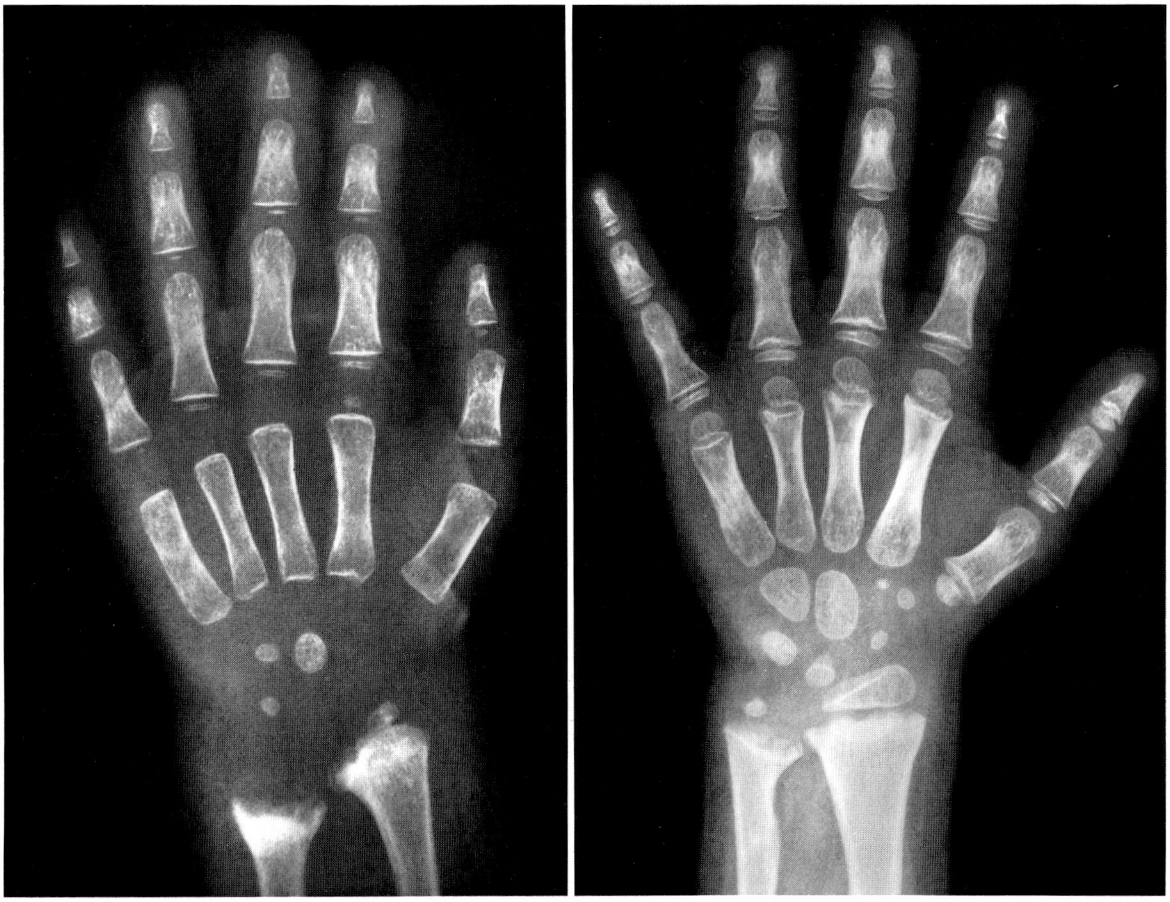

a b

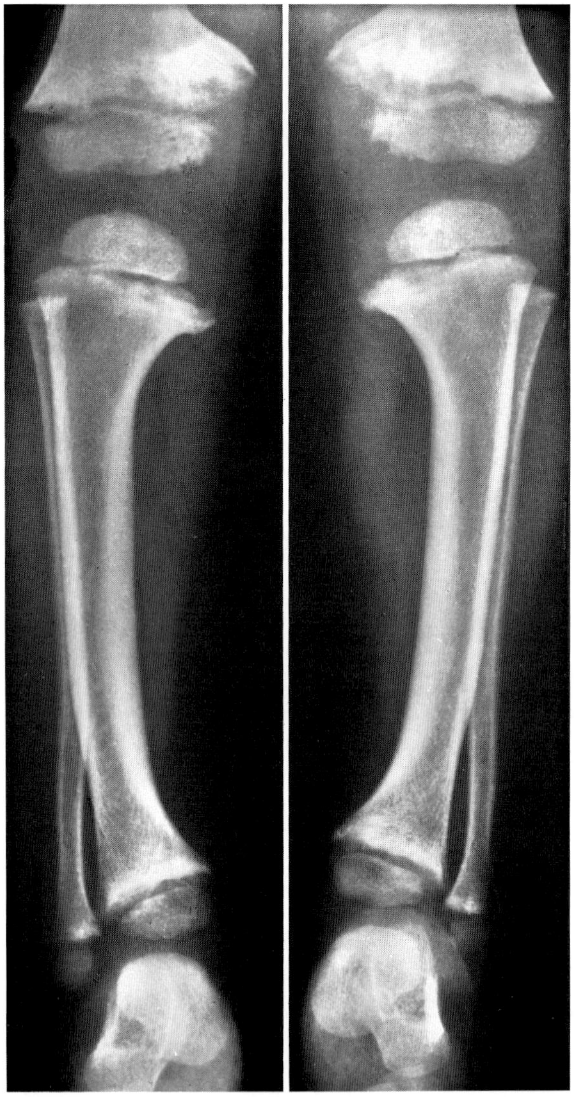

Fig. 3. Metaphyseal chondrodysplasia (Schmid type) in a 4-year-old boy. Flared and irregular femoral and tibial metaphyses, both legs bowed

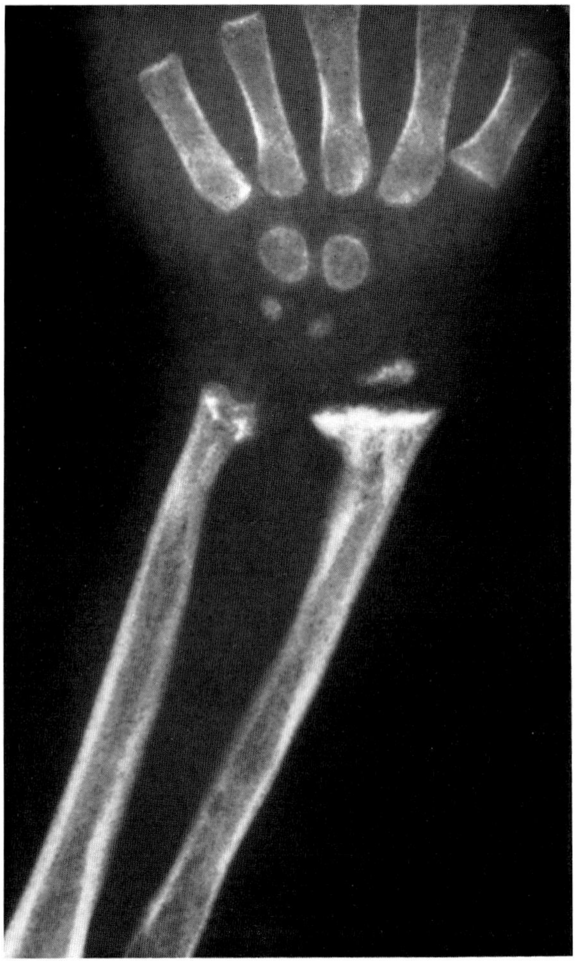

Fig. 4. Disturbed skeletal growth after radiotherapy. Irregular demarcation of radial and ulnar metaphyses, widening of radial growth plate and sclerosis of metaphysis

1.1.11 Multiple Epiphyseal Dysplasia

Synonym: dysplasia epiphysialis multiplex

The term multiple epiphyseal dysplasia includes a heterogenous group of conditions with the main finding of an epiphyseal affection. This affection produces a not very prominent shortness of stature. Inheritance is autosomal dominant, although some cases of autosomal recessive inheritance have been reported. The abnormalities in the hand are very variable, ranging from slight irregularities of the epiphyses to marked irregularities of the epiphyses with brachydactyly. Thiemann's disease is perhaps not a separate disease but one of the disorders within this entity. This disease has been described in males between the ages of 10 and 20 years [1–3]. In multiple epiphyseal dysplasia the spine is usually normal.

Radiographic Findings [1–4]

Hand

Epiphyses: ivory or dense
delayed in appearance
thin

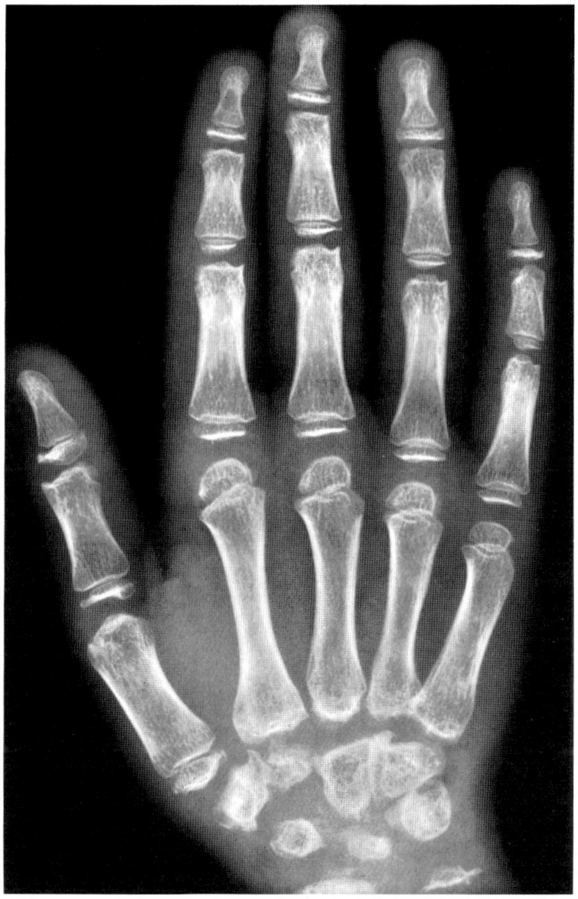

Fig. 1. Multiple epiphyseal dysplasia in a 10-year-old girl. Delayed maturation of irregular carpals, irregular distal ends of proximal phalanges, thinned and slightly dense epiphyses

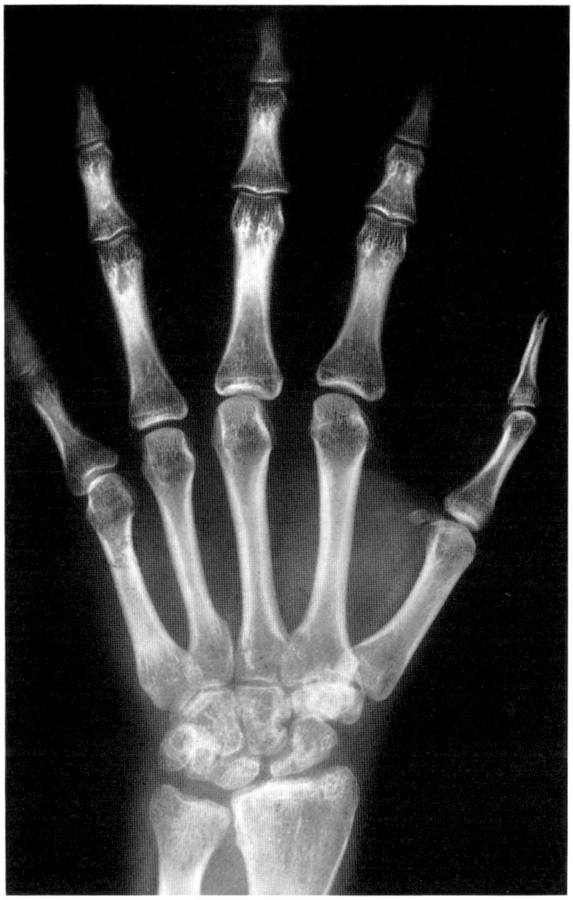

Fig. 2. Multiple epiphyseal dysplasia in an adult man. Brachydactyly of middle phalanges of second and fifth fingers, irregular and small carpals, slight deformation of distal radius and ulna

fragmented
irregular
Metaphyses widened and somewhat cupped
Shortened and thickened tubular bones
Hypoplastic and irregular carpals
Delayed carpal maturation
Increased carpal angle
V-shaped deformity of wrist
Occasional brachydactyly

Other Sites
Foot: hypoplasia of tarsals
brachydactyly
Long tubular bones: epiphyseal abnormalities with coxa vara, genu vara, genu valga
Spine: mild platyspondylisis
anterior wedging of vertebral bodies

Differential Diagnosis

Chondrodysplasia punctata (Sect. 1.1.2)
Diastrophic dysplasia (Sect. 1.1.4)
Mucopolysaccharidosis (Sect. 6.1.1)
Cretinism (Sect. 7.2.1)
Spondyloepiphyseal dysplasia
Spondylometaphyseal dysplasia
Pseudoachondroplasia

References

1 Maudsley RH (1955) Dysplasia epiphysialis multiplex. J Bone Joint Surg [Br] 37b:228–234
2 Poznanski AK, Holt JF (1971) The carpals in congenital malformation syndromes. AJR 112:443–459
3 Felman AH (1969) Multiple epiphyseal dysplasia. Radiology 93:119–125
4 Berg PK (1966) Dysplasia epiphysialis multiplex. AJR 97:31–38

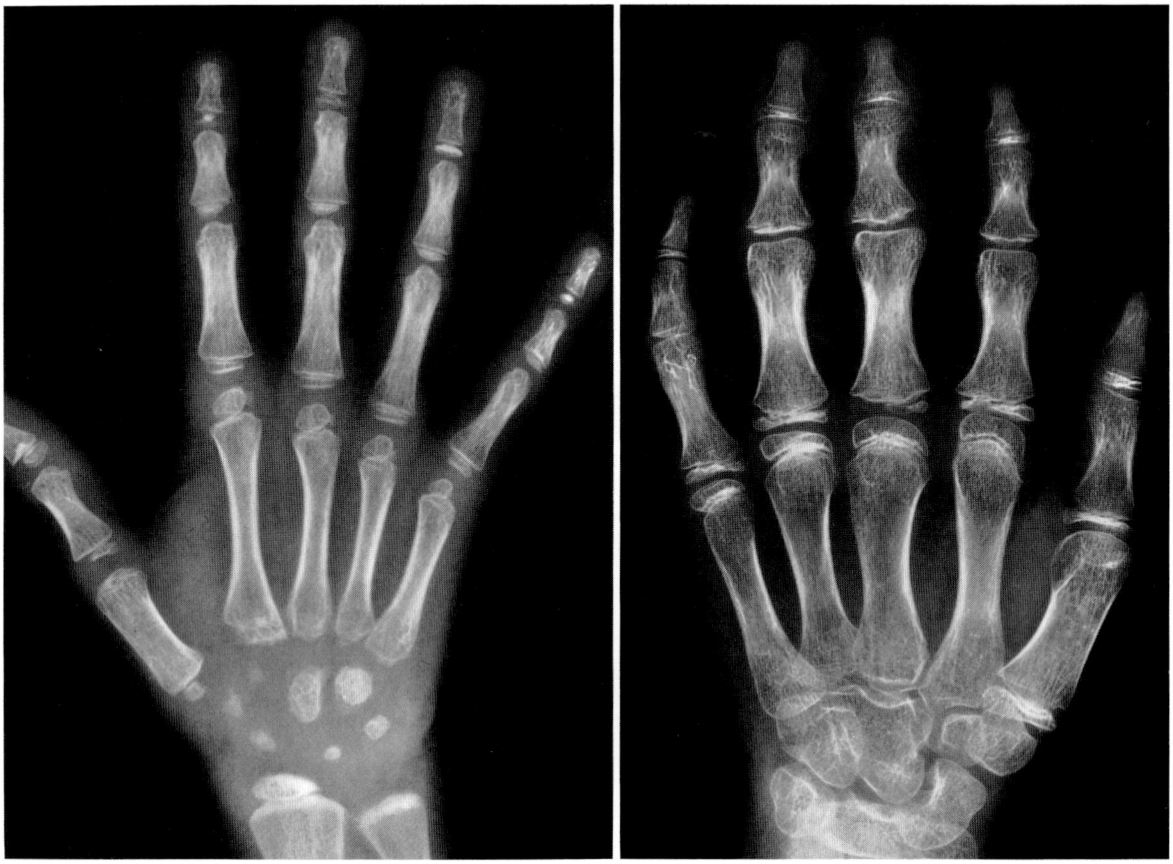

a b

Fig. 3a, b. Multiple epiphyseal dysplasia. **a** In a 10-year-old boy: Delayed skeletal maturation. Dense distal epiphyses of second, fourth, and fifth fingers, thinning of epiphyses at other sites. **b** In another 10-year-old boy: Thinning and fragmentation of epiphyses, comparatively short and thick phalanges and metacarpals

Fig. 4. Multiple epiphyseal dysplasia in a 10-year-old ▷ girl. Significant epiphyseal abnormalities in femur and tibia, irregular ossification of patella

Fig. 5. Spondyloepiphyseal dysplasia in a 16-year-old boy. Dense epiphyses in most of the phalanges. The vertebral bodies presented severe platyspondylisis

Fig. 6. A 9-year-old girl. Familial multiple ivory and dense epiphyses, mostly situated at the usual sites. The additional dense epiphyses in several of the middle phalanges suggest the diagnosis of multiple epiphyseal dysplasia rather than Thiemann's disease. Except for similar abnormalities at the toes, no other skeletal abnormalities were present. The epiphyses of all the long bones were normal

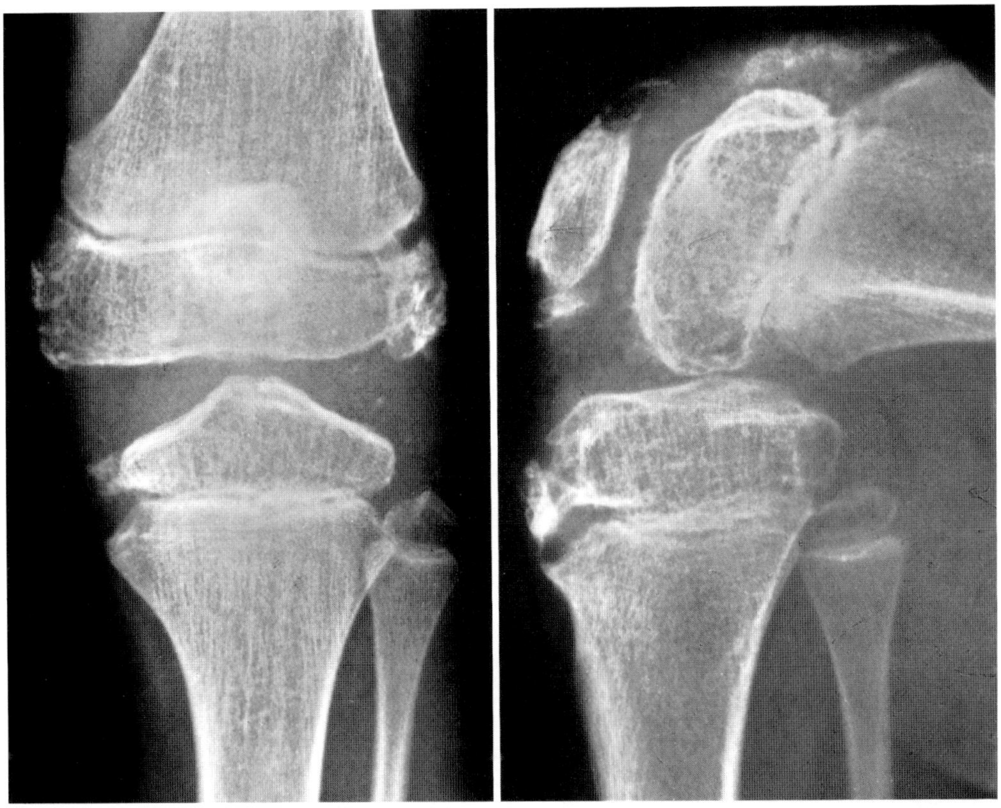

4

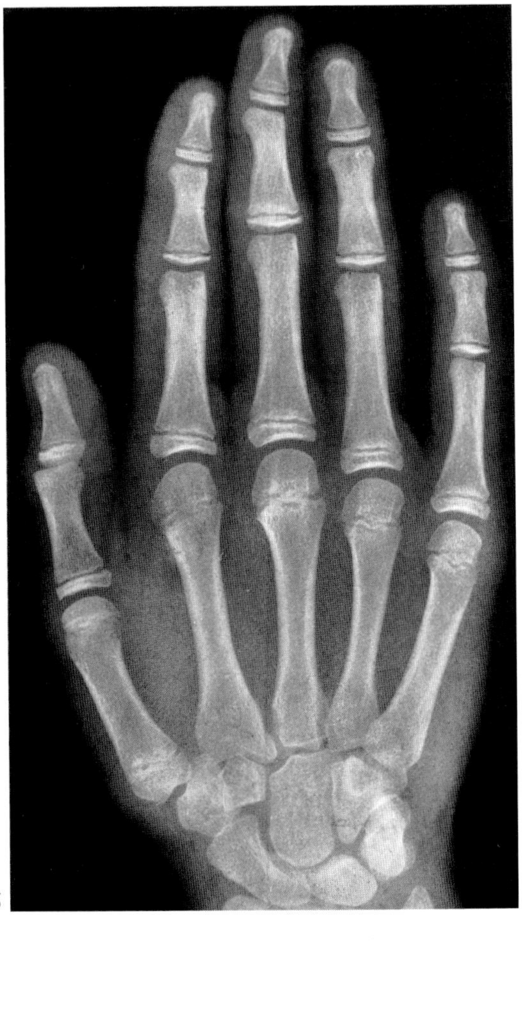

5

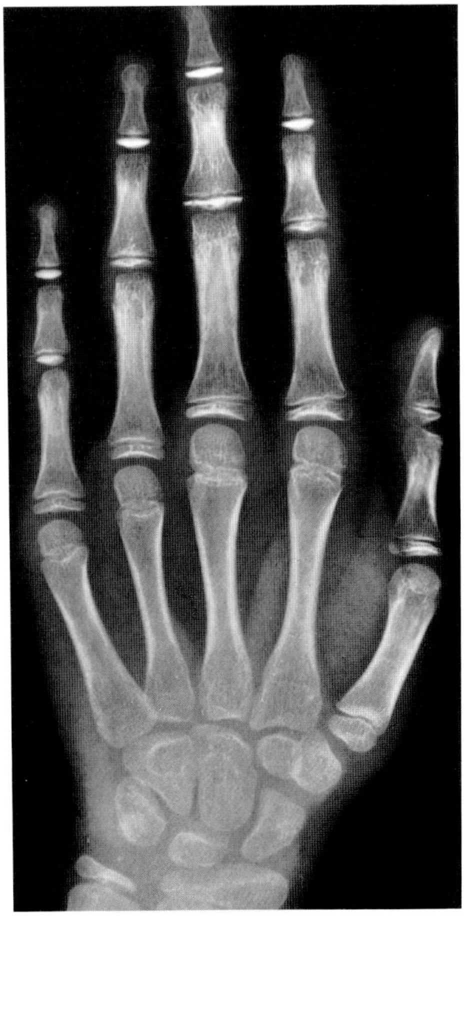

6

1.1.12 Trichorhinophalangeal Syndrome

Synonym: Giedion's syndrome

This usually autosomal dominant inherited syndrome is characterized by bulbous nose, hand changes, and hypoplasia or slow growth of the hair. Sometimes the patient's stature is shortened and mental retardation is present.

Radiographic Findings [1, 2]

Hand

Cone-shaped epiphyses (Giedion type 12), particularly in middle phalanges, with central portion fused with remainder of shaft
Ivory epiphyses in distal phalanges
Brachydactyly
Curvature of fingers

Other Sites

Foot: findings similar to hand abnormalities
Pelvis: osteonecrosis of hips

Differential Diagnosis

Other disorders with cone-shaped epiphyses (Sect. 2.2.9)

References

1 Gorlin RJ, Cohen MM Jr, Wolfson J (1969) Tricho-rhino-phalangeal syndrome. Am J Dis Child 118:595–599
2 Giedion A, Burdea M, Fruchter Z, Meloni T, Trose V (1973) Autosomal dominant transmission of the tricho-rhino-phalangeal syndrome. Report of 4 unrelated families, a review of 60 cases. Helv Paediatr Acta 28:249–256

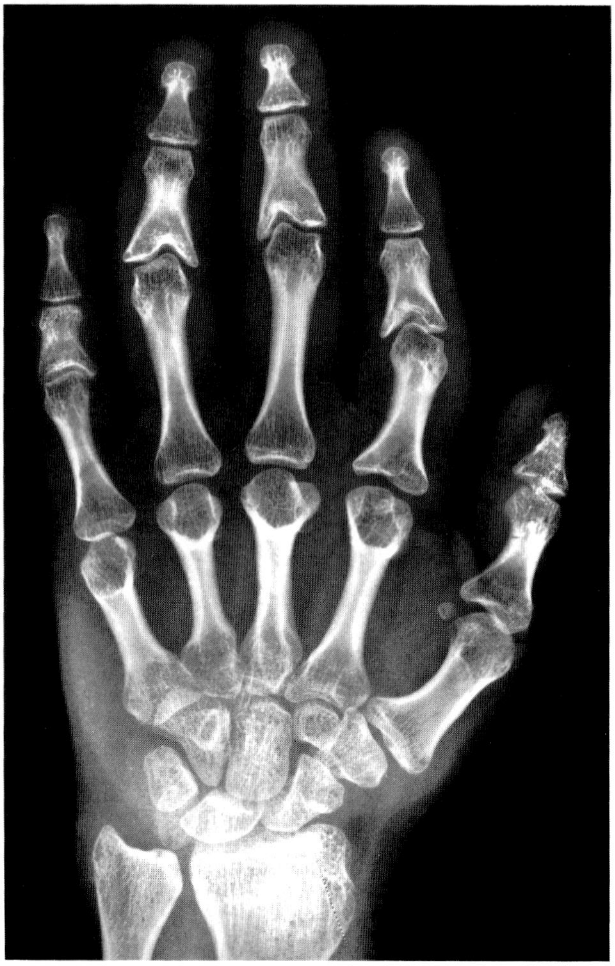

Fig. 1. Trichorhinophalangeal syndrome in an 18-year-old woman. Widening of proximal end of middle phalanges with curving of affected fingers, brachydactyly of middle phalanges and of distal phalanges of first and third fingers

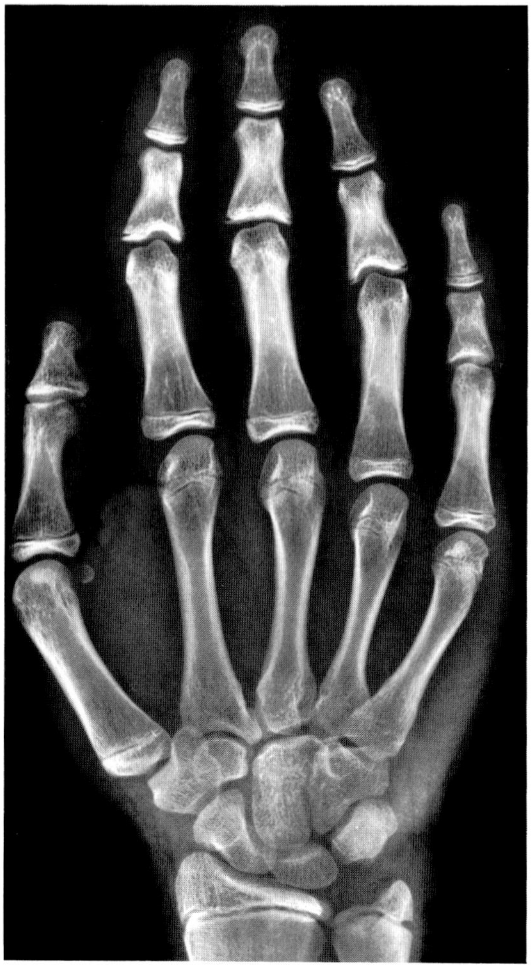

Fig. 2. Trichorhinophalangeal syndrome in a 17-year-old boy. Characteristic abnormalities of the middle phalanges: the proximal ends of these shortened phalanges are slightly widened. A bulbous nose and osteonecrosis of the hips were other findings in this patient

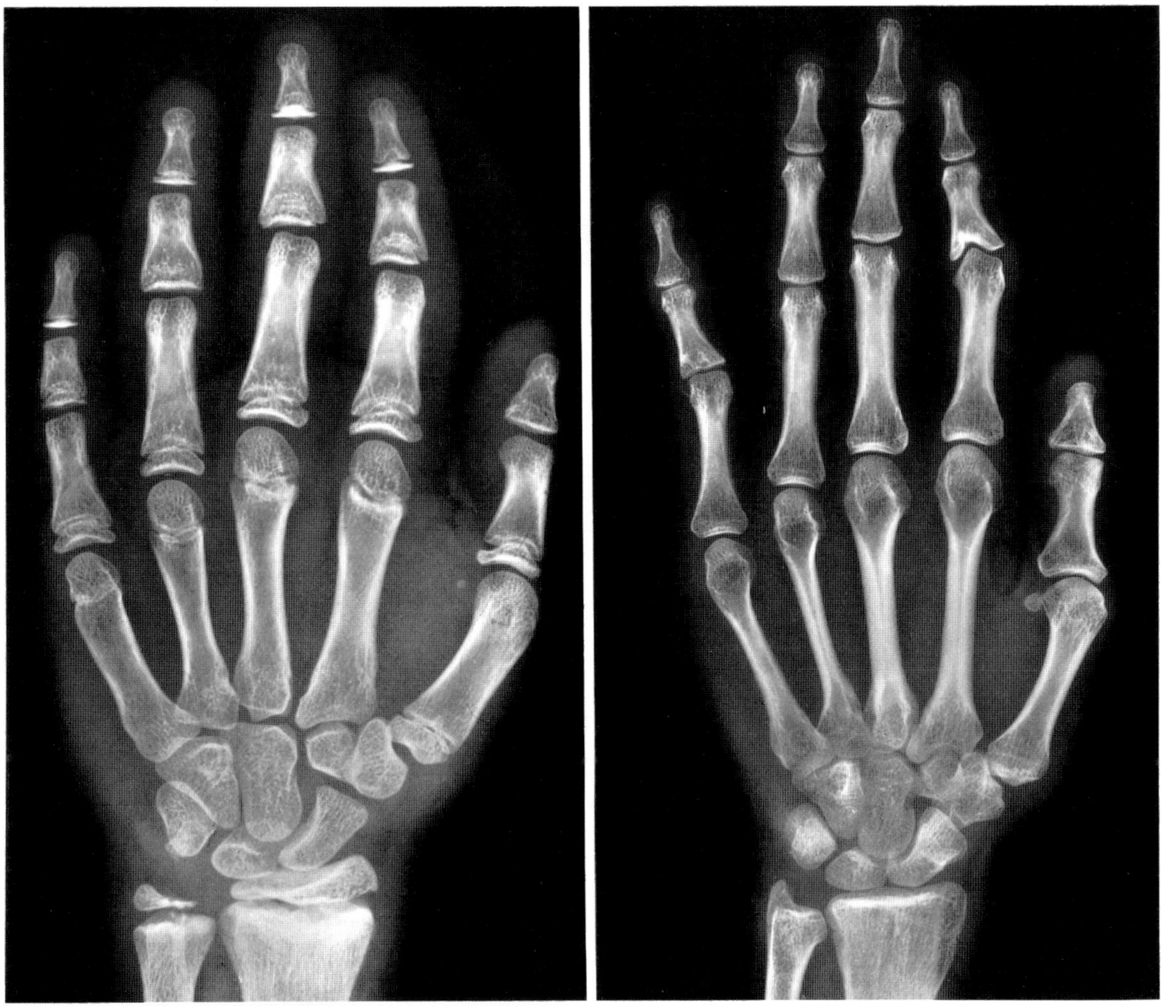

a b

Fig. 3a, b. Trichorhinophalangeal syndrome **a** In a 13-year-old boy: Cone-shaped epiphyses in most fingers, ivory distal epiphyses, shortening of middle phalanges and of distal phalanx of thumb. Slight irregularity and flattening of distal epiphyses of radius and ulna. **b** In a 25-year-old woman: Widening of middle phalanx of second finger, additional brachydactyly of distal phalanx of thumb and middle phalanx of fifth finger

1.2 Abnormalities of Density of Cortical Diaphyseal Structure and/or Metaphyseal Modeling

1.2.1 Osteogenesis Imperfecta

The osseous manifestations of osteogenesis imperfecta are caused by deficient activity of periosteal and endosteal osteoblastic activity. The reduced periosteal activity disturbs the circumferential growth of the bones. To a lesser degree, failure of endochondral bone formation is important too. The synthesis of collagen matrix is involved, associated with disturbance in the mineralization of bone.

Classification

Osteogenesis imperfecta can be classified into four types on the basis of clinical and radiographic findings and mode of inheritance [1–4]:

Type I, autosomal dominant: *osteogenesis imperfecta with blue sclerae* (mild long bone disease)
Findings: blue sclerae, easy bruising, impaired hearing and deafness, arcus corneae
Spine: scoliosis
Skull: abnormal dentinogenesis
Long tubular bones: fractures, hypermobile joints

Type II, autosomal recessive: *lethal perinatal osteogenesis imperfecta* (Vrolik's type)
Findings: stillbirth or death soon after birth
Long bones: multiple fractures, bowing and shortening of limbs, crumpled appearance
Skull: wormian bones, osteopenia
Thorax: beading of ribs

Type III, autosomal recessive: *progressively deforming osteogenesis imperfecta with normal sclerae* (severe long bone disease)
Findings: faintly blue or white sclerae
Long tubular bones: fractures usually present at birth, marked bone fragility, increasing deformity of limbs, ligamentous laxity
Spine: progressive kyphoscoliosis
Skull: abnormal dentinogenesis (yellowish-brown teeth)

Type IV, autosomal dominant: *osteogenesis imperfecta with normal sclerae* (individuals with marked shortening of stature and/or skeletal deformity, as well as patients with only a slight handicap, are encountered in this group)
Findings: variable age of onset of fractures (from birth to adult life)
Long tubular bones, spine: variable deformity
Skull: abnormal dentinogenesis

Radiographic Findings [2–5]

Hand
Severe osteoporosis
Slender tubular bones
Thin cortex
Coarsening of bony trabeculae
Fractures (uncommon)

Other Sites
Ribs and long tubular bones (thin bone type):
- osteoporosis
- thinning of cortex
- multiple fractures
- deformation, bowing
- slender bones
- poor trabeculation of spongiosa

Ribs and long tubular bones (thick bone type):
- deformation, bowing
- crumpled bones
- abundant callus formation
- congenital fractures
- longitudinal compression (telescoping)

Skull: wormian bones
- enlarged sinuses
- bulging in temporal and occipital regions
- abnormal dentition

Spine: scoliosis
- platyspondylisis

Pelvis: protrusio acetabuli

Fig. 1. Osteogenesis imperfecta type II in a 1-day-old boy. Shortening of upper limb, some telescoping of humerus, multiple congenital fractures ▷

Fig. 2. Osteogenesis imperfecta type I or type IV in a 2-year-old girl. Very thin metacarpal cortices, some coarsening of trabeculae especially in distal radius and ulna

Fig. 3. Osteogenesis imperfecta type II in a stillborn baby. Numerous fractures in skeleton, telescoping of long tubular bones, beading of ribs

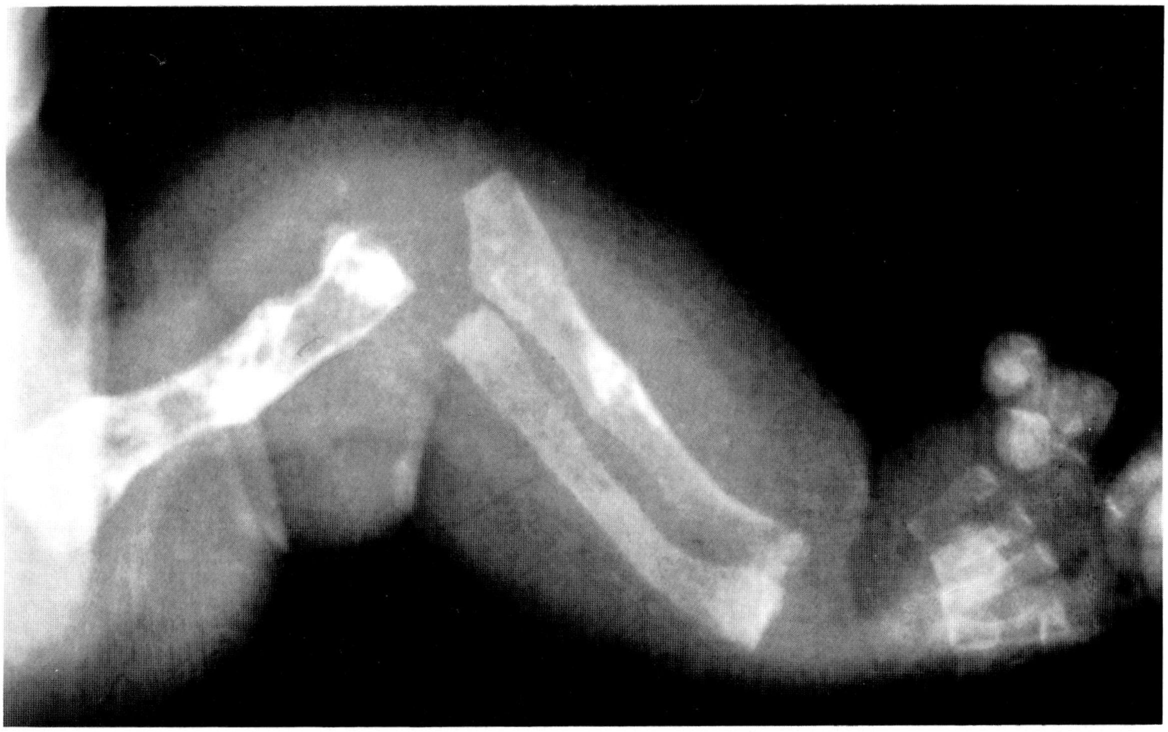

1

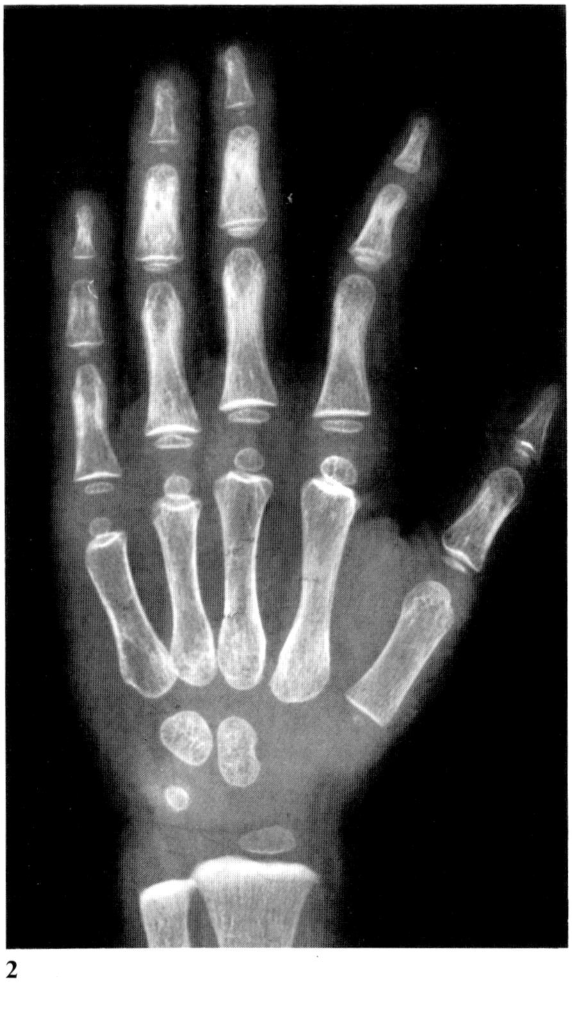

2

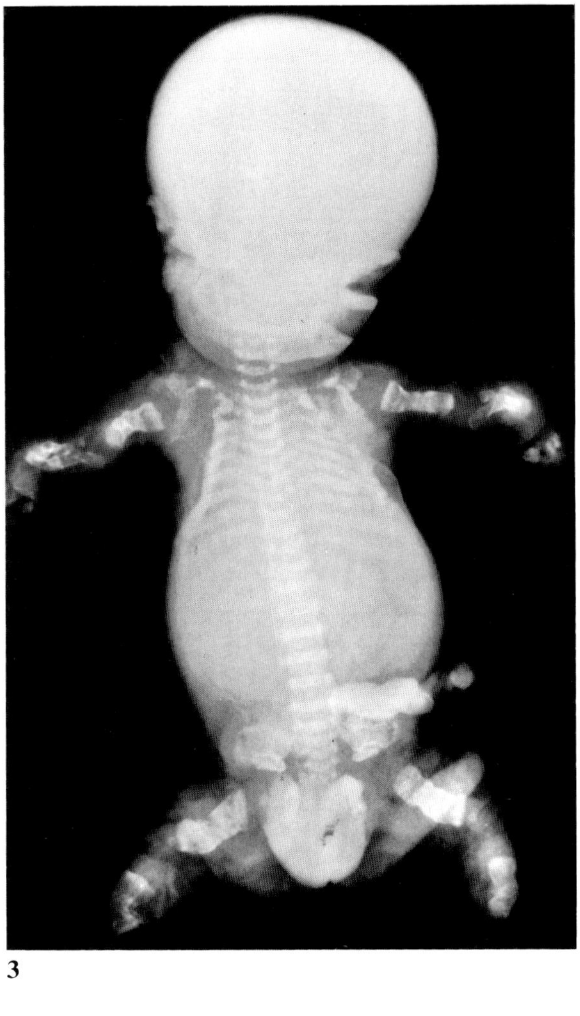

3

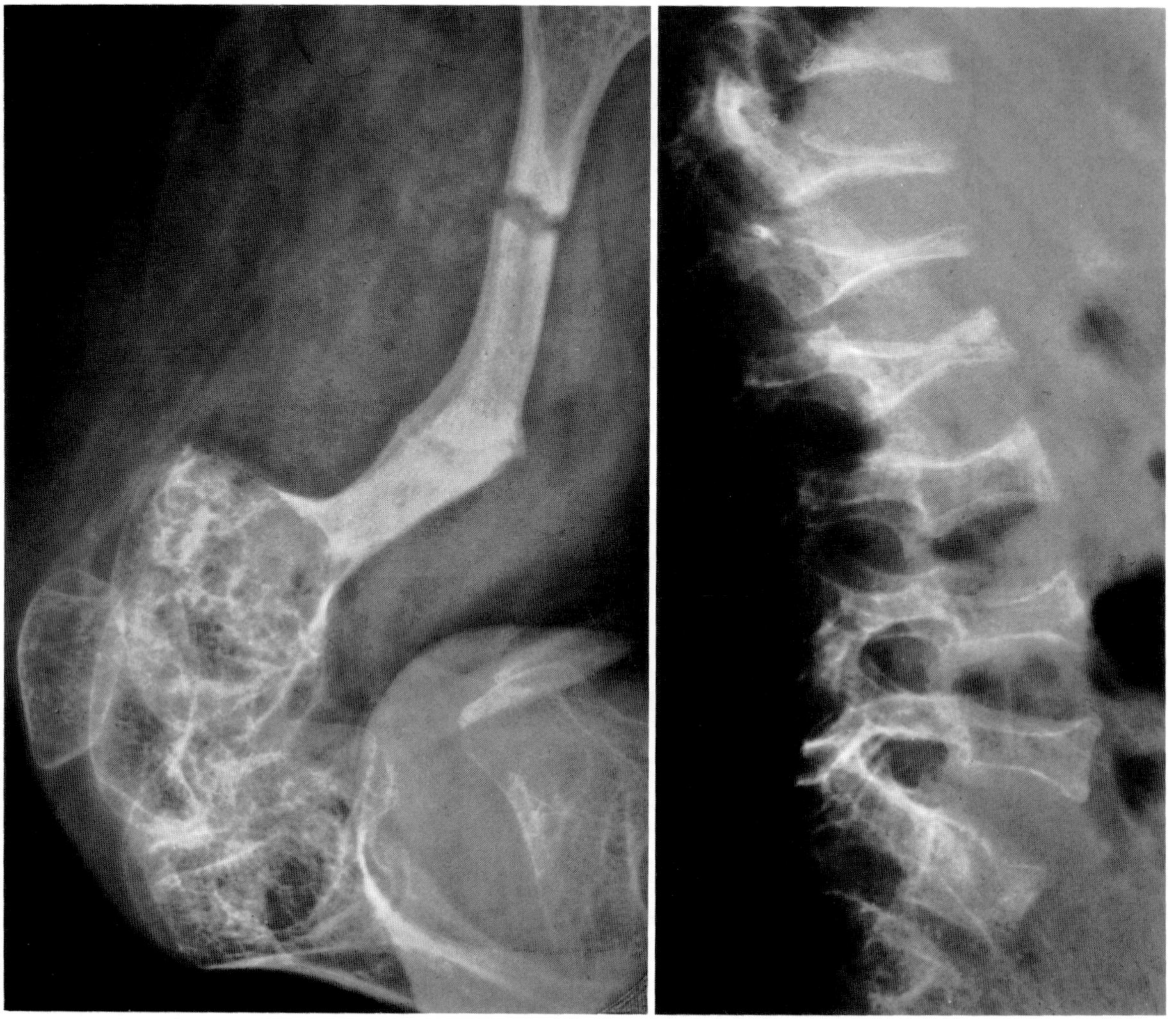

Fig. 4a, b. Osteogenesis imperfecta. **a** In a 15-year-old girl: Bizarre bowing of lower limb with coarsening of trabecular bone structures. Femur presents recent fracture. Probably type III. **b** In a 5-year-old boy: Severe osteoporosis of spine resulting in platyspondylisis. Probably type IV

Differential Diagnosis

Idiopathic juvenile osteoporosis [6]
Battered child syndrome
Congenital insensivity to pain
Hypophosphatasia
Cushing's disease

References

1 Sillence DO, Rimoin DL, Danks DM (1979) Clinical variability in osteogenesis imperfecta – variable expressivity or genetic heterogeneity. In: Bergsma D (ed) Birth defects. Liss, New York, pp 113–119 (Original Article Series, vol 15)
2 Fairbank T (1951) Atlas of general affections of the skeleton. Livingstone, Edinburgh
3 Clemens D, Benz HJ (1979) Osteogenesis imperfecta cystica (Fairbank) – eine Sonderform der Osteogenesis imperfecta congenita (Vrolik). Fortschr Geb Röntgenstr Nuklearmed Ergänzungsband 131:72–77
4 Spranger JW, Langer L, Wiedemann HR (1974) Bone dysplasias: An atlas of constitutional disorders of skeletal development. Saunders, Philadelphia
5 Greenfield GB (1979) Radiology of bone disease. Lippincott, Philadelphia
6 Stöver B, Ball F, Walther A (1974) Idiopathische juvenile Osteoporose. Fortschr Geb Röntgenstr Nuklearmed Ergänzungsband 121:435–444

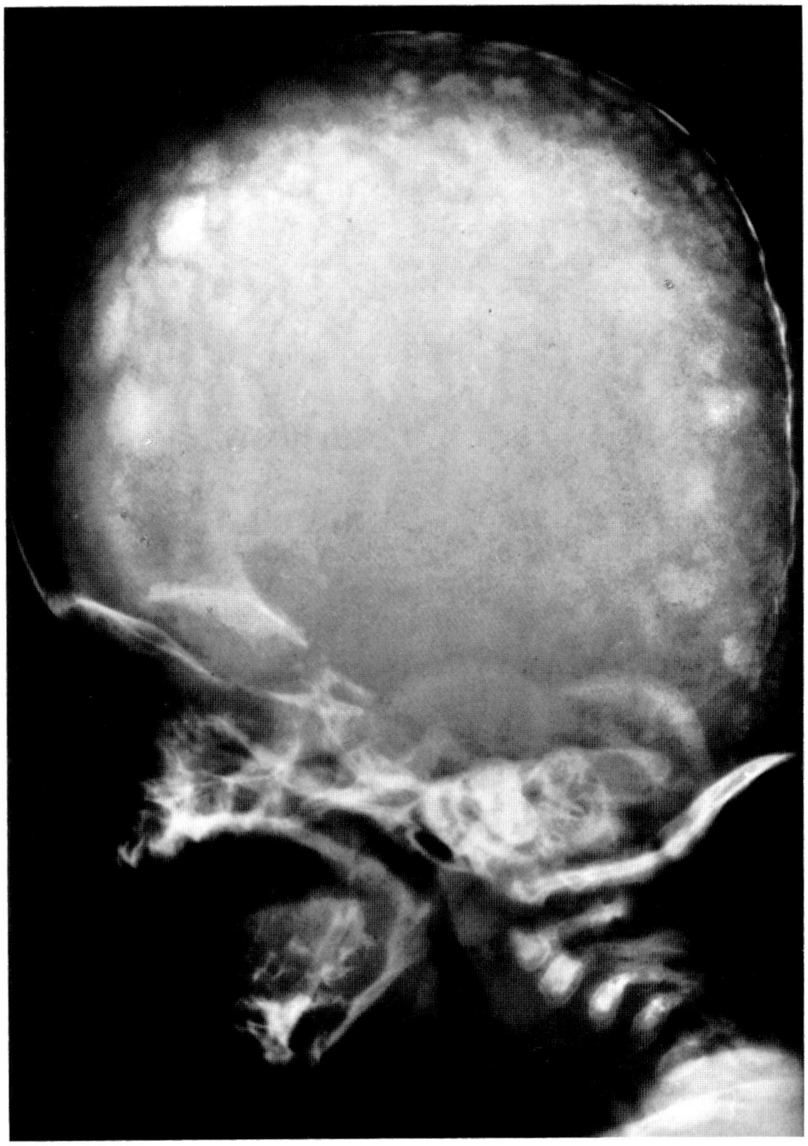

Fig. 5. Osteogenesis imperfecta type II in a 2-week-old baby. Multiple wormian bones in skull

1.2.2 Osteopetrosis

Synonyms: Albers-Schönberg disease, marble-bone disease

There are two forms of osteopetrosis:

1. *Precocious manifestation*: Autosomal recessive disorder characterized by failure to thrive, hepatosplenomegaly, anemia, bone sclerosis, and death. The majority of victims succumb before the end of the first year of life, mostly from recurrent infections [1, 2].
2. *Delayed manifestation*: Autosomal dominant benign form, usually not recognizable in the neonate [1, 2].

The failure of osteoclastic resorption results in excessive masses of unresorbed calcified cartilage and osteoid. These structures obliterate the bone marrow spaces, crowding out the hematopoetic cells. Alternating bands of sclerosis and lucency in the growing bones are often present (bone-in-bone aspect). In the lethal form, signs of rickets may be associated [3]. The bones become brittle and fractures can occur.

Radiographic Findings [1–5]

Hand

Dense sclerosis (metaphyseal)
Alternating bands of sclerosis and translucency (bone-in-bone aspect)
Diminished marrow space of tubular bones
Abnormal metaphyseal modeling
Signs of rickets
Periosteal bone reaction

Other Sites

Long tubular bones: modeling failure in metaphyses
brittleness and density
alternating bands of sclerosis and translucency (bone-in-bone aspect)
fractures
Spine: subchondral sclerosis
alternating bands of sclerosis and translucency (bone-in-bone aspect)
Skull: sclerosis

Differential Diagnosis

Pyknodystosis (Sect. 1.2.3)
Endosteal hyperostosis D (Sect. 1.2.7)
Hypervitaminosis D (Sect. 6.2.2)
Lead poisoning (Sect. 7.5.2)
Sclerosteosis [5]

References

1 Loria Cortes R, Quesada-Calvo E, Cordero-Chavem C (1977) Osteopetrosis in children. A report of 26 cases. Pediatrics 91:43–50
2 Yu JS, Oates RK, Walsh KH, Stuckey SJ (1971) Osteopetrosis. Arch Dis Child 46:257–263
3 Milgram JW, Muraly J (1982) Osteopetrosis. A morphological study of twenty-one cases. J Bone Joint Surg [Am] 64a:912–929
4 Beighton P, Horan F, Hamersma H (1977) A review of the osteopetroses. Postgrad Med J 53:507–516
5 Beighton P, Cremin BJ, Hamersma H (1976) The radiology of sclerosteosis. Br J Radiol 49:934–938

Fig. 1. Osteopetrosis in an 8-month-old boy. Dense tubular bones with signs of rickets. Periosteal bone formation and abnormal modeling. Small bands of lucency in the metaphyses as well as proximally in the metacarpals. Delayed skeletal maturation ▷

Fig. 2. Same patient as Fig. 1. Typical bone-in-bone aspect and very dense bone structures. Marrow spaces in tubular bones severely diminished

Fig. 3. Osteopetrosis. Increased bone density, particularly in metaphyseal areas. Bone-in-bone aspect

Fig. 4. Osteopetrosis in a stillborn baby. Characteristic radiographic findings

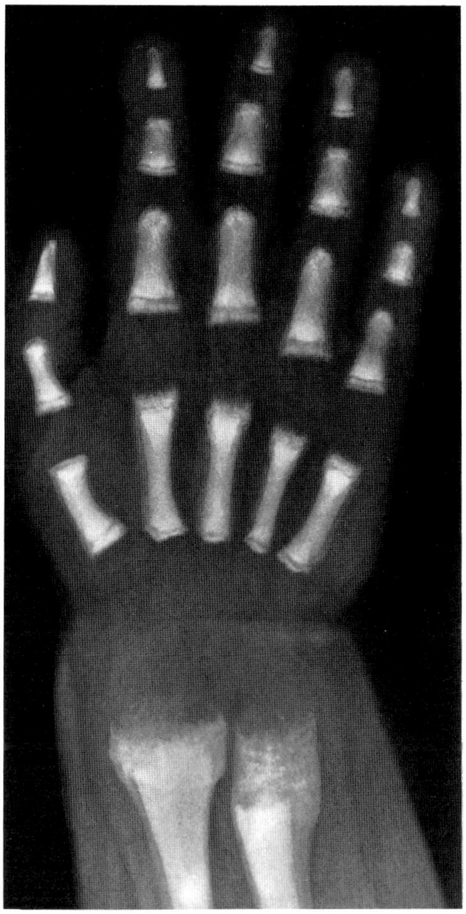

1

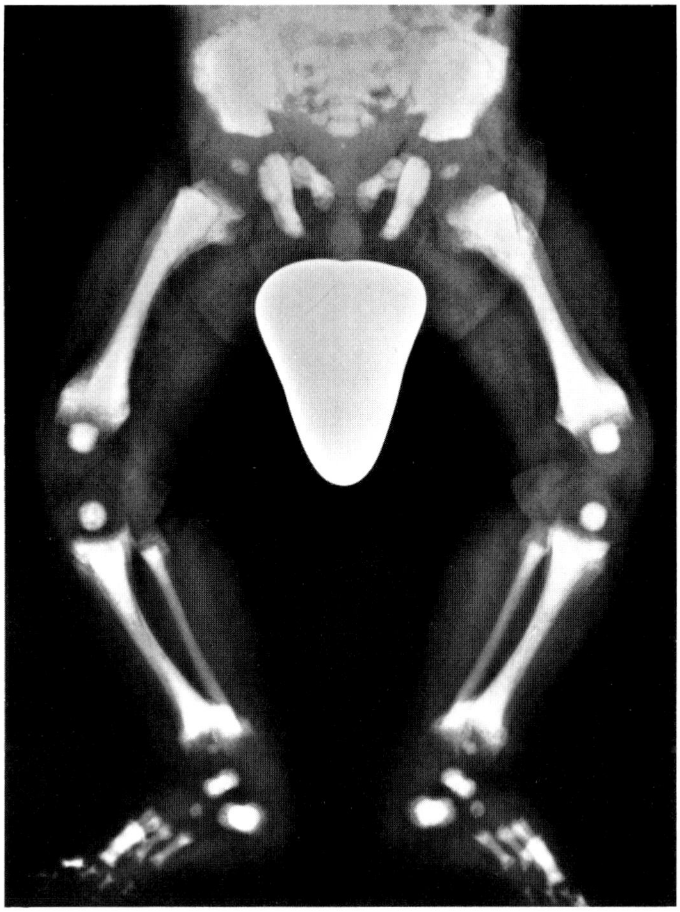

2

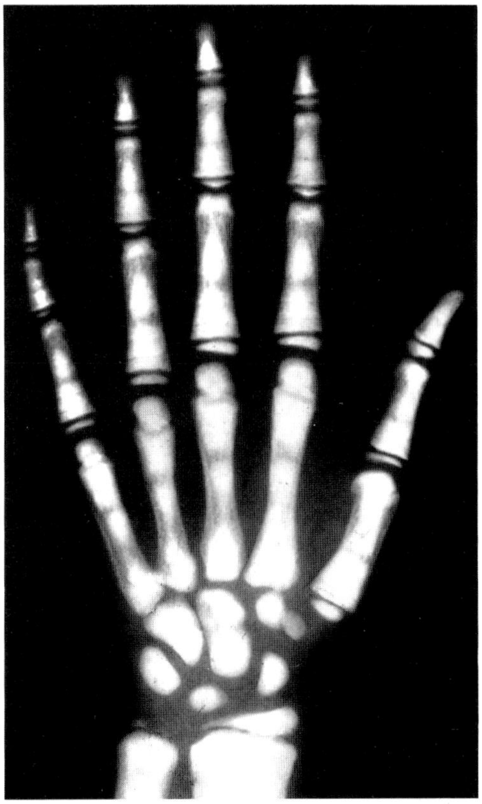

3

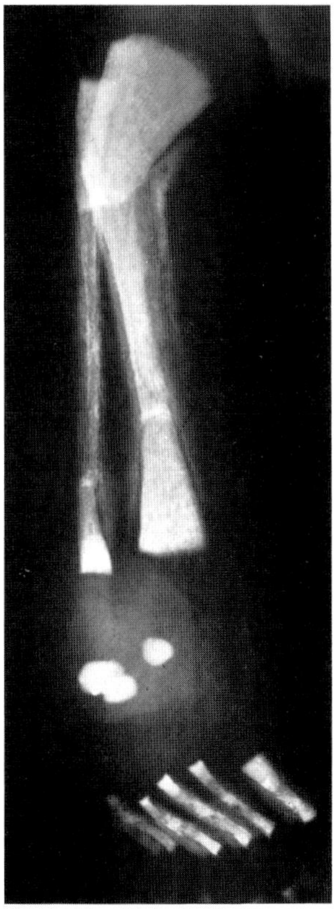

4

1.2.3 Pyknodysostosis

This autosomal recessive disorder is characterized by short stature and dense bones presenting an increased tendency to fracture. Healing of these fractures is not delayed, but resulting deformities are frequently encountered.

Radiographic Findings [1–4]

Hand

Increased bone density
Brachydactyly, especially of distal phalanges
Osteolysis of distal phalanges
Madelung's deformity

Other Sites

Long tubular bones: increased bone density
  fragility
  coxa vara and valga
Skull: large skull with prominent forehead
  absence of frontal sinuses
  delayed closure of sutures and fontanelles
  hypoplasia of jaw bones
  wormian bones
  dental abnormalities
Spine: kyphoscoliosis
  "spool-shaped" vertebral bodies

Differential Diagnosis (Fig. 3)

Cleidocranial dysplasia (Sect. 1.1.8)
Osteopetrosis (Sect. 1.2.2)
Pachydermoperiostosis (Sect. 1.2.8)
Idiopathic phalangeal acro-osteolysis (Sect. 3.1)
Hypervitaminosis D (Sect. 6.2.2)
Sclerosteosis [5]
Progressive diaphyseal dysplasia

References

1 Elmore SM (1967) Pycnodysostosis: a review. J Bone Joint Surg [Am] 49a:153–162
2 Shiraiski S (1971) Pycnodysostosis. Acta Orthop Scand 42:227–243
3 Dusenberry JF Jr, Kane JJ (1967) Pycnodysostosis. Report of three new cases. AJR 99:717–723
4 Steinbach HL, Gold RH, Preger L (1975) Roentgen appearance of the hand in diffuse disease. Year Book Medical Publishers, Chicago
5 Cremin BJ (1979) Sclerosteosis in children. Pediatr Radiol 8:173–177

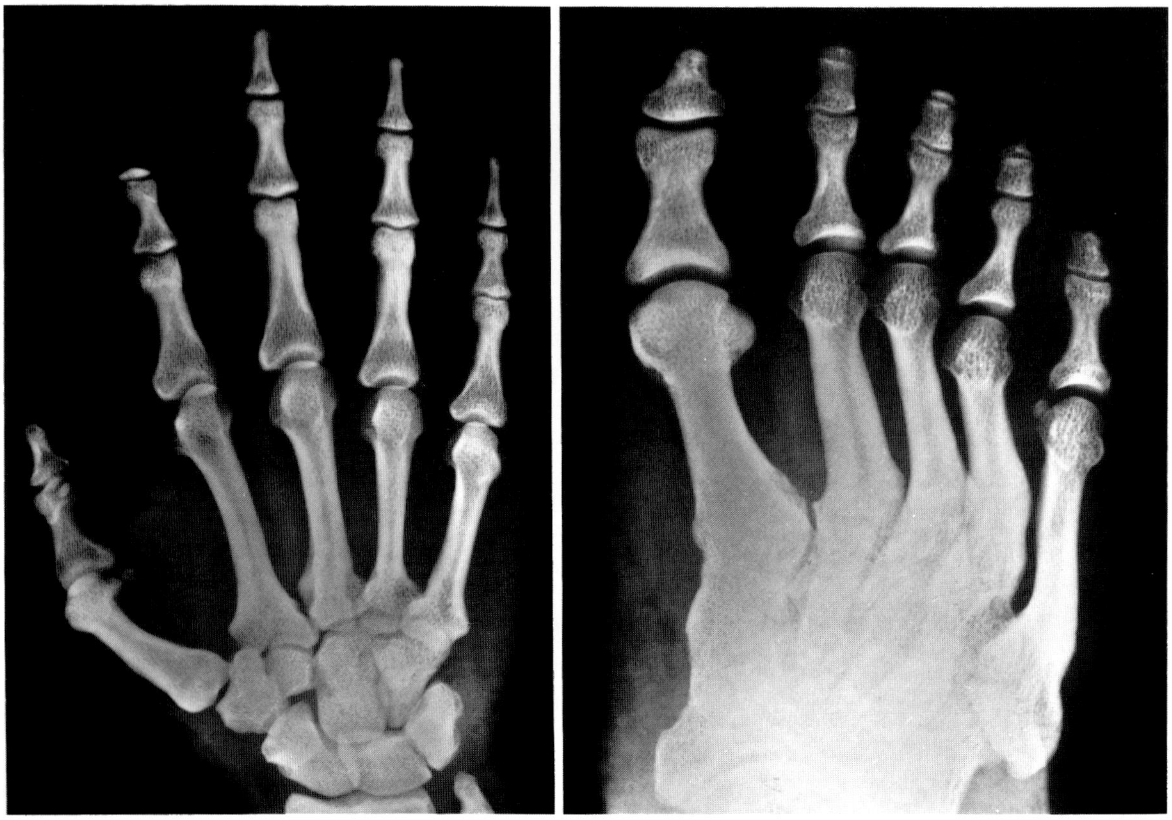

a b

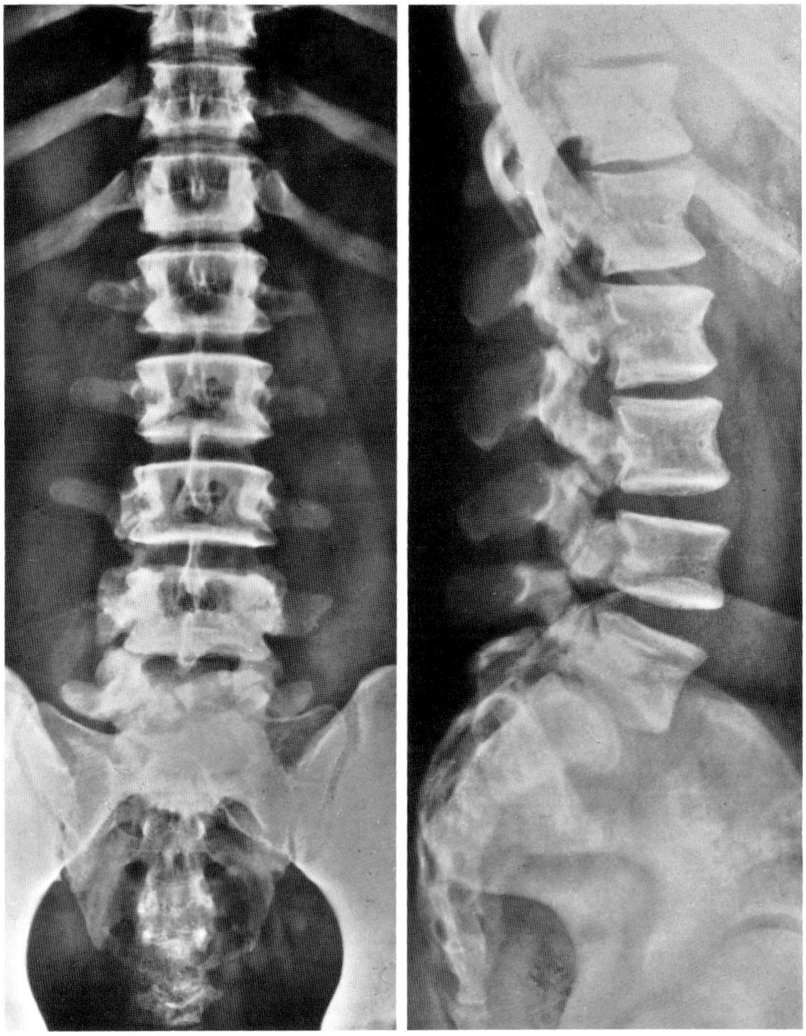

Fig. 2. Pyknodysostosis. "Spool-shaped" lumbar vertebral bodies below level of T 12

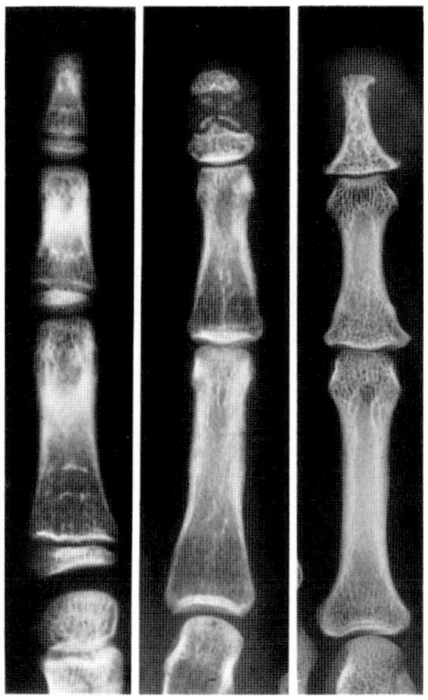

3a b c

Fig. 3. Differential diagnosis. **a** Hypervitaminosis D. Small transverse bands of increased density in metaphyseal areas. **b** Phalangeal acro-osteolysis Hadju-Cheney syndrome. **c** Pachydermoperiostosis: Tuft erosion, normal bone density

◁ **Fig. 1a, b.** Pyknodysostosis in a 30-year-old man. **a** Right hand: Increased bone density, short tubular bones, osteolysis of distal phalanges. **b** Right foot: Same abnormalities

1.2.4 Osteopoikilosis

Synonyms: osteopathia condensans disseminata, spotted bones

Osteopoikilosis is an uncommon familial condition characterized by punctate or short linear bone densities. Sometimes a mixed type of osteopoikilosis and osteopathia striata is present [1]. Patients with this innocuous disorder are usually asyptomatic. Solitary bone islands can be regarded as minimal manifestations of osteopoikilosis. Cutaneous lesions (fibrocollagenous infiltration) are found in approximately 25% of cases [2, 3].

Radiographic Findings [1–6]

Numerous well-defined punctate or short linear bone densities with a predilection for epiphyseal and metaphyseal regions of long tubular bones, carpal bones, pelvis, and scapulae.

Differential Diagnosis

Osteoblastic metastases
Tuberous sclerosis (Sect. 7.1.2)
Mastocytosis (Sect. 7.6.7)

Associated Disorders [1–3, 5]

Osteopathia striata (Sect. 1.2.5)
Melorheostosis (Sect. 1.2.6)

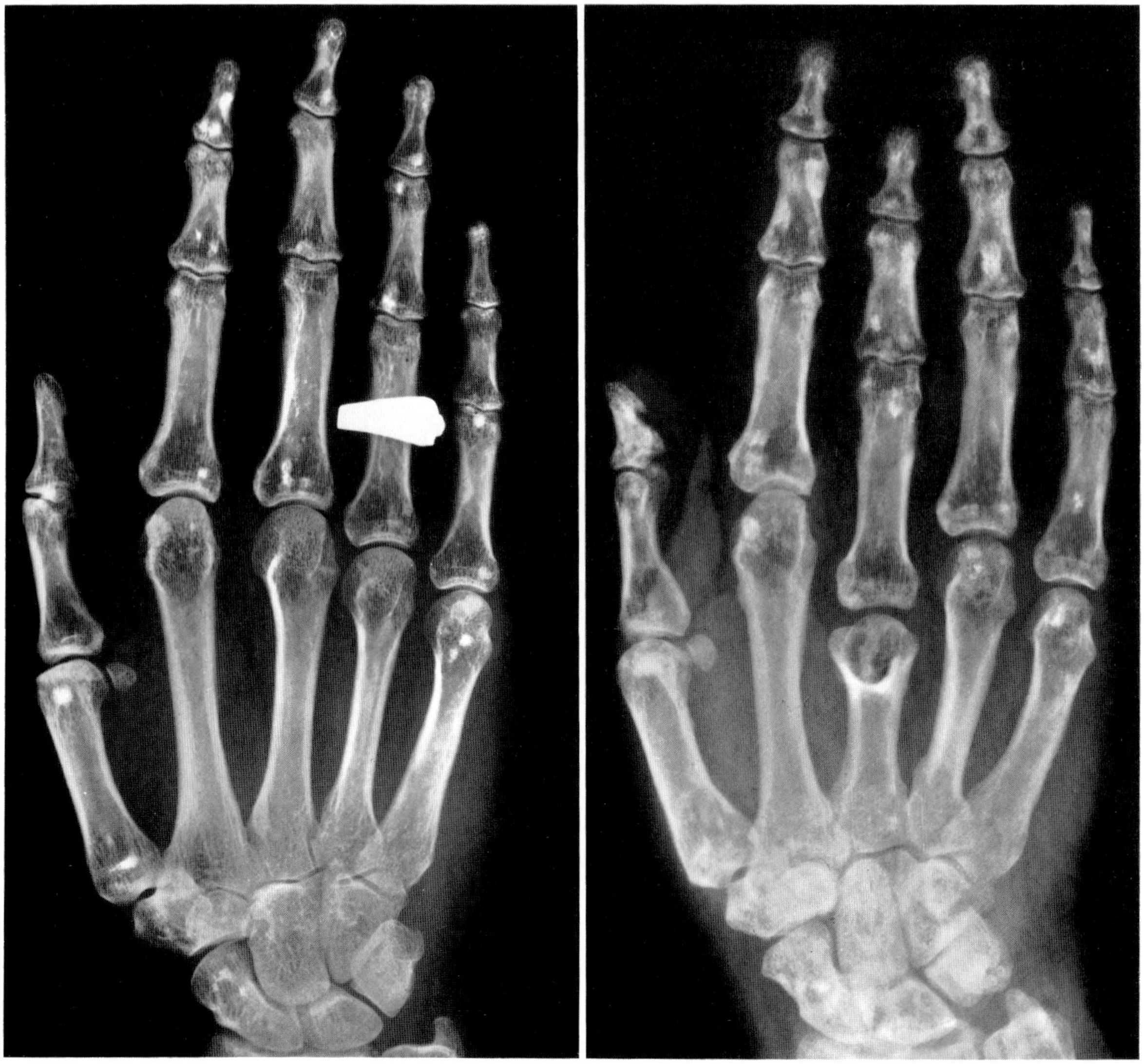

a b

Fig. 1a, b. Osteopoikilosis. **a** In an adult woman: Multiple small densities in the hand. **b** In a 44-year-old woman: Associated shortening of the third metacarpal and the distal phalanx of the thumb. The right hand of this patient presented a short fifth metacarpal

Gardner's syndrome
Hyperostosis frontalis interna
Focal dermal hypoplasia
Neurofibromatosis
Hemangioma

References

1 Schnyder PA (1980) Osseous changes of osteopathia striata associated with cranial sclerosis. Skeletal Radiol 5:19–22
2 Lippelt C, Petzel H (1982) Dermatofibrosis lenticularis disseminata mit Osteopoikilie (Buschke-Ollendorff Syndrom). Radiologe 22:553–561
3 Resnick D, Niwayama G (1981) Diagnosis of bone and joint disorders. Saunders, Philadelphia
4 Jonasch E (1955) 12 Fälle von Osteopoikilie. Fortschr Geb Röntgenstr Nuklearmed Ergänzungsband 82:344–353
5 Melnick JC (1959) Osteopathia condensans disseminata (osteopoikilosis). Study of a family of 4 generations. AJR 82:229–238
6 Walker GF (1964) Mixed sclerosing bone dystrophies. Two case reports. J Bone Joint Surg [Br] 46b:546–552

1.2.5 Osteopathia Striata

Synonym: Voorhoeve's disease

In osteopathia striata linear sclerotic streaks of bone are encountered, especially in the long tubular bones. The hand bones are usually quite normal. This condition may be associated with osteopoikilosis [1, 3, 5], melorheostosis [3, 5], focal dermal hypoplasia [3, 5], and cranial sclerosis [1–4]. Osteopathia striata in combination with basal skull sclerosis is probably a new autosomal dominant entity.

The presentation of osteopathia striata in a study of 45 cases [5] could be classified as follows:

Group 1 ($n=13$): uncomplicated osteopathia striata (autosomal dominant inheritance)
Group 2 ($n=23$): association with other bony abnormalities (15 osteopoikilosis; 3 partial osteopetrosis; 2 melorheostosis; 3 progressive diaphyseal dysplasia)
Group 3 ($n=9$): associated with focal dermal hypoplasia

Radiographic Findings [6]

Hand
The hand bones are usually normal but tiny linear sclerotic densities can be present

Other Sites
Long tubular bones: sclerotic streaks
Pelvis: linear sclerotic densities
Skull: cranial sclerosis, mostly thickening of skull base
high-arched palate
dental abnormalities
Spine: thoracolumbar scoliosis
spondylolisthesis L5-S1

Differential Diagnosis

Osteopetrosis (Sect. 1.2.2)
Melorheostosis (Sect. 1.2.6)
Paget's disease (Sect. 6.2.9)
Ollier's disease (Sect. 7.4.1.3)
Fibrous dysplasia (Sect. 7.4.3.1)
Fluorosis (Sect. 7.5.1)
Osteoblastic metastases

References

1 Schnyder PA (1980) Osseous changes of osteopathia striata associated with cranial sclerosis. An autosomal dominant entity. Skeletal Radiol 5:19–22
2 Horan FT, Beighton PH (1978) Osteopathia with cranial sclerosis. An autosomal dominant entity. Clin Genet 13:201–206
3 Knockaert D, Dequeker J (1979) Osteopathia striata and focal dermal hypoplasia. Skeletal Radiol 4:223–227
4 Boer SM de, Gool AV van (1974) Schedel- en gebitsafwijkingen bij een patiënt met osteopathia striata. Ned Tijdschr Geneeskd 118:1373–1380
5 Larrégue M, Michel Y, Maroteaux J, Fauré C (1973) L'osteopathie striée et dysmorphies squelettiques associées dans l'hypoplasie dermique en aires. Rev Rhum Mal Osteoartic 6:415–423
6 Gehweiler JA, Bland WR, Carden TS Jr, Daffner RH (1973) Osteopathia striata – Voorhoeve's disease. Review of the roentgen manifestations. AJR 118:450–455

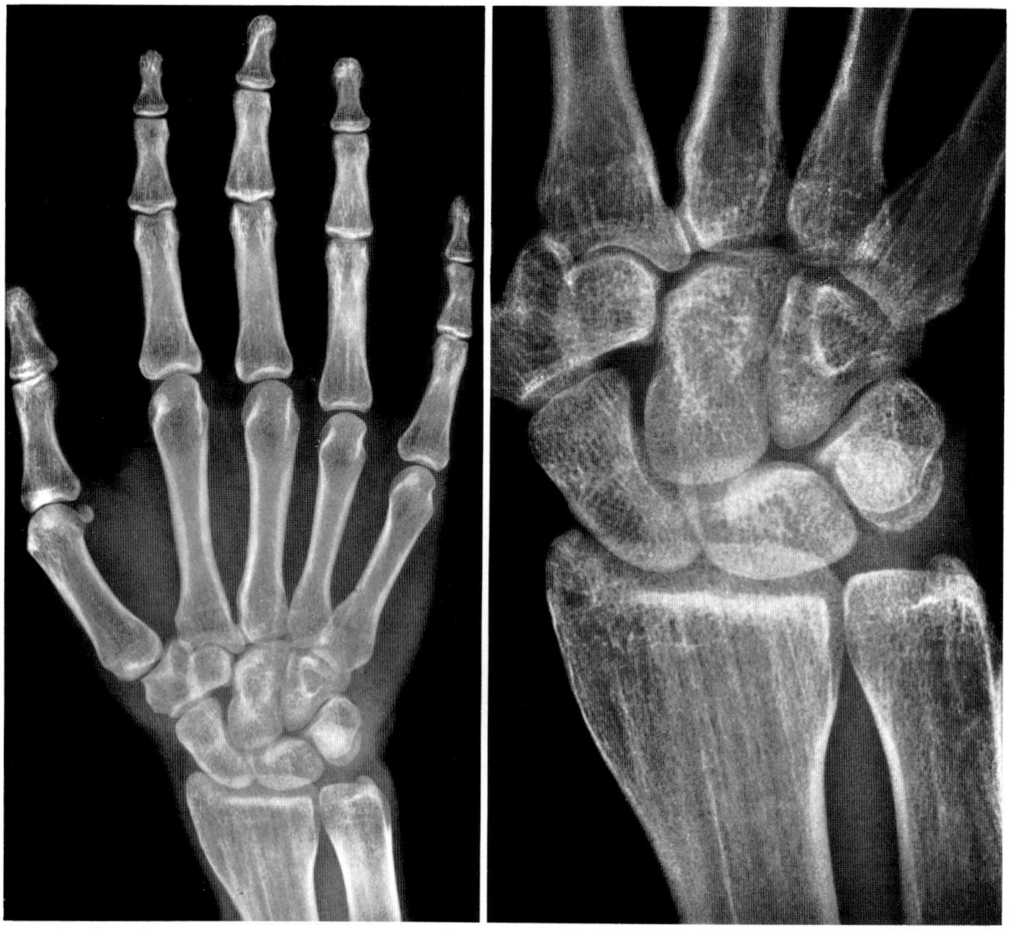
1a b

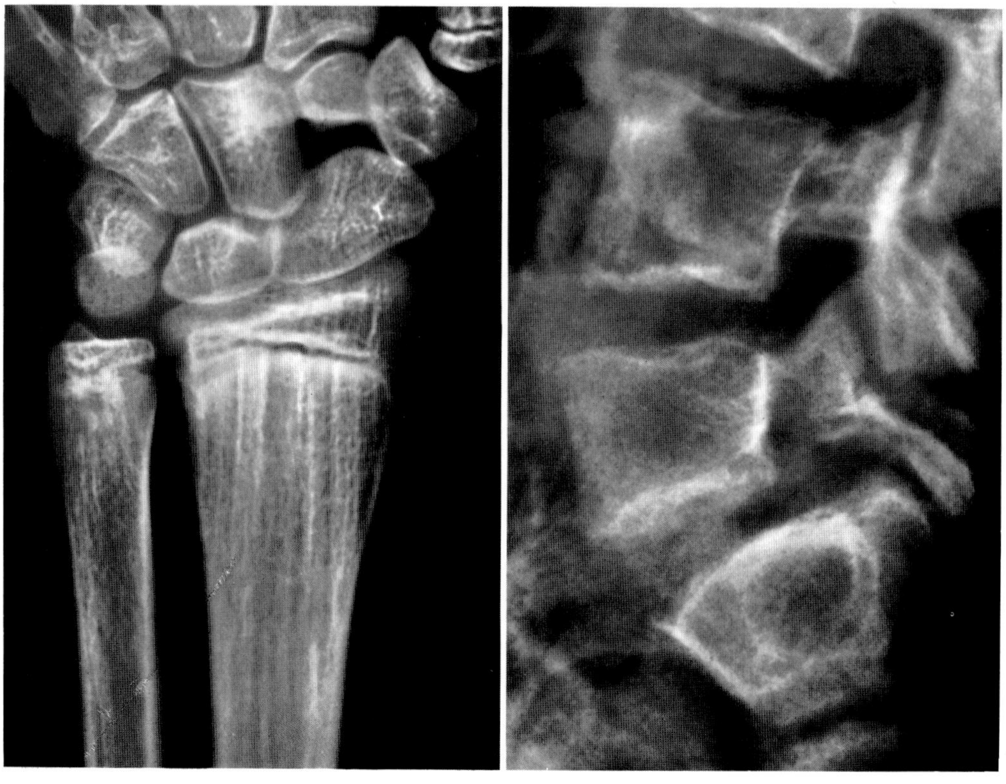
2a b

◁ **Fig. 1 a, b.** Osteopathia striata in a 23-year-old woman. Cranial sclerosis, rather dense vertebral bodies, dental abnormalities. Some streaks of dense bone in distal radius (**b**) and in several proximal phalanges

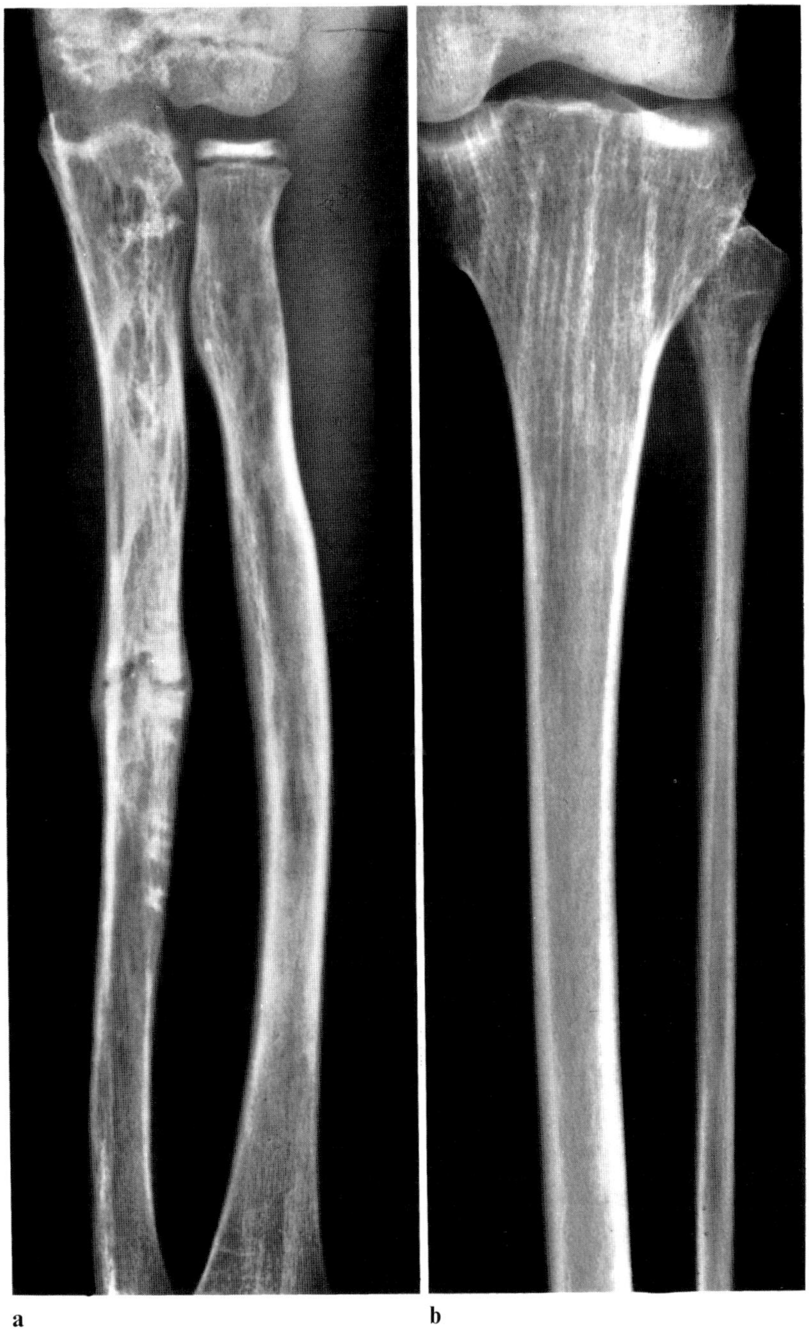

Fig. 3 a, b. Osteopathia striata. **a** In an 11-year-old boy: Longitudinal sclerotic streaks of bone, particularly within fractured ulna. **b** In a 28-year-old woman: Linear sclerotic streaks of bone within tibia

◁ **Fig. 2 a, b.** Osteopathia striata in a 14-year-old girl. Skull thickening, hypoplasia of dens, spondylolisthesis of fifth lumbar vertebral body. **a** Significant dense streaks in radius. **b** Spondylolisthesis of fifth lumbar vertebral body

1.2.6 Melorheostosis

In melorheostosis there is probably a sensory nerve supply to skeletal structures, related to spinal segments. The radiation of referred pain could be explained in terms of sclerotomes, or zones of the skeleton supplied by individual spinal sensory nerves [1]. It has been supposed that melorheostosis may be a late result of a segmental sensory nerve lesion. Frequently, the skeletal abnormalities are accompanied by lesions of the soft tissues in the same sclerotome. Nevi, hemangiomas, arteriovenous malformations, fibrotic contractures, and even periarticular ossification of soft tissue can be present [2]. Melorheostosis can be totally asymptomatic, or the patient may complain of chronic pain.

Radiographic Findings

Juxtacortical and/or endosteal streaks of hyperostosis along the long axis of some tubular hand bones in the region of a distinct sclerotome. The carpal bones may also be hyperostotic.

Differential Diagnosis

Osteopathia striata (Sect. 1.2.5)
Tuberous sclerosis (Sect. 7.1.2)
Neurofibromatosis (Sect. 7.1.2)

a

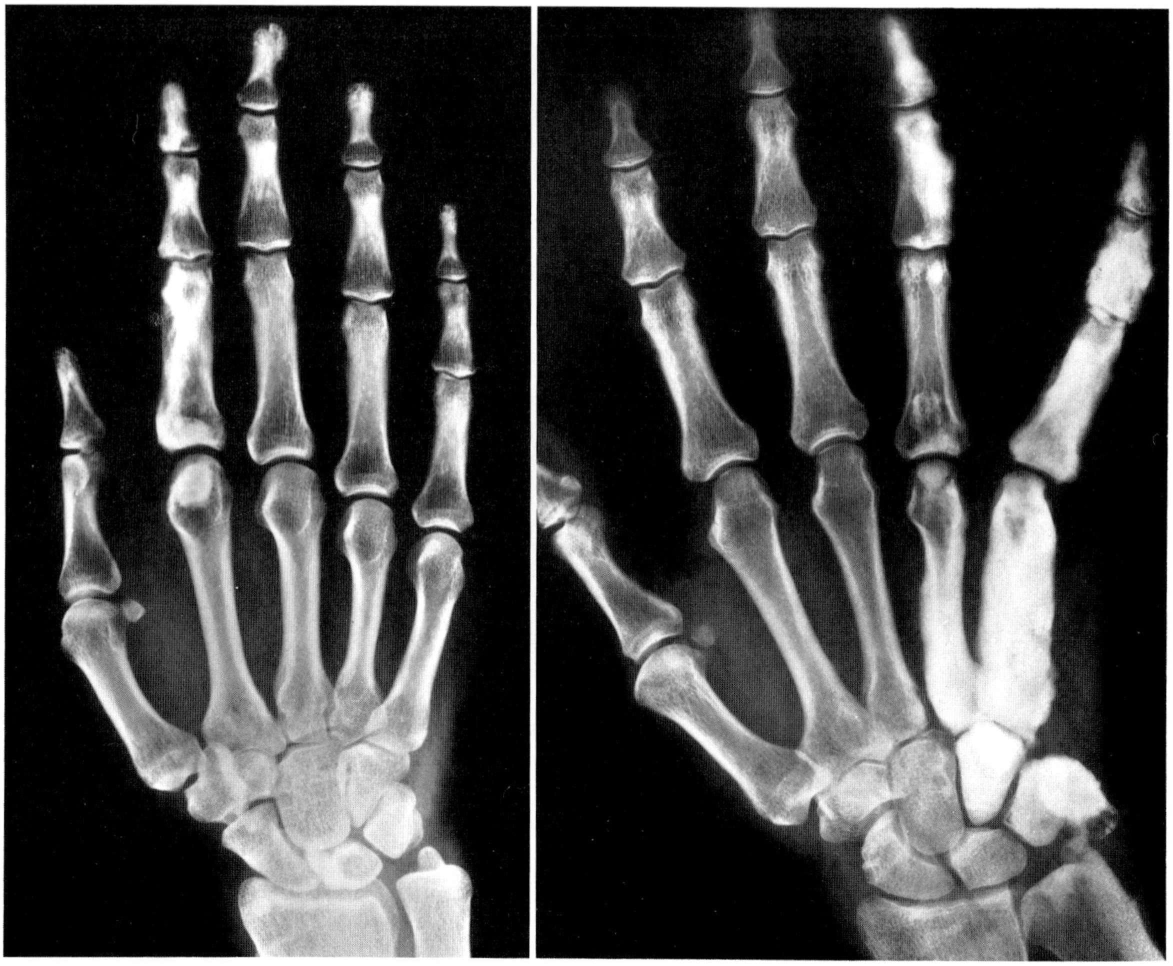

b

Fig. 1 a, b. Melorheostosis. **a** In a 33-year-old woman: Linear hyperostotic densities in second finger, other densities in second metacarpal, trapezium, scaphoid, and lunate. Lesions correspond well with C6 sclerotome. **b** In a 50-year-old man: Significant hyperostotic densities in fourth and fifth rays, additional densities in ulnar carpals, ossification in soft tissue between ulna and pisiform. Abnormalities correspond with C8 sclerotome

Associated Disorders [3]

Osteopoikilosis (Sect. 1.2.4)
Osteopathia striata (Sect. 1.2.5)
Tuberous sclerosis, neurofibromatosis (Sect. 7.1.2)
Linear scleroderma
Hemangiomas

References

1 Murray RO, McCredic J (1979) Melorheostosis and the sclerotomes: a radiological correlation. Skeletal Radiol 4:57–71
2 Morris JM, Samilson RL, Corley CL (1963) Melorheostosis. Review of the literature and report of an interesting case with a nineteen-year follow-up. J Bone Joint Surg [Am] 45:1191–1197
3 Resnick D, Niwayama G (1981) Diagnosis of bone and joint diseases. Saunders, Philadelphia

1.2.7 Endosteal Hyperostosis

Synonyms: Hyperostosis corticalis generalisata familiaris, van Buchem's disease, generalized cortical hyperostosis

Endosteal hyperostosis [1] occurs in two forms: autosomal dominant (WORTH [2]) and autosomal recessive (VAN BUCHEM [3]). Endosteal hyperostosis usually presents in late childhood with progressive enlargement of the mandible, prominence of the forehead, and a broad nasal bridge; however, the patients may remain asymptomatic. Intellect and habitus are normal. Cranial nerve compression by encroachment of the foramina at the skull base is the cause of neurological features (particularly facial palsy). Cranial nerve complications are predominantly present in the van Buchem form, less common in the Worth form.

Radiographic Findings [1–7]

Hand
Hyperostosis and diaphyseal thickening of tubular bones
Tuft erosion (unusual)
Normal carpals
Normal epiphyseal region

Other Sites
Skull: sclerotic calvarium
sclerotic skull base
patent air sinuses
Mandible: hyperostosis
increased mandibular angle
Spine: some degree of sclerosis
Chest: coarse trabecular pattern or diffuse sclerosis in clavicles, ribs, and scapulae
Long tubular bones: increased cortical thickening and sclerosis in diaphyses
usually normal modeling
diminution of medullary cavity
bony excrescences on shafts

Differential Diagnosis

Sclerosteosis [4]
Craniodiaphyseal dysplasia [4, 8]
Craniometaphyseal dysplasia [4]
Frontometaphyseal dysplasia [4, 9, 10]
Familial hyperphosphatasia
Paget's disease (Sect. 6.2.9)

References

1 Special report (1978) International nomenclature of constitutional diseases of bone. AJR 131:352–354
2 Worth HM, Wollin DG (1966) Hyperostosis corticalis generalisata congenita. J Can Assoc Radiol 17:67–72
3 Van Buchem FSP, Hadders HN, Hansen JF, Woldring MG (1962) Hyperostosis corticalis generalisata. Report of seven cases. Am J Med 33:387–395
4 Beighton P, Cremin BJ (1980) Sclerosing bone dysplasias. Springer, Berlin Heidelberg New York
5 Owen RH (1976) Van Buchem's disease (hyperostosis corticalis generalisata). Br J Radiol 49:126–132
6 Spranger JW, Langer LO, Wiedemann HR (1974) Bone dysplasias. An atlas of constitutional disorders of skeletal development. Saunders, Philadelphia
7 Gorlin RJ, Glass L (1977) Autosomal dominant osteosclerosis Radiology 125:547–553
8 Wemmer U, Böttger E (1978) Die kraniometaphysäre Dysplasie (Jackson). Fortschr Geb Röntgenstr Nuklearmed Ergänzungsband 128:66–69
9 Moss AA, Mainzer F (1970) Osteopetrosis: an unusual cause of terminal tuft erosion. Radiology 97:631–632
10 Kleinsorge H, Böttger E (1977) Das Gorlin-Cohen-Syndrom (fronto-metaphysäre Dysplasie). Fortschr Geb Röntgenstr Nuklearmed Ergänzungsband 127:451–458

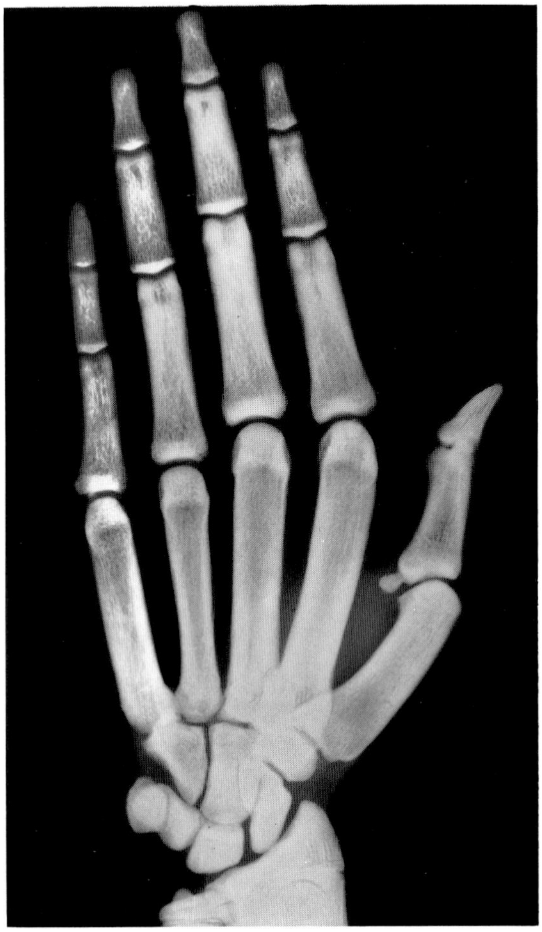

Fig. 1. Endosteal hyperostosis (VAN BUCHEM) in a 17-year-old male. Undermodeled tubular bones with cortical thickening, normal carpals. Additional findings: large mandible, sclerosis of skull, unilateral facial palsy. Decompression of the appropriate facial nerve was performed. Although the undermodeling of the tubular bones is more characteristic for sclerosteosis, the absence of syndactyly, nail hypoplasia, normal dental occlusion, and the descend make van Buchem's disease more likely

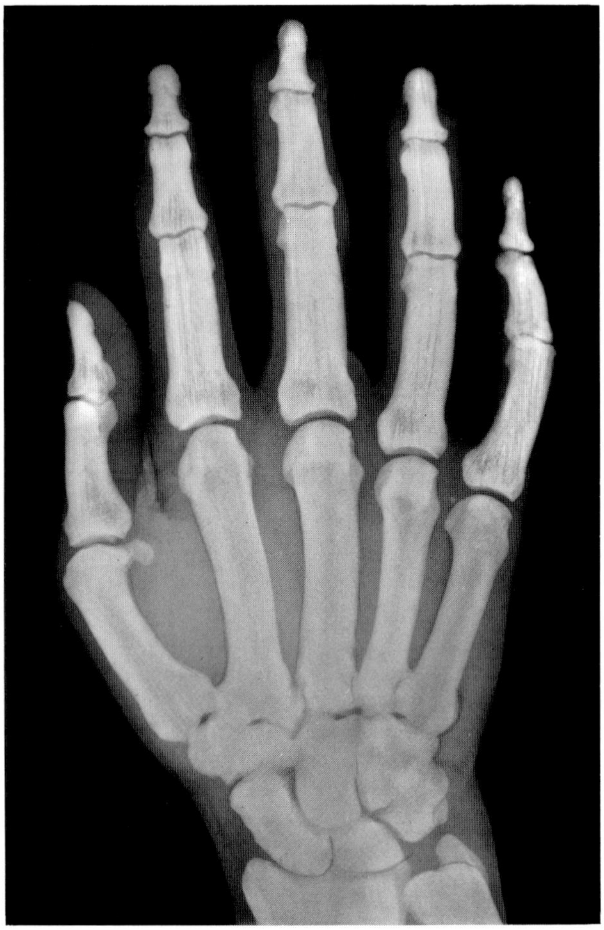

Fig. 2. Endosteal hyperostosis (VAN BUCHEM) in a 53-year-old man with sclerosis of the skull and without neurological features. Particularly the metacarpals and the proximal phalanges are widened and undermodeled. The long bones of this patient presented the same abnormalities

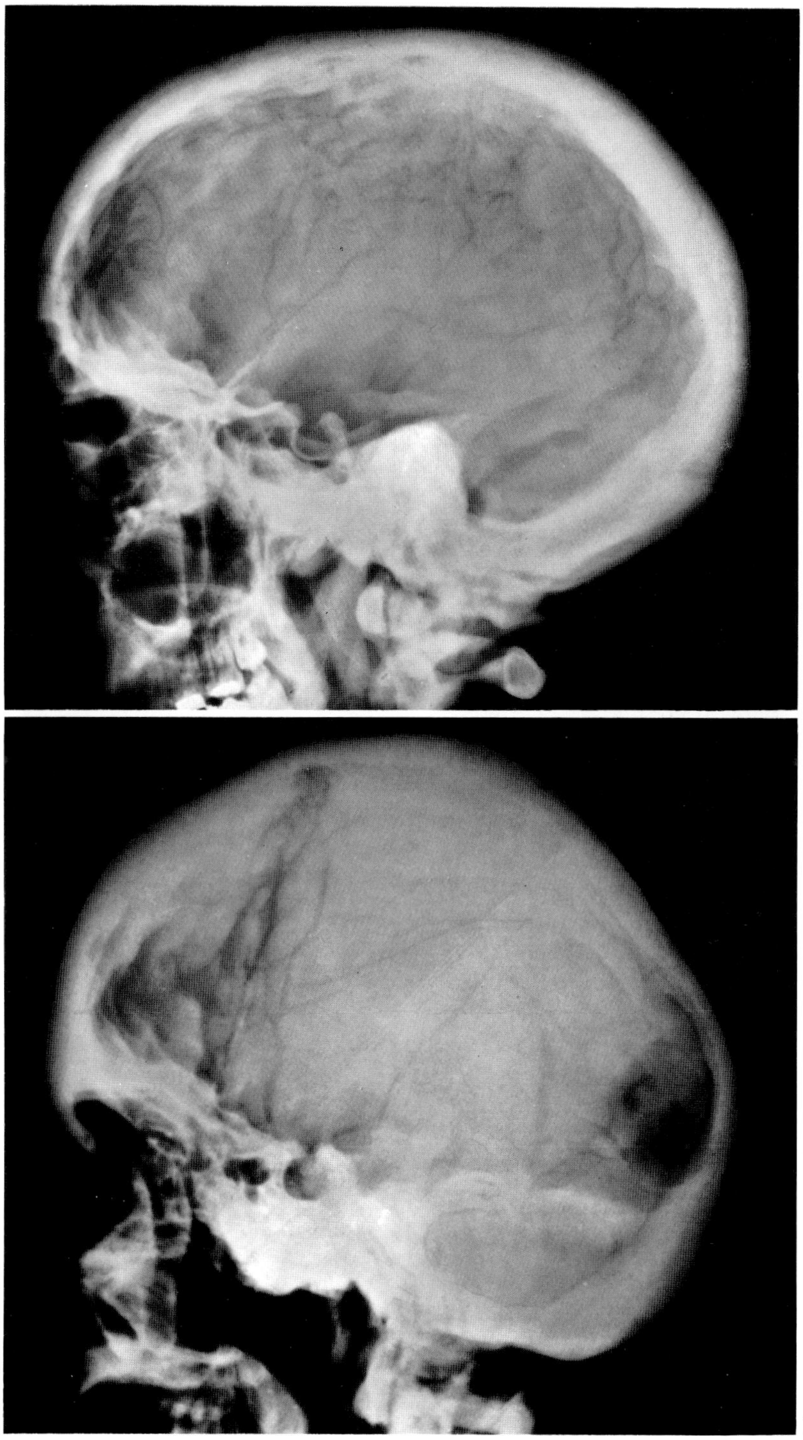

a

b

Fig. 3a, b. Endosteal hyperostosis (van Buchem). **a** In a 17-year-old male: Significant hyperostosis of calvarium and skull base. **b** In a 48-year-old man: Remarkable hyperostosis of calvarium and skull base. The tubular bones of the hand presented with cortical thickening and widening due to undermodeling

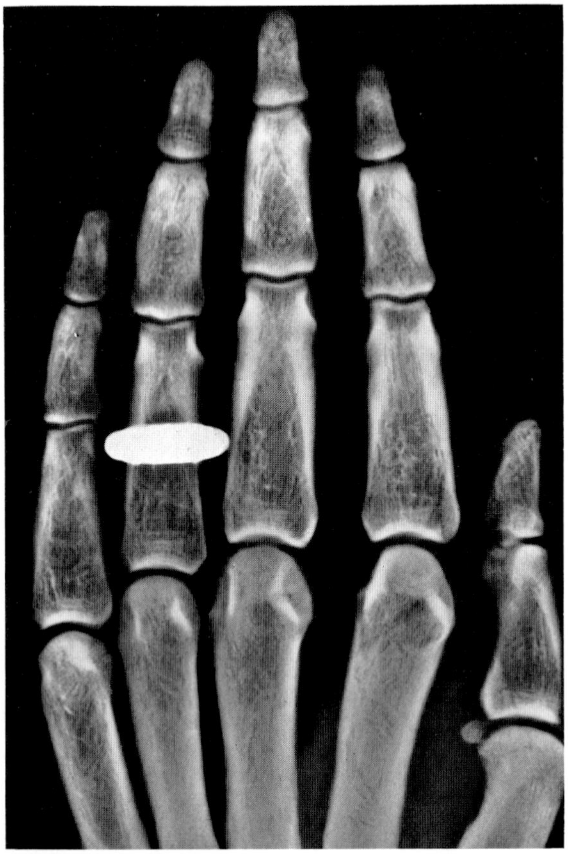

Fig. 4. Endosteal hyperostosis (VAN BUCHEM) in an adult man. Increased density of tubular bones by diaphyseal thickening

Fig. 5a, b. Same patient as Fig. 4. **a** Right shoulder: Increased density of skeleton. **b** Mandible: Hyperostosis and increased mandibular angle

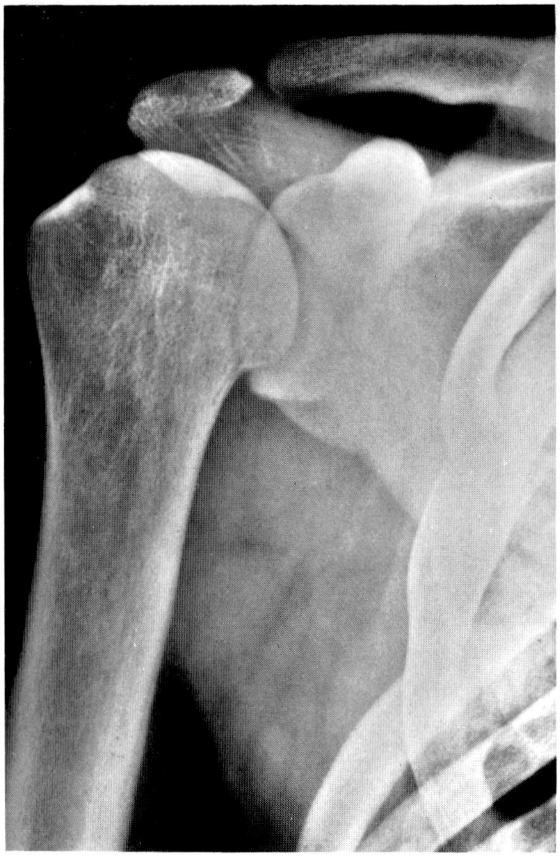

a

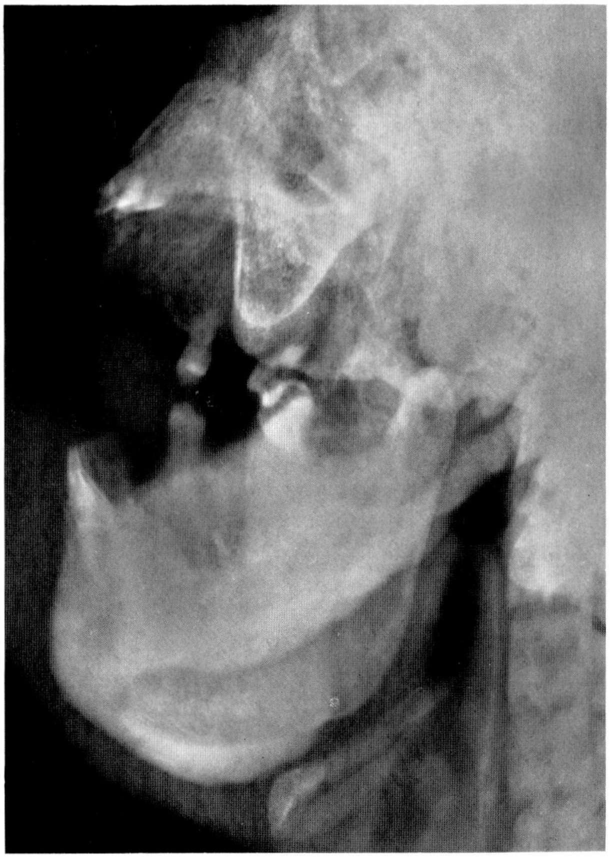

b

1.2.8 Pachydermoperiostosis

Synonyms: idiopathic hypertrophic osteoarthropathy, Touraine-Solente-Golé syndrome, familial acromegaloid osteosis, osteodermatopathia hypertrophicans

This autosomal dominant hereditary self-limiting disorder with variability in expression has a predilection for males. After presentation, mostly in adolescence, the abnormalities progress for a period of about 10 years. In the complete syndrome, clubbing of fingers and toes, thickening and oiliness of the skin, hyperhidrosis, and periostitis are present. Occasionally, there is intermittent swelling or pain of the large joints. The abnormalities are probably the result of a decrease in peripheral blood flow. Arteriography shows vascular stasis, tortuosity, and segmental narrowing of the small arteries [1].

Radiographic Findings [2–4]

Hand
Clubbing of fingers distal to distal interphalangeal joints
Acro-osteolysis
Periostitis

Other Sites
Foot: clubbing of toes
acro-osteolysis
periostitis
Long tubular bones: periostitis in distal ends
Skull: wormian bones

Differential Diagnosis

Periostitis of multiple bones
Acromegaly (Sect. 7.2.2)
Osteomyelitis (Sect. 7.3.3)
Fluorosis (Sect. 7.5.1)
Hypertrophic osteoarthropathy (Pierre-Marie-Bamberger) (Sect. 7.6.8)
Thyroid acropachy (Sect. 7.6.8)
Leukemia (Sect. 7.6.8)
Venous stasis
Infantile cortical hyperostosis
Trauma
Hypervitaminosis A

Differential Diagnosis

Acro-osteolysis (Sect. 3.1)

References

1 Rimoin DL (1965) Pachydermoperiostosis (idiopathic clubbing and periostitis). N Engl J Med 272:923–931
2 Guyer PB, Brunton FJ, Wren MWG (1978) Pachydermoperiostosis with acroosteolysis. Report of five cases. J Bone Joint Surg [Br] 60b:219–223
3 Lazarus JH, Galloway JK (1973) Pachydermoperiostosis. AJR 118:308–313
4 Harbison JB, Nice CM (1971) Familial pachydermoperiostosis presenting as an acromegaly-like syndrome. AJR 112:532–536

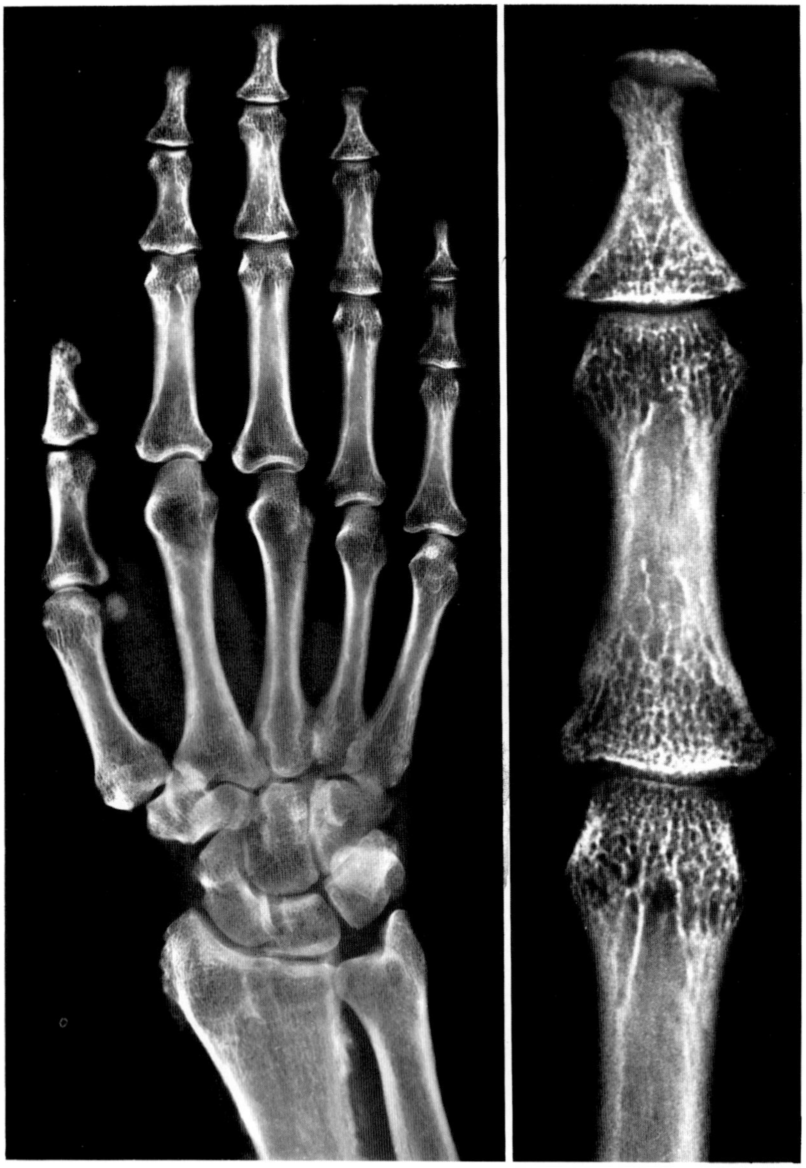

a b

Fig. 1a, b. Pachydermoperiostosis in a 21-year-old man. Acro-osteolysis, periosteal new bone formation of radius. Other abnormalities: wormian bones and hyperhidrosis

Fig. 2a, b. Pachydermoperiostosis. **a** In a 21-year-old man: Osteolysis of tuft of thumb and thickening of first, second, and third metacarpals by periosteal new bone formation. **b** In his 23-year-old sister: Acro-osteolysis of tufts ▷

Fig. 3a, b. Pachydermoperiostosis. **a** In a 1-year-old boy: Clubbing of great toe and deformation of distal phalanx. **b** In same patient as Fig. 2b. Acro-osteolysis of toes

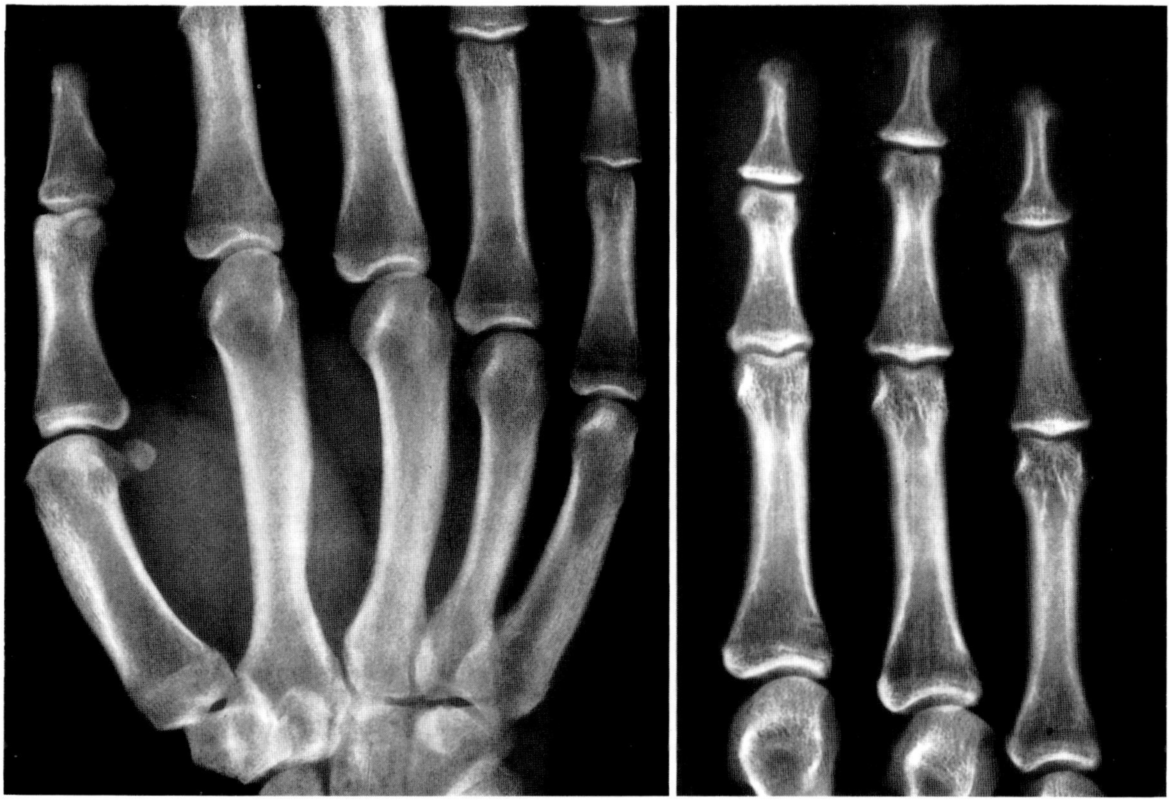

2a b

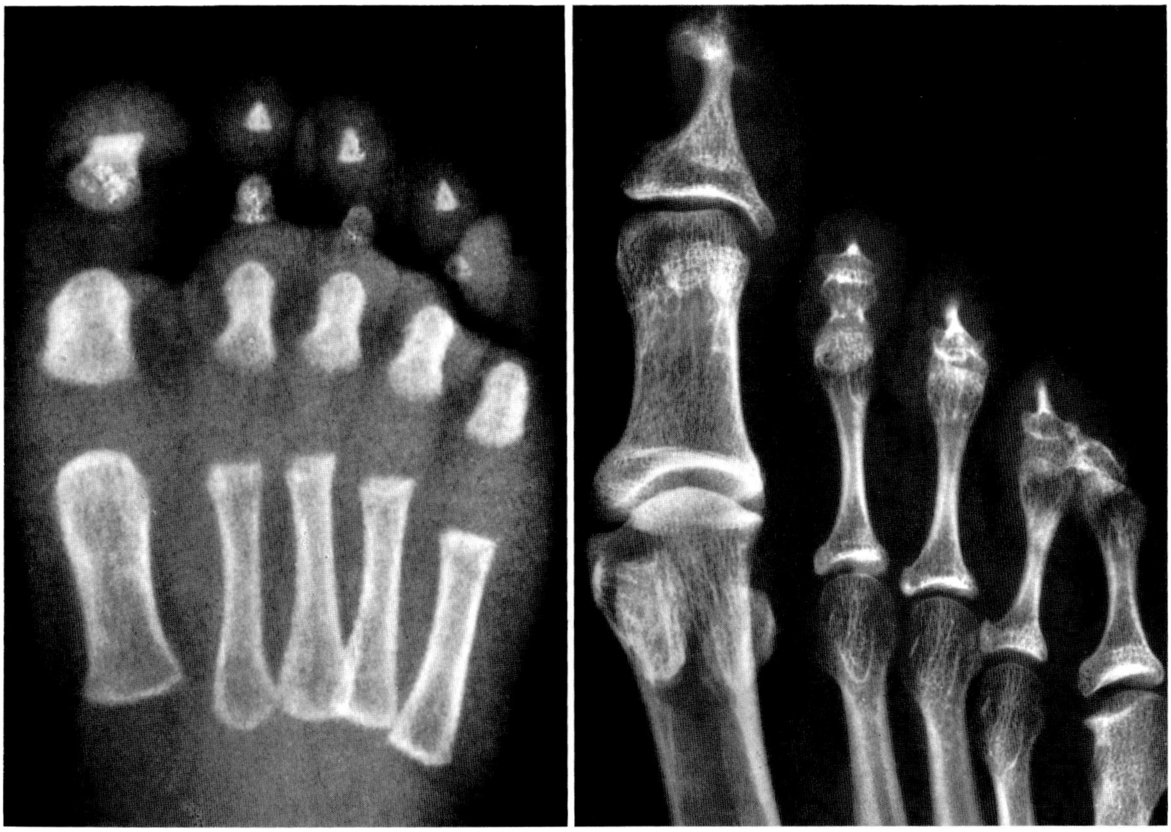

3a b

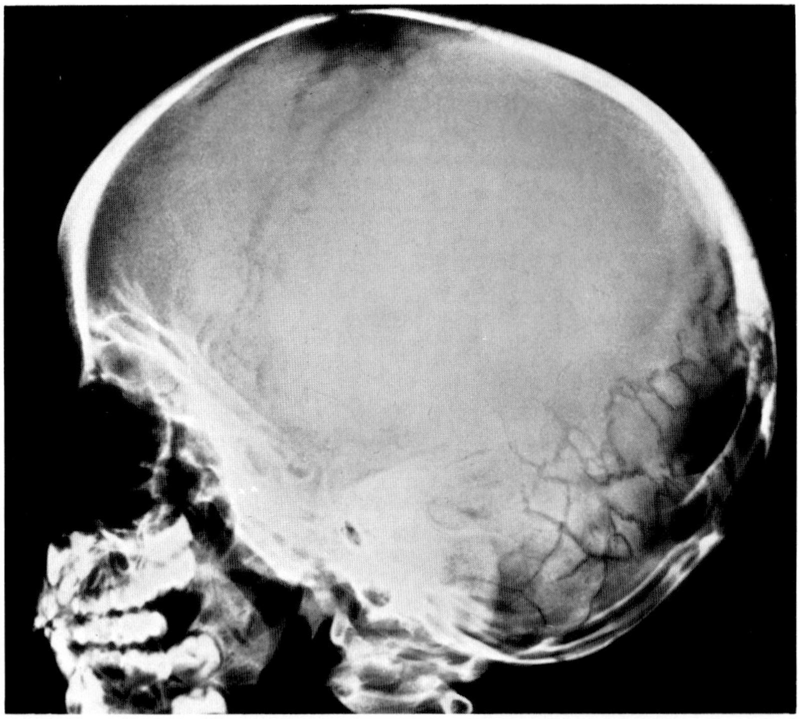

Fig. 4. Pachydermoperiostosis in a 3-year-old boy: Wormian bones

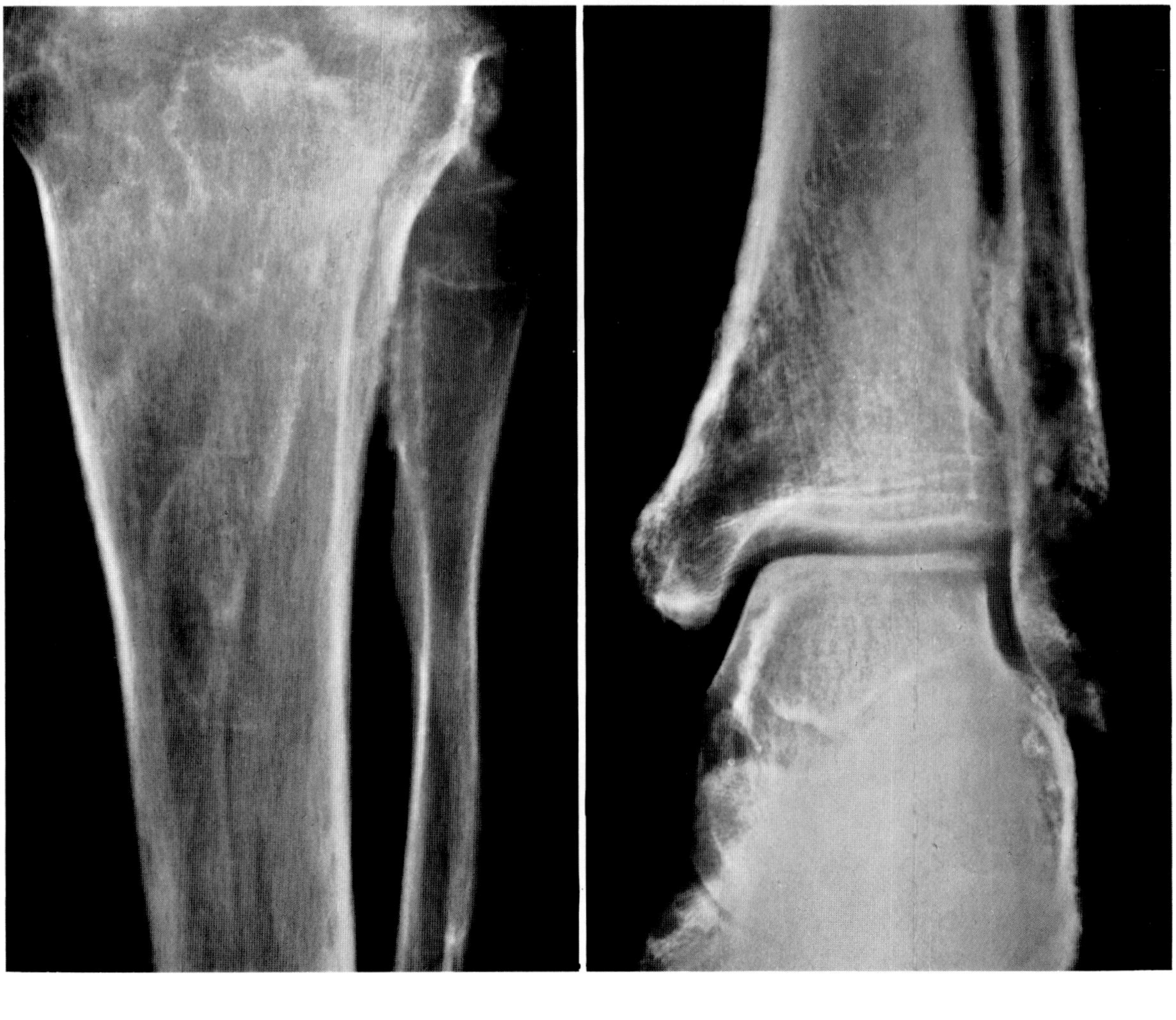

a b

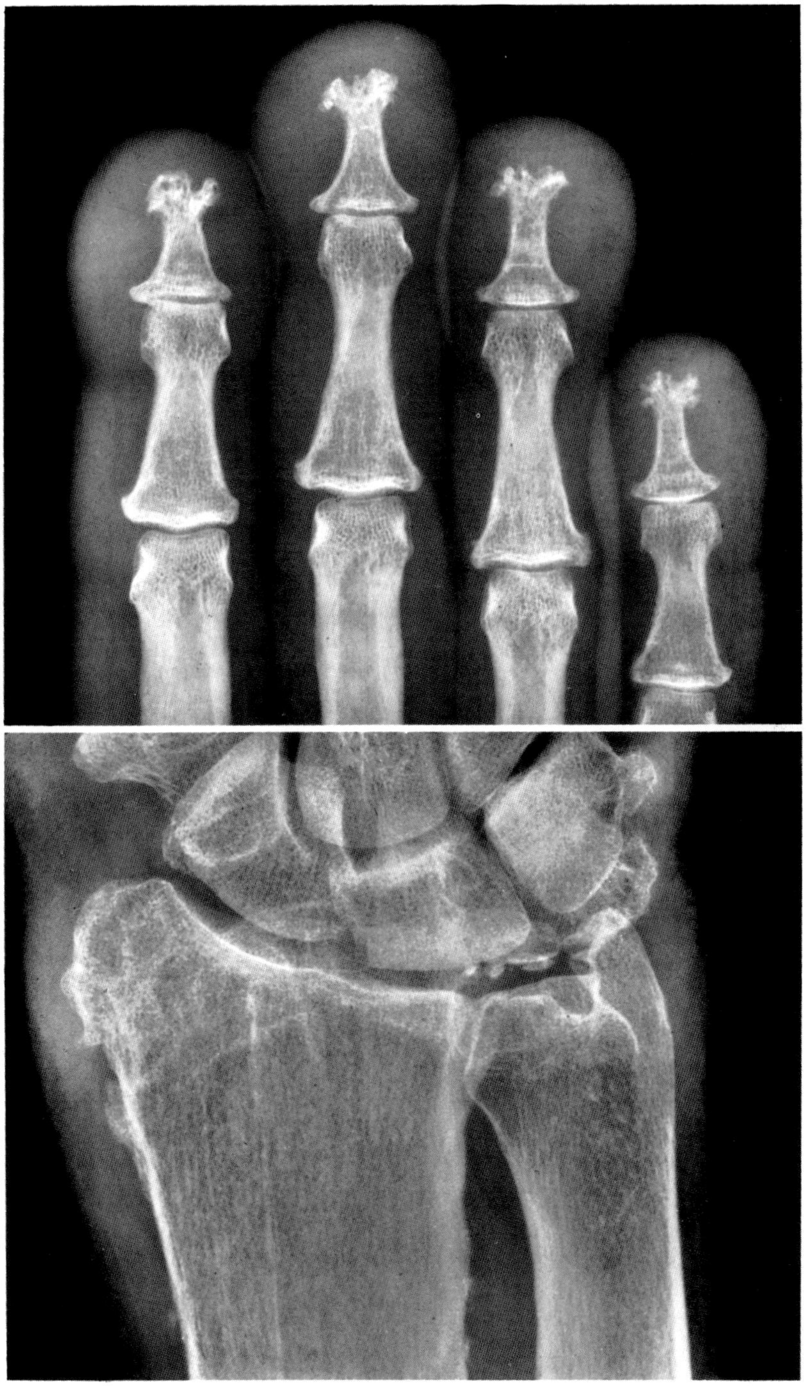

a

b

Fig. 6a, b. Pachydermoperiostosis in an adult man. **a** Clubbing of fingers and osteolysis of tufts. **b** Extensive periosteal new bone formation along radius and widening of radial metaphysis

◁ **Fig. 5a, b.** Pachydermoperiostosis. **a** In same patient as Fig. 2b: Periosteal bone apposition along tibia and fibula. **b** In a 50-year-old man: Periosteal apposition along distal tibia and fibula

2 Dysostoses (Malformation of Individual Bones Singly or in Combination)

2.1 Dysostoses with Cranial and Facial Involvement

2.1.1 Acrocephalosyndactyly and Acrocephalopolysyndactyly

The different types of acrocephalosyndactyly and acrocephalopolysyndactyly (Carpenter's syndrome) are characterized by the combination of premature fusion of the cranial sutures (craniosynostosis) and malformations of the hands and feet.

Differential Diagnosis

Rubinstein-Taybi syndrome (Sect. 2.2.18)
Laurence-Moon-Biedl-Bardet syndrome

Radiographic Findings [1–9]

	CARPENTER	APERT (type I), APERT-CROUZON (type II)	SAETHRE CHOTZEN (type III)	WAARDENBURG (type IV)	PFEIFFER (type V)	SUMMIT
Hand						
Thumb: broad, short	±	+ +		+	+	
short proximal phalanx	+	+ (or absent)		+	(triangular, trapezoid)	
short distal phalanx		+				
double ossification center proximal phalanx	+					
Syndactyly (osseous or cutaneous)	cut. mild 3–4 fingers	cut. + oss. 2–4 fingers	occasion. cut.	mild		±
Short middle phalanges	triangular	+		+	+ thumb	+
Symphalangism		+				
Metacarpal fusion		+				
Carpal fusion		hamate, capitate				
Bifid distal phalanges				2–3 fingers		
Foot						
Great toe: duplication		occasion.				
broad, short	+	+			+	+
Syndactyly (osseous or cutaneous)	cut.	cut. + oss.				± oss.
Short middle phalanges	+	+		+	+	±
Symphalangism		+				
Metatarsal fusion		1–2 rays				
Polydactyly (preaxial)	+					
Oligodactyly				+		
Skull						
Acrocephaly	severe	severe	mild	mild	mild	mild
Asymmetry			+			
Hypoplasia of mandible	+			+		
Hypoplasia of maxilla		+	+		+	
Inheritance	aut. rec.	aut. dom.	aut. dom.	?	aut. dom.	aut. rec.

References

1 Temtamy SA (1960) Carpenter's syndrome: acrocephalopolysyndactyly. An autosomal recessive syndrome. J Pediatr 69:111–120
2 Spranger JW, Langer LO, Wiedemann HR (1974) Bone dysplasias: an atlas of constitutional disorders of skeletal development. Saunders, Philadelphia
3 Poznanski AK, Garn SM, Holt JF (1971) The thumb in the congenital malformation syndromes. Radiology 100:115–129
4 Palacios E, Schimke RN (1969) Craniosynostosis-syndactylism. AJR 106:144–155
5 Hoover GH, Flatt AE, Weiss MW (1970) The hand and Apert's syndrome. J Bone Joint Surg 52-A:878–895
6 Duggan CA, Keener EB, Gay BB Jr (1970) Secondary craniosynostosis. AJR 109:277–281
7 Bartsocas CS, Weber AL, Crawford JD (1970) Acrocephalosyndactyly Type III, Chotzen's syndrome. J Pediatr 77:267–272
8 Saldino RM, Steinbach HL, Epstein CJ (1977) Familial acrocephalosyndactyly (Pfeiffer syndrome). AJR 116:609–622
9 Zippel H, Schüler KH (1969) Dominant vererbte Akrozephalosyndaktylie (ACS). Fortschr Geb Röntgenstr Nuklearmed Ergänzungsband 110:234–245

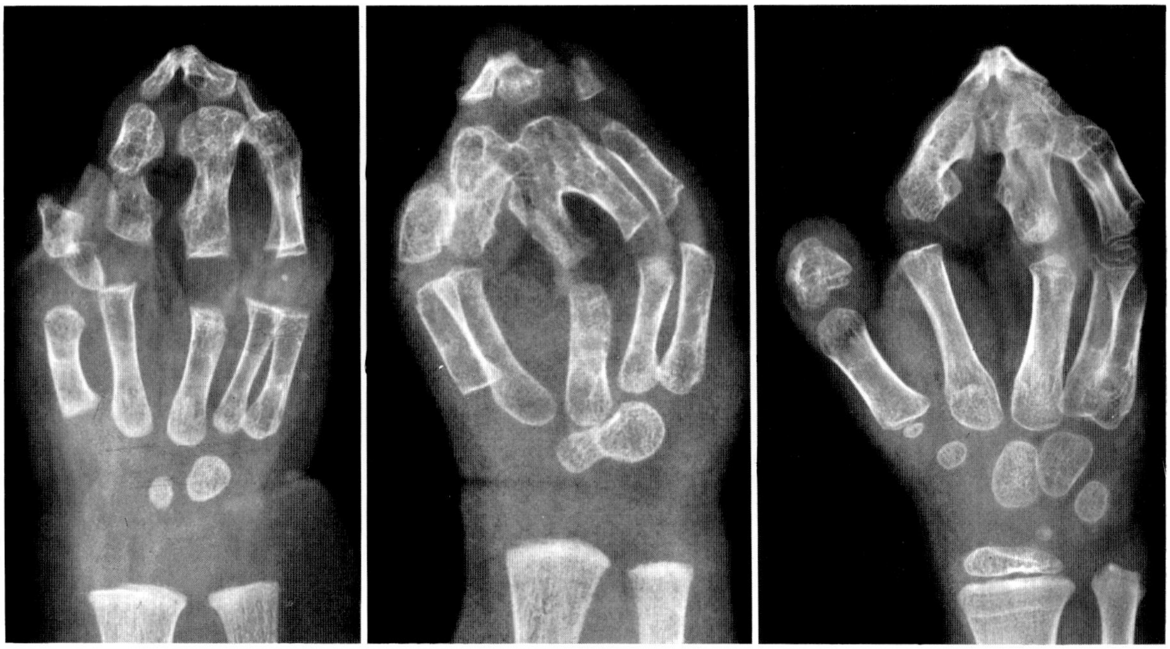

a b c

Fig. 1a–c. Acrocephalosyndactyly (Apert, type I). **a** In an 8-month-old girl: Short and broad thumb with short, hypoplastic proximal phalanx, symphalangism, cutaneous and osseous fusion of second, third, and fourth fingers, cutaneous syndactyly only of fifth finger. **b** In a 1-year-old girl: Short and broad thumb with large, deformed proximal phalanx, symphalangism, cutaneous and osseous fusion of second, third, and fourth fingers, cutaneous syndactyly only of fifth finger, carpal fusion between hamate and capitate. **c** In a 5-year-old boy: Short and broad thumb with only one deformed phalanx, fusion of fourth and fifth metacarpals, severe cutaneous and osseous syndactyly

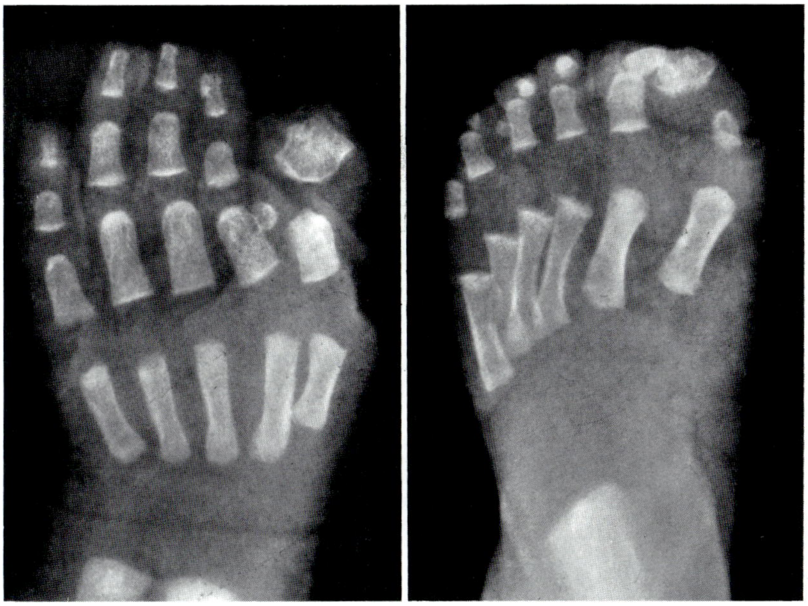

a b

Fig. 2a, b. Acrocephalopolysyndactyly (Carpenter's syndrome). **a** Broad thumb with abnormal distal phalanx and double ossification center of proximal phalanx, cutaneous syndactyly of second and third fingers. The other hand presented the same abnormalities. **b** Right foot: Preaxial polydactyly and syndactyly of big toe and second toe

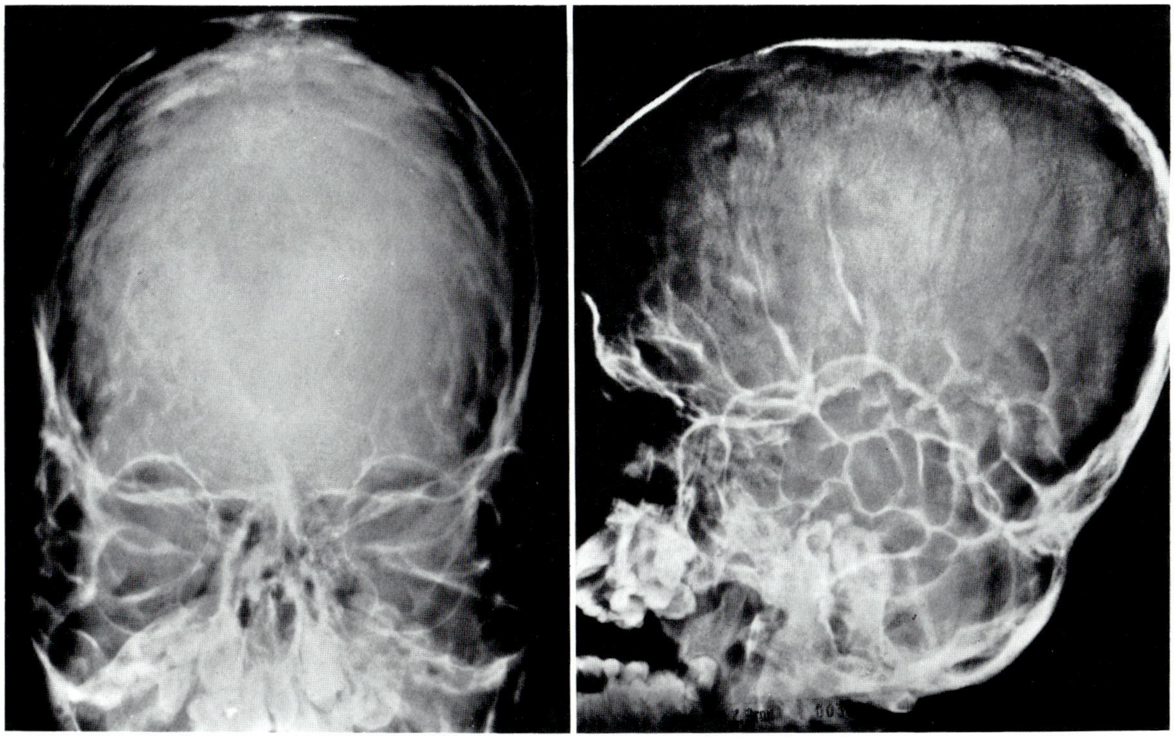

a b

Fig. 3a, b. Acrocephalosyndactyly (Apert, type I) in an 11-year-old boy. Large, tower-shaped skull, hypoplastic maxilla

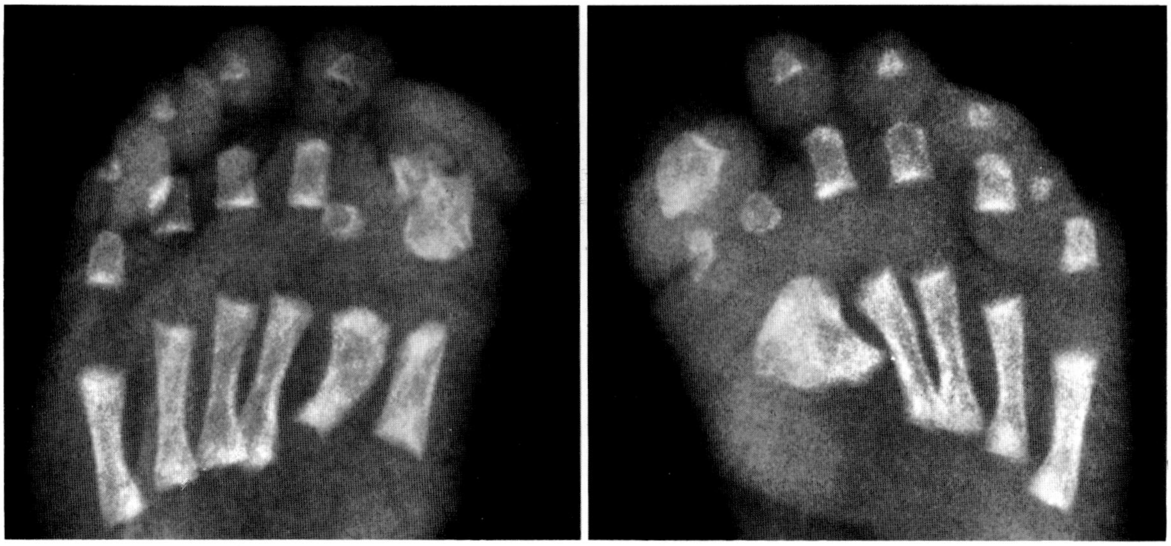

a b

Fig. 4a, b. Acrocephalopolysyndactyly (Carpenter's syndrome). Short and deformed big toes, preaxial polydactyly in both feet, broad, triangular first metatarsal in right foot (**b**)

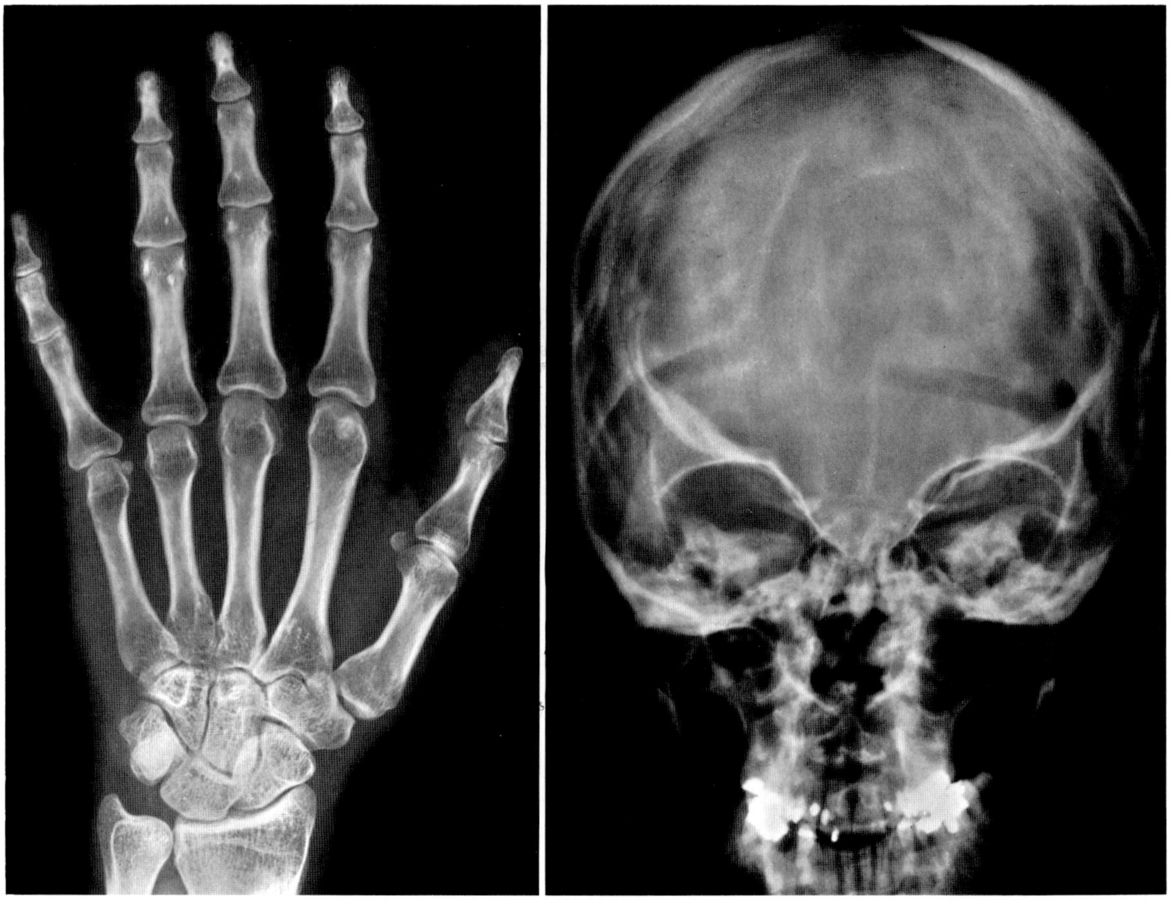

a b

Fig. 5a, b. Acrocephalosyndactyly (SAETHRE CHOTZEN, type III) in a 28-year-old woman. The hand bones are normal (**a**) and the skull presents a significant asymmetry (**b**)

2.1.2 Basal Cell Nevus Syndrome

Synonym: Gorlin's syndrome

This autosomal dominant hereditary disorder is characterized by the presence of multiple basal cell nevi, from which basal cell carcinoma may develop. Associated abnormalities are found in the jaws (odontogenic cysts), ribs, eyes, gastrointestinal tract, and urogenital tract. A broad nasal root, prominent supraorbital ridges, hypertelorism, prognathism, and frontal and temporal bossing are other typical clinical features.

Radiographic Findings [1–4]

Hand

Brachymetacarpia in fourth ray (or third, fourth, and fifth rays)
Flame-shaped translucencies in phalanges
Less common features: short phalanges of thumb
polydactyly
syndactyly
arachnodactyly

Other Sites

Skull: calcifications in dura (lamellar), falx cerebri, bridging of sella turcica
hypertelorism
Mandible: well-defined odontogenic cysts
Spine: block vertebrae
incomplete segmentation
spina bifida occulta
kyphoscoliosis
Thorax: cervical ribs
bifid ribs
rib synostosis
hypoplasia of scapula
Foot: abnormalities analogous to those in hand
Long tubular bones: widespread osteolytic lesions

Differential Diagnosis

Other conditions with brachymetacarpia (Sect. 2.2.11)
(Pseudo)pseudohypoparathyroidism (Sect. 6.1.2)
Tuberous sclerosis (Sect. 7.1.2.1)
Hyperlipoproteinemia (Sect. 7.1.5)
Sarcoidosis (Sect. 7.3.12)
Metastatic fat necrosis (Sect. 7.6.4)

References

1 Gorlin RJ, Goltz RW (1960) Multiple nevoid basal-cell epithelioma, jaw cysts and bifid rib. A syndrome. N Engl J Med 262:908–912
2 Becker MH, Kopf AW, Laude A (1967) Basal nevus syndrome. Its roentgenographic significance. Review of the literature and report of four cases. AJR 99:817–825
3 Mc Evoy BF, Gatzek H (1969) Multiple nevoid basal cell carcinoma syndrome: radiological manifestations. Br J Radiol 42:24–28
4 Blinder G, Barki Y, Pezt M, Bar-Ziv B (1984) Widespread osteolytic lesions of the long bones in basal cell nevus syndrome. Skeletal Radiol 12:196–198

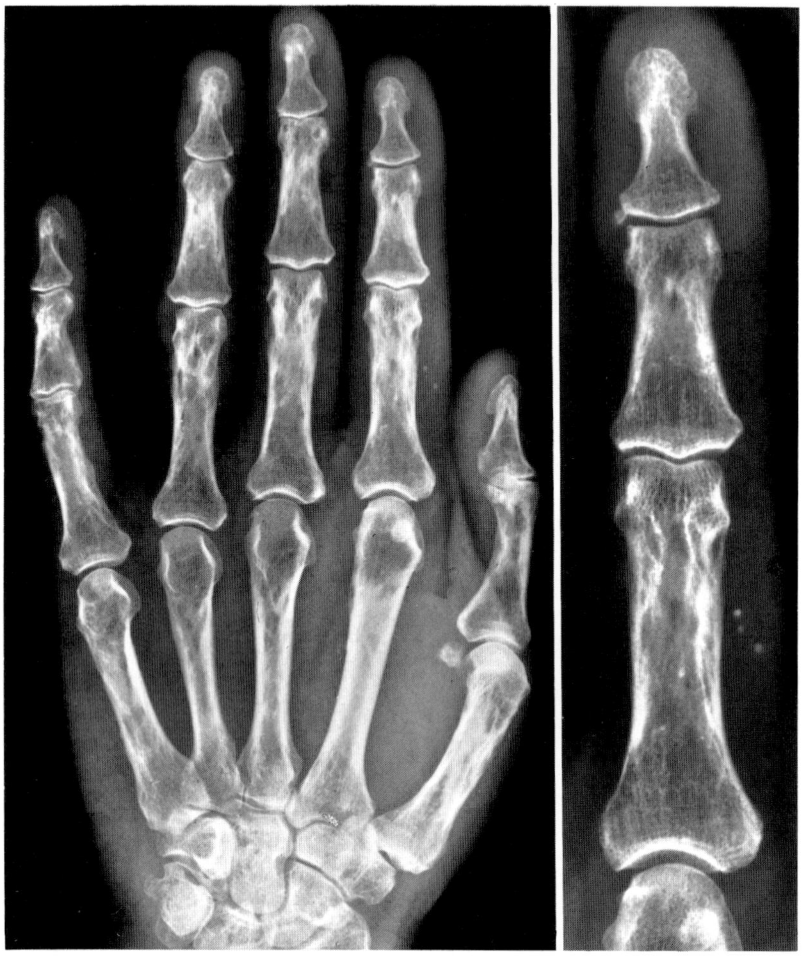

a b

Fig. 1 a, b. Basal cell nevus syndrome in a 68 year old woman. Flame-shaped lucencies in the tubular bones of right hand (**a**) several distinct soft tissue calcifications in second finger (**b**)

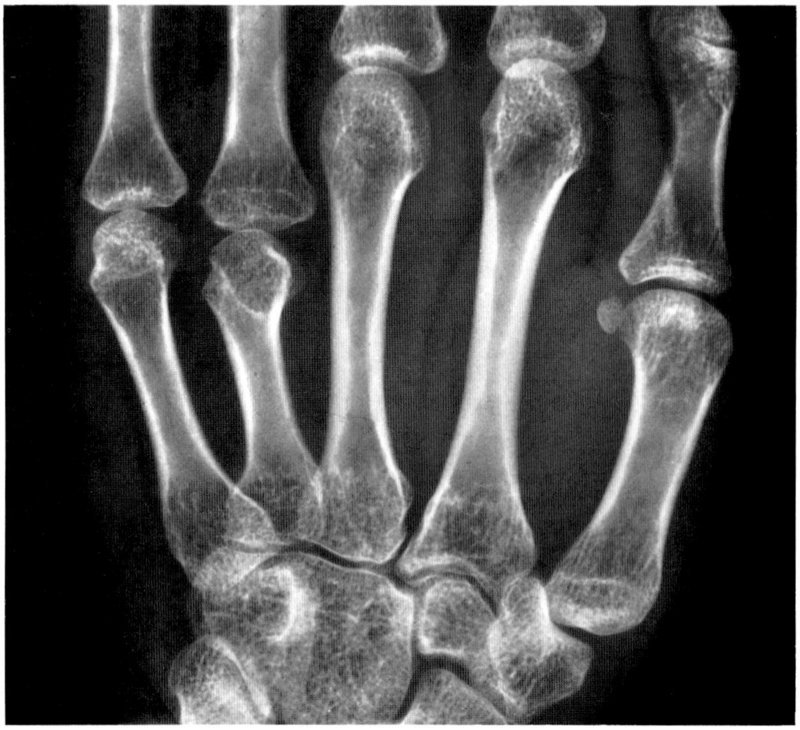

Fig. 2. Basal cell nevus syndrome in a 26-year-old man. Left hand: Short fourth metacarpal, fifth metacarpal only slightly hypoplastic

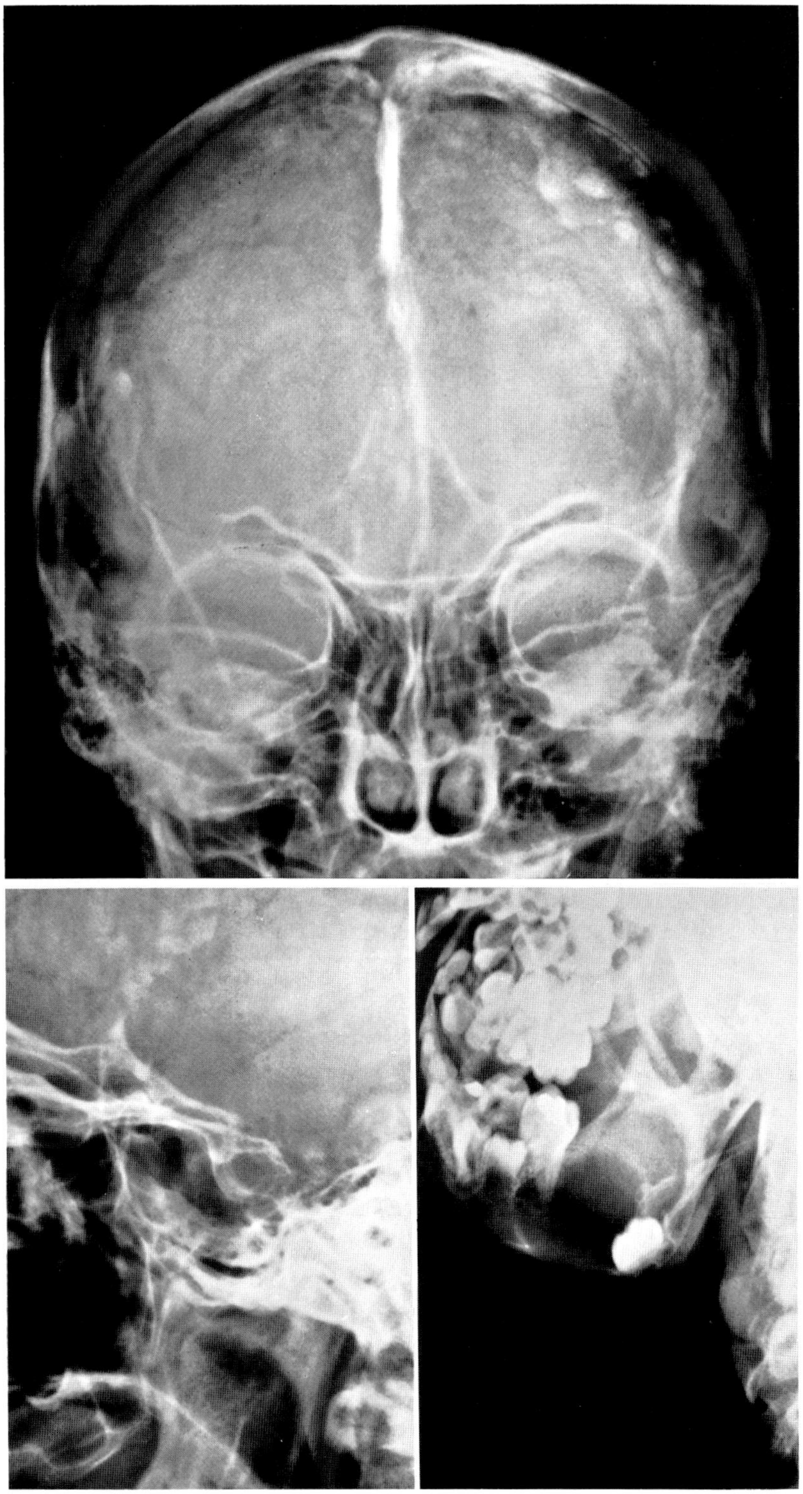

a

b c

Fig. 3a–c. Basal cell nevus syndrome. **a, b** In a 39-year-old woman: Extensive calcification of falx cerebri and dura, bridging of sella turcica. **c** In a 10-year-old girl: Well-defined odontogenic mandibular cyst

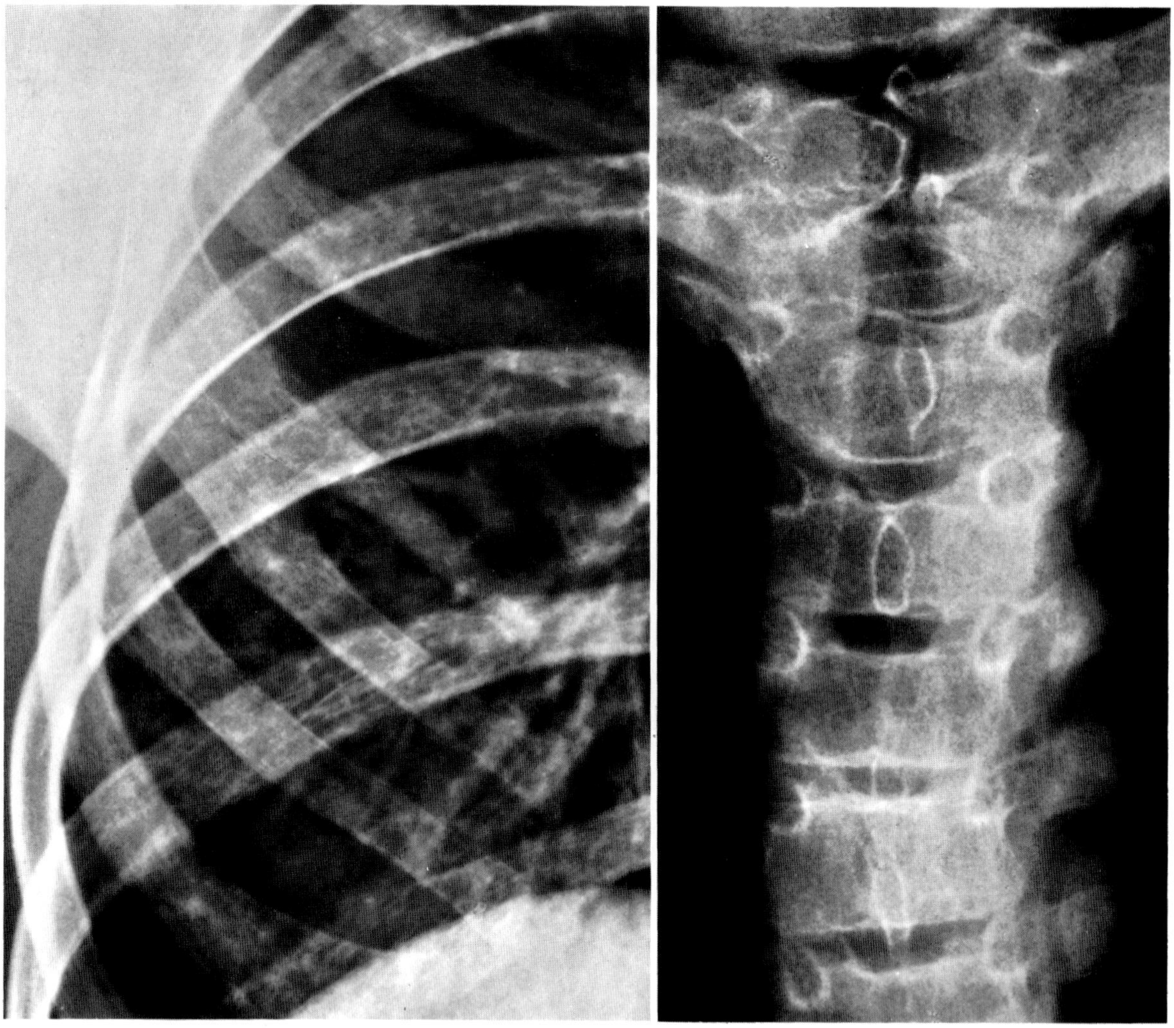

a b

Fig. 4a, b. Basal cell nevus syndrome in a 10-year-old girl. **a** Bifid fourth rib. **b** Spina bifida in first and second vertebral arches of thoracic spine

2.2 Dysostoses with Predominant Involvement of Extremities

2.2.1 Radial Dysplasia

Radial dysplasia may be sporadic or caused by autosomal dominant inheritance. The incidence is about 1:30,000 [1]. The clinical and radiographic findings vary widely: in some patients only slight hypoplasia of the hand is present, while in others aplasia of the radial side of the forearm and hand may be encountered. A number of abnormalities and syndromes are associated with radial dysplasia.

Associated Abnormalities

Hand
Ulnar dysplasia
Central dysplasia
Triphalangism of thumb
Carpal fusion
Polydactyly
Brachydactyly
Syndactyly

Other Sites
Cleft palate
Congenital heart disease
Spina bifida
Klippel-Feil deformity

Renal abnormalities
Esophageal atresia
Ear abnormalities

Associated Disorders [2]

Holt-Oram syndrome (Sect. 2.2.19)
Fanconi's anemia [3, 4]
Thrombocytopenia absent radius syndrome [5]
Vater syndrome [6]
Rokitansky-Küster-Hauser syndrome [7].
Cornelia de Lange's syndrome (Sect. 5.1)
Thalidomide deformity
Dyschondrosteosis [8]
Mesomelic dwarfism [9]
Seckel's syndrome [10]
Chondroectodermal dysplasia (Sect. 1.1.6)
Ring D syndrome [18]
Trisomy 18 (Sect. 4.1)
Trisomy 13 [11]
Craniosynostosis
Acrofacial dysostosis [12]

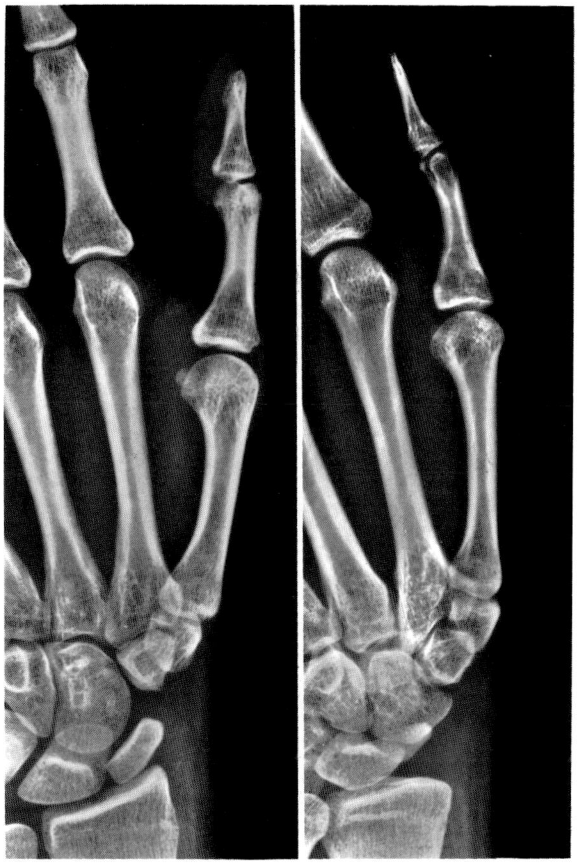

Fig. 1a, b. Rokitansky-Küster-Hauser syndrome, in two patients. Hypoplasia and abnormally placed carpals at radial side of the hand, slender first metacarpals

References

1 Birch-Jensen A (1949) Congenital deformities of the upper extremities. Andelsbogtrykkeriet, Odense
2 Poznanski AK (1984) The hand in radiologic diagnosis. Saunders, Philadelphia
3 Minagi H, Steinbach HL (1966) Roentgen appearance of anomalies associated with hypoplastic anemias of childhood: Fanconi's anemia and congenital hypoplastic anemias (erythrogenesis imperfecta). AJR 97:100–109
4 Juhl JH, Wesenberg RL, Gwinn JL (1967) Roentgenographic findings in Fanconi's anemia. Radiology 89:646–653
5 Dignan PStJ, Mauer AM, Frantz C (1967) Phocomelia with congenital hypoplastic thrombocytopenia and myeloid leukemoid reactions. J Pediatr 70:561–573
6 Quan L, Smith DW (1973) The Vater association, vertebral defects, anal atresia, TE fistula with esophageal atresia, radial and renal dysplasia. A spectrum of associated defects. J Pediatr 82:104–107
7 Kords H (1976) Rokitansky-Küster-Syndrom (Vaginal-Aplasie, rudimentärer Uterus) kombiniert mit Nierenaplasie, Phokomelie und multiplen Skelett-Fehlbildungen im Sinne eines Klippel-Feil-Syndroms. Geburtshilfe Frauenheilkd 36:672–677
8 Kozlowski K, Zychowicz C (1971) Dyschondrosteosis. Acta Radiol 11:459–465
9 Silverman FN (1973) Mesomelic dwarfism. In: Kaufmann HJ (ed) Intrinsic diseases of bones. Karger, Basel, pp 546–562 (Progress in pediatric radiology, vol 4)
10 Harper RG, Orti E, Baker RK (1967) Birdheaded dwarfs (Seckel's syndrome). A familial pattern of developmental, dental, skeletal, genital and central nervous system anomalies. J Pediatr 70:799–804
11 James AE Jr, Delcourt CL, Atkins L, Janower ML (1969) Trisomy 13–15. Radiology 92:44–49
12 Weyers H (1952) Über eine korrelierte Mißbildung der Kiefer und Extremitätenaksen (dysostosis acrofacialis). Fortschr Geb Röntgenstr Nuklearmed Ergänzungsband 77:562–567

a b c d e

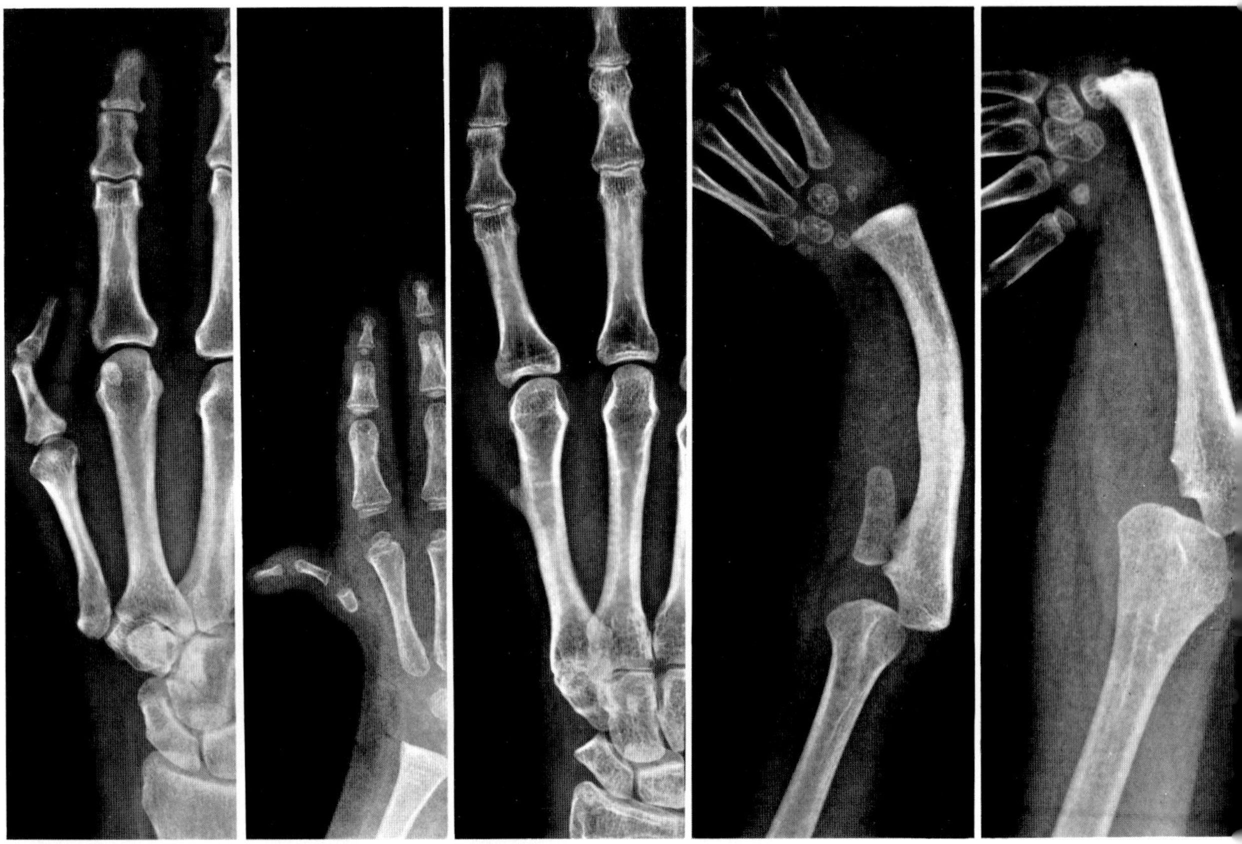

Fig. 2a–e. Radial dysplasia. **a** Slight hypoplasia of first metacarpal. **b** Hypoplasia of first metacarpal and thumb. **c** Absent thumb and abnormal radially placed carpals (Fanconi's anemia). **d** Absent thumb and hypoplasia of radius. **e** Thumb present but radius absent (thrombocytopenia absent radius syndrome)

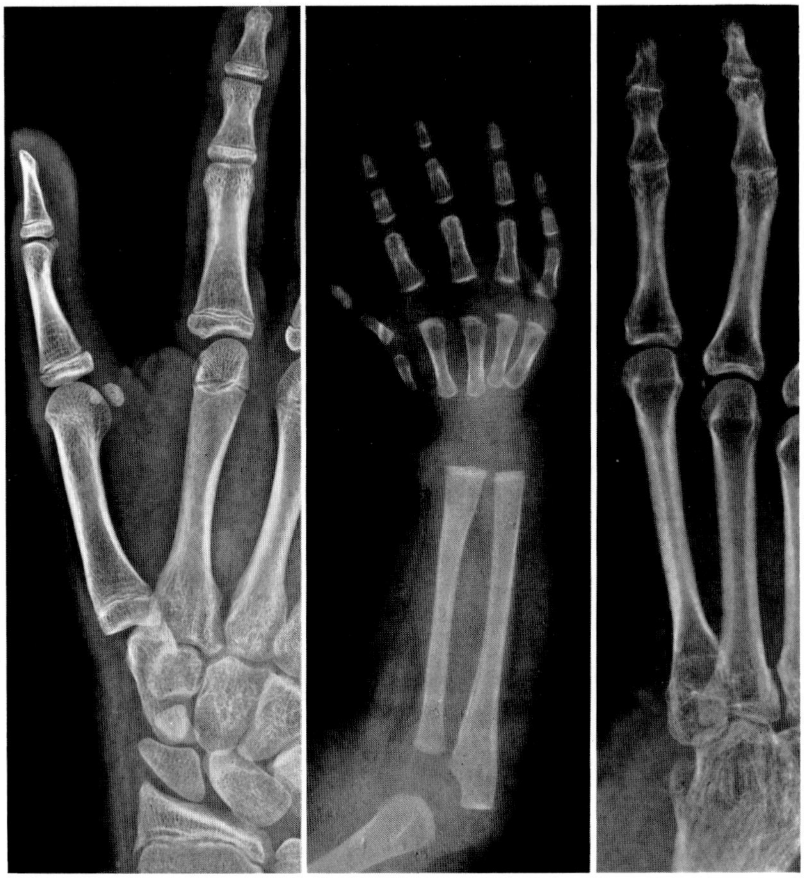

a b c

Fig. 3a–c. Radial dysplasia. **a** Holt-Oram syndrome: Abnormal radially placed carpals, os centrale carpi. **b** Vater syndrome: Hypoplastic thumb and first metacarpal. **c** Fanconi's anemia: Absent radius and carpal fusion

2.2.2 Ulnar Dysplasia

Ulnar dysplasia is a rare disorder ranging from slight hypoplasia of the ulnar digits to (very rarely) absence of the entire ulna [1]. Most cases are sporadic, and a certain number of syndromes are associated [2].

Associated Abnormalities of Hand and Forearm

Radial dysplasia
Central dysplasia
Carpal fusion
Symphalangism
Syndactyly
Radio-ulnar synostosis
Radiohumeral synostosis [3]
Luxation of radial head

Associated Disorders [2]

Symphalangism (Sect. 2.2.12)
Cornelia de Lange's syndrome (Sect. 5.1)
Acrofacial dysostosis [4]
Nievergelt's syndrome

References

1 Walter E, Eibach E (1978) Die Ulnaaplasia. Fortschr Geb Röntgenstr Nuklearmed Ergänzungsband 129:55–57
2 Poznanski AK (1984) The hand in radiologic diagnosis. Saunders, Philadelphia
3 Ogden JA, Watson HK, Bohne W (1976) Ulnar dysplasia. J Bone Joint Surg 50-A:467–472
4 Weyers H (1952) Ueber eine korrelierte Mißbildung der Kiefer und Extremitätenaksen (dysostosis acrofacialis). Fortschr Geb Röntgenstr Nuklearmed Ergänzungsband 77:562–567

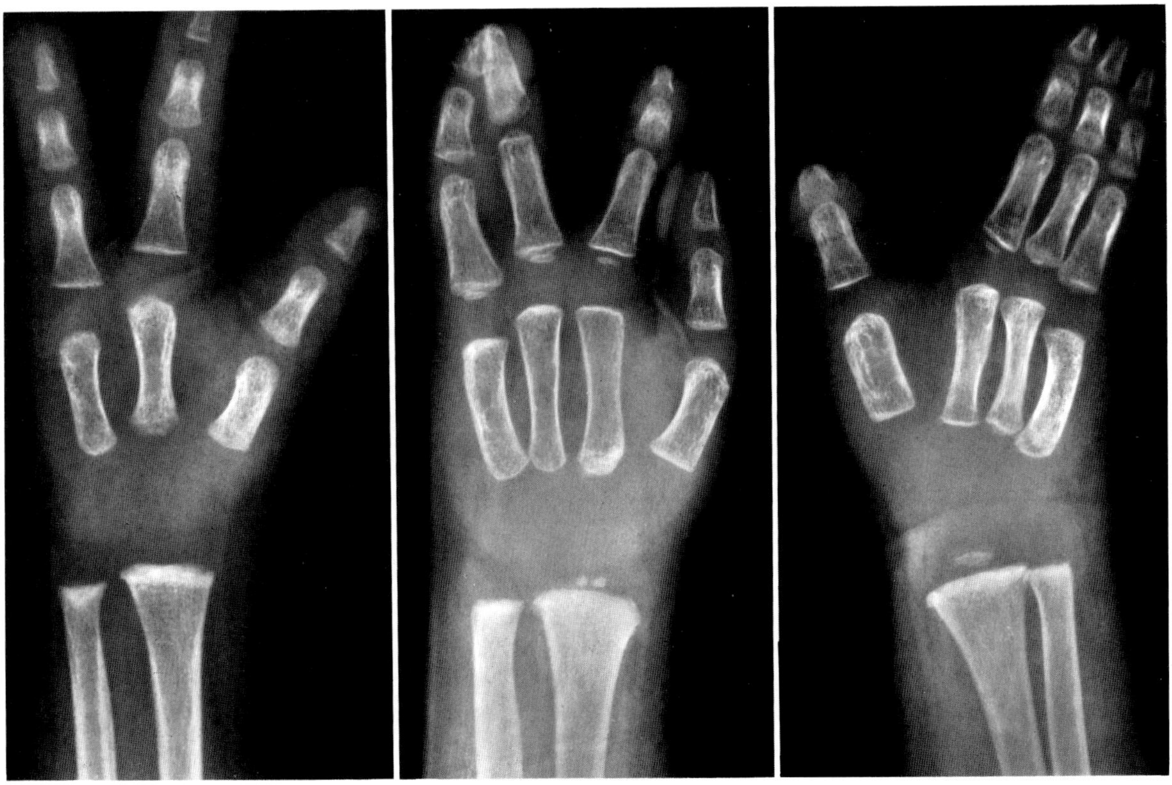

a b c

Fig. 1 a–c. Ulnar dysplasia in two children. **a** Absence of fourth and fifth digits and metacarpals. **b, c** In a 2-year-old girl: Both hands abnormal, significant syndactyly

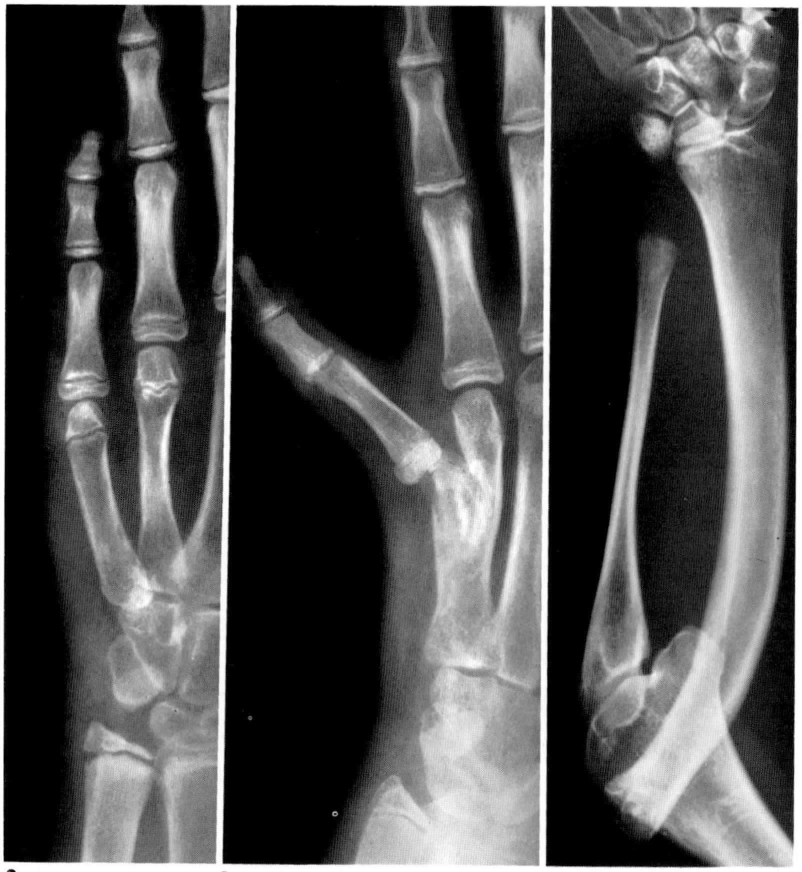

2a b c

Fig. 2a–c. Ulnar dysplasia. **a** In a 16-year-old boy. Cornelia de Lange's syndrome: Hypoplasia of middle and distal phalanges of fifth finger. **b** In a 17-year-old boy: Slight hypoplasia of fifth finger, fusion of fourth and fifth metacarpals. **c** In a 17-year-old girl: Ulnar hypoplasia, bowing of radius, luxation of radial head, carpal fusion (scaphoid-trapezium)

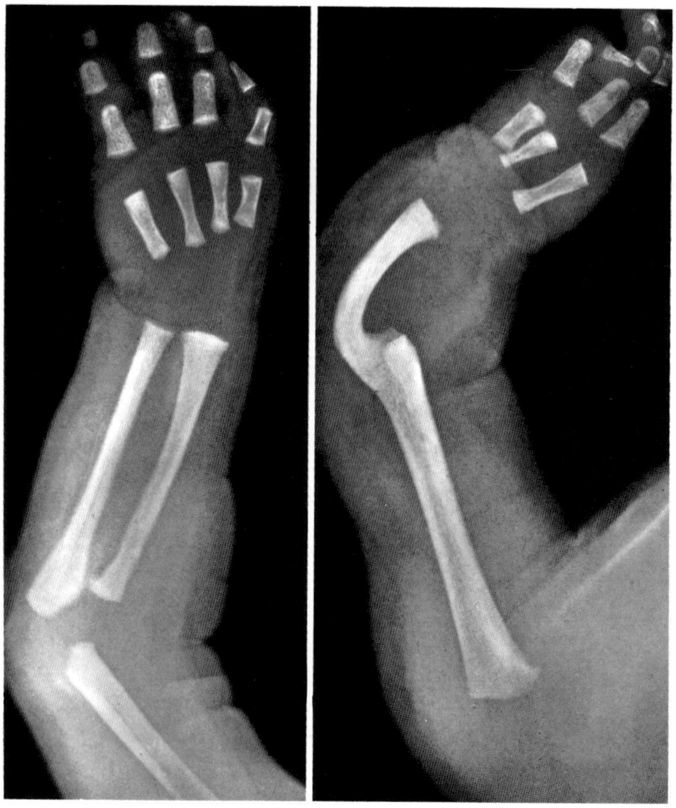

3a b

Fig. 3a, b. Bilateral ulnar dysplasia in a 1-day-old girl. **a** Fifth finger of left hand is absent. **b** Right hand and forearm are severely hypoplastic, radius and humerus are synostotic

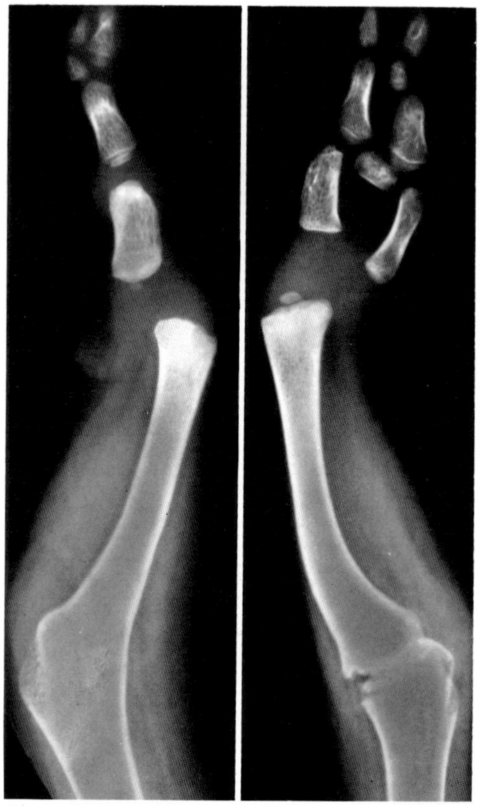

4a b

Fig. 4a, b. Ulnar dysplasia in a 4-year-old boy. Severe ulnar dysplasia of both hands and forearms, associated central dysplasia, radiohumeral synostosis in one elbow (**a**)

2.2.3 Central Dysplasia

Synonyms: split hand, lobster claw, cleft hand

The incidence of central dysplasia is 1:90,000. This anomaly is probably hereditary with variable penetrance [1–3]. The unilateral or bilateral abnormalities present symmetrically or asymmetrically. Frequently, similar foot abnormalities are associated.

Associated Abnormalities

Hand
Radial dysplasia
Ulnar dysplasia
Syndactyly
Absent carpals
Carpal fusion

Other Sites [1, 2, 4]
Split foot
Cleft palate
Deafness
Cataract
Cyclopia
Congenital nystagmus and fundal changes
Anonychia
Imperforate anus
Congenital heart disease

Differential Diagnosis

Amniotic bands (Sect. 2.2.4)
Terminal transverse defects (Sect. 2.2.5)

References

1 Poznanski AK (1984) The hand in radiologic diagnosis. Saunders, Philadelphia
2 Temtamy SA, McKusick VA (1978) The genetics of hand malformations. Liss, New York
3 Temtamy SA (1966) Genetic factors in hand malformations. Thesis. Johns Hopkins University. Baltimore
4 Warkany J (1971) Congenital malformations: notes and comments. Year Book Medical Publishers, Chicago

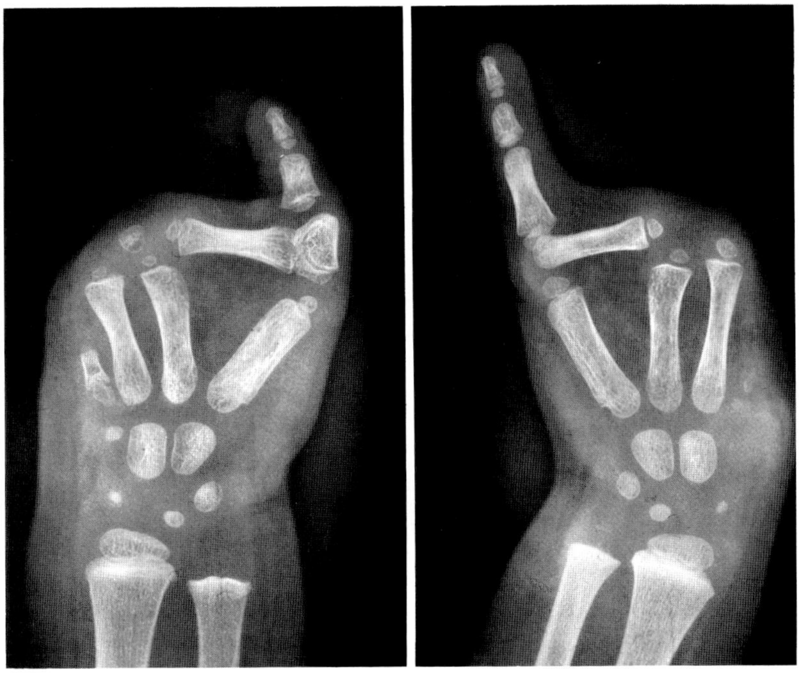

Fig. 1a, b. Central dysplasia and radial dysplasia. Bizarre deformation a b

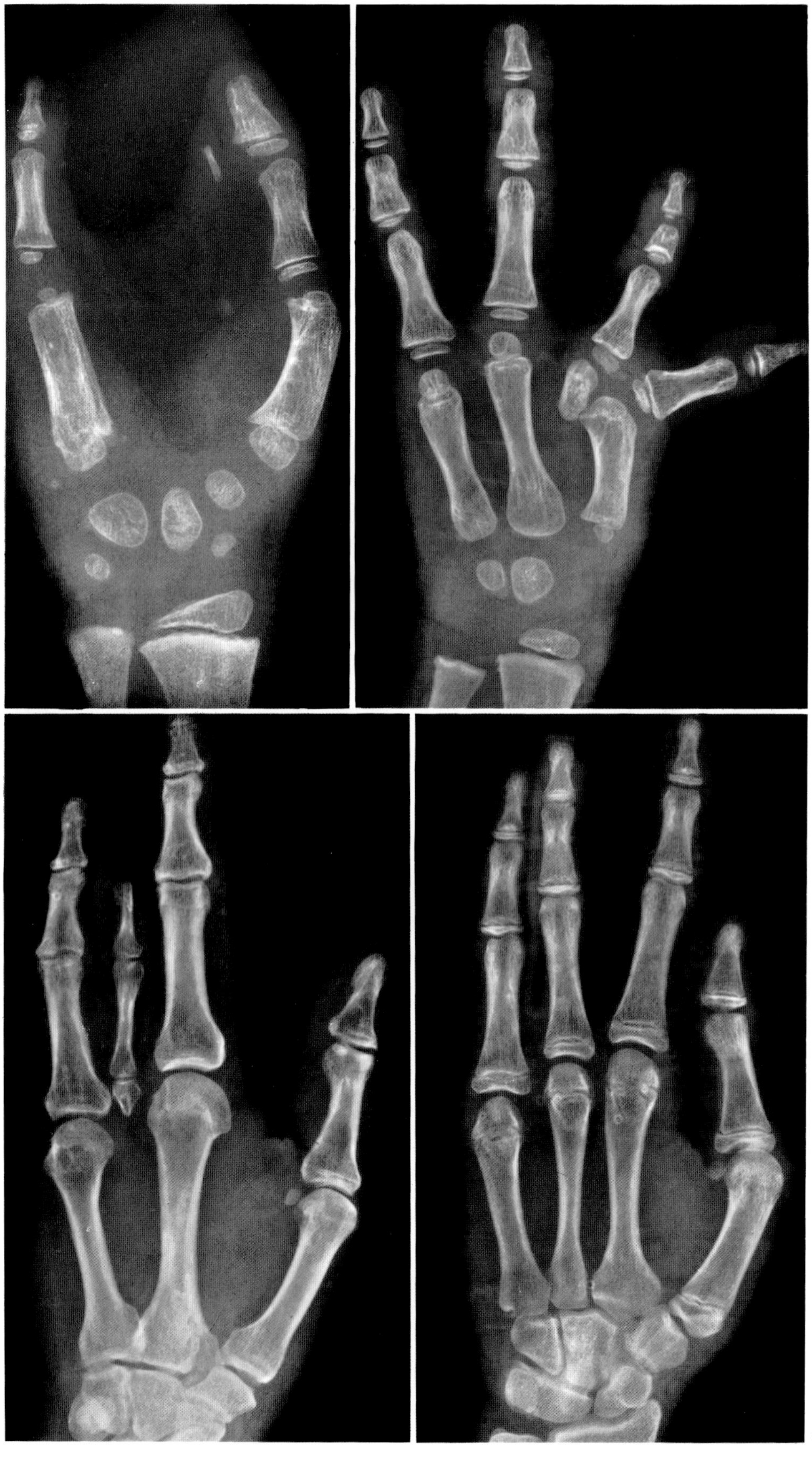

a b c d

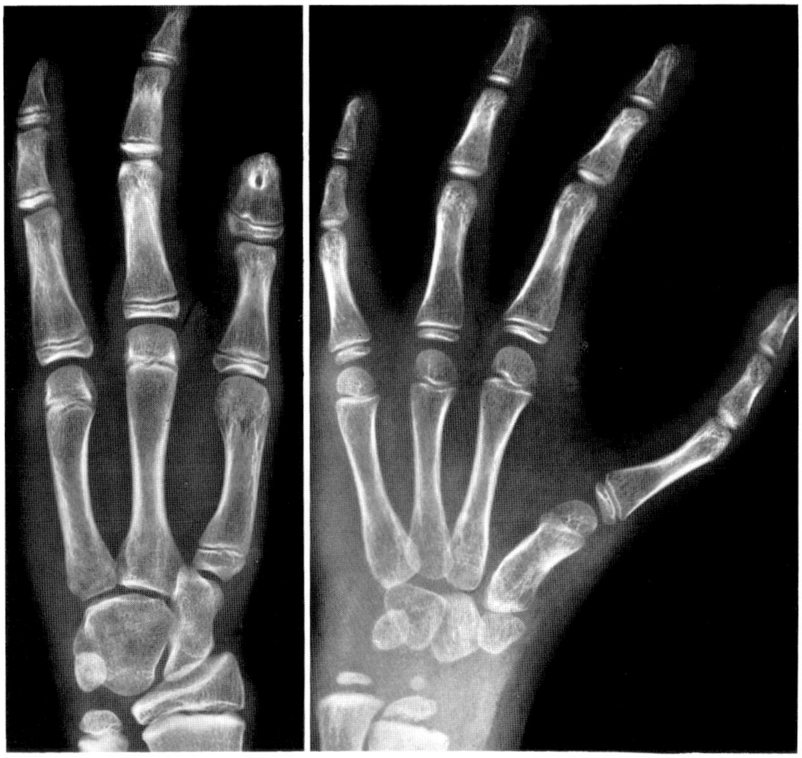

a b

Fig. 3. Central dysplasia. **a** Three-finger hand: Bifid distal phalanx of thumb with a central defect, carpal fusion. **b** Pseudo-central dysplasia after previous pollicization surgery for thumb aplasia

◁ **Fig. 2a–d.** Central dysplasia. **a** Only two digits are present. **b** Abnormal position of the thumb, otherwise mainly central dysplasia. The fourth and fifth digits are normal. **c** Hypoplastic fourth digit. The second finger is probably absent. **d** The second finger is probably absent together with the trapezoid

2.2.4 Amniotic Bands

Synonym: Streeter's bands

Amniotic bands are sporadic and have an incidence of 1:10,000–45,000 births [1, 2]. Their name reflects the fact that intrauterine constriction bands developed by a damaged amnion are thought to be the cause. Encircling of parts of the hand are frequently present. Occasionally there is soft tissue distension distal to the rings and hypoplasia of the distal elements.

Radiographic Findings [4]

Digits encircled by constriction rings in soft tissue
Syndactyly
Autoamputation of phalanges, fingers, or even whole hand
Sometimes: dumbbell-formed phalangeal bones, brachydactyly similar to Bell type B (see Sect. 2.2.11), carpal fusion

Associated Abnormalities

Club foot
Cleft palate and lip [3]

Differential Diagnosis

Terminal transverse defects (Sect. 2.2.5)

References

1 Poznanski AK (1984) The hand in radiologic diagnosis. Saunders, Philadelphia
2 Pillay VK, Hesketh KT (1965) Intrauterine amputations and annular limb defects in Singapore. J. Bone Joint Surg 47-B:514–519
3 Patterson TJS (1961) Congenital ring-constrictions. Br J Plast Surg 14:1–31
4 Baker CJ, Rudolph AJ (1971) Congenital ring constrictions and intrauterine amputations. Am J Dis Child 121:393–400

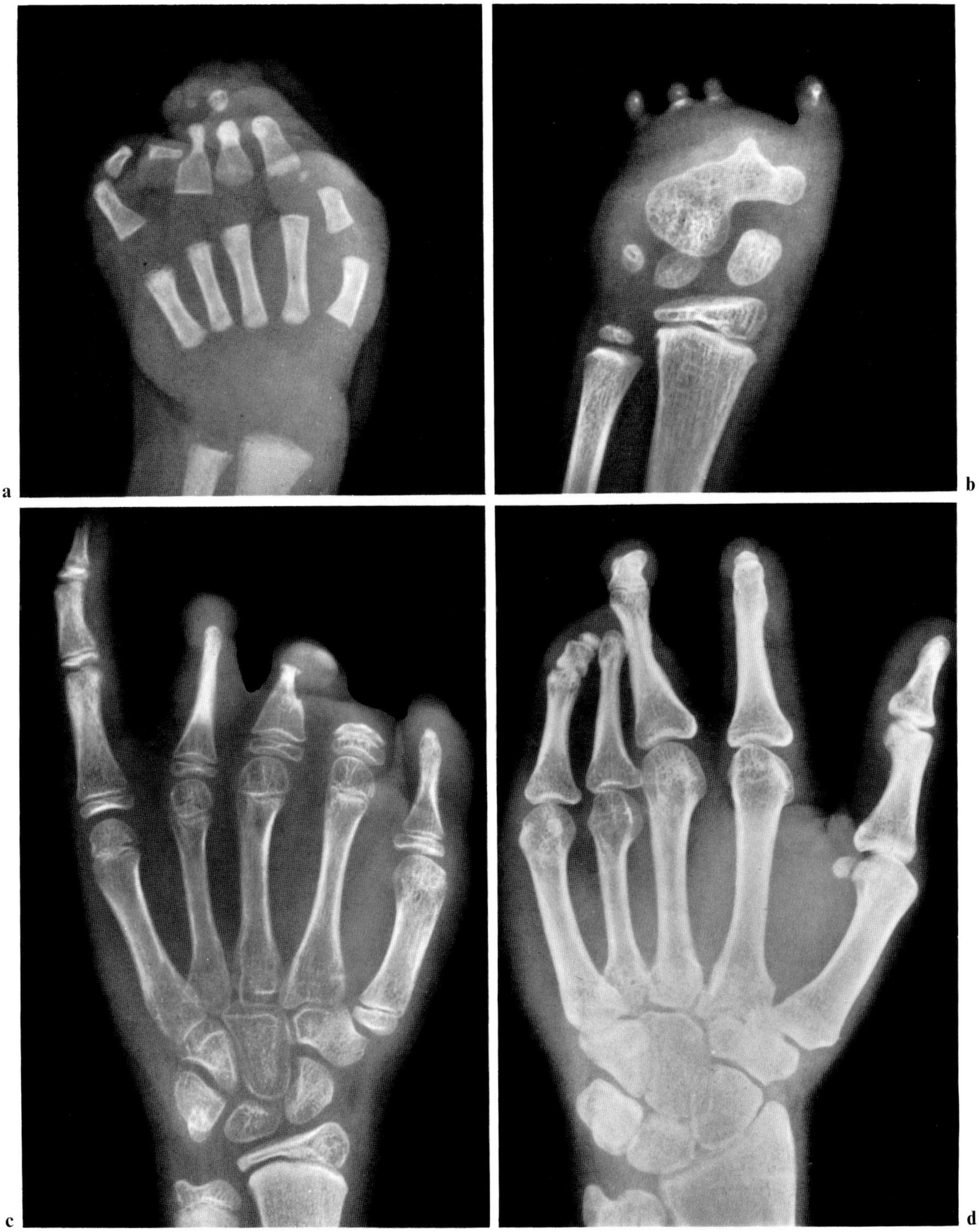

Fig. 1 a–d. Amniotic bands. **a** In a 3-month-old girl: Syndactyly of three fingers, constriction rings, dumbbell-formed fourth proximal phalanx. **b** In a 9-year-old girl: Constriction rings, small ossification centers in deformed fingers, carpal fusion. Other hand normal. **c** In a 10-year-old girl: Fifth finger normal, other fingers deformed. **d** In an 18-year-old man: Constriction rings, syndactyly, diabolo-formed third proximal phalanx. Thumb normal

2.2.5 Terminal Transverse Defects

Synonym: ectrodactyly

Terminal transverse defects are usually sporadic and present as unilateral abnormalities. Autoamputation is not likely. Probably the missing limbs have never been formed [1]. The defects can be divided into aphalangism (missing phalanges), adactyly (missing fingers), acheiria (missing hand), and acheiropodia (missing hand and foot).

Radiographic Findings

Absence of bones in hand or forearm (depending on degree of severity)
Smooth and flat distal end of limb
Syndactyly
Occasionally: soft tissue calcification, foot abnormalities, symphalangism
Sometimes: brachydactyly similar to Bell type B (see Sect. 2.2.11)

Differential Diagnosis

Amniotic bands (Sect. 2.2.4)

Associated Disorders

Cornelia de Lange's syndrome (Sect. 5.1)
Aglossia-adactyly [2]
Ankyloglossia superior [3]
Hanhart's syndrome
Möbius' syndrome [4]

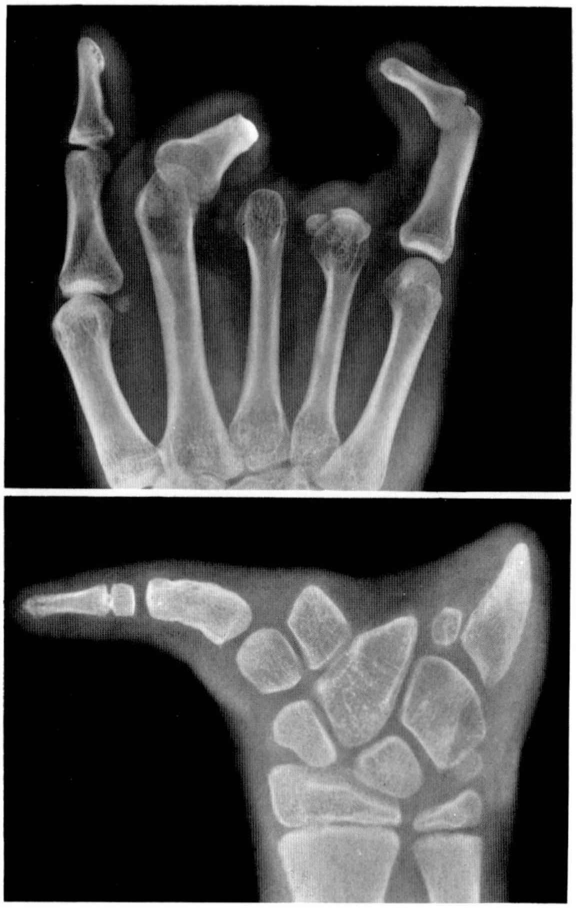

a
b

Fig. 1 a, b. Terminal transverse defects. **a** In a 17-year-old female: Normal thumb, other fingers all abnormal, third finger completely absent. **b** In an 11-year-old girl: Smooth distal delineation of soft tissues, deformed terminal bones

References

1 Poznanski AK (1984) The hand in radiologic diagnosis. Saunders, Philadelphia
2 Kelln EE, Bennett CG, Klingberg WG (1968) Aglossia adactylia syndrome. Am J Dis Child 116:549–552
3 Wilson RA, Kliman MR, Hardyment AF (1963) Ankyloglossia superior (palato-glossal adhesion) in the newborn infant. Pediatrics 31:1051–1054
4 Hanission AS, Furte F, Hayes WT, Duncan JM (1970) Moebius syndrome in twins. Am J Dis Child 120:472–475

2.2.6 Accessory Carpals

Accessory carpal bones are encountered in approximately 1.6% of normal individuals [1]. Only the os styloideum and the os centrale carpi are of clinical significance. The os styloideum can be traumatized (carpe Bossu) and the os centrale carpi is sometimes associated with congenital malformation syndromes (HOLT-ORAM, LARSEN, otopalatodigital, hand-foot-uterus) [2–4].

Disorders with Supernumerary Carpals [4]

Diastrophic dysplasia (Sect. 1.1.4)
Chondroectodermal dysplasia (Sect. 1.1.6)
Larsen's syndrome (Sect. 1.1.9)
Holt-Oram syndrome (Sect. 2.2.19)
Turner's syndrome (Sect. 4.3)
Hand-foot-uterus syndrome
Otopalatodigital syndrome
Dyschondrosteosis

Differential Diagnosis

Post-traumatic bony fragments
Soft tissue calcifications (Sect. 6.2.7)

References

1 O'Rahilly R (1953) Survey of carpal and tarsal anomalies. J Bone Joint Surg 35-A:626–642
2 Bassöe E, Bassöe HH (1955) The styloid bone and carpe Bossu disease. AJR 74:886–888
3 Köhler A, Zimmer EA (1968) Borderlands of the normal and early pathology in skeletal roentgenology, 3rd edn. Grune and Stratton, New York
4 Poznanski AK (1984) The hand in radiologic diagnosis. Saunders, Philadelphia

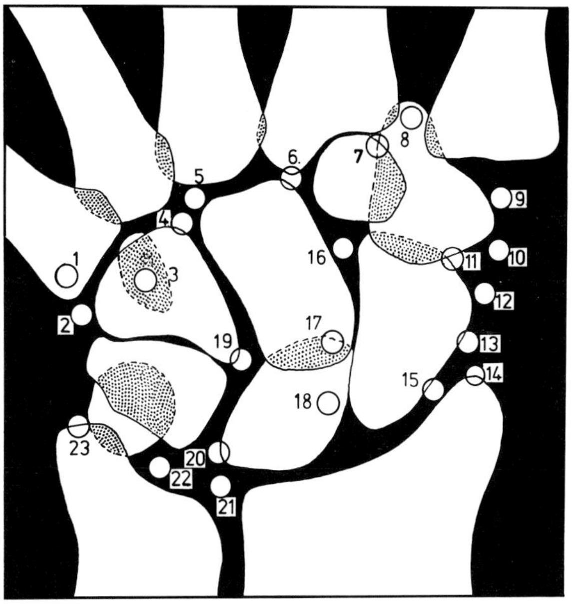

Fig. 1. Accessory carpals [3]. *1* Os vesalianum; *2* os ulnare externum; *3* os hamuli proprium; *4* os capitatum secundarium; *5* ossiculum Gruberi; *6* os styloideum; *7* os trapezoides secundarium; *8* os trapezium secundarium; *9* os paratrapezium; *10* ossification in bursa or tendon; *11* os epitrapezium; *12* os radiale externum; *13* bony fragment after fracture; *14* persistent ossification center of distal radial epiphysis or os radiostyloideum [1]; *15* os paranaviculare; *16* os centrale carpi; *17* os hypolunatum; *18* os epilunatum; *19* os epipyramis; *20* accessory carpal between lunatum and triquetrum; *21* accessory carpal in radio-ulnar joint; *22* os triangulare; *23* persistent ossification center of distal ulnar epiphysis or os ulnostyloideum [1]

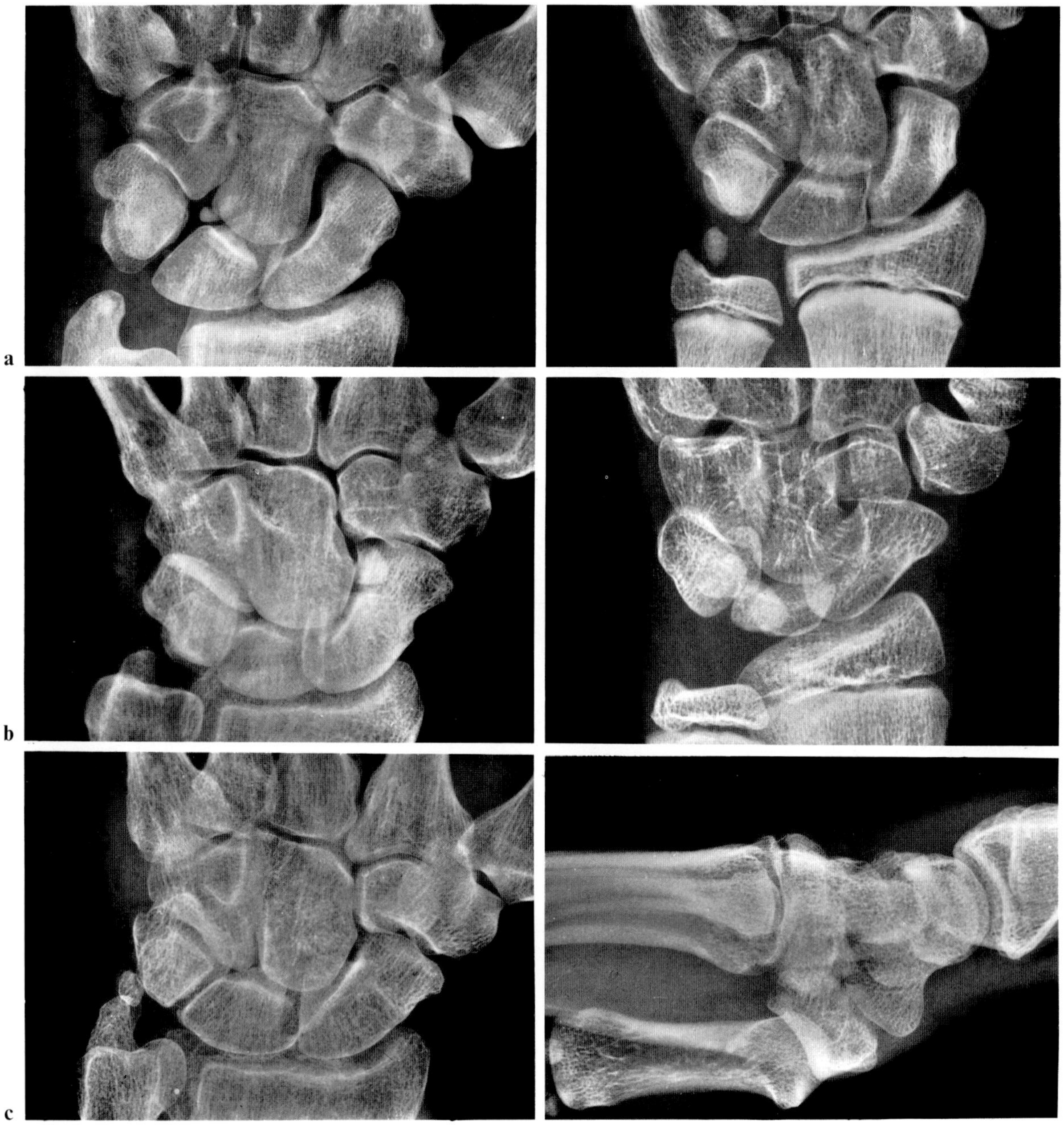

Fig. 2a–f. Accessory carpals. **a** Os epipyramis; **b** os centrale carpi; **c** persistent ossification center or os ulnostyloideum; **d** os triangulare; **e** double ossification centers of os lunatum; **f** os styloideum

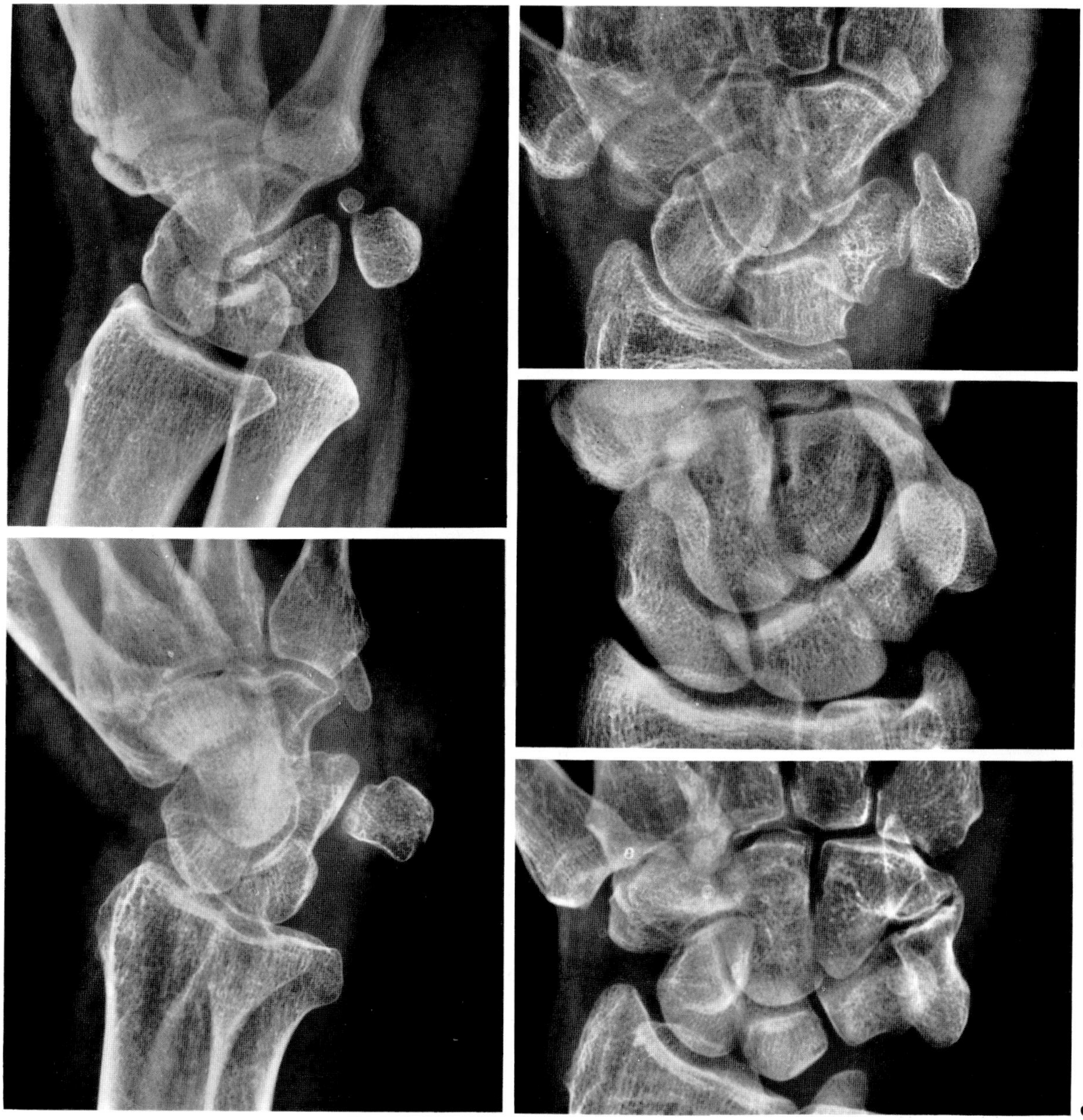

Fig. 3a–e. Variability between pisiform and hamate. **a** Small ossicle between pisiform and hamate; **b** ossicle adjacent to hamate (os hamuli proprium?); **c** small pisiform exostosis; **d** large pisiform exostosis without fusion with hamate; **e** articulation between a large pisiform and hamate

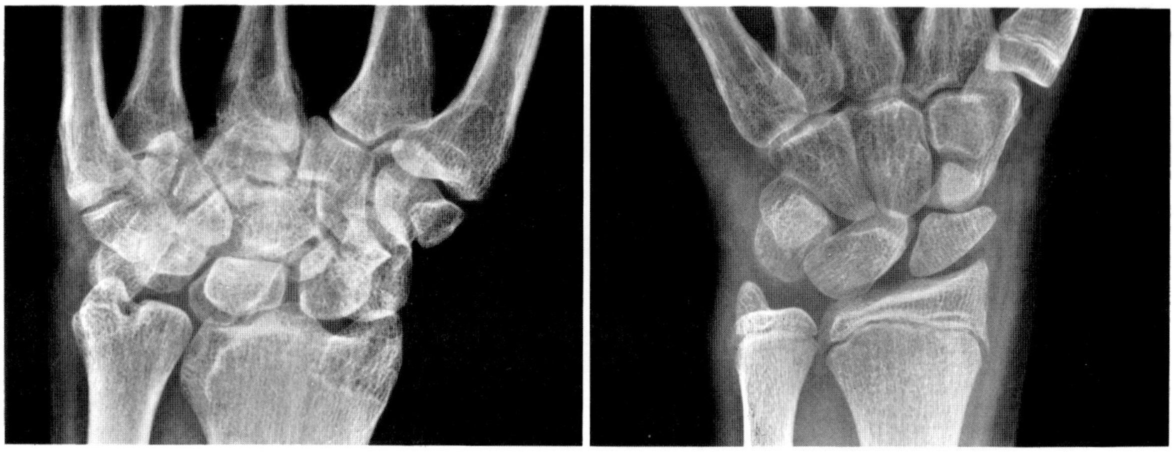

a b

Fig. 4a, b. Syndromes with supernumerary carpals. **a** Larsen's syndrome; **b** Holt-Oram syndrome, os centrale carpi, abnormal configuration of scaphoid and trapezium

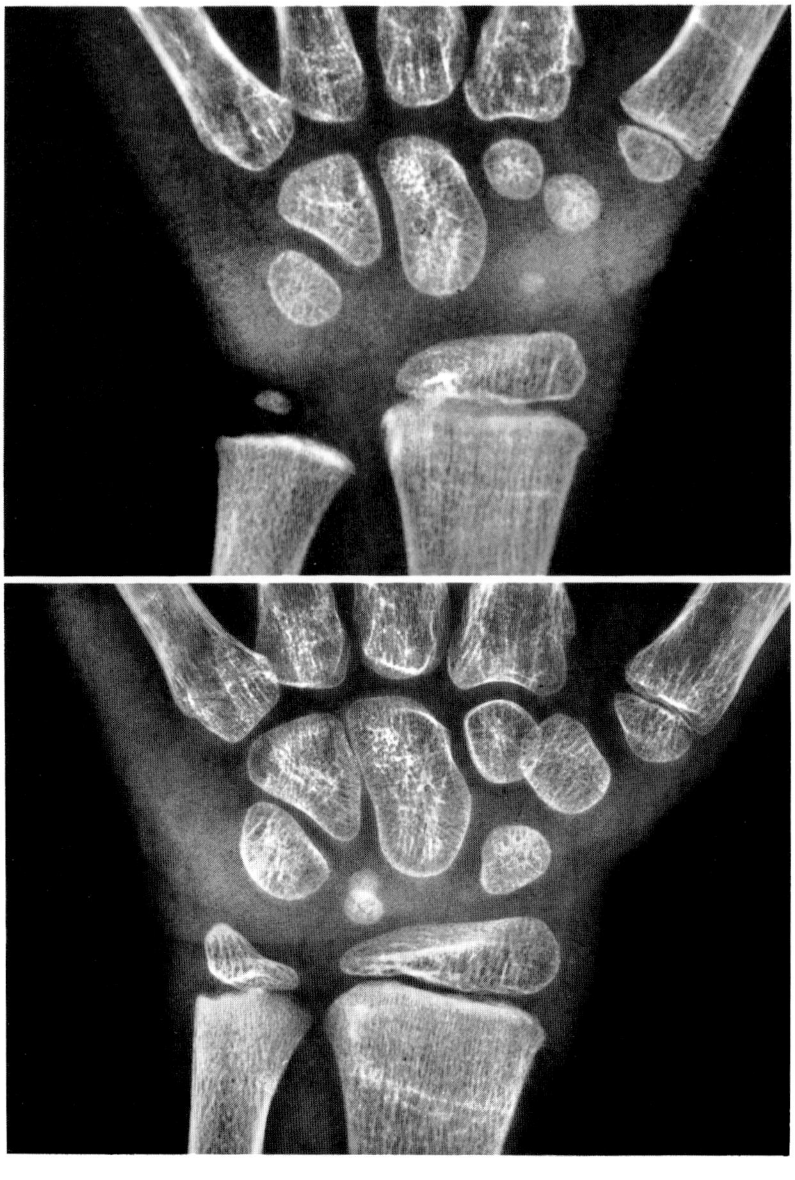

a b

Fig. 5a–b. Double ossification centers of lunate. **a** Delayed appearance of lunate. **b** After 2 years, double ossification centers. This may be seen in normal individuals, but also in some malformation syndromes

2.2.7 Carpal Fusion

Carpal fusion in the same row is usually an isolated anomaly. Carpal fusion across the rows is usually associated with congenital malformation syndromes.

Incidence [1, 2]

Triquetrum-lunate fusion	1‰–80‰
Capitate-hamate fusion	0.3‰–7.5‰
Trapezium-trapezoid fusion	0.2‰
Capitate-trapezoid fusion	very rare
Pisiform-hamate fusion	very rare
Trapezium-scaphoid fusion	very rare [3]
Fusion of multiple carpals	very rare
Proximal to distal row fusions	very rare

Associated Abnormalities (Fig. 3)

Radial dysplasia (Sect. 2.2.1)
Ulnar dysplasia (Sect. 2.2.2)
Central dysplasia (Sect. 2.2.3)
Amniotic bands (Sect. 2.2.4)
Polydactyly (Sect. 2.2.13)
Triphalangeal thumb (Sect. 2.2.15)
Tarsal fusion
Radio-ulnar synostosis

Acquired Carpal Fusion (Fig. 5)

Pyogenic arthritis (Sect. 7.3.2)
Rheumatoid arthritis (Sect. 7.3.4)
Rheumatoid arthritis in infancy (Sect. 7.3.5)
Tuberculosis (Sect. 7.3.9)
After surgery

Associated Disorders [1]

Diastrophic dysplasia (Sect. 1.1.4)
Chondroectodermal dysplasia (Sect. 1.1.6)
Fanconi's anemia (Sect. 2.2.1 [3])
Dyschondrosteosis (Sect. 2.2.1 [8])
Otopalatodigital syndrome (Sect. 2.2.8 [5])
Noonan's syndrome (Sect. 2.2.11 [9])
Hand-foot-uterus syndrome (Sect. 2.2.11 [30])
Holt-Oram syndrome (Sect. 2.2.19)
Acrocephalosyndactyly (Sect. 2.1.1)
Turner's syndrome (Sect. 4.3)
Cornelia de Lange's syndrome (Sect. 5.1)
Arthrogryposis multiplex congenita (Sect. 7.1.1)
Dermatomyositis
Lieberberg's syndrome
Alport's syndrome

References

1 Poznanski AK (1984) The hand in radiologic diagnosis. Saunders, Philadelphia
2 Cope JR (1974) Carpal coalition. Clin Radiol 25:261–266
3 Dawe C, Wynne-Davies R, Fulford GE (1982) Clinical variation in dyschondrosteosis. A report on 13 individuals in 8 families. J Bone Joint Surg 64-B:377–381
4 Seibert-Daiker FM (1975) Anlage eines Os hypolunatum beiderseits mit kongenitaler Konkreszenz des Scaphoideum und Trapezium. Fortschr Geb Röntgenstr Nuklearmed Ergänzungsband 122:463–465

a b c

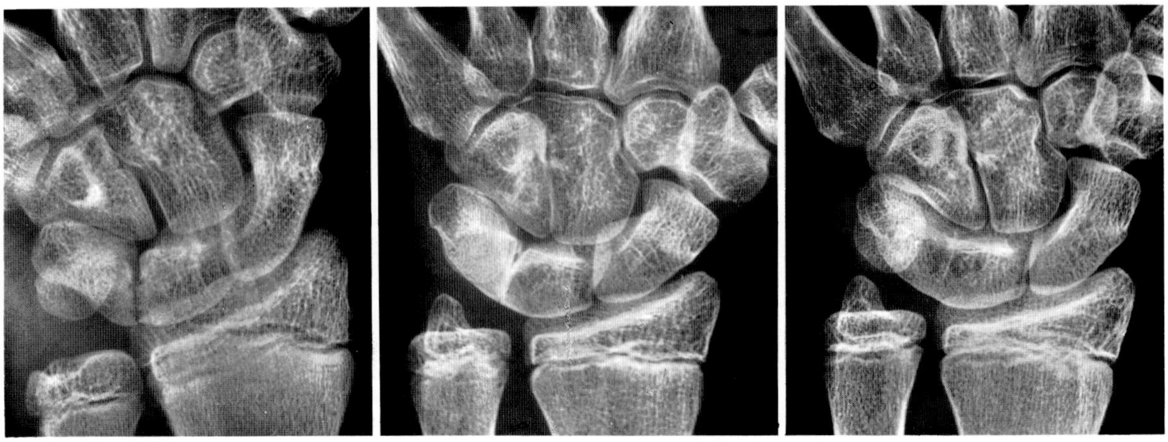

1

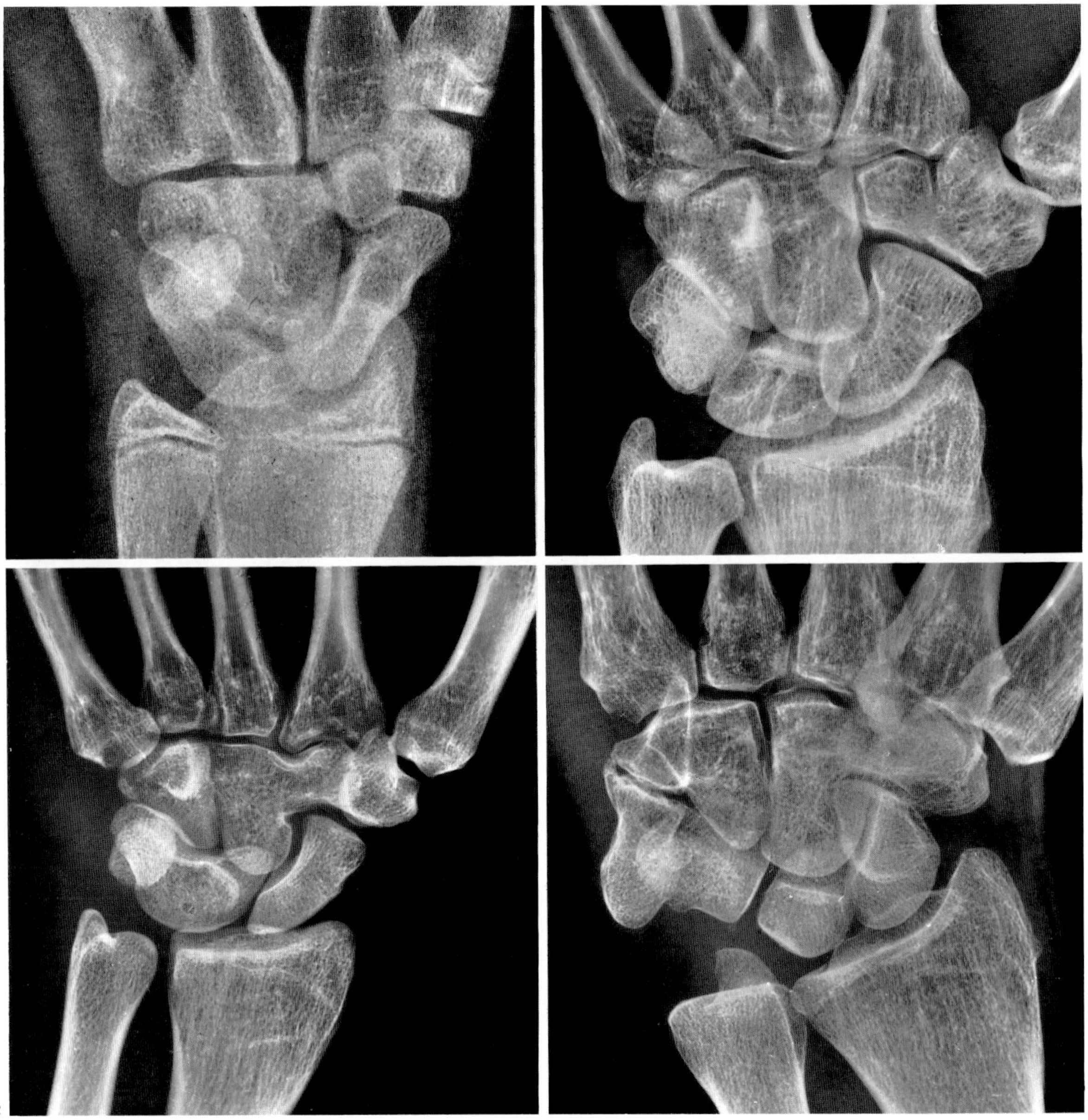

a b

c d

2

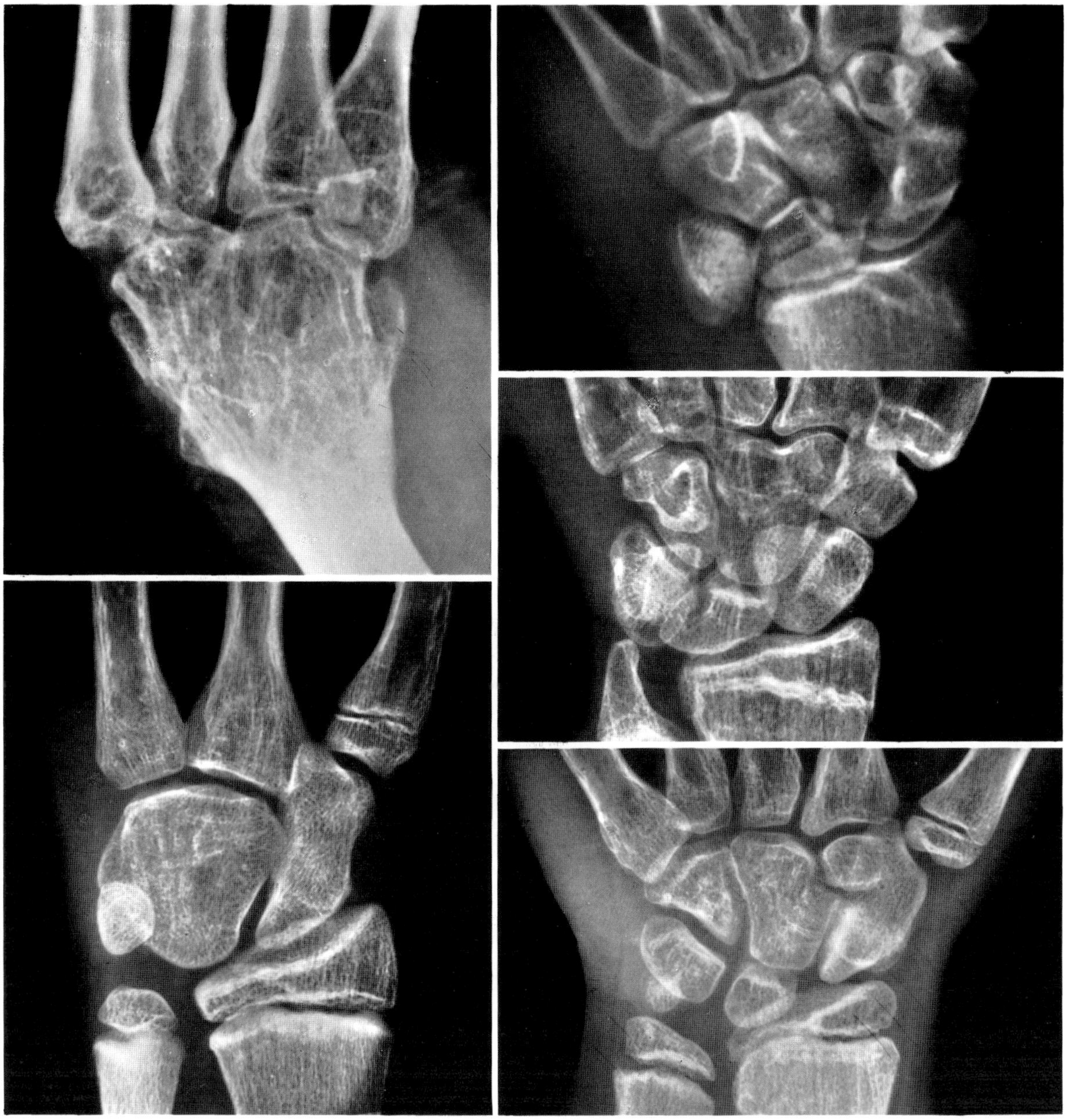

Fig. 3. a Radial dysplasia and carpal fusion (Fanconi's anemia). **b** Central dysplasia and carpal fusion. **c** Ulnar dysplasia: trapezium-scaphoid fusion. **d** Noonan's syndrome: capitate-trapezoid fusion. **e** Turner's syndrome: trapezium-scaphoid fusion

◁ **Fig. 1 a–c.** Triquetrum-lunate fusion. **a** Small cleft between triquetrum and lunate. **b** Partial fusion. **c** Complete fusion

Fig. 2. a Capitate-hamate fusion. **b** Trapezium-trapezoid fusion. **c** Capitate-trapezoid fusion, associated with triquetrum-lunate fusion. **d** Small cleft between pisiform and hamate

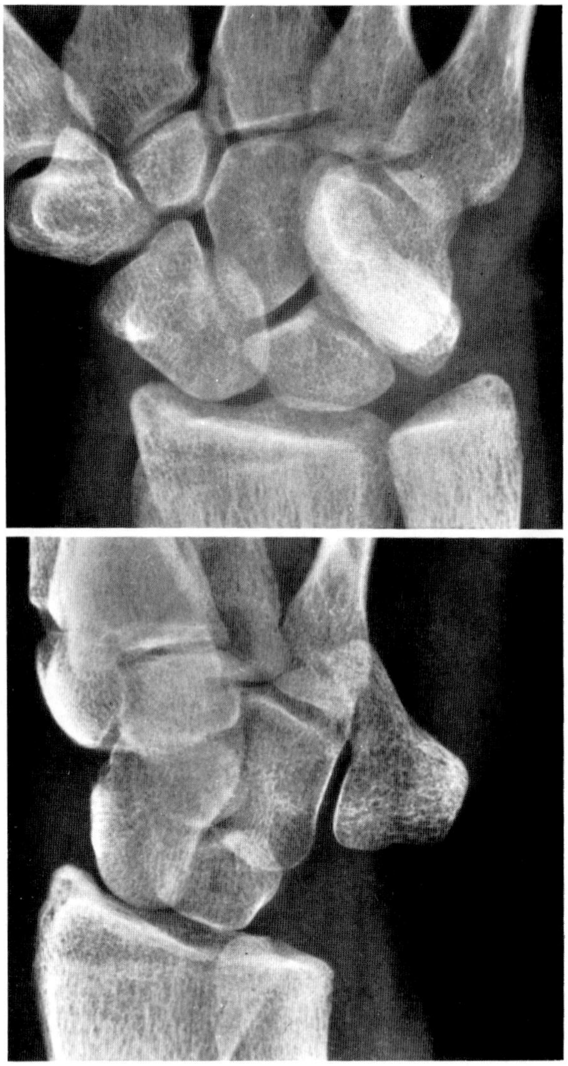

Fig. 4. Carpal fusion (hamate-pisiform-triquetrum) and triphalangeal thumb in a 22-year-old woman with interstitial nephritis and perception deafness (Alport's syndrome)

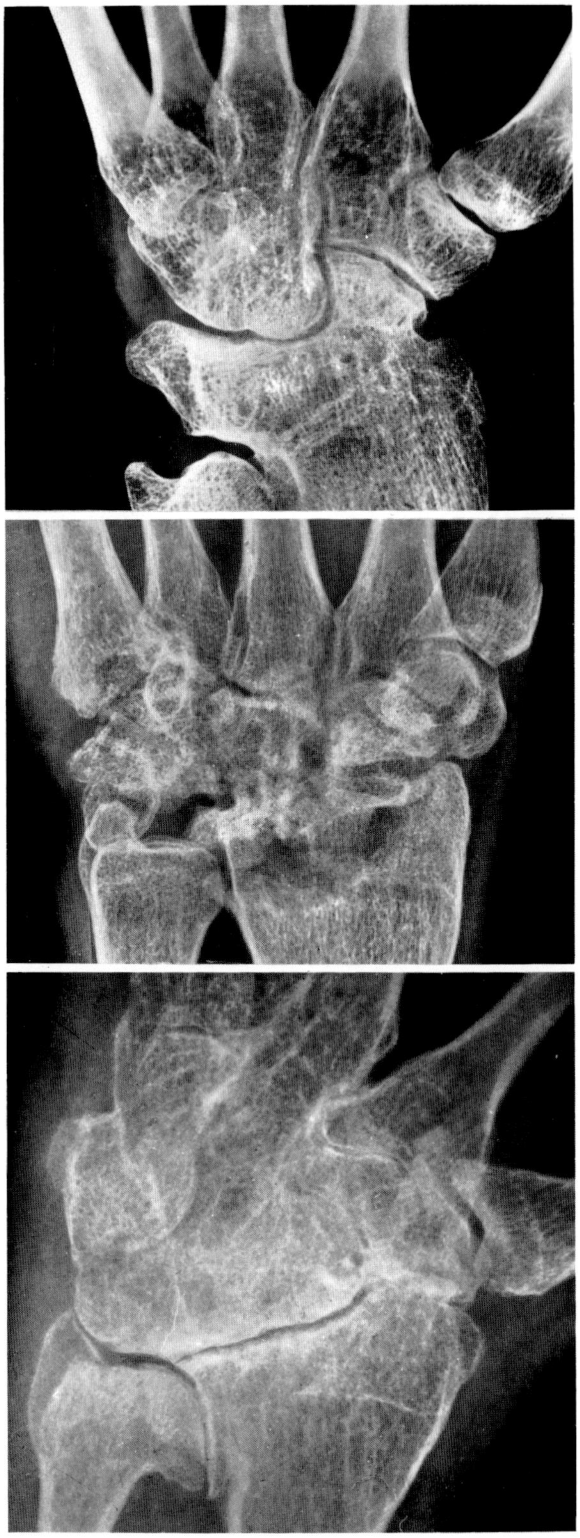

a

b

c

Fig. 5 a–c. Acquired carpal fusion. **a** Juvenile rheumatoid arthritis. **b** Tuberculosis of wrist. **c** Rheumatoid arthritis

2.2.8 Carpal Angle

The carpal angle is formed by the intersection of the line tangent to the scaphoid and lunate and the line tangent to the lunate and triquetrum. Above the age of 14 years, the following values are found [1, 2]:

	Mean	S.D.
White male	133.8°	9.8°
White female	129.6°	8.7°
Black male	141.7°	9.5°
Black female	138.6°	8.7°

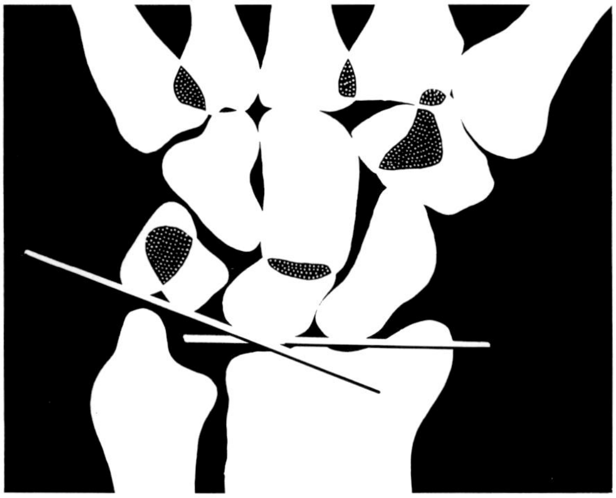

Fig. 1. Measurement of carpal angle

Associated Disorders with Decreased Carpal Angle [1]

Radial dysplasia (Sect. 2.2.1)
Rokitansky-Küster-Hauser syndrome (Sect. 2.2.1 [7])
Turner's syndrome (Sect. 4.3)
Mucopolysaccharidosis (Sect. 6.1.1)
Dyschondrosteosis [3, 4]
Madelung's deformity

Associated Disorders with Increased Carpal Angle [1]

Diastrophic dysplasia (Sect. 1.1.4)
Multiple epiphyseal dysplasia (Sect. 1.1.11)
Trisomy 21 (Sect. 4.2)
Pfeiffer's mucopolysaccharidosis (Sect. 6.1.1)
Arthrogryposis multiplex congenita (Sect. 7.1.1)
Otopalatodigital syndrome [5]
Frontometaphyseal dysplasia [6]

References

1 Poznanski AK (1984) The hand in radiologic diagnosis. Saunders, Philadelphia
2 Harper HAS, Poznanski AK, Garn GM (1974) The carpal angle in American populations. Invest Radiol 9:217–221
3 Langer LO Jr (1965) Dyschondrosteosis; heritable bone dysplasia with characteristic roentgenographic features. AJR 95:178–188
4 Dawe C, Wynne-Davies R, Fulford GE (1982) Clinical variation in dyschondrosteosis. A report of 13 individuals in 8 families. J Bone Joint Surg 64-B:377–381
5 Poznanski AK, McPherson RI, Gorlin RJ, Garn SM, Nagy JM, Gall JC Jr, Stern AM, Dijkman DJ (1973) The hand in the oto-palato-digital syndrome. Ann Radiol (Paris) 16:203–209
6 Kassner EG, Haller JO, Reddy H, Mitarotundo A, Katz I (1976) Frontometaphyseal dysplasia: evidence for autosomal dominant inheritance. AJR 127:927–933

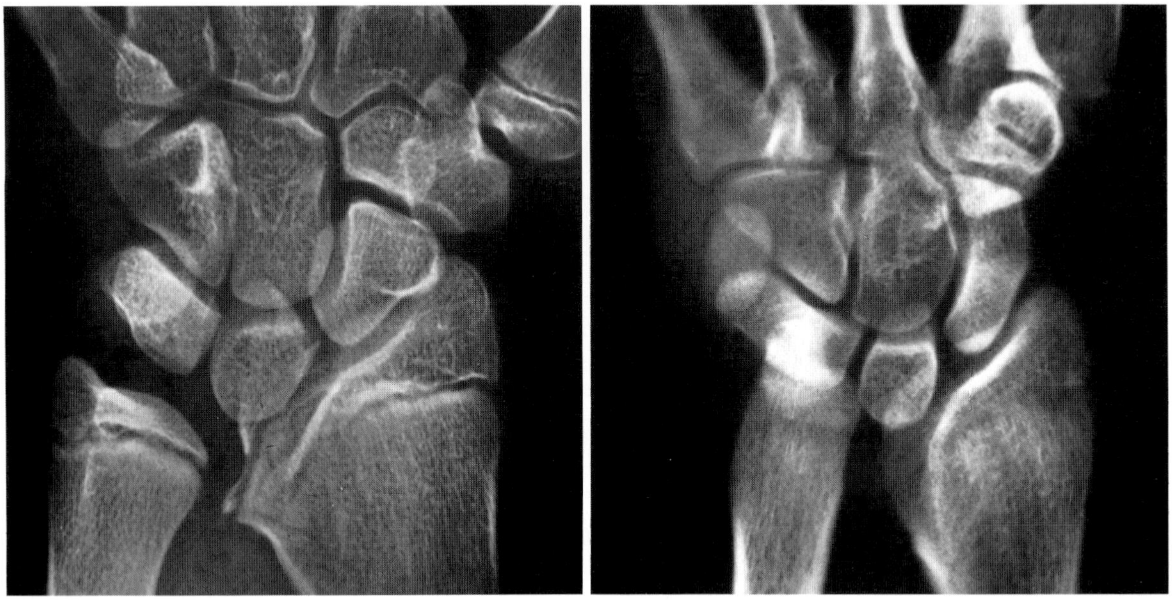

a b

Fig. 2a, b. Madelung's deformity. **a** In a 14-year-old boy: Decreased carpal angle (106°) and abnormal arrangement of carpals in proximal row. **b** In a 15-year-old girl: Decreased carpal angle (108°). The lunate seems to be caught in the cleft between the radius and the ulna. The scaphoid is somewhat displaced in a distal direction, and the triquetrum is relatively large

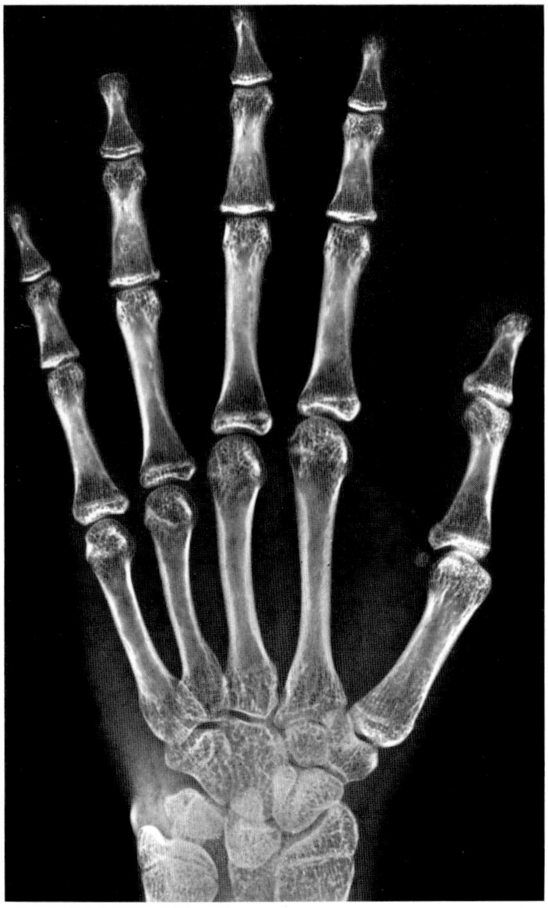

Fig. 3. Turner's syndrome in an 18-year-old woman. Madelung's deformity of wrist, abnormal arrangement of proximal row of carpals. Carpal angle 112°

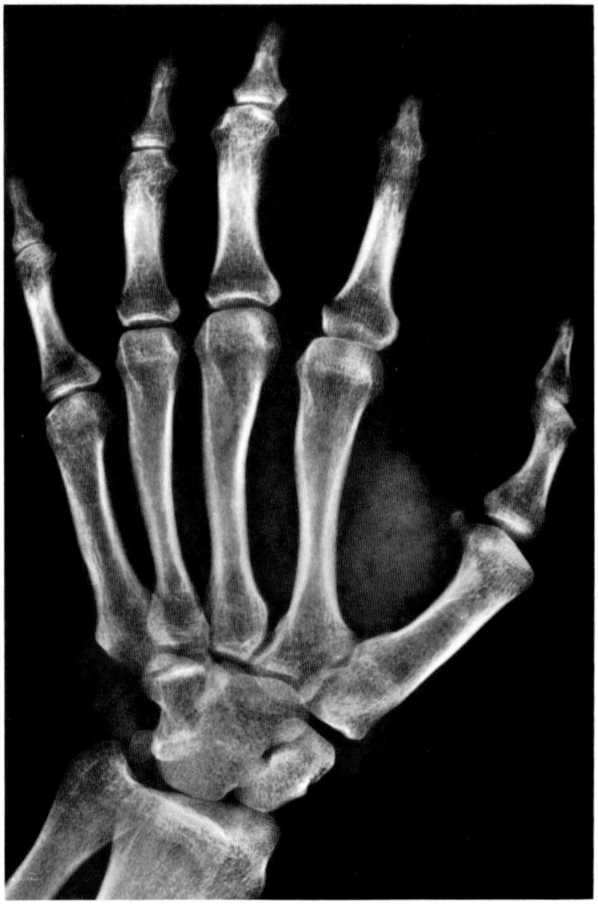

Fig. 4. Arthrogryposis multiplex congenita in a 29-year-old man. Fusion of carpals, increased carpal angle

Cone-Shaped Epiphyses in Normal and Abnormal Children [1]

Finger	Phalanx	Normal	Abnormal
1	Distal	+	+
	Proximal	–	+
2	Distal	+	+
	Middle	+	+
	Proximal	–	+
3	Distal	+	+
	Middle	–	+
	Proximal	–	+
4	Distal	±	+
	Middle	–	+
	Proximal	–	+
5	Distal	±	+
	Middle	+	+
	Proximal	–	+

2.2.9 Cone-Shaped and Bracket-Shaped Epiphyses

GIEDION made a classification of 38 different types of cone-shaped epiphyses, some of which seem to be pathognomonic for certain congenital malformation syndromes [1, 2]. Cone-shaped epiphyses associated with ivory epiphyses in the same hand may be found in trichorhinophalangeal syndrome (Sect. 1.1.12), Seckel's syndrome, and Cockayne's syndrome.

Associated Conditions [3]

Achondroplasia (Sect. 1.1.3)
Chondroectodermal dysplasia (Sect. 1.1.6)
Asphyxiating thoracic dysplasia (Sect. 1.1.7)
Cleidocranial dysplasia (Sect. 1.1.8)

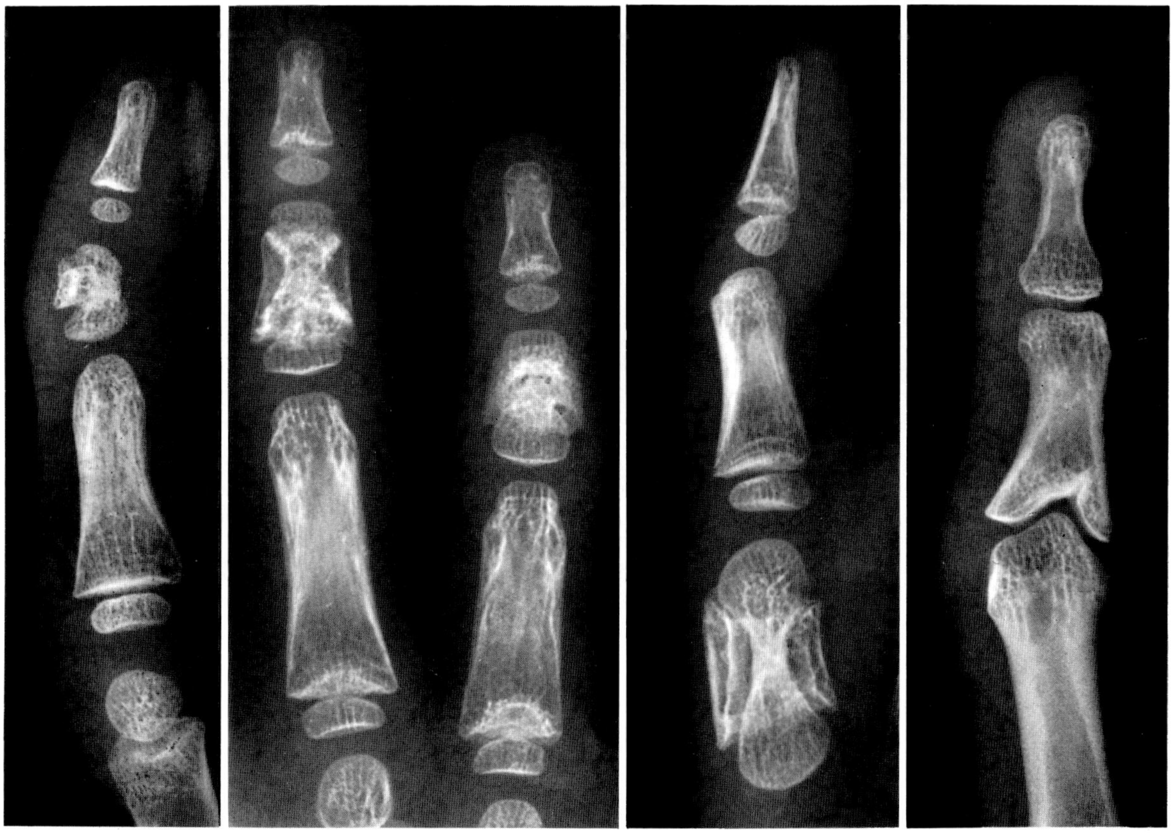

a b c d

Fig. 1a–d. Several types of cone-shaped and bracket-shaped epiphyses. **a** Middle phalanx of fifth finger: This abnormality may be present in otherwise normal individuals, and mostly causes brachydactyly or clinodactyly. **b** In a 5-year-old boy: The abnormalities seem to be bracket-shaped epiphyses in a patient with cleidocranial dysplasia. **c** Bracket-shaped epiphysis in first metacarpal bone. **d** 25-year-old woman: Deformation of middle phalanx accompanying trichorhinophalangeal syndrome

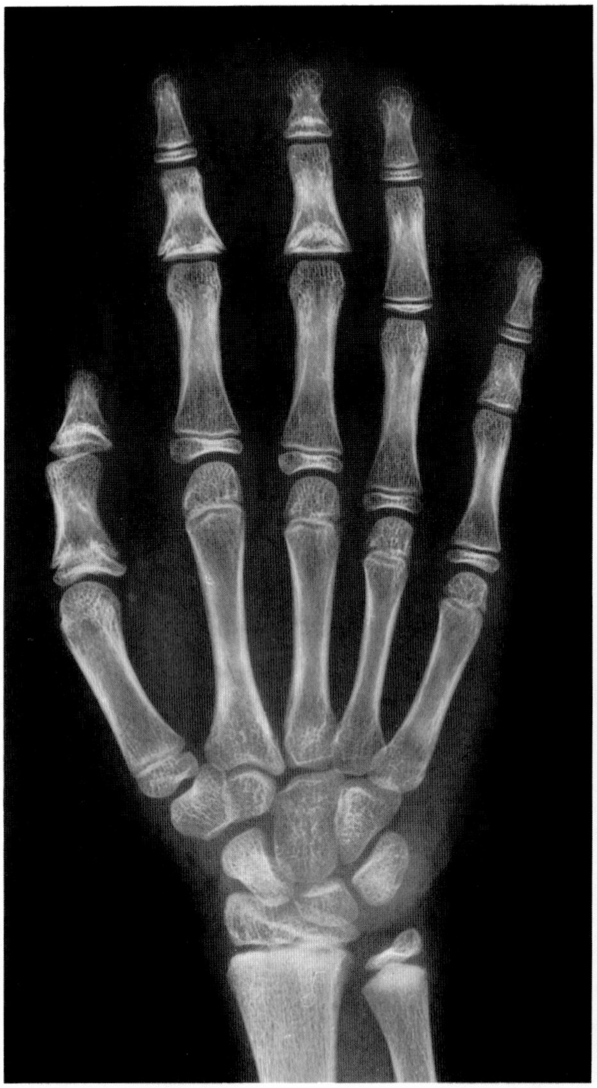

a

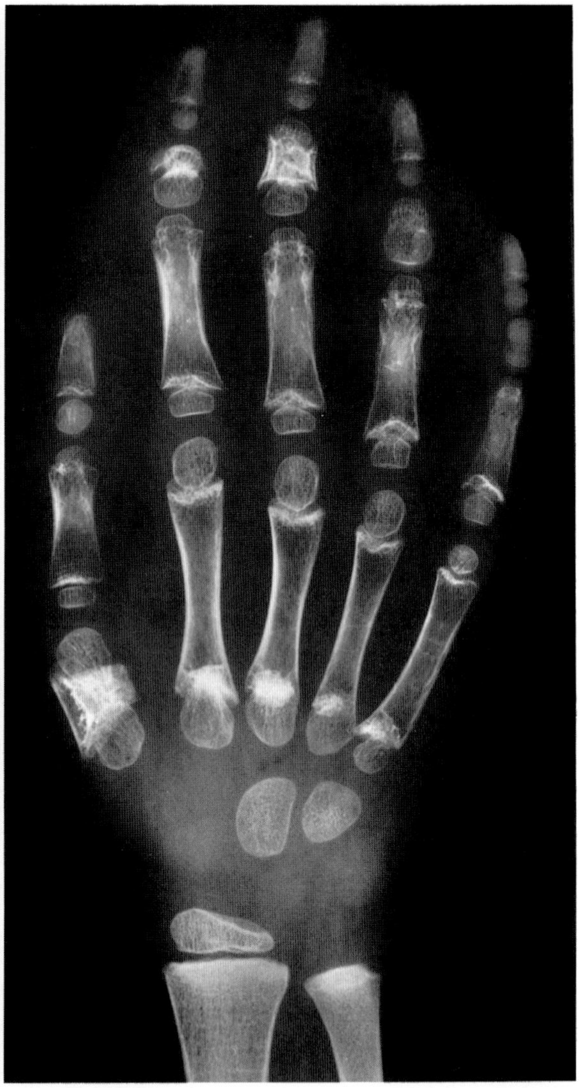

b

Fig. 2a, b. Cone-shaped epiphyses. **a** In a 13-year-old girl with trichorhinophalangeal syndrome: Cone-shaped epiphyses in distal phalanges of first and third fingers, proximal phalanx of thumb, middle phalanges of second, third, and fifth fingers. **b** In a 9-year-old boy with cleidocranial dysplasia: Multiple cone-shaped and bracket-shaped epiphyses in fingers, pseudoepiphyses in metacarpals

Trichorhinophalangeal syndrome (Sect. 1.1.12)
Peripheral dysostosis [4]
Acrodysostosis [4]
Seckel's syndrome [5]
Saldino-Mainzer syndrome [6]
Sickle cell anemia [7]
Kashin-Beck disease
Cockayne's syndrome

Bracket-Shaped Epiphyses

In a bracket-shaped epiphysis the cylindrically formed epiphyseal plate encircles the axis of the bone. This may be a normal variety in the middle phalanx of the fifth digit, but may also be encountered in diastrophic dysplasia (Sect. 1.1.4), Rubinstein-Taybi syndrome (Sect. 2.2.18) [3], and cleidocranial dysplasia (Sect. 1.1.8).

References

1 Giedion A (1965) Cone-shaped epiphyses (CSE). Ann Radiol (Paris) 8:135–145
2 Giedion A (1967) Cone-shaped epiphyses of the hands and their diagnostic value. The tricho-rhino-phalangeal syndrome. Ann Radiol (Paris) 10:322–329

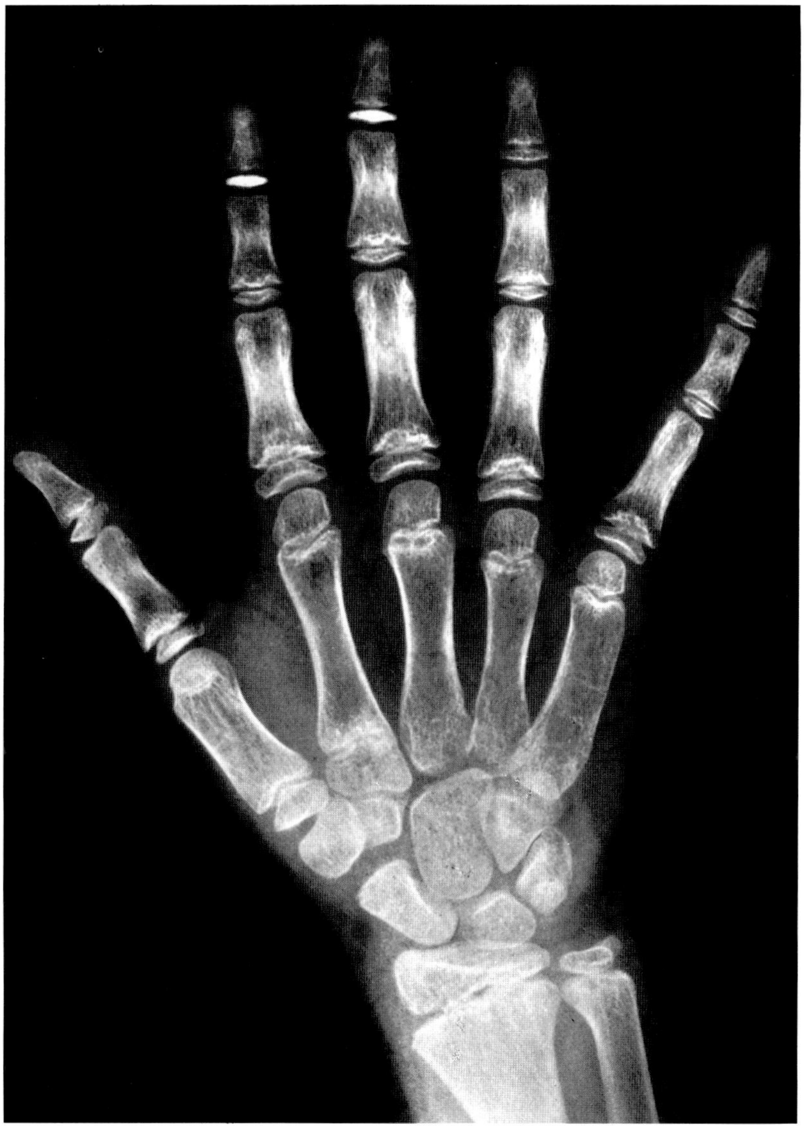

Fig. 3. Cone-shaped epiphyses associated with ivory epiphyses. Pseudoepiphysis in base of second metacarpal. No clinical evidence of trichorhinophalangeal syndrome, Seckel's syndrome, or Cockayne's syndrome

3 Poznanski AK (1984) The hand in radiologic diagnosis. Saunders, Philadelphia
4 Giedion A (1976) Acrodysplasia. Peripheral dysostosis, acrodysostosis and Thiemann's disease. Clin Orthop 114:107–115
5 Poznanski AK, Iannaccone G, Pasquino AM, Boscherini B (1983) Radiological findings in the hand in Seckel syndrome (bird-headed dwarfism). Pediatr Radiol 13:19–24
6 Saldino RM, Mainzer F (1971) Cone-shaped epiphyses (CSE) in siblings with hereditary renal disease and retinitis pigmentosa. Radiology 98:39–45
7 Reynolds J (1965) The roentgenological features of sickle cell disease and related hemoglobinopathies. Thomas, Springfield

2.2.10 Ivory Epiphyses

Ivory epiphyses are solid epiphyses without visible trabecular bone structure. As time goes on they become less dense, and later on they fuse normally with the metaphyses. The occurrence of these normal variants is most common between the age of 4 and 10 years. The incidence in individuals below the age of 16 years is 0.35%. The distal phalanges of the second and fifth fingers are most often affected. In one study [1], the 86 cases of ivory epiphyses were broken down as follow:

Second distal phalanx	31
Third distal phalanx	10
Fourth distal phalanx	5
Fifth distal phalanx	37
Fifth middle phalanx	3

At other sites, dense epiphyses are usually not of the ivory type but display trabecular structures. In these cases additional abnormalities can be present.

Associated Hand Abnormalities

Retardation of skeletal maturation (especially of phalangeal epiphyses)
Slight shortening of tubular bones
Occasionally cone-shaped epiphyses. Ivory epiphyses together with cone-shaped epiphyses in the same hand are described in trichorhinophalangeal syndrome (Sect. 1.1.12), Seckel's syndrome, and Cockayne's syndrome

Associated Disorders

Multiple epiphyseal dysplasia (Sect. 1.1.11)
Thiemann's disease (Sect. 1.1.11)

a
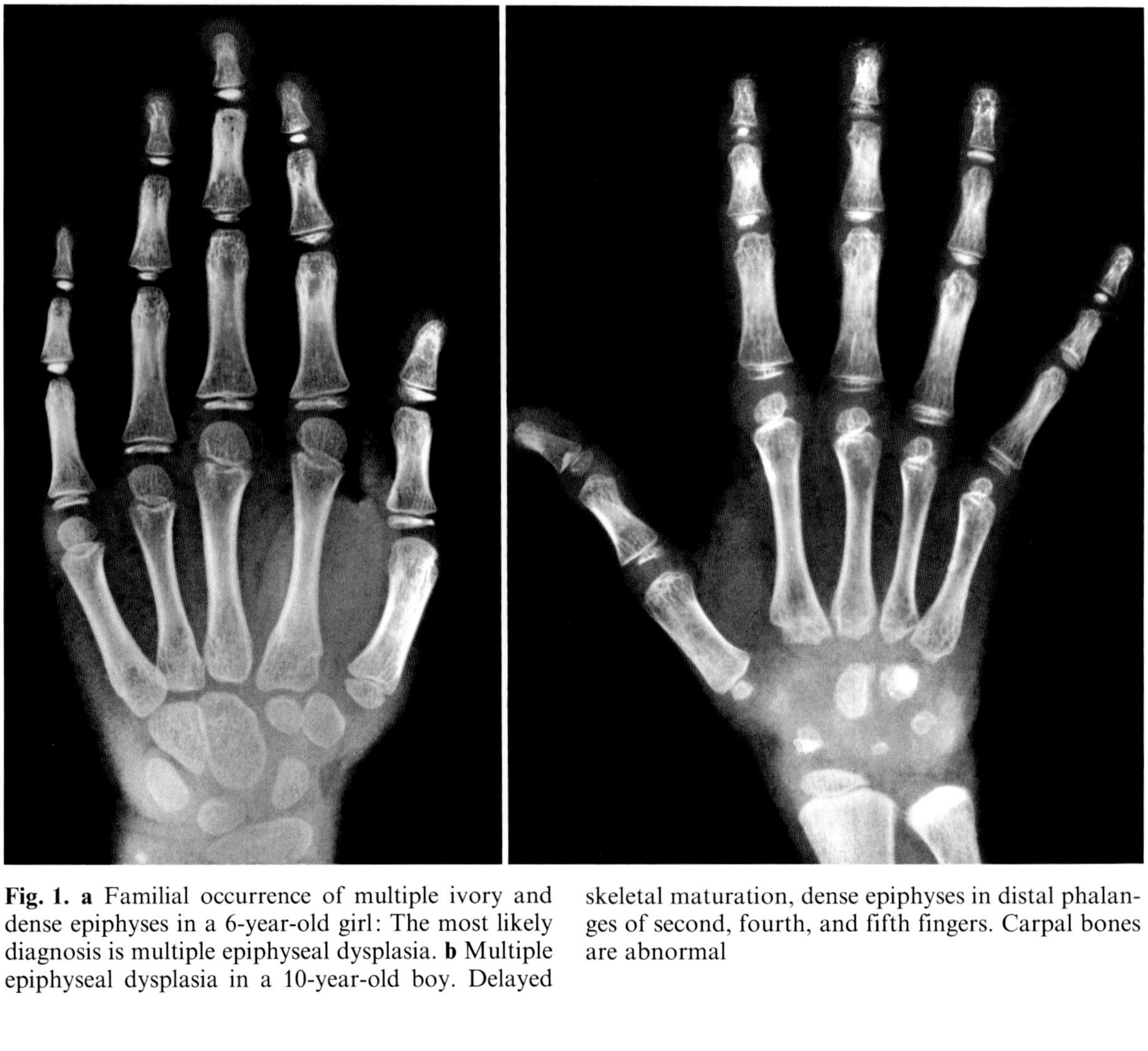
b

Fig. 1. a Familial occurrence of multiple ivory and dense epiphyses in a 6-year-old girl: The most likely diagnosis is multiple epiphyseal dysplasia. **b** Multiple epiphyseal dysplasia in a 10-year-old boy. Delayed skeletal maturation, dense epiphyses in distal phalanges of second, fourth, and fifth fingers. Carpal bones are abnormal

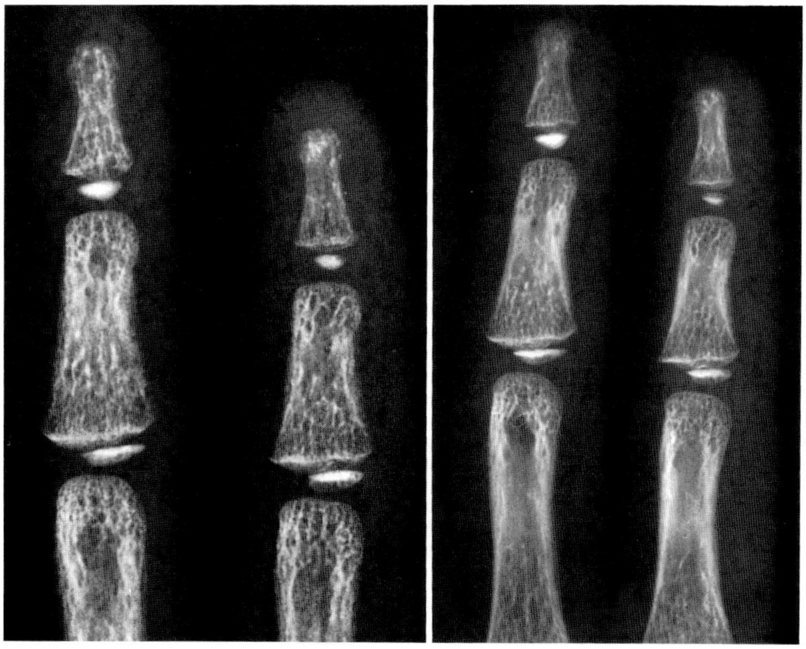

a b

Fig. 2a, b. Renal rickets in a 6-year-old girl. **a** Ivory epiphyses in distal phalanges and dense epiphyses in middle phalanges. Signs of subperiosteal bone resorption due to secondary hyperparathyroidism. **b** After 3 months of treatment the signs of secondary hyperparathyroidism are diminished

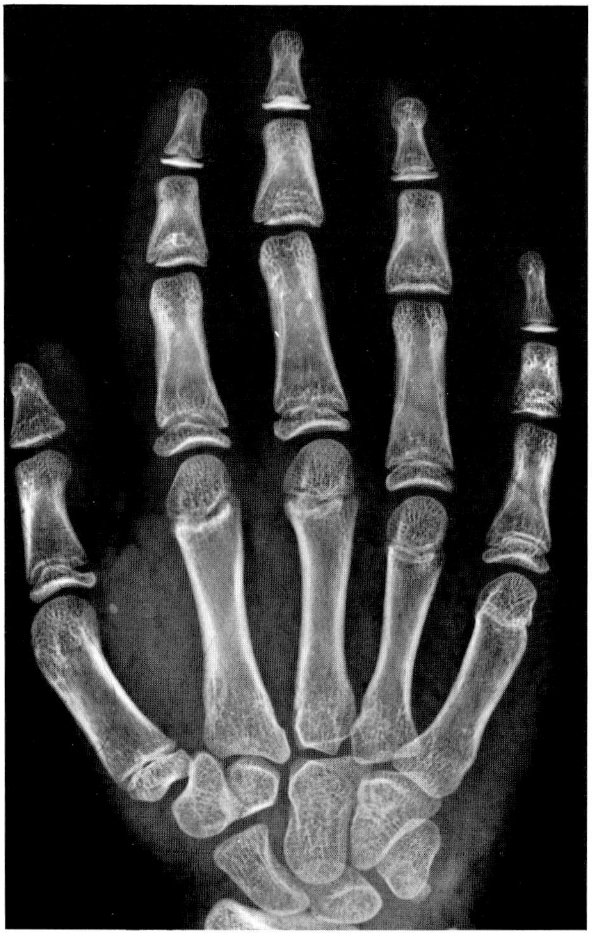

Fig. 3. Trichorhinophalangeal syndrome in a 13-year-old boy. Combination of cone-shaped epiphyses and ivory epiphyses

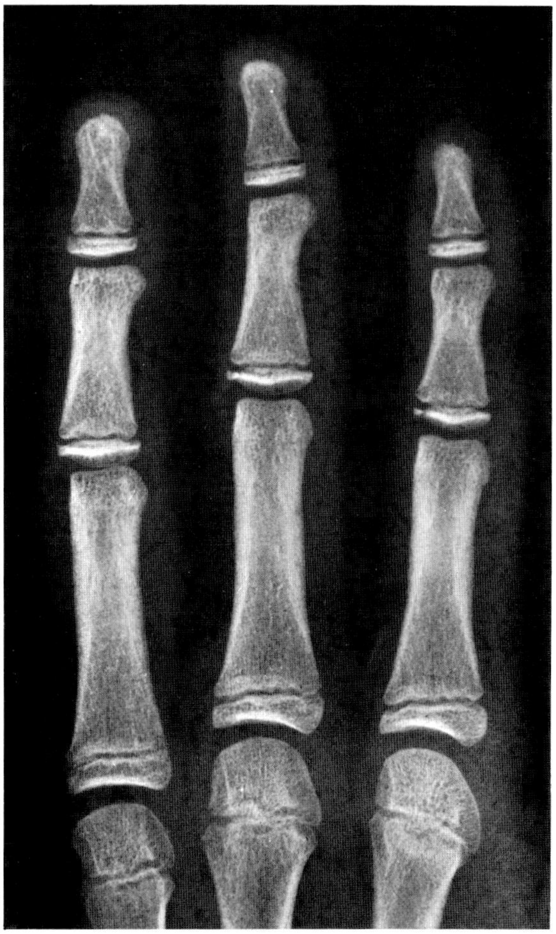

Fig. 4. Spondyloepiphyseal dysplasia in a 16-year-old boy. Dense epiphyses in almost all phalanges, some fragmentation of epiphyses in middle phalanges of second and third fingers

Trichorhinophalangeal syndrome (Sect. 1.1.12)
Trisomy 18 (Sect. 4.1)
Mucopolysaccharidosis (Sect. 6.1.1)
Hypothyroidism (Sect. 6.1.2)
Rickets (Sect. 6.2.1)
Renal osteodystrophy (Sect. 6.2.4)
Seckel's syndrome [2]
Cockayne's syndrome
Acrodysplasia [3]
Mucolipidosis III
Spondyloepiphyseal dysplasia

References

1 Kuhns LR, Poznanski AK, Harper HAS, Garn SM (1973) Ivory epiphyses. Radiology 109:643–648
2 Poznanski AK, Iannaccone G, Pasquino AM, Boscherini B (1983) Radiological findings in the hand in Seckel's syndrome (bird-headed dwarfism). Pediatr Radiol 13:19–24
3 Giedion A (1976) Acrodysplasia. Peripheral dysostosis and Thiemann's disease. Clin Orthop 114:107–115

2.2.11 Brachydactyly and Brachymetacarpia

Shortening of tubular bones in the hand may be congenital (hypoplasia) or acquired (tumor, arthritis, osteomyelitis, sickle cell anemia, surgery). Congenital hypoplasia of the tubular bones in the hand can be subdivided into four groups:
1. Distal phalanges (brachytelephalangy)
2. Middle phalanges (brachymesophalangy)
3. Proximal phalanges
4. Metacarpals (brachymetacarpia)

Brachydactyly is classified by Bell on the basis of anatomy and heredity into seven types (Fig. 1). A certain overlap between these types is frequently seen.

Measurements

Length of hand bones: birth to 15 months (Table 1) [1, 5].
Standards for metacarpal and phalangeal length and variability (Tables 2, 3) [2].
Relative slenderness: metacarpal index (Fig. 2) [3].

Hypoplasia of Distal Phalanges

For acquired shortening of the distal phalanges, see Sect. 3.1.

Associated Abnormalities [5]:
Hypoplastic nails
Hypoplasia of middle phalanges (Bell type B)

Associated Disorders [5]

Chondroectodermal dysplasia (Sect. 1.1.6)
Asphyxiating thoracic dysplasia (Sect. 1.1.7)
Cleidocranial dysplasia (Sect. 1.1.8)
Larsen's syndrome (Sect. 1.1.9)
Poland's syndrome (Sect. 2.2.17)
Laurence-Moon-Biedl-Bardet syndrome
Trisomy 18 (Sect. 4.1)
Arthrogryposis multiplex congenita (Sect. 7.1.1) [31]
Coffin-Siris syndrome [21]
Rüdinger's syndrome [22]
Trisomy 13 [23]
Zimmerman-Laband syndrome [24]
Keutel's syndrome [29]
Myotonic dystrophy [31]
Liebenberg's syndrome

Distal Phalanx of Thumb
Synonyms: stub thumb, murderer thumb's, Bell type D brachydactyly

A short and broad distal phalanx of the thumb is rather often present as an isolated finding with autosomal dominant inheritance in otherwise normal individuals.

Associated Disorders

Rubinstein-Taybi syndrome (Sect. 2.2.18)
Acrocephalosyndactyly and acrocephalopolysyndactyly (Sect. 2.1.1)
Hand-foot-uterus syndrome [30]
Diastrophic dysplasia (Sect. 1.1.4)
Otopalatodigital syndrome [13]

Table 1. Lengths of the hand bones in males and females (newborn to 15 months). Measurements include the epiphyses. From GEFFERTH [1]

Bones		Newborn		2 Wk. to $2^1/_2$ Mo.		Over $2^1/_2$ Mo. to $4^1/_2$ Mo.		Over $4^1/_2$ Mo. to 7 Mo.		Over 7 Mo. to 11 Mo.		Over 11 Mo. to 15 Mo.	
		Mean	S.D.	Mean	S.D.	Mean	S.D.	Mean	S.D.	Mean	S.D.	Mean	S.D.
Males													
Distal	5	4.5	0.5	4.8	0.6	5.0	0.4	5.3	0.9	5.8	0.7	6.3	0.6
	4	5.5	0.5	5.4	0.6	6.0	0.6	6.3	0.5	6.7	0.4	7.3	0.7
	3	5.6	0.5	5.3	0.9	5.9	0.7	6.3	0.8	6.5	0.6	7.1	0.9
	2	5.1	0.5	4.7	0.4	5.0	0.5	5.5	0.7	5.8	0.5	6.4	0.7
	1	5.9	0.5	6.5	0.5	6.8	0.6	7.3	0.4	7.7	0.7	8.9	0.9
Mid	5	5.5	0.5	5.9	0.7	6.1	0.4	6.8	1.0	7.5	1.0	7.7	1.0
	4	7.5	0.5	8.6	1.1	8.7	0.9	9.9	0.8	10.3	0.8	11.4	1.0
	3	7.9	0.5	8.5	1.1	9.2	0.7	10.2	0.9	11.1	1.0	11.6	1.1
	2	6.5	0.6	6.9	0.7	7.2	0.6	8.1	0.8	8.5	0.7	9.3	1.1
Proximal	5	8.5	0.6	9.5	1.0	10.0	1.0	11.0	1.3	12.1	1.0	13.1	1.1
	4	10.8	0.5	12.1	1.3	12.9	1.3	14.0	1.0	15.5	1.0	16.9	1.4
	3	11.7	0.6	12.8	1.2	13.5	1.0	14.9	0.9	16.0	1.2	18.0	1.3
	2	10.3	0.5	11.7	1.4	12.0	0.8	13.7	1.1	14.7	1.0	16.1	1.4
	1	7.3	0.6	8.3	0.9	8.9	0.7	9.7	1.0	10.7	0.7	11.6	1.0
Metacarpal	5	11.2	0.6	12.7	0.9	13.2	1.2	14.3	1.2	15.8	1.2	17.1	1.1
	4	12.7	0.6	14.1	1.0	14.8	1.4	15.9	1.2	17.7	1.1	19.2	1.1
	3	14.2	0.8	15.8	1.5	16.5	1.0	18.3	2.3	19.7	1.6	21.3	1.2
	2	14.5	0.5	16.4	1.4	17.0	1.4	19.0	1.5	20.3	1.6	22.4	1.4
	1	9.4	0.8	10.6	1.4	11.9	0.9	12.3	1.8	13.5	1.2	14.6	1.4
Females													
Distal	5	4.6	0.6	4.6	0.6	4.9	0.4	5.4	0.8	5.7	0.6	5.9	0.6
	4	5.2	0.5	5.6	0.9	5.9	0.7	6.2	0.9	6.9	0.4	7.6	0.6
	3	5.3	0.6	5.4	0.7	5.8	0.7	6.3	0.7	6.5	0.7	7.5	0.8
	2	4.8	0.7	5.0	0.4	5.2	0.8	5.7	0.6	5.8	0.9	6.4	0.8
	1	6.0	0.4	6.4	0.6	6.8	0.7	7.5	0.6	8.4	0.6	9.4	1.0
Mid	5	5.6	0.5	5.5	0.5	6.2	0.6	6.6	0.7	7.5	0.8	7.9	1.1
	4	7.3	0.9	8.0	0.9	8.8	1.7	9.8	1.0	10.8	0.7	11.9	1.4
	3	7.5	0.8	8.1	1.9	9.2	0.7	9.9	0.8	11.3	1.0	12.3	1.4
	2	6.4	0.6	6.8	1.0	7.5	1.0	8.2	0.8	8.6	0.8	9.9	0.6
Proximal	5	8.5	0.8	9.0	0.9	10.3	0.6	11.2	1.0	12.5	1.0	13.3	1.8
	4	10.8	0.7	11.8	0.8	12.8	1.0	14.2	1.1	16.1	1.8	18.1	1.8
	3	11.3	0.8	12.3	1.3	13.6	2.4	15.2	1.3	16.8	1.2	19.2	1.3
	2	10.4	0.6	11.1	1.1	12.5	0.8	13.5	1.0	15.0	1.4	17.3	1.6
	1	7.5	0.6	8.0	1.0	9.0	0.9	9.6	1.6	11.1	1.2	12.3	1.0
Metacarpal	5	11.7	1.0	12.2	1.3	13.7	1.0	15.2	1.3	16.7	1.7	18.3	2.1
	4	12.8	1.1	13.3	1.2	14.9	1.0	16.9	1.2	18.7	1.7	20.2	1.4
	3	14.3	0.9	15.3	1.3	17.3	1.5	19.2	1.4	20.6	1.6	22.9	2.8
	2	14.8	1.3	15.6	1.0	17.8	1.9	19.5	1.6	21.7	1.9	24.5	3.0
	1	9.5	0.5	10.3	0.7	11.4	1.0	12.6	1.0	14.0	1.4	15.6	1.1

Table 2. Standards for metacarpal and phalangeal lengths and variability (age 2–10 years). After GARN et al. [2]

Bones		2		3		4		5		6		7		8		9		10	
		Mean	S.D.	Mean	S.D.	Mean	S.D.	Mean	S.D.	Mean	S.D.	Mean	S.D.	Mean	S.D.	Mean	S.D.	Mean	S.D.
Males																			
Distal	5	8.8	–	8.4	0.6	9.0	0.7	9.9	0.6	10.7	0.6	11.4	0.8	12.2	0.9	12.6	1.0	13.5	0.9
	4	9.2	0.7	9.9	0.8	10.5	0.8	11.5	0.9	12.3	0.9	13.1	1.0	13.9	1.0	14.4	1.0	15.3	1.2
	3	8.7	0.9	9.5	0.8	10.2	0.8	11.1	0.8	11.8	0.9	12.7	1.0	13.4	1.0	14.0	1.0	14.8	1.2
	2	8.2	0.5	8.8	1.1	9.1	0.8	10.1	0.9	10.8	0.9	11.6	1.0	12.4	1.0	13.0	1.0	13.7	1.1
	1	11.1	0.6	12.3	0.8	13.2	1.0	14.4	0.9	15.4	0.9	16.5	1.0	17.4	1.0	17.9	1.2	19.0	1.2
Middle	5	8.8	0.9	9.8	0.8	10.6	1.0	11.2	1.0	12.0	1.0	12.7	1.1	13.5	1.1	14.3	1.2	15.0	1.2
	4	13.5	0.9	14.5	1.0	15.8	0.9	16.7	0.9	17.7	1.0	18.7	1.1	19.8	1.1	20.9	1.3	21.6	1.4
	3	14.1	0.8	15.1	1.1	16.5	1.0	17.6	1.0	18.7	1.1	19.8	1.2	20.9	1.2	22.0	1.4	22.9	1.4
	2	11.2	0.8	12.3	1.1	13.5	1.0	14.4	0.9	15.3	1.0	16.1	1.1	17.1	1.1	18.1	1.2	18.8	1.2
Proximal	5	16.1	0.7	17.8	0.9	19.2	1.0	20.6	1.0	21.8	1.0	23.0	1.1	24.2	1.3	25.2	1.5	26.4	1.5
	4	20.5	0.9	22.8	1.0	24.7	1.2	26.4	1.2	27.9	1.3	29.5	1.4	31.0	1.6	32.3	1.9	33.9	1.8
	3	21.8	1.0	24.2	1.1	26.3	1.4	28.1	1.4	29.8	1.4	31.5	1.6	33.2	1.8	34.7	2.2	36.1	1.9
	2	19.5	1.0	21.9	1.2	23.7	1.3	25.4	1.4	26.8	1.5	28.3	1.6	29.7	1.8	31.4	1.9	32.5	1.9
	1	15.2	–	15.9	1.1	17.2	1.1	18.3	1.2	19.6	1.2	20.8	1.3	21.8	1.3	23.1	1.5	24.2	1.4
Metacarpal	5	23.9	1.0	26.3	1.5	28.9	1.9	32.1	2.2	34.6	2.2	36.7	2.1	38.8	2.5	40.6	2.5	42.7	2.9
	4	25.5	1.1	28.9	1.5	31.7	2.1	35.0	2.5	37.9	2.7	40.1	2.5	42.2	3.1	44.1	2.8	46.5	3.5
	3	28.6	1.3	32.3	1.8	35.6	2.3	39.3	2.8	42.6	2.9	45.3	2.8	47.6	3.5	49.8	3.0	52.3	3.7
	2	30.6	1.5	34.5	1.7	37.9	2.3	41.6	2.7	44.9	2.9	47.7	2.8	50.2	3.4	52.6	3.0	55.0	3.9
	1	19.6	1.3	22.0	1.2	24.1	1.6	26.7	1.6	29.0	1.7	30.9	1.8	32.7	2.1	34.4	2.1	36.3	2.3
Females																			
Distal	5	7.8	0.6	8.4	0.6	9.1	0.7	9.9	0.7	10.6	0.8	11.4	0.9	12.1	1.0	12.7	1.1	13.5	1.2
	4	9.1	0.7	9.9	0.7	10.6	0.8	11.5	0.9	12.4	1.0	13.2	1.1	14.0	1.1	14.4	1.2	15.5	1.4
	3	8.8	0.7	9.9	0.8	10.2	0.7	11.1	0.9	12.2	1.3	12.7	1.1	13.5	1.1	14.1	1.1	15.0	1.4
	2	8.0	0.8	8.6	0.7	9.4	0.7	10.1	0.8	10.9	0.9	11.7	1.0	12.3	1.1	13.1	1.1	13.8	1.4
	1	11.3	0.8	12.5	0.8	13.2	0.8	14.4	1.0	15.4	1.1	16.3	1.2	17.3	1.3	17.8	1.3	19.0	1.6
Middle	5	9.0	1.2	9.8	1.1	10.5	1.1	11.2	1.1	12.2	1.2	12.9	1.3	13.6	1.4	14.2	1.4	15.2	1.6
	4	13.5	0.9	14.9	1.0	15.8	1.1	16.9	1.2	18.1	1.3	19.1	1.4	20.1	1.4	20.9	1.5	22.2	1.7
	3	14.2	0.9	15.6	1.1	16.6	1.2	17.9	1.2	19.2	1.3	20.3	1.4	21.4	1.4	22.1	1.6	23.6	1.8
	2	11.6	0.9	12.8	1.0	13.6	1.1	14.8	1.1	16.0	1.2	16.8	1.3	17.8	1.4	18.1	1.5	19.6	1.7
Proximal	5	16.3	1.0	17.9	1.1	19.1	1.1	20.6	1.3	22.0	1.4	23.1	1.6	24.4	1.6	25.2	1.6	27.1	2.0
	4	20.7	1.1	22.9	1.3	24.6	1.3	26.3	1.5	28.2	1.7	29.7	1.9	31.2	2.0	32.4	2.0	34.5	2.4
	3	22.2	1.2	24.5	1.3	26.4	1.4	28.3	1.8	30.4	1.8	32.1	2.0	33.7	2.2	35.0	2.2	37.3	2.6
	2	20.1	1.2	22.3	1.3	24.0	1.8	25.8	1.7	27.7	1.7	29.2	1.9	30.7	2.0	31.5	2.4	34.0	2.4
	1	14.9	1.0	16.3	1.1	17.2	1.3	18.8	1.3	20.2	1.3	21.4	1.5	22.7	1.6	23.5	2.0	25.5	2.1
Metacarpal	5	23.7	1.5	26.9	2.1	29.4	1.8	32.6	2.0	35.1	2.1	37.2	2.4	39.4	2.5	40.8	2.5	43.8	2.8
	4	26.0	1.9	29.6	2.7	32.2	2.0	35.6	2.5	38.4	2.7	40.5	2.8	43.1	3.0	44.3	2.8	47.5	3.5
	3	29.4	2.1	33.4	2.9	36.3	2.2	40.3	2.7	43.3	3.1	45.8	3.1	48.7	3.2	49.9	3.2	53.6	3.8
	2	31.3	1.9	35.2	2.7	38.2	2.3	42.2	2.7	45.6	3.2	48.1	3.3	51.2	3.3	52.6	3.4	56.6	4.1
	1	19.9	1.6	22.7	1.6	24.8	1.7	27.3	1.8	29.6	1.9	31.5	2.0	33.5	2.1	34.8	2.4	37.4	2.6

Table 3. Standards for metacarpal and phalangeal lengths and variability (age 11 years to adult). After GARN et al. [2]

Bones		11		12		13		14		15		16		17		18		Adults	
		Mean	S.D.	Mean	S.D.	Mean	S.D.	Mean	S.D.	Mean	S.D.	Mean	S.D.	Mean	S.D.	Mean	S.D.	Mean	S.D.
Males																			
Distal	5	14.2	0.9	15.0	0.9	15.8	0.9	16.8	1.0	17.6	1.1	17.9	1.0	18.1	1.0	18.1	1.2	18.7	1.3
	4	16.1	1.2	17.0	1.3	17.8	1.4	18.8	1.3	19.6	1.4	20.0	1.3	20.3	1.3	20.0	1.3	20.5	1.2
	3	15.6	1.2	16.4	1.2	17.1	1.3	18.2	1.3	19.0	1.4	19.3	1.4	19.5	1.3	19.4	1.3	20.1	1.2
	2	14.3	1.1	15.0	1.0	15.7	1.4	16.7	1.2	17.5	1.2	17.8	1.3	18.2	1.3	18.1	1.3	18.8	1.4
	1	19.7	1.2	20.6	1.3	21.7	1.4	22.8	1.3	24.1	1.4	24.5	1.4	24.9	1.4	24.8	1.5	25.2	1.4
Middle	5	15.7	1.4	16.5	1.5	17.5	1.5	18.9	1.6	19.9	1.4	20.4	1.4	20.6	1.4	21.0	1.4	21.6	1.6
	4	22.6	1.5	23.6	1.5	24.8	1.7	26.5	1.6	27.7	1.5	28.4	1.5	28.7	1.4	29.1	1.5	29.6	1.6
	3	24.0	1.4	24.9	1.4	26.3	1.6	28.0	1.5	29.2	1.5	30.0	1.6	30.2	1.6	30.6	1.8	31.1	1.8
	2	19.8	1.8	20.4	1.3	21.6	1.6	23.2	1.5	24.3	1.5	25.0	1.5	25.3	1.4	25.6	1.7	26.1	1.6
Proximal	5	27.6	1.7	28.9	2.0	30.5	2.4	32.9	2.4	34.7	2.0	35.6	1.8	36.1	1.8	35.9	2.0	36.3	2.0
	4	35.3	2.0	37.0	2.4	38.8	2.8	41.6	2.8	43.7	2.6	44.9	2.3	45.4	2.2	45.2	2.5	45.5	2.3
	3	37.8	2.3	39.5	2.6	41.5	2.9	44.4	2.8	46.6	2.5	47.8	2.4	48.3	2.3	48.2	2.7	48.5	2.6
	2	33.9	2.1	35.5	2.4	37.2	2.6	39.8	2.6	41.8	2.2	42.8	2.0	43.3	2.1	43.4	2.4	43.7	2.2
	1	25.4	1.6	26.7	2.0	28.5	2.2	30.9	2.2	32.9	1.8	33.8	1.5	34.6	2.6	34.7	1.8	35.0	1.9
Metacarpal	5	44.6	2.8	47.1	3.2	49.1	4.0	52.2	3.9	55.4	3.6	57.1	2.8	57.9	2.5	57.5	2.9	58.0	3.0
	4	48.4	3.1	51.0	3.7	53.1	4.6	56.4	4.5	59.5	4.1	61.5	3.7	62.6	3.1	61.7	3.4	62.1	3.5
	3	54.6	3.4	57.3	4.0	59.5	5.1	63.1	4.9	66.7	4.4	68.7	4.1	69.7	3.3	69.0	3.7	69.0	3.8
	2	57.3	3.5	60.6	3.9	63.3	5.1	67.1	4.8	70.6	4.3	73.2	3.8	74.2	2.9	73.9	3.5	73.7	3.8
	1	38.2	2.4	40.2	2.7	42.5	3.0	45.1	2.8	47.6	2.6	48.8	2.3	49.5	2.1	49.4	2.7	49.6	2.9
Females																			
Distal	5	14.2	1.3	15.0	1.3	15.4	1.3	15.6	1.3	15.9	1.4	15.9	1.4	16.2	1.3	16.0	1.2	16.2	1.2
	4	16.2	1.4	17.1	1.4	17.6	1.2	17.9	1.3	18.0	1.4	18.0	1.3	18.1	1.4	17.9	1.3	18.0	1.3
	3	15.8	1.3	16.6	1.4	17.1	1.4	17.3	1.3	17.6	1.5	17.5	1.4	17.6	1.4	17.4	1.3	17.7	1.3
	2	14.4	1.3	15.2	1.5	15.7	1.5	15.8	1.5	16.1	1.6	16.0	1.6	16.3	1.5	16.2	1.3	16.6	1.3
	1	20.0	1.7	20.9	1.7	21.4	1.6	21.7	1.6	22.0	1.7	22.0	1.7	22.1	1.8	22.0	1.6	22.1	1.6
Middle	5	16.2	1.7	17.2	1.7	17.9	1.8	18.1	1.6	18.4	1.7	18.5	1.7	18.5	1.9	18.6	1.7	18.7	1.7
	4	23.4	1.8	24.7	1.8	25.7	1.9	25.9	1.6	26.3	1.8	26.4	1.8	26.5	1.9	26.3	1.8	26.4	1.7
	3	24.9	1.9	26.2	1.9	27.2	2.0	27.5	1.7	28.1	1.8	28.0	1.9	28.0	1.8	27.8	1.8	27.9	1.7
	2	20.6	1.8	21.8	1.9	22.7	1.8	23.0	1.8	23.5	1.8	23.3	1.9	23.4	1.9	23.1	1.6	23.2	1.6
Proximal	5	28.7	2.1	30.5	2.2	31.9	2.2	32.3	2.1	32.9	2.2	32.8	2.3	32.8	2.3	32.5	2.0	32.5	1.9
	4	36.5	2.5	38.8	2.6	40.3	2.5	40.9	2.3	41.5	2.5	41.6	2.6	41.7	2.6	41.1	2.2	40.8	2.4
	3	39.5	2.7	41.7	2.8	43.5	2.8	44.1	2.4	44.8	2.6	44.8	2.7	44.8	2.5	44.2	2.4	44.0	2.3
	2	35.9	2.6	38.0	2.6	39.5	2.6	39.9	2.4	40.6	2.6	40.6	2.6	40.7	2.6	39.9	2.3	40.0	2.3
	1	27.2	2.3	29.2	2.4	30.6	2.2	31.1	1.9	31.8	2.0	31.7	2.1	31.9	2.2	31.3	1.9	31.4	2.0
Metacarpal	5	46.3	2.9	48.7	2.9	50.8	2.8	52.1	2.8	52.6	3.0	52.8	3.0	53.0	2.7	52.0	2.7	51.9	3.6
	4	50.2	3.8	52.8	3.7	55.1	3.6	56.2	3.6	56.9	3.6	57.2	3.9	57.2	3.5	56.1	2.9	56.0	3.5
	3	56.5	4.0	59.5	4.2	62.1	4.0	63.4	3.9	63.9	3.9	64.3	4.0	64.5	4.0	63.2	3.4	62.6	4.0
	2	59.9	4.3	63.2	4.4	66.2	4.2	67.4	3.9	68.1	4.2	68.6	4.3	68.9	4.1	67.5	3.4	66.9	4.3
	1	39.7	3.0	42.0	3.0	43.8	2.7	44.4	2.5	45.3	2.4	45.0	2.8	45.0	2.6	44.6	2.2	44.2	2.6

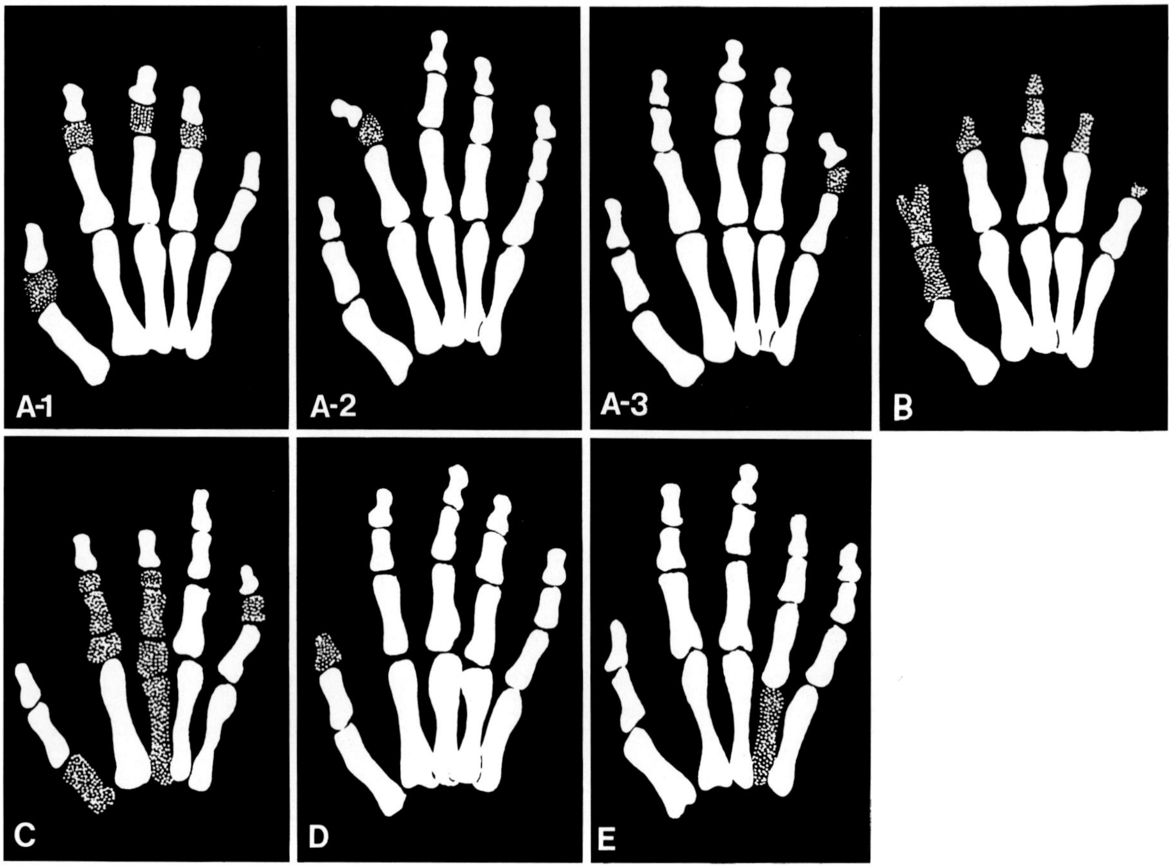

Fig. 1. Bell's classification of brachydactyly. Modified from POZNANSKI [5]

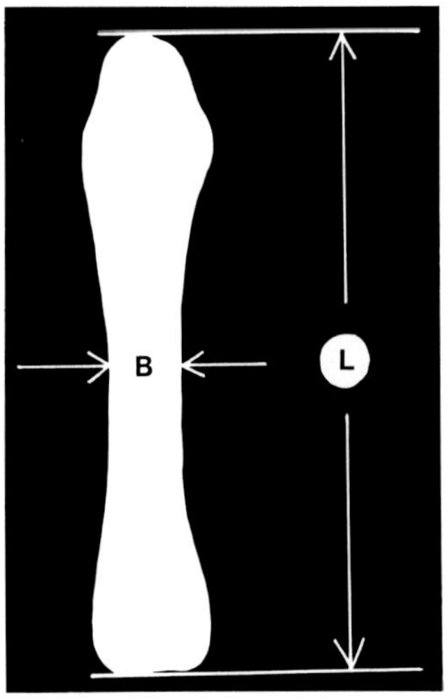

Fig. 2. Relative slenderness (RS) of metacarpals.

$$RS = \frac{\text{length of metacarpal, L}}{\text{breadth at midpoint, B}}$$

$$\text{Metacarpal index} = \frac{RS2 + RS3 + RS4 + RS5}{4}$$

Metacarpal index	Men		Women	
Normal values	Mean	Range	Mean	Range
Right	6.8	5.9–7.6	7.7	6.3–8.9
Left	7.0	6.0–8.0	7.8	6.8–9.0

Modified from PARISH [3]

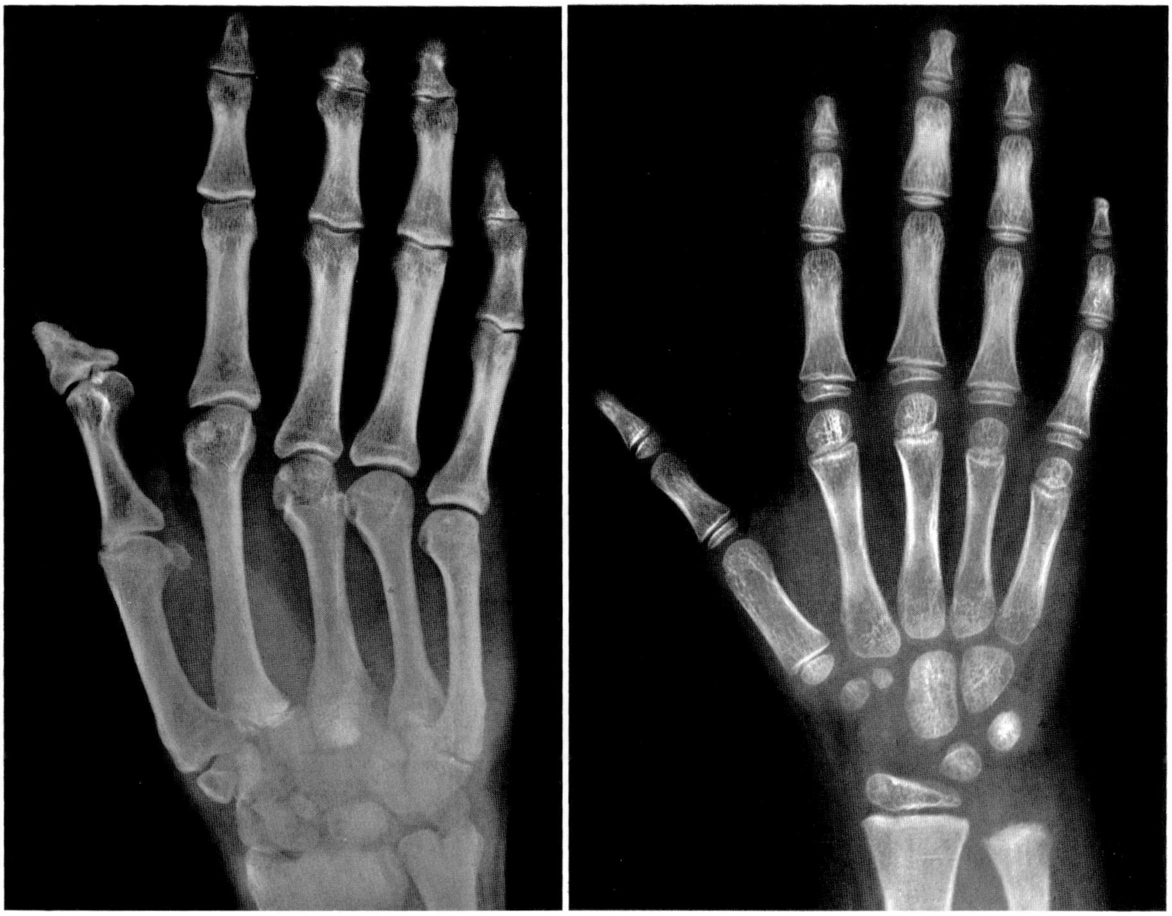

a b

Fig. 3a, b. Brachytelephalangy. **a** Larsen's syndrome: Hypoplasia of distal phalanges of first to fourth digits, rather long middle phalanges. **b** Laurence-Moon-Biedl-Bardet syndrome: Hypoplasia of the distal phalanges is one of the radiographic findings in this syndrome. Other hand abnormalities may occur, such as postaxial polydactyly, shortening of the metacarpals, and shortening of the middle phalanx of the fifth digit

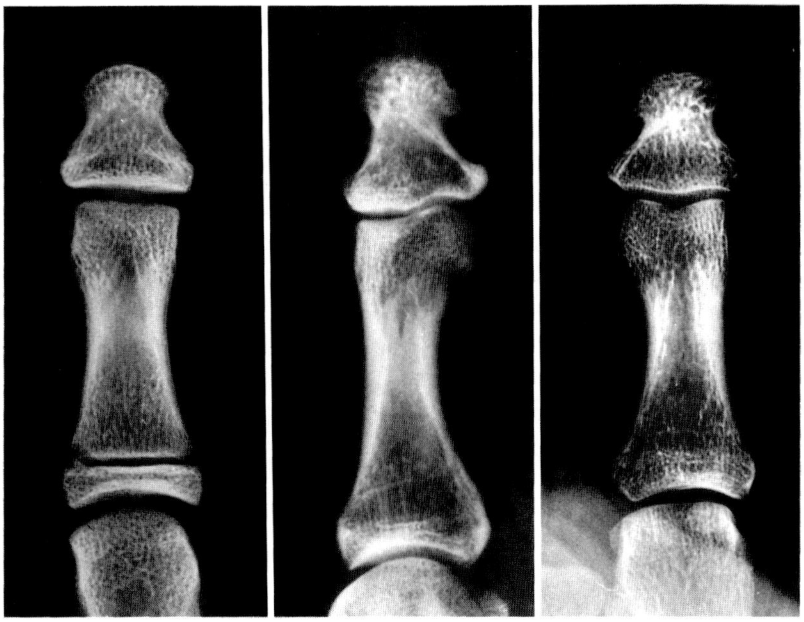

a b c

Fig. 4a–c. Three different patients with a short and broad distal phalanx of the thumb

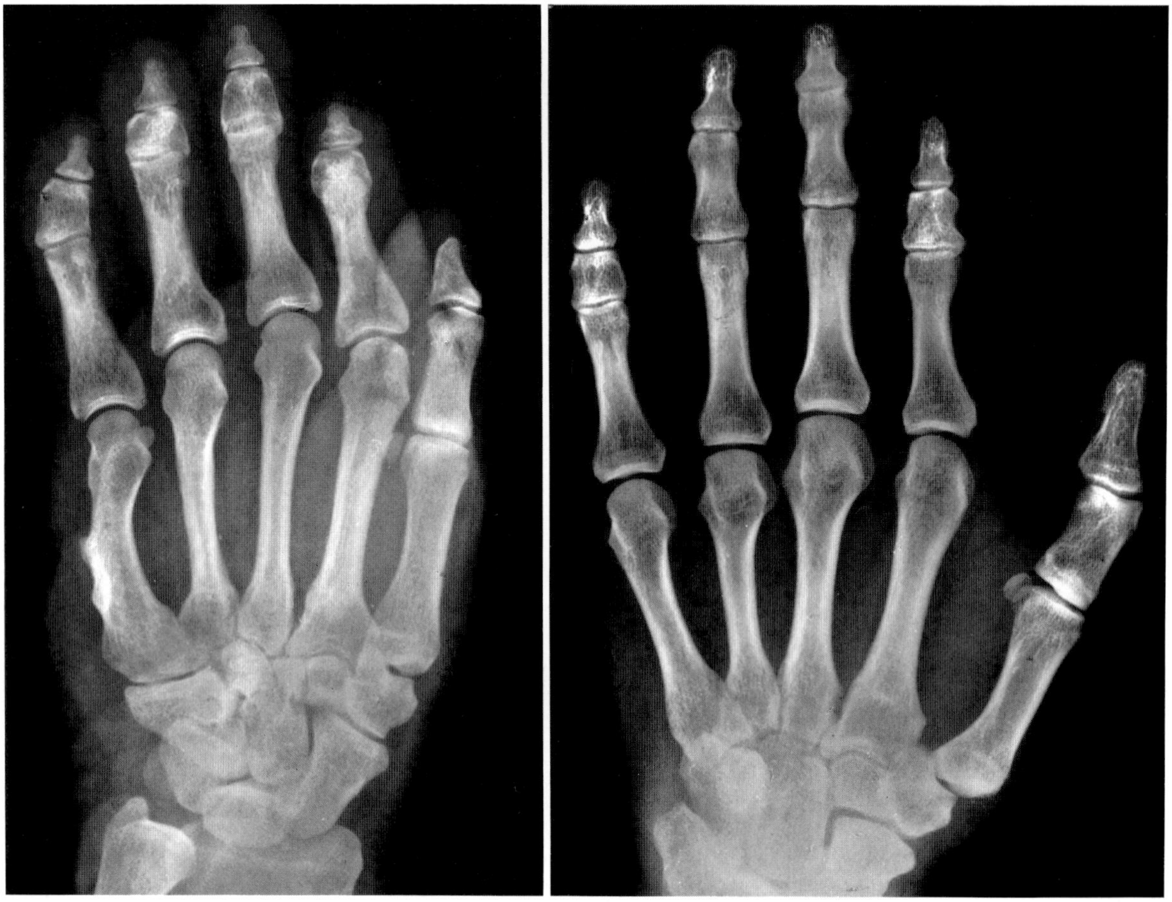

a b

Fig. 5a, b. Brachymesophalangy. **a** Chondroectodermal dysplasia in a 50-year-old man: Previous amputation of a postaxial digit, hypoplastic middle and distal phalanges with hypoplastic nails, accessory carpal between hamate and capitate. **b** Poland's syndrome in a 27-year-old man: Hypoplasia of all middle phalanges and proximal phalanx of thumb, distal phalanges of second to fifth fingers also hypoplastic

Hypoplasia of Middle Phalanges

Hypoplasia of the middle phalanges may occur in only one digit or in several digits of the same hand.

In Several Digits

Associated Abnormalities [4, 5]
Hypoplasia of metacarpals (Bell type C)
Hypoplasia of proximal phalanx of thumb (Bell type A1)
Hypoplasia of the distal phalanges (Bell type B)
Syndactyly
Symphalangism

Associated Disorders [5]

Acrocephalosyndactyly and acrocephalopolysyndactyly (Sect. 2.1.1)
Cleidocranial dysplasia (Sect. 1.1.8)
Poland's syndrome (Sect. 2.2.17)
Trichorhinophalangeal syndrome (Sect. 1.1.12)
Chondroectodermal dysplasia (Sect. 1.1.6)
Oculodentodigital dysplasia [7]
Orodigitofacial syndrome [6]
Myotonic dystrophy [31]

Hypoplasia of Middle Phalanx of Fifth Finger
Hypoplasia of the middle phalanx of the fifth finger is the most frequent abnormality in the hand. The hypoplastic phalanx may be straight, but in many cases the radial part is shorter than the ulnar part (clinodactyly). The abnormality is commonly present as an isolated and normal variant, without clinical significance.

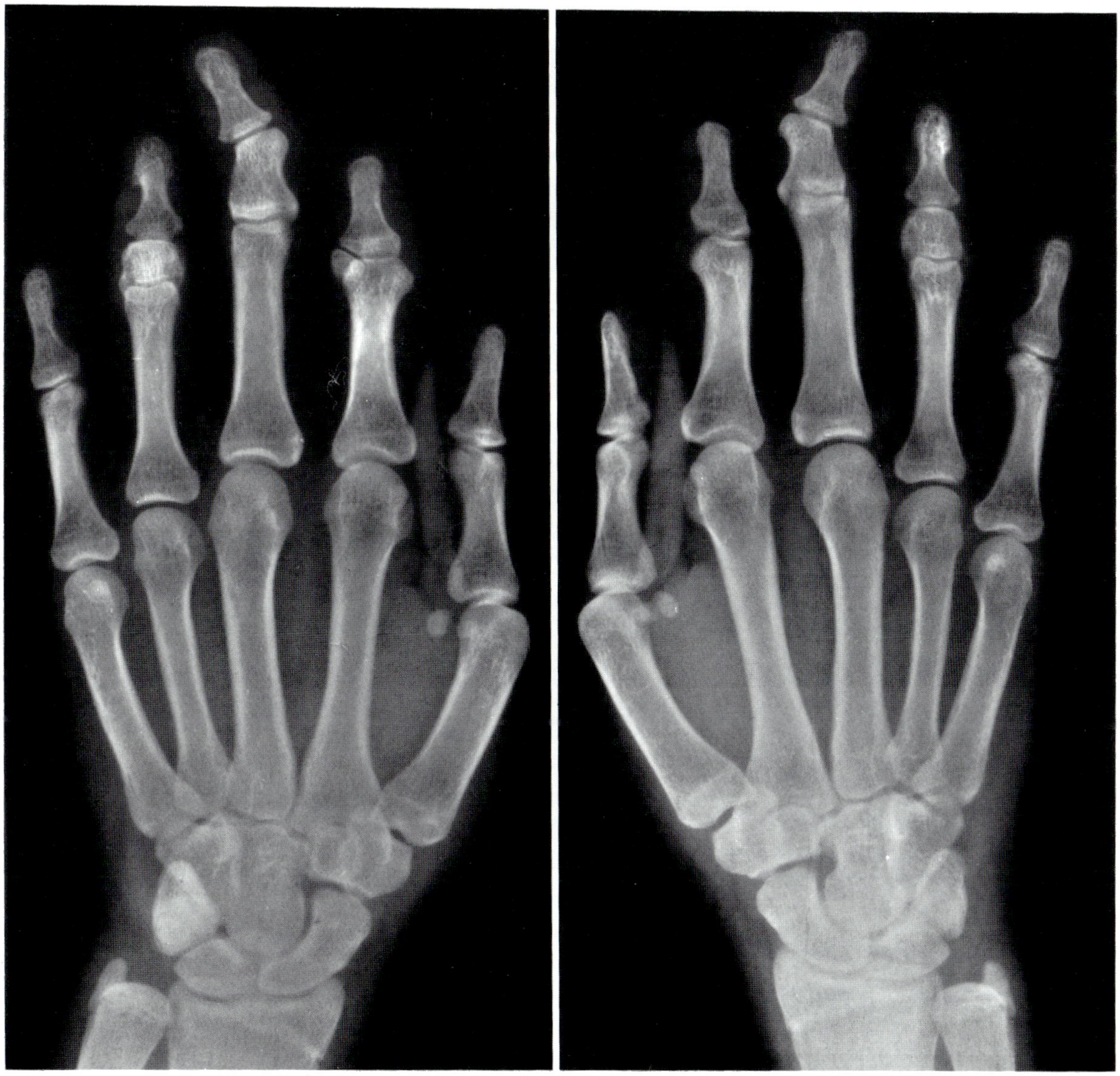

a b

Fig. 6a, b. Oculodentodigital dysplasia in a 16-year-old girl: Both hands affected patient suffering from microphthalmia and operated on for syndactyly. Radiographs present severe shortening and tapering of fingers with short or even absent middle phalanges. Nails were present. Additional findings in this dysplasia: clinodactyly, camptodactyly, osteoporosis, abnormalities of foot, hypoplastic enamel of teeth

Associated Abnormalities [5]
Cone-shaped epiphysis in same phalanx
Symphalangism
Brachymesophalangy
Brachytelephalangy

Disorders Involving Fifth Finger Brachymesophalangy [5, 8]:
Trichorhinophalangeal syndrome (Sect. 1.1.12)
Acrocephalosyndactyly and acrocephalopolysyndactyly (Sect. 2.1.1)
Poland's syndrome (Sect. 2.2.17)
Rubinstein-Taybi syndrome (Sect. 2.2.18)
Holt-Oram syndrome (Sect. 2.2.19)
Trisomy 18 (Sect. 4.1)
Trisomy 21 (Sect. 4.2)
Turner's syndrome (Sect.4.3)
Marfan's syndrome (Sect. 5.2)
Fibrodysplasia ossificans progressiva (Sect. 7.1.3)
Oculodentodigital dysplasia [7]
Otopalatodigital syndrome [13]
Orodigitofacial syndrome [6]

a b c

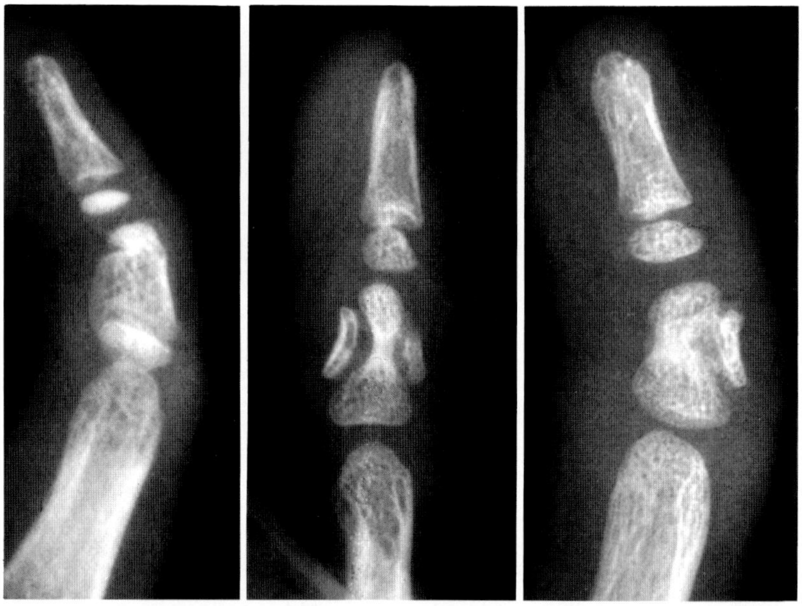

Fig. 7a–c. Clinodactyly. **a** In a 7-year-old boy: Pseudoepiphysis in middle phalanx, ivory epiphysis in distal phalanx. **b, c** In a 9-year-old boy: Abnormal ossification of middle phalanx with a bracket-shaped epiphysis. Epiphyseal plate encircles axis of bone

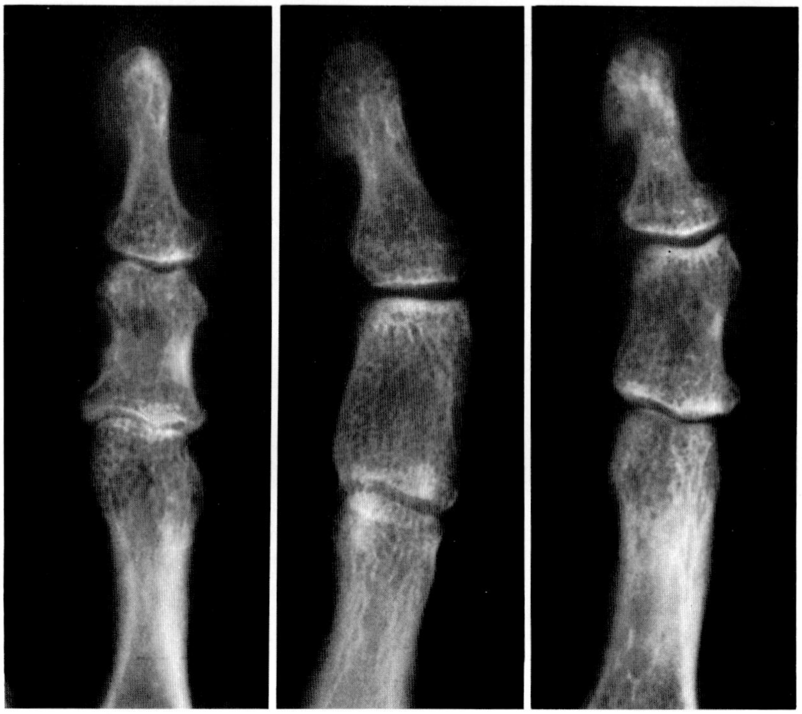

a b c

Fig. 8a–c. Fifth finger brachymesophalangy and clinodactyly. **a** Straight hypoplastic middle phalanx; **b, c** clinodactyly

Treacher-Collins syndrome [14]
Nail-patella syndrome [16]
Laurence-Moon-Biedl-Bardet syndrome
Noonan's syndrome [9]
Thrombocytopenia absent radius syndrome [11]
Goltz syndrome (focal dermal hypoplasia) [12]
Popliteal pterygium syndrome [17]
Seckel's syndrome [15]
Russell-Silver syndrome [10]
Ankyloglossia superior [18]
XXXXY syndrome [19]
XXXXX syndrome [20]
Cri du chat syndrome
Bloom's syndrome

a 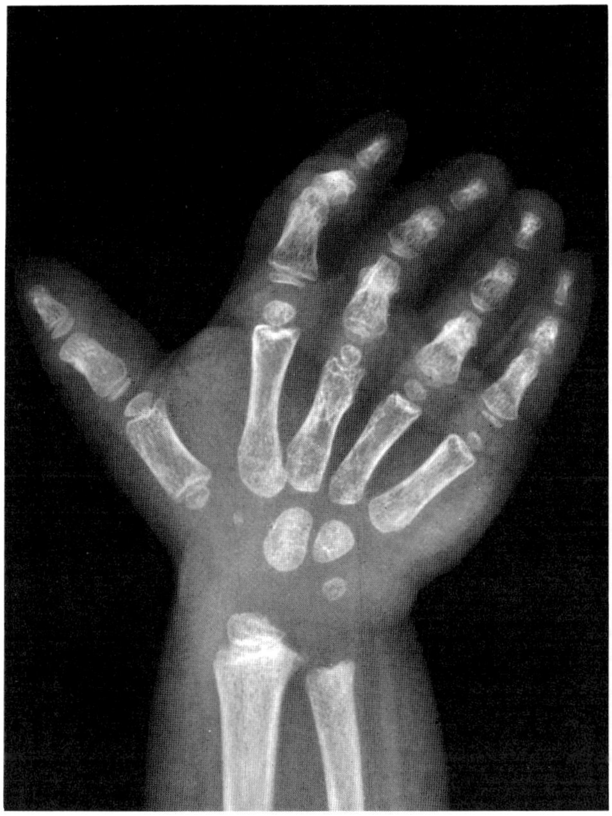 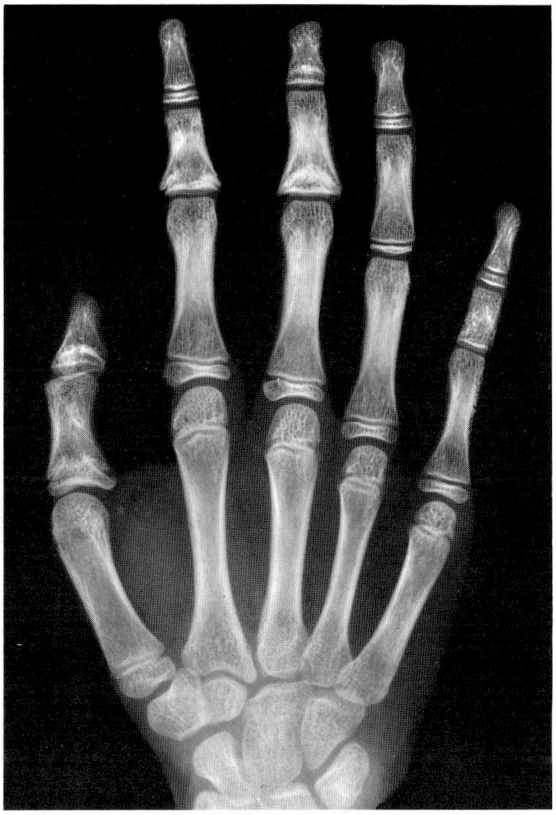 b

Fig. 9a, b. Two syndromes with fifth finger brachymesophalangy. **a** Orodigitofacial syndrome type II in a 4-year-old girl: This patient presents with shortening of the third and fourth metacarpals and camptodactyly of the second and third fingers. The bone structure in the above-mentioned metacarpals and in several phalanges is slightly abnormal, and cortical irregularities are present. **b** Trichorhinophalangeal syndrome in a 13-year-old girl: Typical cone-shaped epiphyses in thumb and second and third fingers

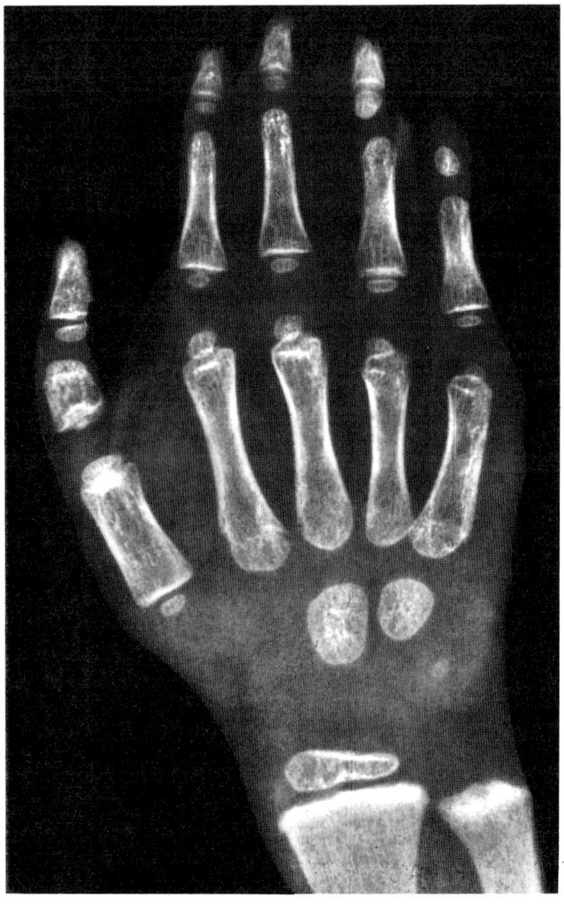

Fig. 10. Unclassified abnormalities in a 4-year-old boy. Hypoplasia of proximal phalanx of thumb associated with syndactyly, hypoplastic nails, and absence of middle phalanges in other fingers. Elongation of proximal phalanges of second to fifth fingers

Hypoplasia of Proximal Phalanges

Hypoplasia of the proximal phalanges seems always to be associated with other anomalies of the hand bones.

Associated Abnormalities [5]
Brachymesophalangy
Brachymetacarpia
Symphalangism

Disorders Involving Hypoplasia of Proximal Phalanx of Thumb [5]
Diastrophic dysplasia (Sect. 1.1.4)
Acrocephalosyndactyly and acrocephalopolysyndactyly (Sect. 2.1.1)
Basal cell nevus syndrome (Sect. 2.1.2)
Radial dysplasia (Sect. 2.2.1)
Rubinstein-Taybi syndrome (Sect. 2.2.18)
Fibrodysplasia ossificans progressiva (Sect. 7.1.3)
Hand-foot-uterus syndrome [25, 30]

Disorder Involving Hypoplasia of Proximal Phalanges in Several Fingers
Diastrophic dysplasia (Sect. 1.1.4)

Hypoplasia of Metacarpals

Brachymetacarpia may also be acquired.

Abnormalities Associated with Hypoplasia of Metacarpals
Brachymesophalangy
Hypoplasia of proximal phalanges
Radial dysplasia
Ulnar dysplasia
Anomalies of carpals

Hypoplasia of First Metacarpal
Hypoplasia of the first metacarpal may be found as an isolated anomaly, combined with other hypoplastic metacarpals and phalanges (Bell type C), or as a component of radial dysplasia.

Syndromes Involving Hypoplasia of First Metacarpal [5]
Cleidocranial dysplasia (Sect. 1.1.8)
Juberg-Hayward syndrome [25]
Radial dysplasia (Sect. 2.2.1)
Cornelia de Lange's syndrome (Sect. 5.1)
Fibrodysplasia ossificans progressiva (Sect. 7.1.3)
Diastrophic dysplasia (Sect. 1.1.4)
Hand-foot-uterus syndrome [25, 30]

Hypoplasia of Third to Fifth Metacarpals
Hypoplasia of the fourth metacarpal is common. In a number of cases it is combined with hypoplasia of the third and/or fifth metacarpal and is a hereditary form of brachydactyly (Bell types A-1, C, and E) [5, 8].

Disorders Involving Hypoplasia of Third to Fifth Metacarpals
Achondroplasia and hypochondroplasia (Sect. 1.1.3)
Larsen's syndrome (Sect. 1.1.9)
Multiple epiphyseal dysplasia (Sect. 1.1.11)
Trichorhinophalangeal syndrome (Sect. 1.1.12)
Basal cell nevus syndrome (Sect. 2.1.2)
Ulnar dysplasia (Sect. 2.2.2)
Turner's syndrome (Sect. 4.3)
(Pseudo)pseudohypoparathyroidism (Sect. 6.1.2)
Multiple cartilaginous exostoses (Sect. 7.4.1)
Peripheral dysostosis [28]
Dyschondrosteosis [27]
Orodigitofacial syndrome [6]
Cockayne's syndrome [26]
Russel-Silver syndrome [10]
Cri du chat syndrome
Biedmond's syndrome
Klinefelter's syndrome
Bixler's syndrome
Beckwith-Wiedeman syndrome
Cryptodontic brachymetacarpia

References

1 Gefferth K (1972) Metrische Auswertung der kurzen Röhrenknochen der Hand von der Geburt bis zum Ende der Pubertät: Längenmaße. Acta Paediat Hung 13:117–124
2 Garn SM, Hertzog KP, Poznanski AK, Nagy JM (1972) Metacarpophalangeal length in the evaluation of skeletal malformation. Radiology 105:375–381
3 Parish JG (1960) Skeletal syndromes associated with arachnodactyly. Proc R Soc Med 53:515–518
4 Bell J (1951) On brachydactyly and symphalangism. In: Penrose LS (ed) The treasury of human inheritances. Cambridge University Press, Cambridge, vol 5, pp 1–31

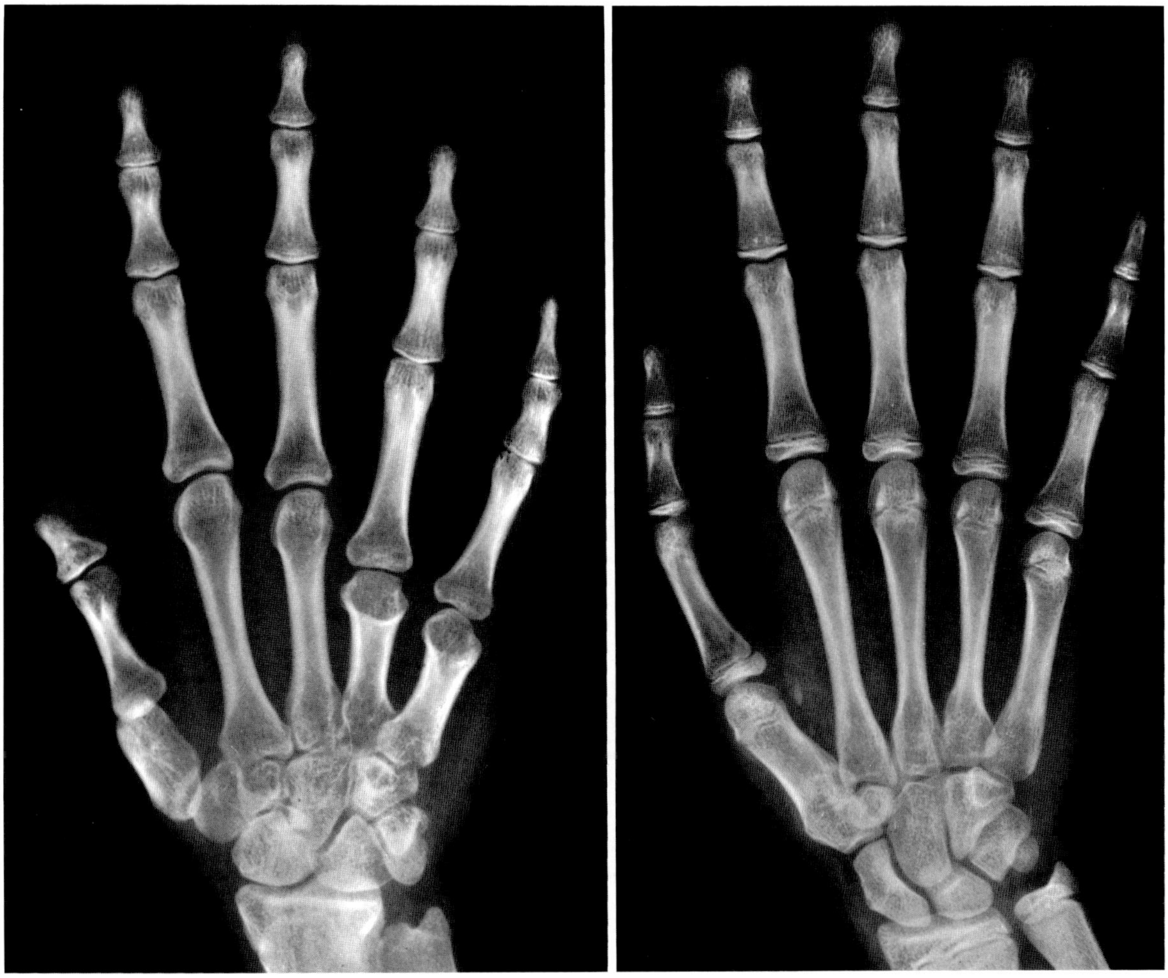

a b

Fig. 11. a Probable hand-foot-uterus syndrome in a 17-year-old female: Hypoplasia of first, fourth and fifth metacarpals, clinodactyly, stub thumb, os centrale carpi, abnormal arrangement of carpals. **b** A 14-year-old girl: Triphalangeal thumb and shortened first metacarpal due to surgical intervention

5 Poznanski AK (1984) The hand in radiologic diagnosis. Saunders, Philadelphia
6 Rimoin DL, Edgerton MT (1967) Genetic and clinical heterogeneity in the oral-facial-digital syndromes. J Pediatr 71:94–102
7 Reisner SH, Kott E, Bornstein B, Salinger H, Kaplan I, Gorlin RJ (1969) Oculo-dento-digital dysplasia. Am J Dis Child 118:600–607
8 Reeder MM, Felson B (1975) Gamuts in radiology. Pergamon, Oxford
9 Riggs W Jr (1970) Roentgen findings in Noonan's syndrome. Radiology 96:393–395
10 Moseley JE, Moloshok RE, Freiberger RH (1966) The Silver syndrome: congenital asymmetry, short stature and variations in sexual development. Roentgen features. AJR 97:74–81
11 Dignan PStJ, Mauer AM, Frantz C (1967) Phocomelia with congenital hypoplastic thrombocytopenia and myeloid leukemoid reactions. J Pediatr 70:561–573
12 Ginsburg LD, Sedano HO, Gorlin RJ (1970) Focal dermal hypoplasia syndrome. AJR 110:561–571
13 Poznanski AK, Macpherson RI, Gorlin RJ, Garn SM, Nagy JM, Gall JC Jr, Stern AM, Dijkman DJ (1973) The hand in the oto-palato-digital syndrome. Ann Radiol 16:203–209
14 Stovin JJ, Lyon JA Jr, Clemmens RL (1960) Mandibulo-facial dysostosis. Radiology 74:225–231
15 Harper RG, Orti E, Baker RK (1967) Bird-headed dwarfs (Seckel's syndrome). A familial pattern of developmental dental, skeletal, genital and central nervous system anomalies. J Pediatr 70:799–804
16 Preger L, Miller EH, Winfield JS, Choy SH (1967) Hereditary onycho-osteo-arthro-dysplasia. AJR 100:546–549
17 Gorlin RJ, Sedano HO, Cervenka J (1968) Popliteal pterygium syndrome. A syndrome comprising cleft lip-palate, popliteal and intercrural pterygia, digital and genital anomalies. Pediatrics 41:503–509
18 Wilson RA, Kliman MR, Hardyment AF (1963) Ankyloglossia superior (palato-glossal adhesion) in the newborn infant. Pediatrics 31:1051–1054
19 Houston CS (1967) Roentgen findings in the XXXXY chromosome anomaly. J Can Assoc Radiol 18:258–267

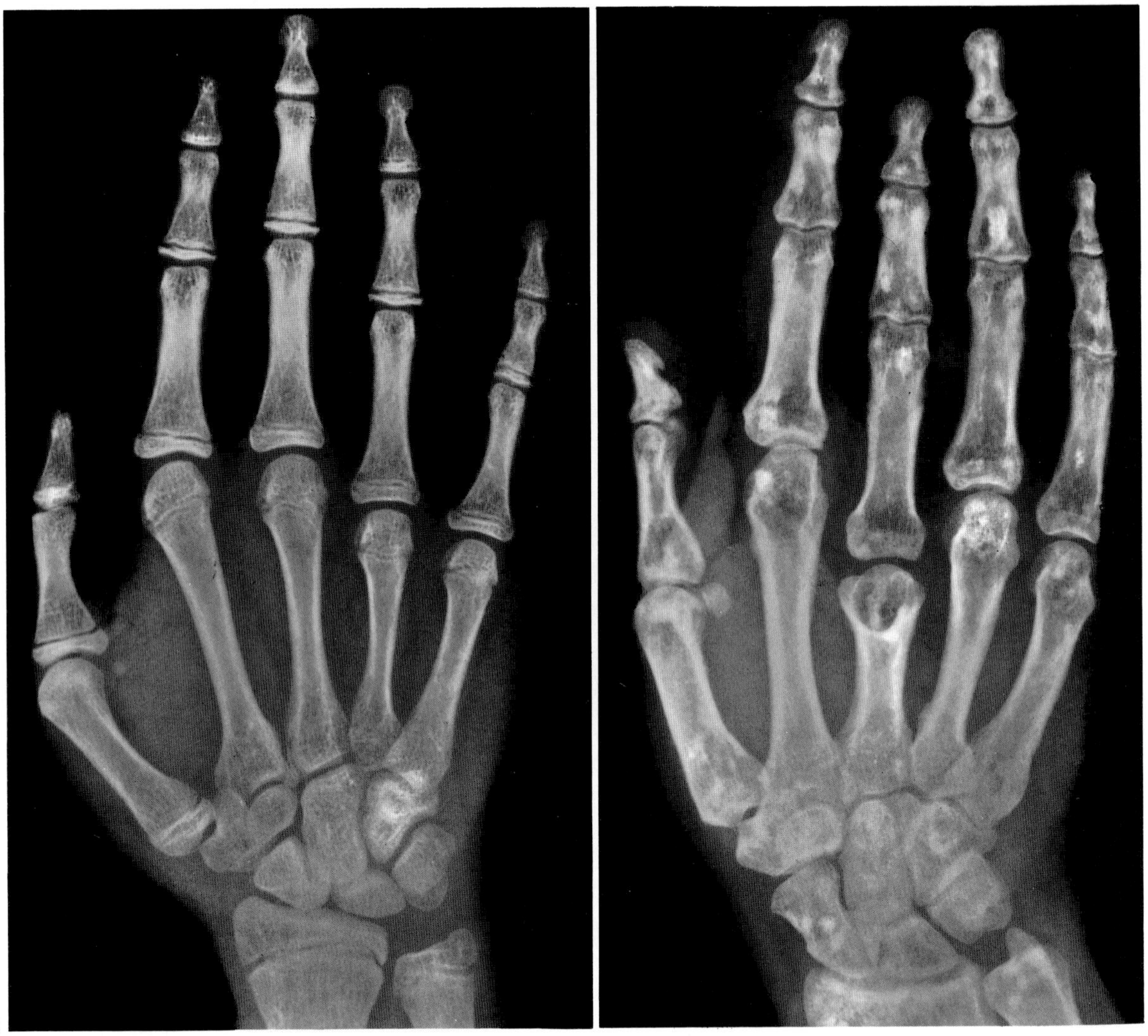

Fig. 12a, b. Brachymetacarpia. **a** Turner's syndrome in a 19-year-old woman: Hypoplasia of fourth metacarpal. **b** Osteopoikilosis in a 44-year-old woman: Hypoplasia of third metacarpal. The other hand of this patient presented an isolated and marked hypoplasia of the fifth metacarpal

20 Sergovich F, Uilenberg C, Pozsonyi J (1971) The 49, XXXXX chromosome constitution: similarities to the 49 XXXXY condition. J Pediatr 78:285–290

21 Coffin GS, Siris E (1970) Mental retardation with absent fifth fingernail and terminal phalanx. Am J Dis Child 119:433–439

22 Rüdinger RA, Schmidt W, Loose DA, Passarge E (1971) Severe developmental failure with coarse facial features, distal limb hypoplasia, thickened palmar creases, bifid uvula and ureteral stenosis. A previously unidentified familial disorder with lethal outcome. J Pediatr 79:977–981

23 James AE Jr, Belcourt CL, Atkins L, Janower ML (1969) Trisomy 13–15. Radiology 92:44–49

24 Laband PF, Habib G, Humphreys GS, Hereditary gingival fibromatosis. Report of an affected family with associated splenomegaly and skeletal and soft tissue abnormalities. Oral Surg 17:339–351

25 Poznanski AK, Garn SM, Holt JF (1971) The thumb in the congenital malformation syndromes. Radiology 100:115–129

26 Riggs W, Seibert J (1972) Cockayne's syndrome. AJR 116:623–633

27 Dawe C, Wynne-Davies R, Fulford GE (1982) Clinical variation in dyschondrosteosis. A report of 13 individuals in 8 families. J Bone Joint Surg 64-B:377–381

28 Giedion A (1976) Acrodysplasia. Peripheral dysostosis, acrodysostose and Thiemann's disease. Clin Orthop 114:107–115

29 Keutel J, Jörgensen G, Gabriel P (1971) Ein neues autosomal rezessiv vererbbares Syndrom. Dtsch Med Wochenschr 96:1676–1681

30 Poznanski AK, Stern AM, Gall JC Jr (1970) Radiographic findings in the hand-foot-uterus syndrome (HFUS). Radiology 95:129–134

31 Lee KF, Lin SR, Hodes PJ (1972) New roentgenologic findings in myotonic dystrophy. AJR 115:179–184

2.2.12 Symphalangism

Symphalangism is fusion of neighbouring phalanges within the same finger. Congenitally, this abnormality may be present as an isolated condition or associated with a number of disorders. The proximal interphalangeal joints of the fingers and the distal interphalangeal joints of the toes are usually affected. Sometimes, however, the proximal interphalangeal joints of the toes are involved.

In congenital symphalangism, the ulnar side of the hand is more commonly involved and the thumb is rarely abnormal [1, 2]. Failure of differentiation of the joint segment is thought to be the pathogenetic factor.

Acquired symphalangism may be caused by one of a number of factors, including arthritis, trauma, and operation.

Associated Abnormalities [1, 3–5]

Hand

Absence of distal and middle phalanges
Syndactyly (cutaneous or osseous)
Carpal fusion
Brachydactyly
Cone-shaped epiphyses
Short first and fifth metacarpals
Clinodactyly
Central dysplasia

Other sites

Foot: symphalangism
  tarsal fusion
  clubfoot
  accessory tarsals
Long tubular bones: fusion of humerus and ulna
Skull: Tower skull

Associated Disorders [1]

Diastrophic dysplasia (Sect. 1.1.4)
Bell's brachydactyly types A and C (Sect. 2.2.11)
Popliteal pterygium syndrome (Sect. 2.2.11 [17])
Symphalangism-surdity syndrome

Symphalangism-Surdity Syndrome

This autosomal dominant syndrome, also known as Vesell's syndrome [6–8], is characterized by conduction deafness (stapedial ankylosis), symphalangism, and strabismus. The radiographs show symphalangism of the proximal interphalangeal joints of the fingers and the interphalangeal joints of the toes (distal or proximal). Associated abnormalities may be found (see above).

References

1 Poznanski AK (1984) The hand in radiologic diagnosis. Saunders, Philadelphia
2 Harle TS, Stevenson JR (1967) Hereditary symphalangism associated with carpal and tarsal fusions. Radiology 89:91–94
3 Strasburger AK, Hawkins MR, Eldridge R, Hargrave RL, McKusick VA (1965) Symphalangism: genetic and clinical aspects. Johns Hopkins Med J 117:108–127
4 Wildervanck LS, Goedhard G, Meijer S (1967) Proximal symphalangism of fingers associated with fusion of the os naviculare and talus and occurrence of two accessory bones in the feet (os paranaviculare and os tibiale externum) in an European-Indonesian Chinese family. Acta Genetica Basel 17:166–177
5 Murakami Y (1975) Nievergelt-Pearlman syndrome with impairment of hearing. J Bone Joint Surg 57-B:367–372
6 Gloede JF, Stenger HH (1974) Symphalangismus, Strabismus und Mittelohrmißbildungen. Humangenetik 22:23–32
7 Vesell ES (1960) Symphalangism, strabismus and hearing loss in mother and daughter. N Engl J Med 263:839–842
8 Theunissen EJJM, Cremers CWRJ (1984) Stapesankylosis as symptom of autosomal dominant symphalangism (in Dutch). Ned Tijdschr Geneeskd 128:712–714

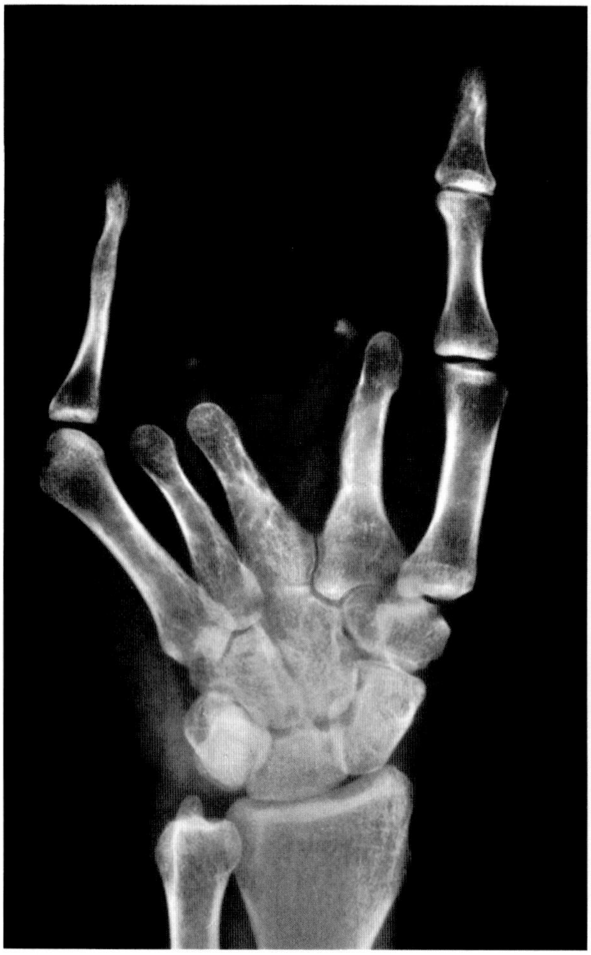

a

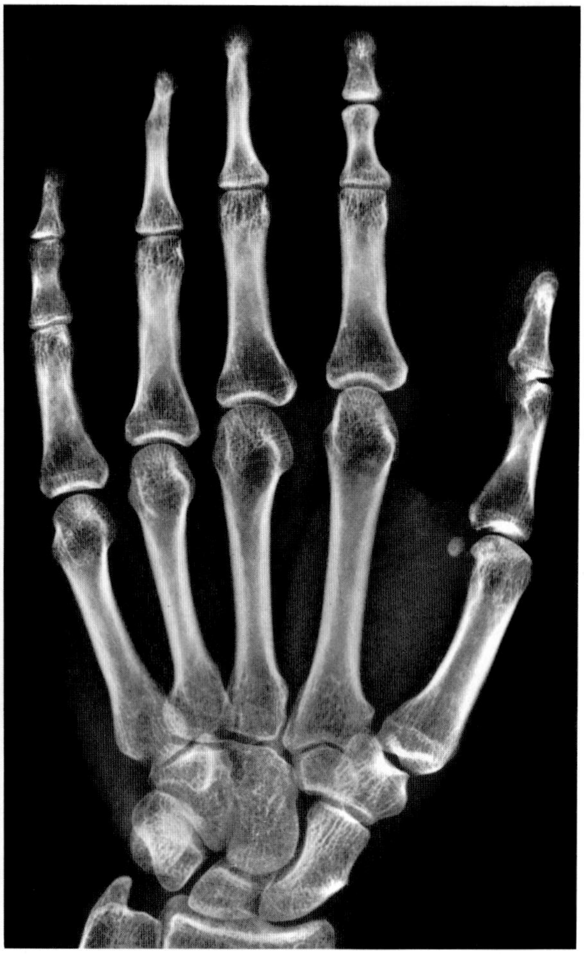

b

Fig. 1a, b. Symphalangism. **a** In a 40-year-old woman: Unilateral central dysplasia with rudimentary ossicles and symphalangism in fifth finger. **b** In a 31-year-old woman: Unilateral symphalangism of distal interphalangeal joints of third and fourth fingers, shortening of middle and distal phalanges in second finger

Fig. 2a, b. Symphalangism-surdity syndrome in a 9-year-old boy with stapedial ankylosis. **a** Symphalangism of proximal interphalangeal joints of fourth and fifth fingers, cone-shaped epiphyses in middle phalanx of index finger and distal phalanx of thumb. **b** Symphalangism of proximal interphalangeal joints of second to fourth toes and distal interphalangeal joint of fifth toe

Fig. 3. Symphalangism-surdity syndrome in a 30-year-old man, father of patient in Fig. 2. Symphalangism of proximal interphalangeal joints of fourth and fifth fingers

Fig. 4. Acquired abnormalities in a 21-year-old female leather worker. The symphalangism of the interphalangeal joints in the index finger and the osteolysis of the tuft are probably caused by recurrent microtrauma and/or recurrent infection. Several years previously this patient had had fractures of the proximal phalanges of the second and third fingers, followed by a severe deformation of the interphalangeal joint of the third finger ▷

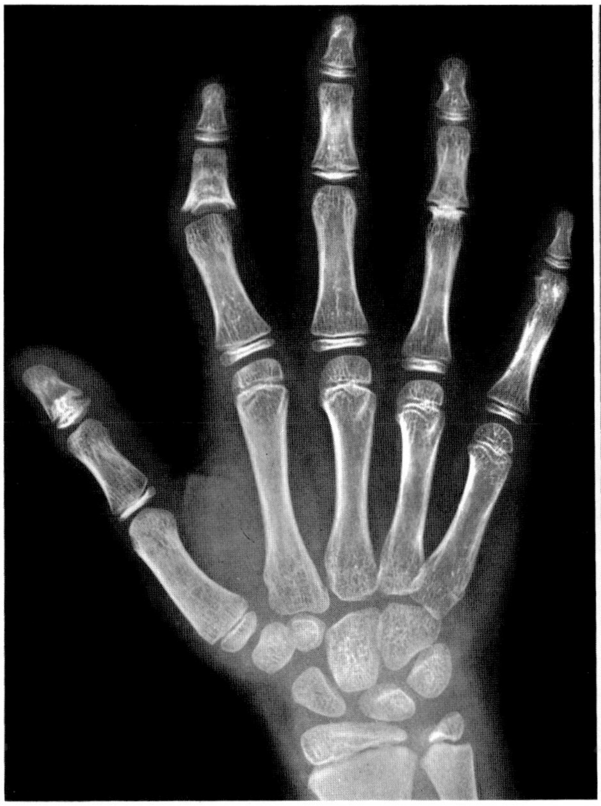

2 a

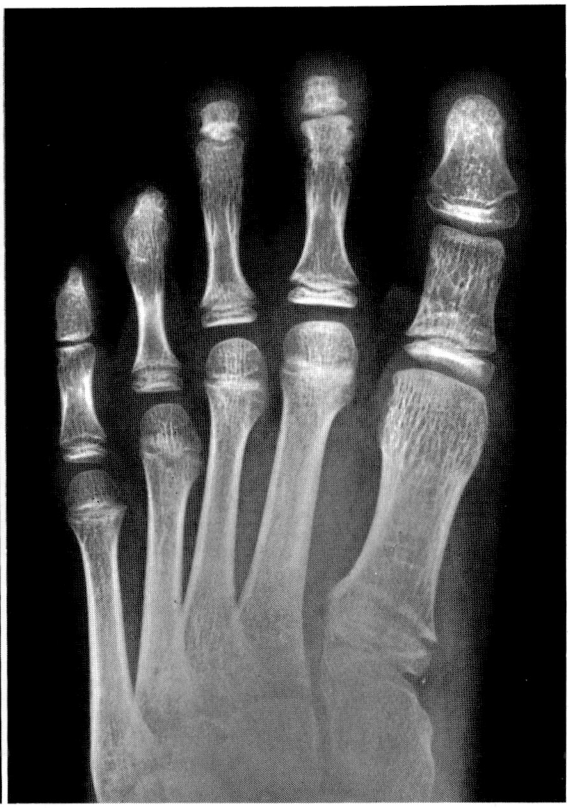

b

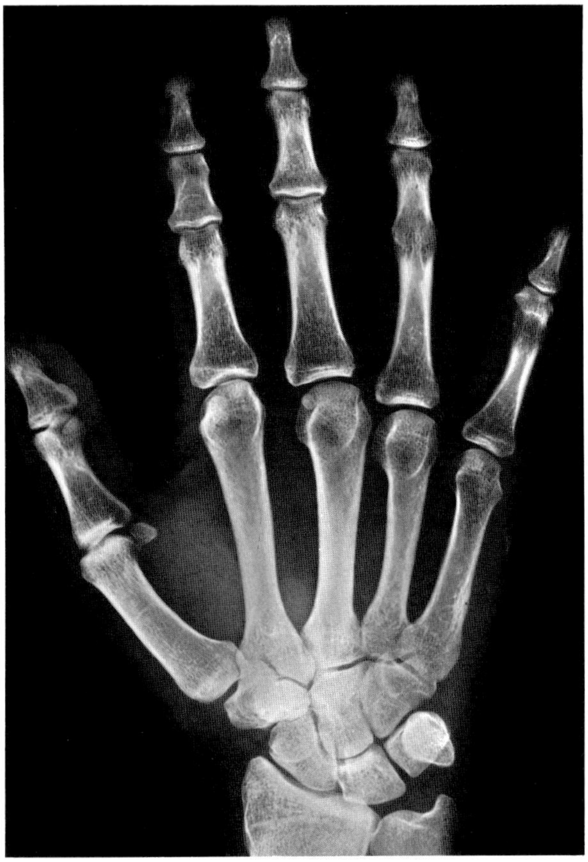

3

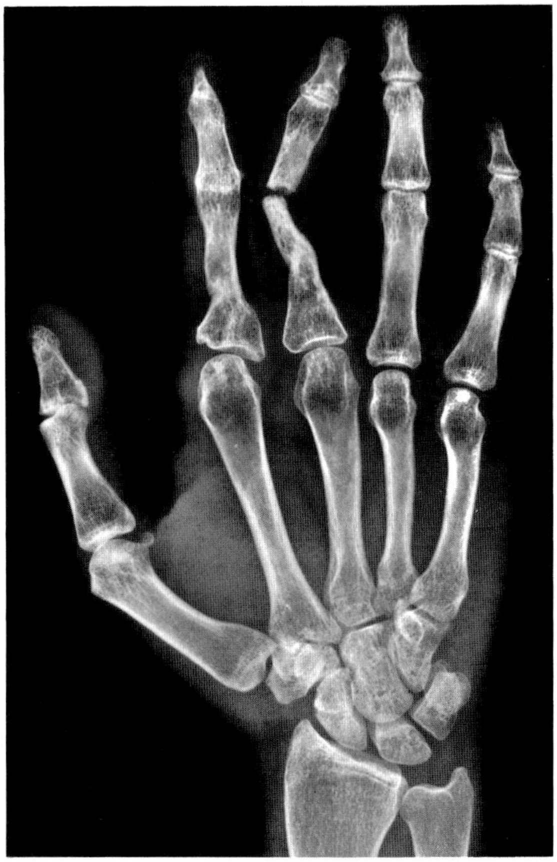

4

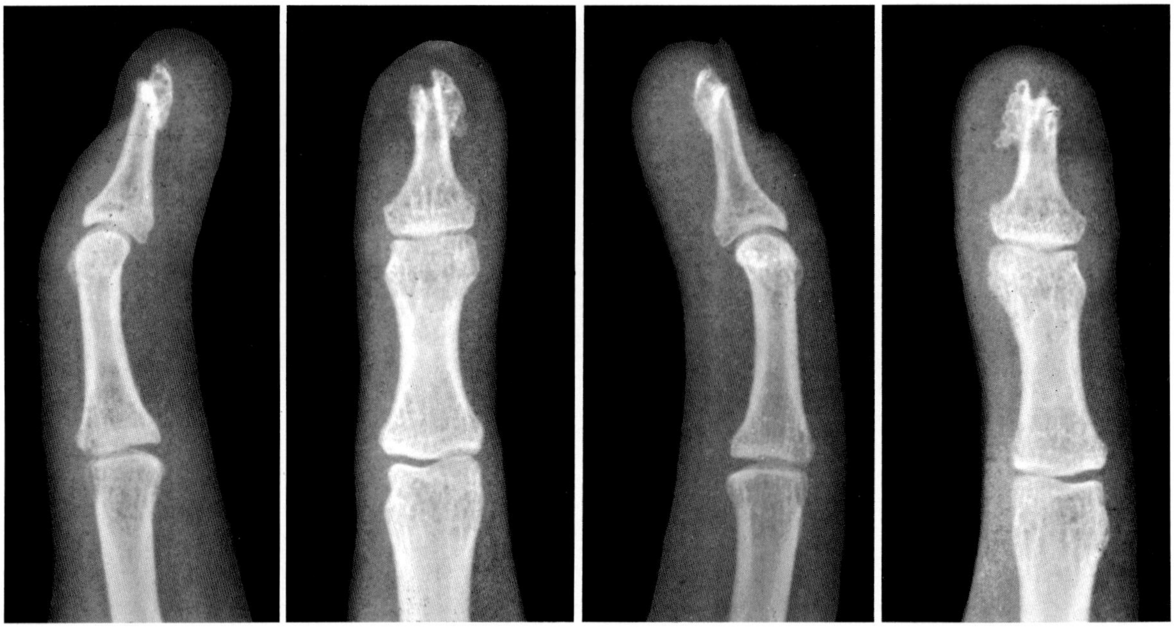

a b c d

Fig. 5a–d. Adult male. **a, b** Left fifth finger; **c, d** right fifth finger. Symmetric abnormalities of proximal interphalangeal joint of both fifth fingers. Flexion of these joints was seriously reduced; diminution of the adjacent soft tissues and some hypoplasia of the articulating bone ends were found. A symmetric defect at the ulnar sides of the tuft was an additional finding. The mother of this patient had the same impaired mobility of the interphalangeal joints of the fifth fingers, but no tuft abnormalities

2.2.13 Polydactyly

The additional digits may be present on the radial side of the hand (preaxial polydactyly) or on the ulnar side (postaxial polydactyly). The second, third, and fourth digits are infrequently involved. The mode of inheritance of polydactyly is not entirely clear. Postaxial polydactyly usually seems to be hereditary in an irregular autosomal dominant pattern [1–3]. Syndactyly and triphalangeal thumb may be additional findings.

Types of Polydactyly [1–3]

1. *Postaxial*
a) Type A: fully developed extra digits. Offspring: polydactyly type A or B.
b) Type B: rudimentary extra digits. Offspring: polydactyly type B.
2. *Preaxial*
a) Thumb polydactyly: usually sporadic. Skeletal abnormalities of thumb vary widely.
b) Polydactyly of triphalangeal thumb.
c) Polydactyly of second finger. This rare deformity is usually associated with some degree of syndactyly.
d) Polysyndactyly. Polydactyly associated with syndactyly is probably an autosomal dominant hereditary anomaly.
3. *Duplication of entire hand*

Associated Hand Abnormalities

Syndactyly
Triphalangeal thumb

Disorders Involving Postaxial Polydactyly [3]

Chondroectodermal dysplasia (Sect. 1.1.6)
Laurence-Moon-Biedl-Bardet syndrome [2].
Meckel's syndrome [5]
Trisomy 13 [2]
Biemond II syndrome [2]
Occasionally: asphyxiating thoracic dystrophy (Sect. 1.1.7)
focal dermal hypoplasia
Mohr's syndrome [6]

Disorders Involving Preaxial Polydactyly [3]

Acrocephalosyndactyly and acrocephalopolysyndactyly (Sect. 2.1.1)
Brachydactyly (Bell type B)
Blackfan-Diamond anemia [4]
Acropectorovertebral dysplasia
Occasionally: Bloom's syndrome [2]
  Holt-Oram syndrome (Sect. 2.2.19)
  Mohr's syndrome [6]
  Fanconi's anemia [7]

References

1 Temtamy SA (1966) Genetic factors in hand malformations. Thesis. Johns Hopkins University, Baltimore
2 Temtamy SA, McKusick VA (1978) The genetics of hand malformations. Liss, New York
3 Poznanski AK (1984) The hand in radiologic diagnosis. Saunders, Philadelphia
4 Aase JM, Smith DW (1969) Congenital anemia and triphalangeal thumbs: a new syndrome. J Pediatr 74:471–474
5 Hsia YE, Bratu M, Herbordt A (1971) Genetics of the Meckel syndrome (dysencephalia splanchnocystica). Pediatrics 48:237–247
6 Rimoin DL, Edgerton MT (1967) Genetic and clinical heterogenicity in the oral-facial-digital syndromes. J Pediatr 71:94–102
7 Poznanski AK, Garn SM, Holt JF (1971) The thumb in the congenital malformation syndromes. Radiology 100:115–129

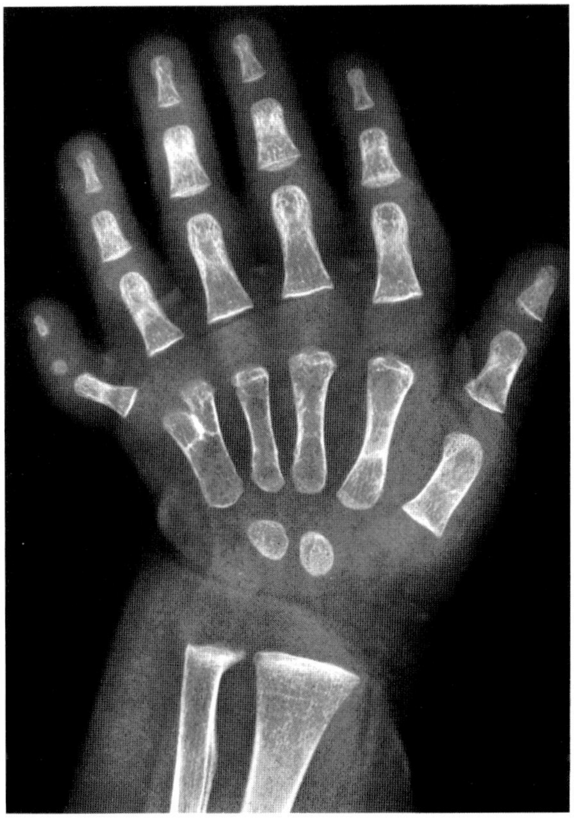

Fig. 1. Postaxial polydactyly type A in a 1-year-old boy. Well-developed digit with partly duplicated fifth metacarpal in left hand

a

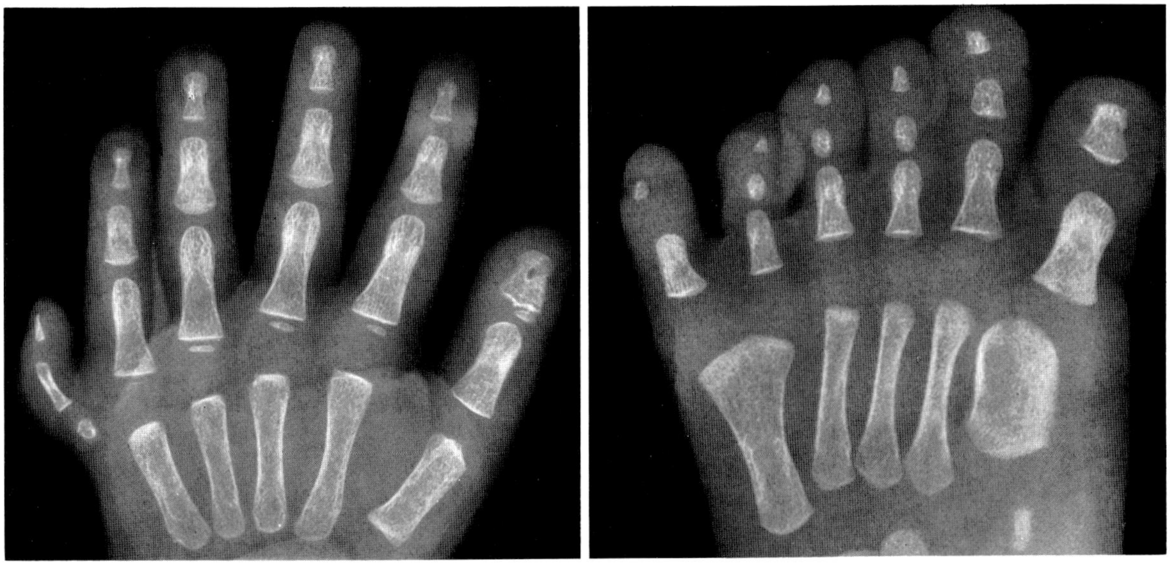

b

Fig. 2a, b. Postaxial polydactyly type B in a 1-year-old girl. **a** Rudimentary digit on ulnar side, bifid distal phalanx of thumb. **b** Both feet presented well-developed extra digits and broad fifth metatarsals. As a rule the extra toes in type B postaxial polydactyly are hypoplastic and rudimentary

3a b

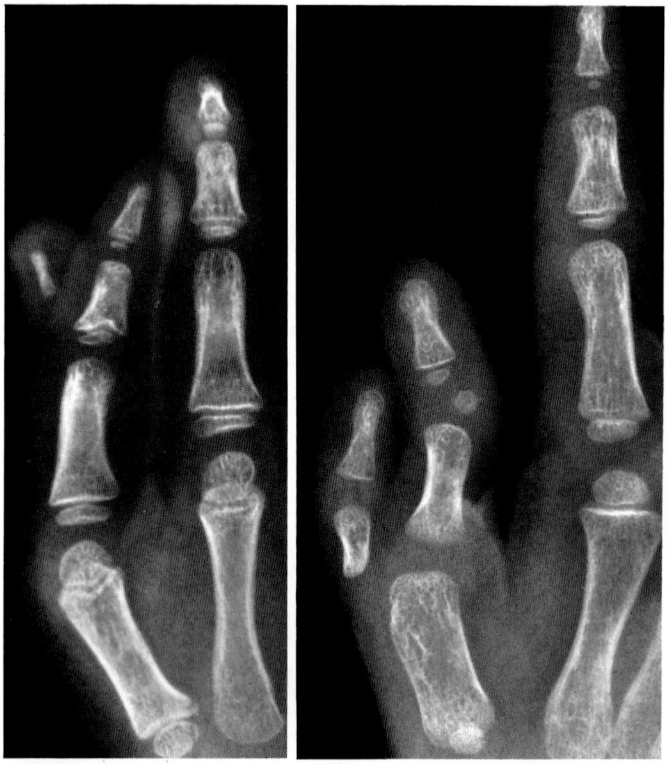

4a b

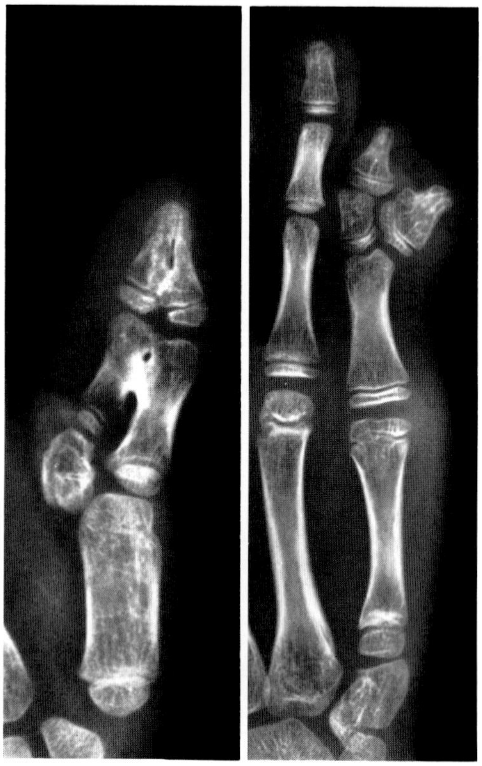

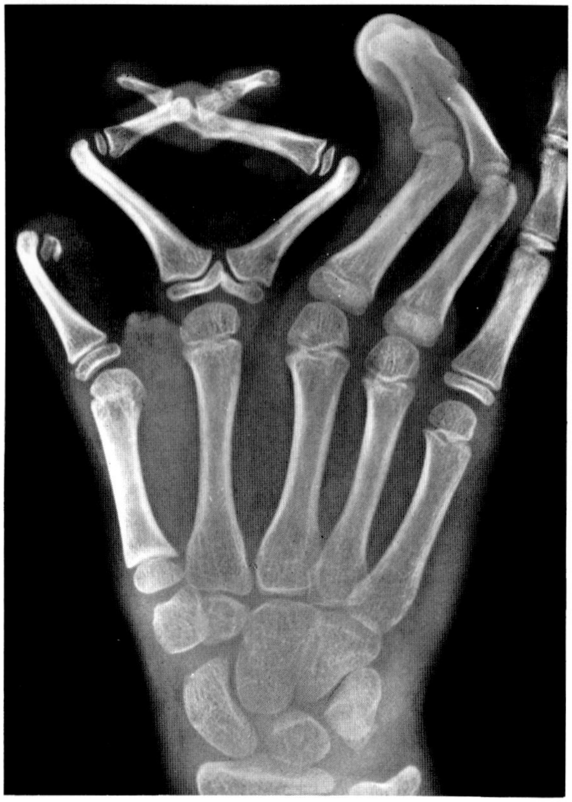

5

Fig. 3a, b. Preàxial polydactyly of thumb. **a** In a 7-year-old girl: Triphalangeal thumb associated with pedunculated rudimentary extra digit. This association is probably a hereditary entity. **b** In a 2-year-old boy: The thumb is probably triphalangeal. The extra digit presents two phalanges and a broad soft tissue connection with the thumb

Fig. 4a, b. Preaxial polydactyly of thumb. **a** In an 8-year-old boy: Duplication of thumb and fusion of corresponding phalanges, broad thumb and first metacarpal. **b** In an 11-year-old boy: Polydactyly of triphalangeal thumb associated with syndactyly between thumb and index finger (polysyndactyly). Remarkable position of extra phalanx in relation to adjacent phalanges of the thumb

Fig. 5. Preaxial polydactyly of index finger in a 9-year-old girl. Duplication of index finger associated with abnormal thumb and syndactyly of third and fourth digits. The other hand presented a triphalangeal thumb and an abnormally developed and curved third finger. Besides these abnormalities of the hands, the patient's feet displayed central dysplasia

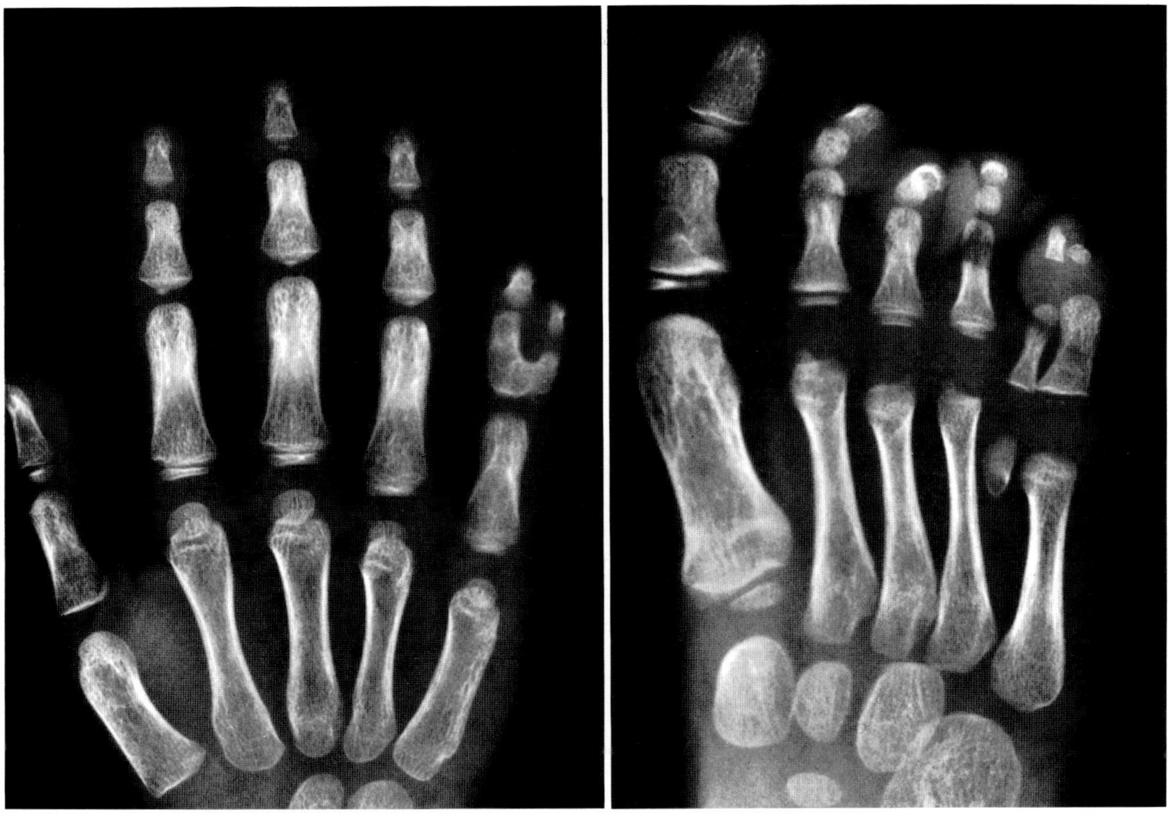

a b

Fig. 6a, b. Postaxial polydactyly associated with syndactyly in a 5-year-old boy. **a** Additional proximal phalanx shows osseous fusion with middle phalanx of fifth finger. **b** Extra toe between the fourth and fifth toes

2.2.14 Syndactyly

Syndactyly is an autosomal dominant anomaly, although sporadic cases have been reported [1]. Either soft tissue involvement or osseous involvement may be present. When only the proximal segments of the digits are involved, the syndactyly is referred to as incomplete, when the entire digits are involved, we speak of complete syndactyly. Syndactyly can also be subdivided according to the digits involved [1, 2]:

Type I Zygodactyly: syndactyly of third and fourth fingers and of second and third toes

Type II Synpolydactyly: syndactyly of third and fourth fingers with partial duplication of these fingers in the web, similar findings in the foot

Type III Syndactyly of fourth and fifth fingers associated with mesophalangy of the fifth finger

Type IV Complete syndactyly of all the fingers

Type V Syndactyly associated with metacarpal and metatarsal fusion

Associated Hand Abnormalities

Triphalangeal thumb
Polydactyly
Duplication of phalanges
Brachydactyly
Carpal fusion
Central dysplasia

Associated Disorders [2]

Acrocephalo(poly)syndactyly (Sect. 2.1.1)
Amniotic bands (Sect. 2.2.4)
Brachydactyly (Bell type B) (Sect. 2.2.11)
Oculodentodigital syndrome (Sect. 2.2.11 [7])
Popliteal pterygium syndrome (Sect. 2.2.11 [17])
Poland's syndrome (Sect. 2.2.13)
Macrodystrophia lipomatosa (Sect. 2.2.16)
Cornelia de Lange's syndrome (Sect. 5.1)
Aarskog's syndrome

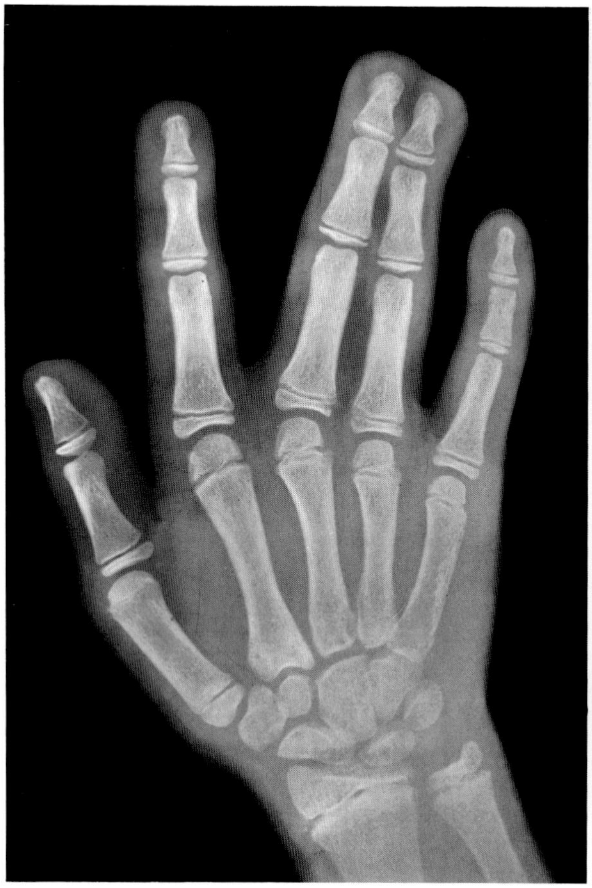

a

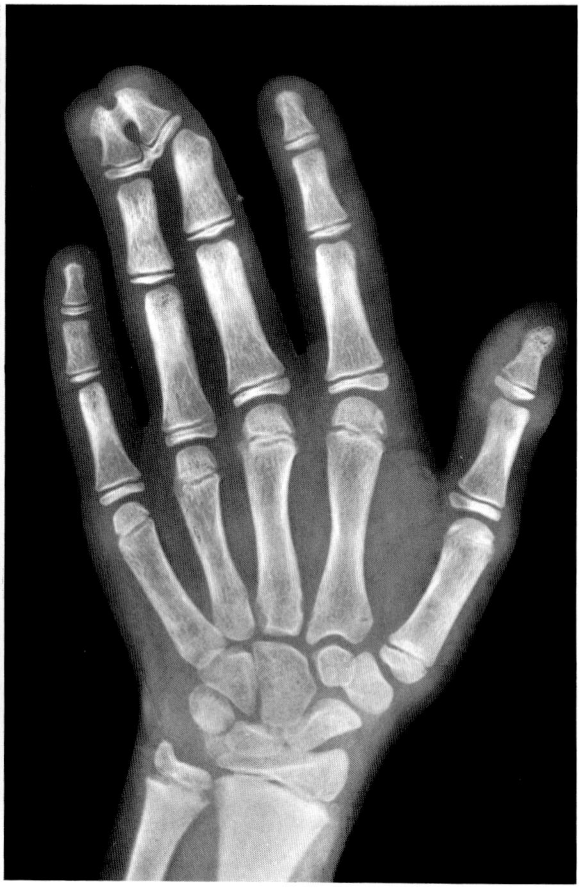

b

Fig. 1 a, b. Syndactyly type I (zygodactyly) in a 12-year-old boy. **a** Left hand: Soft tissue syndactyly. **b** Right hand: Soft tissue and osseous syndactyly

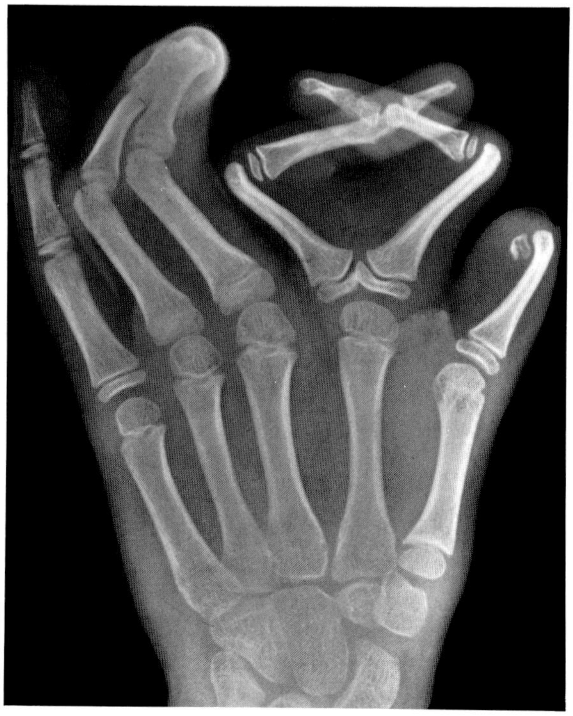

Fig. 2. Syndactyly type II (synpolydactyly) in a 9-year-old girl. Polydactyly of index finger and syndactyly of third and fourth fingers, thumb abnormality with slender proximal phalanx and small rudimentary distal phalanx. Left hand: Triphalangeal thumb and camptodactyly of third finger

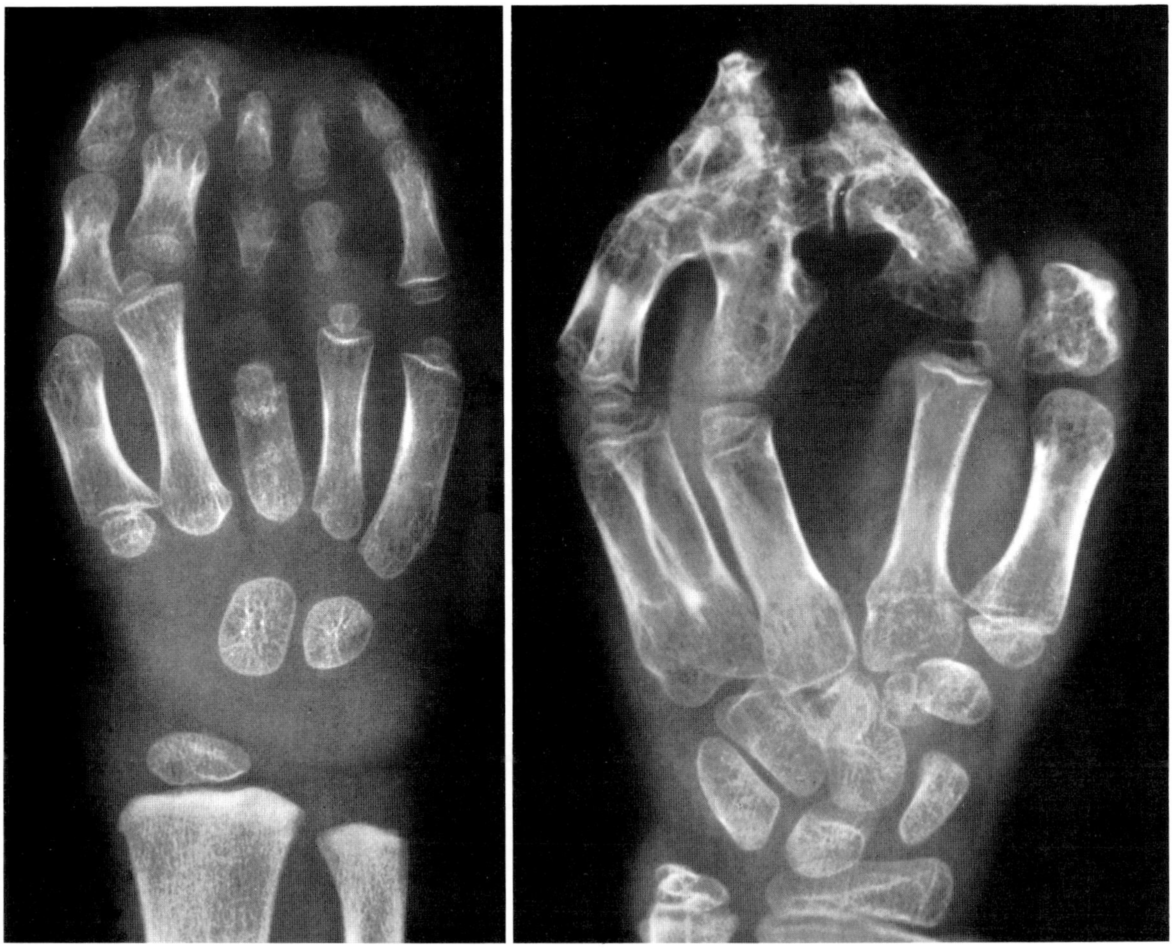

a b

Fig. 3a, b. Syndactyly types IV and V. **a** In a 3-year-old girl: Soft tissue syndactyly of all fingers, central dysplasia, only two phalanges in second to fifth fingers. Other hand normal. **b** In an 11-year-old boy with acrocephalosyndactyly (Apert type): Syndactyly of fingers, fusion of fourth and fifth metacarpals

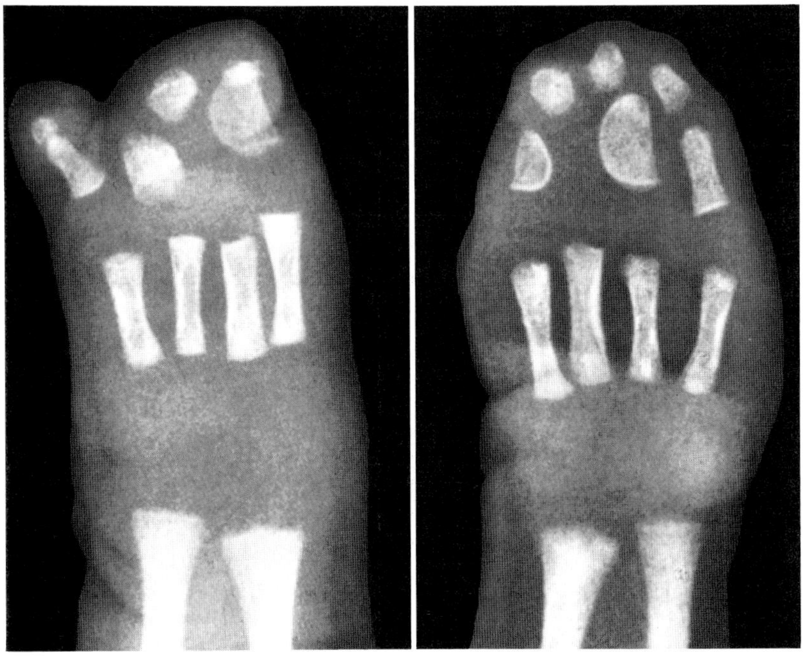

a b

Fig. 4a, b. Syndactyly type IV in a newborn baby with popliteal pterygium syndrome. Syndactyly, hypoplasia, and aplasia of digits, fusion of interphalangeal joints. Pes equinovarus, flat acetabular roofs, and popliteal pterygium are other well-known features of this syndrome

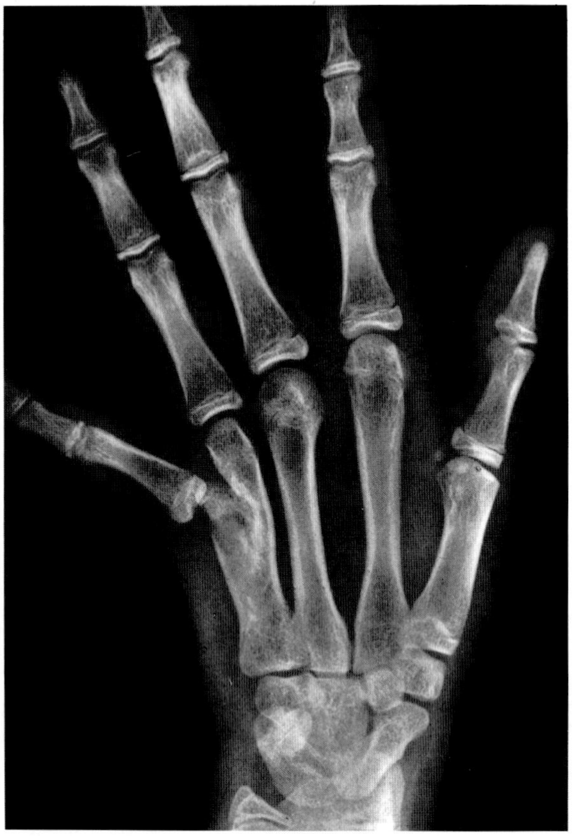

Fig. 5. Syndactyly type V in a 16-year-old boy. Osseous fusion of fourth and fifth metacarpals, incomplete soft tissue syndactyly between third and fourth fingers, hamate-capitate and lunate-triquetrum fusions. This deformity is in fact an example of ulnar dysplasia associated with syndactyly

Acropectorovertebral syndrome
Occasionally: aglossia-adactylia syndrome
ankyloglossia superior syndrome
Bloom's syndrome
Conradi's syndrome
cryptophthalmos-syndactyly syndrome
Fanconi's anemia
Goltz' focal dermal hypoplasia
incontinentia pigmenti
Laurence-Moon-Biedl-Bardet syndrome
Lenz' microphthalmia syndrome
Möbius' syndrome
orofaciodigital syndrome
Pierre-Robin syndrome
Rothmund-Thomson syndrome
Smith-Lemeli-Opitz syndrome
thrombocytopenia absent radius syndrome
trisomy 13
trisomy 18 (Sect. 4.1)

References

1 Temtamy SA (1966) Genetic factors in hand malformations. Thesis. Johns Hopkins University, Baltimore
2 Poznanski AK (1984) The hand in radiologic diagnosis. Saunders, Philadelphia

2.2.15 Triphalangeal Thumb

Synonym: hyperphalangism of thumb

Triphalangeal thumb is a rare, most often solitary malformation. In a number of cases heredity has been established. The additional middle phalanx varies from a wedge-shaped nodule to being well developed [1]. In pseudotriphalangeal thumbs, the epiphysis of the distal phalanx is abnormally large or an abnormal osseous element is present which could be mistaken for a middle phalanx [2].

Radiographic Findings [1–4]

Hand

Extra ossicle – well-developed phalanx, wedge-shaped phalanx, or double ossification center of distal epiphysis (pseudotriphalangism)

Long first metacarpal

Associated Abnormalities

Hand

Duplication of thumb
Polydactyly
Syndactyly
Clinodactyly of thumb
Radial dysplasia of other hand

Other Sites

Arm: radio-ulnar synostosis
absent pectoral muscle
Foot: split foot (central dysplasia) [3]

Associated Disorders [1]

Holt-Oram syndrome (Sect. 2.2.19)
Alport's syndrome (Fig. 4)
Blackfan-Diamond anemia [4]
Juberg-Hayward syndrome [5]
Thalidomide deformities
Townes-Brocks syndrome:

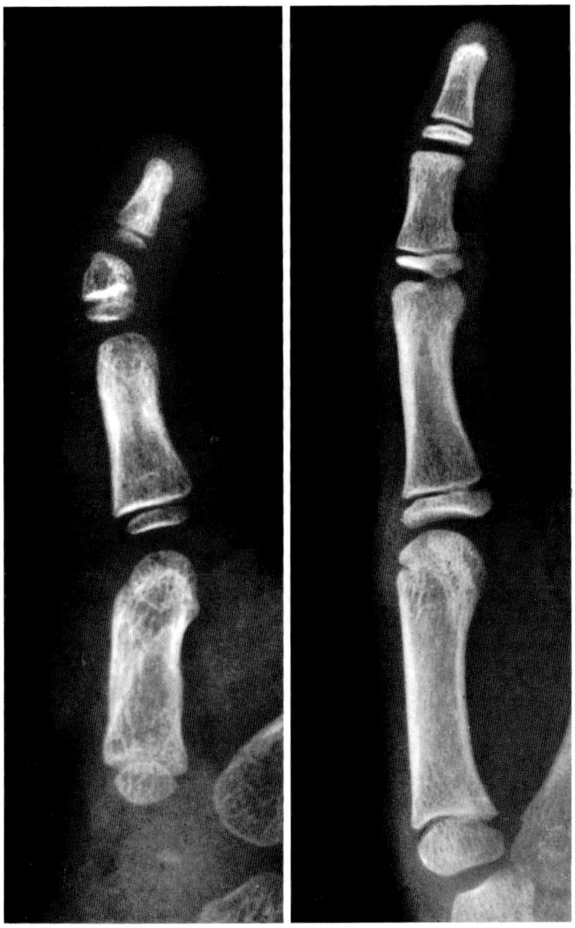

a b

Fig. 1a, b. Triphalangism. **a** In a 3-year-old girl: Small middle phalanx, clinodactyly. **b** In a 9-year-old girl: Well-developed phalanges

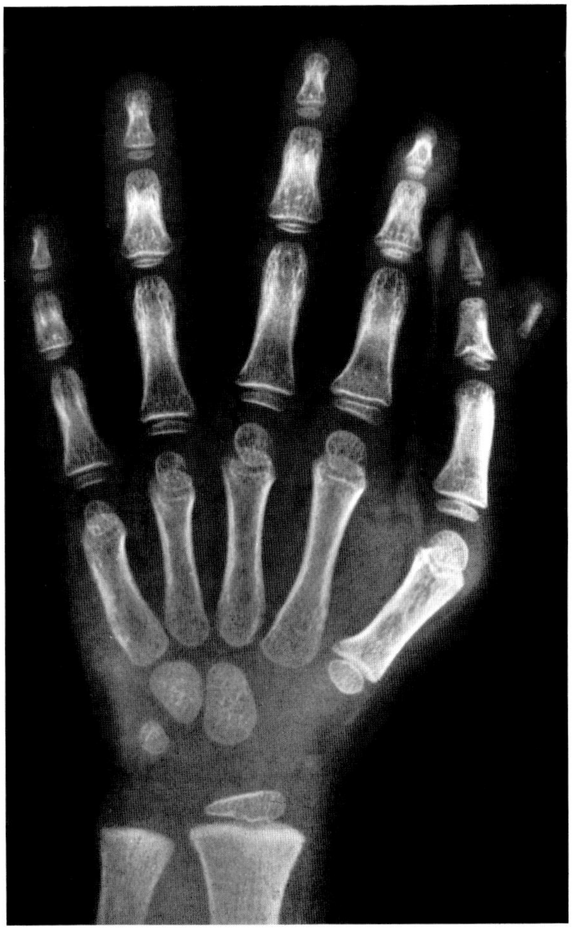

Fig. 2. Triphalangism in a 3-year-old girl associated with preaxial polydactyly

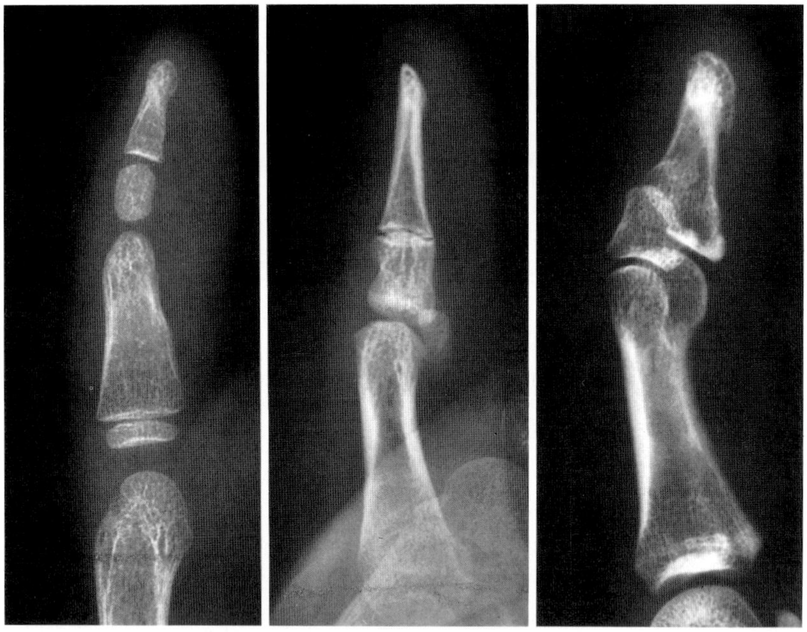

a b c

Fig. 3a–c. Pseudotriphalangism. **a** In a 5-year-old boy: Between the proximal and the distal phalanges of the thumb is an osseous nodule, probably a large epiphysis of the distal phalanx. **b** In same patient at age of 13: Only two phalanges in thumb, large epiphysis of distal phalanx. **c** In a 43-year-old woman: Probably separated and wedge-shaped part of distal epiphysis

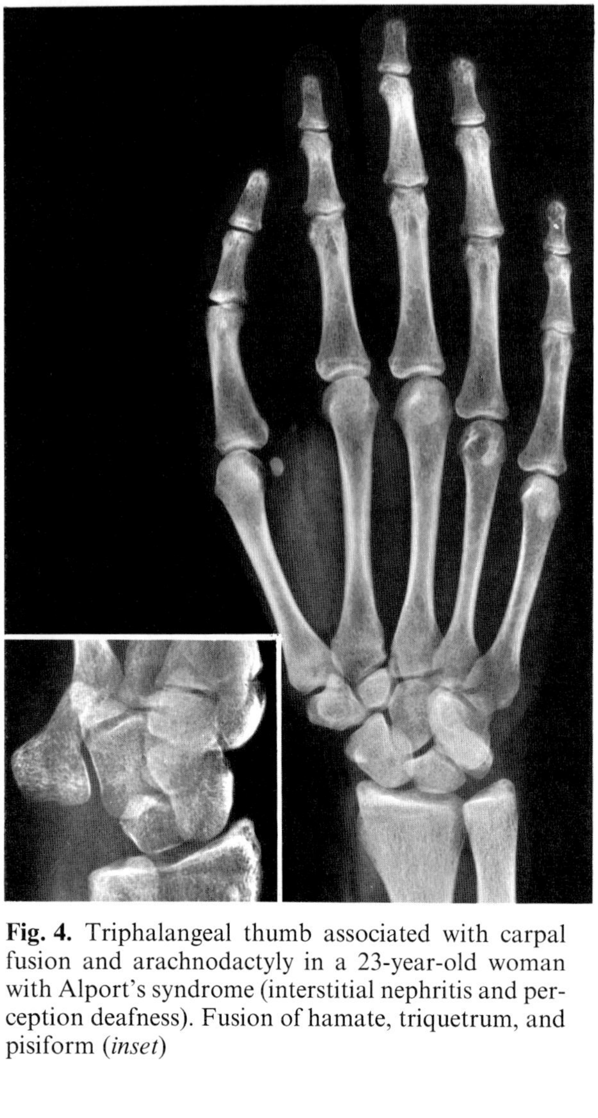

Fig. 4. Triphalangeal thumb associated with carpal fusion and arachnodactyly in a 23-year-old woman with Alport's syndrome (interstitial nephritis and perception deafness). Fusion of hamate, triquetrum, and pisiform (*inset*)

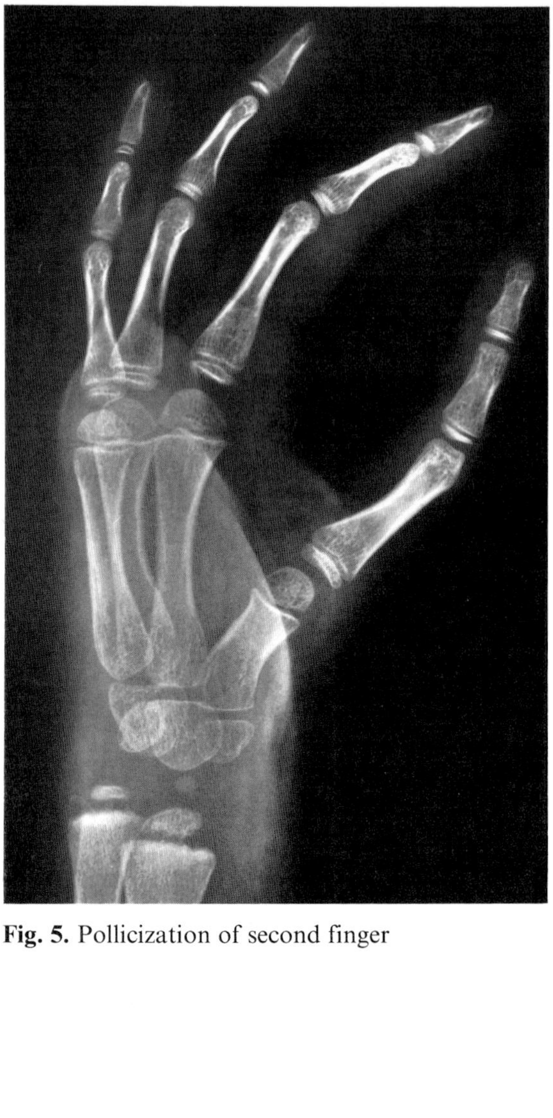

Fig. 5. Pollicization of second finger

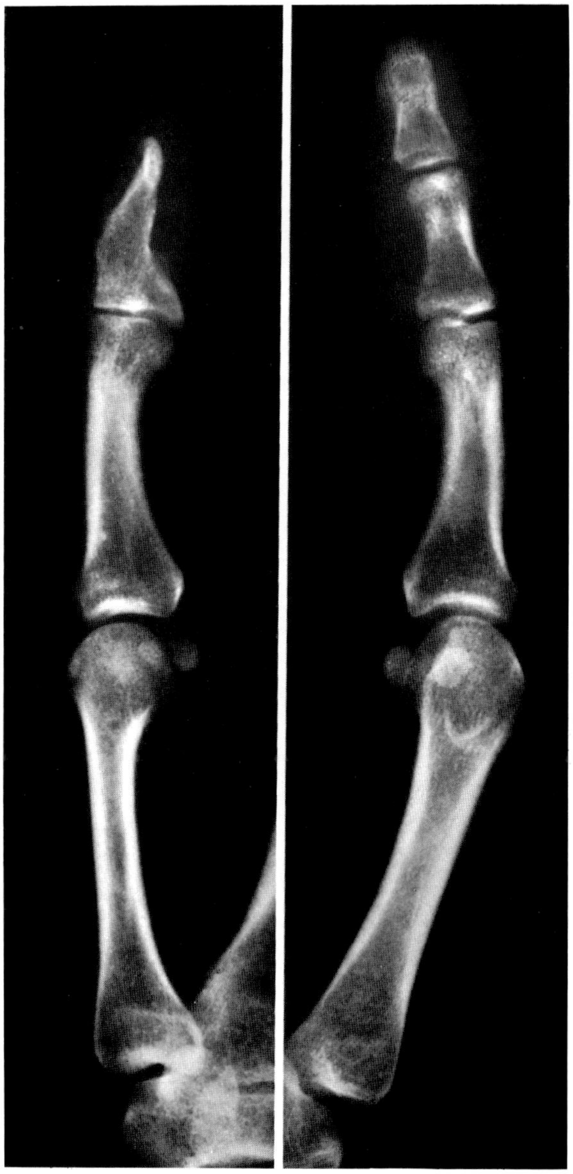

a b

Fig. 6a, b. Townes-Brocks syndrome in an adult man. Triphalangeal thumb (**b**), somewhat enlarged and pointed distal phalanx of contralateral thumb. Deafness and renal dysplasia were other features. His young son presented the same abnormalities and additional findings such as imperforate anus and satyr ears

In this autosomal dominant syndrome, triphalangeal thumbs, satyr ears, sensorineural deafness, imperforate anus, and renal dysplasia are encountered [6, 7]

Occasionally: trisomy 13–15

References

1 Poznanski AK, Garn SM, Holt JF (1971) The thumb in the congenital malformation syndromes. Radiology 100:115–129

2 Theander G, Carstam N (1979) Triphalangism and pseudo-triphalangism of the thumb in children. Acta Radiol 20:223–232

3 Phillips RS (1971) Congenital split foot (lobster claw) and triphalangeal thumb. J Bone Joint Surg 53-B:247–251

4 Aase JM, Smith DW (1969) Congenital anemia and triphalangeal thumbs: a new syndrome. J Pediatr 74:471–474

5 Juberg RC, Haywood JR (1969) A familial syndrome of oral, cranial and digital anomalies. J Pediatr 74:755–761

6 Townes PL, Brocks ER (1972) Hereditary syndrome of imperforate anus with hand, foot and ear anomalies. J Pediatr 81:321–326

7 Walpole IR, Hockey A (1982) Syndrome of imperforate anus, abnormalities of hands and feet, satyr ears, and sensorineural deafness. J Pediatr 100:250–252

2.2.16 Macrodystrophia Lipomatosa (Progressiva)

Synonym: Megalodactyly

Macrodystrophia lipomatosa is a nonhereditary congenital disorder characterized by overgrowth of all the mesenchymal elements of a digit with a disproportionate increase in the fibroadipose tissue. Usually one of the adjacent digits in the hand or foot is also involved, and the abnormalities can be unilateral or bilateral. Both the skeletal structures and the soft tissues (skin, fingernails, subcutaneous fat, vessels, and tendons) are involved due to infiltration of the mesenchymal structures by adipose tissue. A relation with neurofibromatosis has been suggested [1]. The most common sites of macrodystrophia lipomatosa are the second and third fingers, corresponding to the territory of the median nerve. The fifth finger is rarely involved [2, 3].

Radiographic Findings

Long and broad phalanges, splayed distal ends
Soft tissues: enlargement, mottled translucencies
Clinodactyly
Symphalangism
Syndactyly
Polydactyly
Osteoarthrosis

Differential Diagnosis

Neurofibromatosis (Sect. 7.1.2)
Angiodysplasia (Sect. 7.1.4)
Lymphangioma
Dactylitis (Sect. 7.3)

References

1 Goldman AB, Kaye JJ (1977) Macrodystrophia lipomatosa: Radiographic diagnosis. AJR 128:101–105
2 Barsky AJ (1967) Macrodactyly. J Bone Joint Surg 49-A:1255-1266
3 Moore BH (1944) Macrodactylism and associated peripheral nerve changes associated with congenital deformities. J Bone Joint Surg 26:282–290

Fig. 1a, b. Two patients with local gigantism of third finger ▷

Fig. 2. a Macrodystrophia lipomatosa of third finger with clinodactyly. **b** Local gigantism of fifth finger with clinodactyly. Soft tissue enlargement ▷

Fig. 3. Macrodystrophia lipomatosa in a 1-year-old boy. Local gigantism of fourth and fifth digits with syndactyly of distal phalanges. Marked enlargement of soft tissues

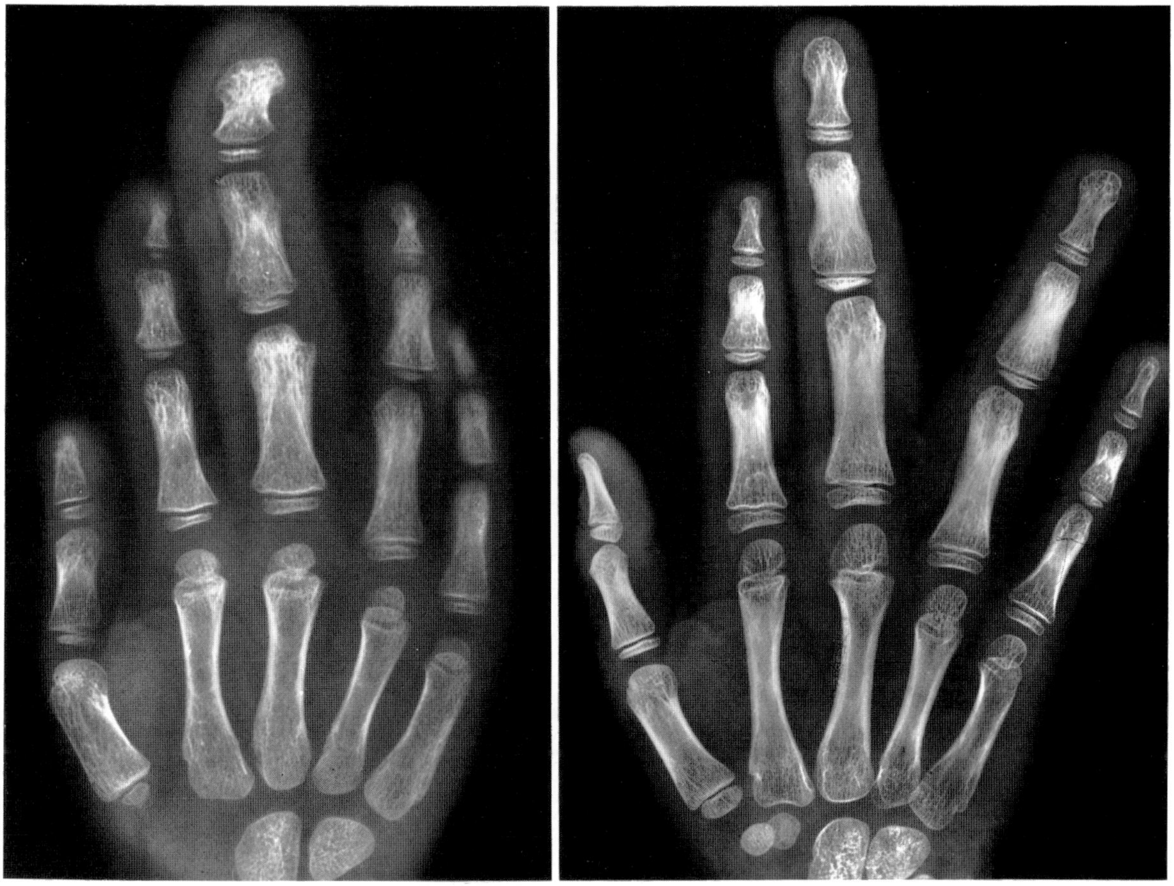

1 a b

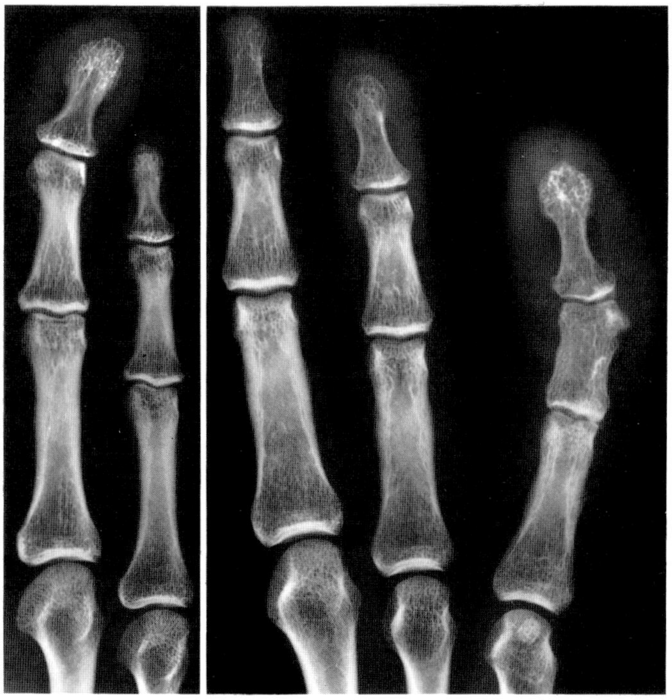

2 a b

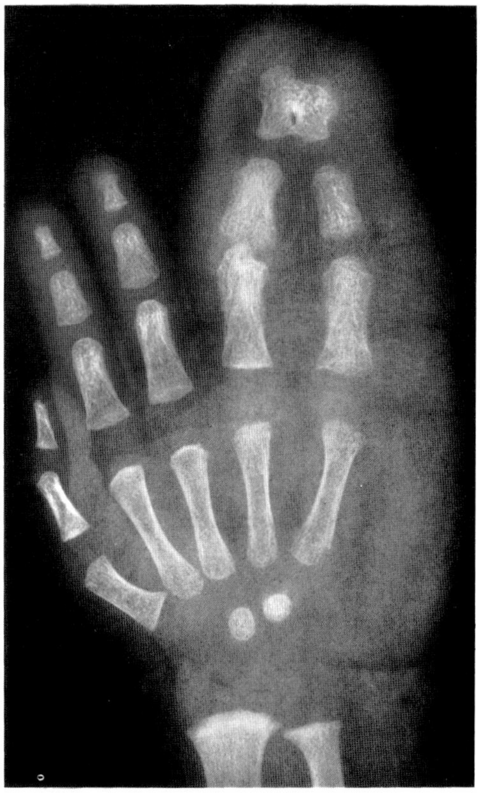

3

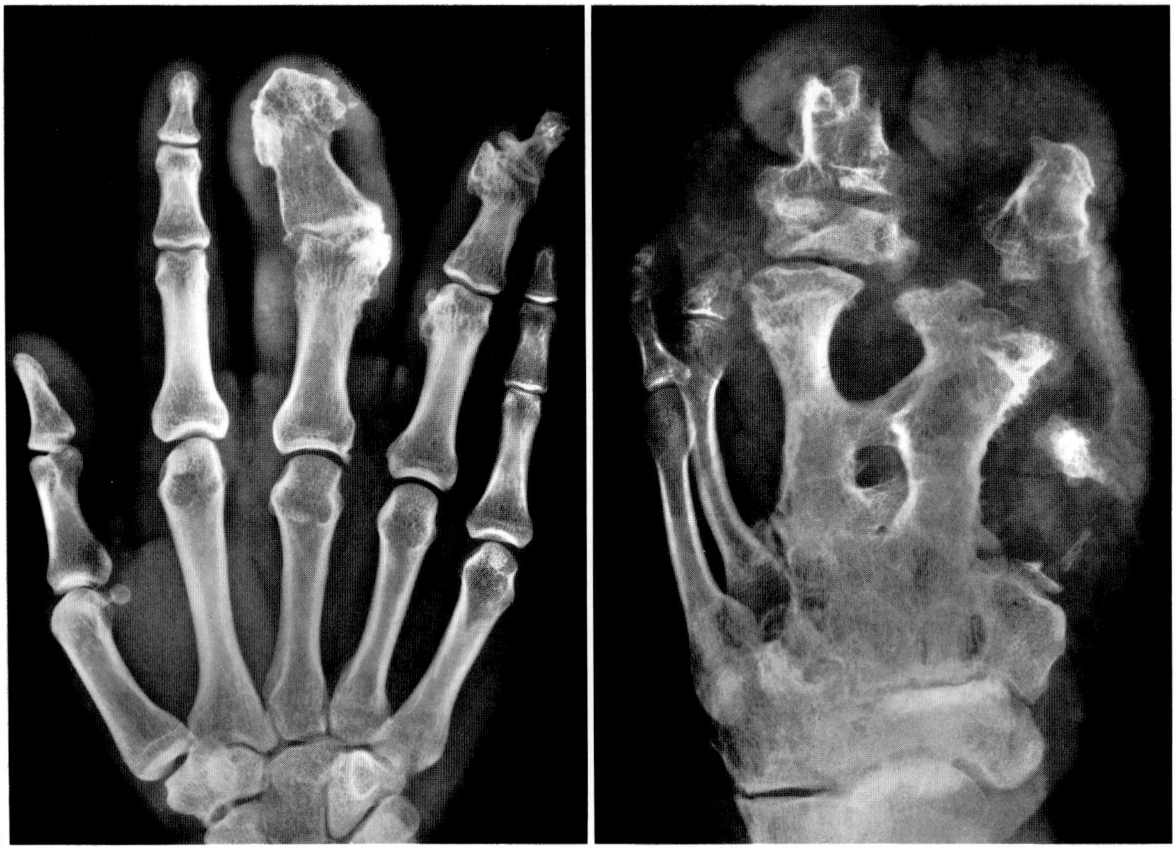

a b

Fig. 4 a, b. Macrodystrophia lipomatosa. **a** In a 26-year-old man: Third and fourth fingers are involved. Only two phalanges in third finger, with distal phalanx hugely enlarged. Mottled translucencies in soft tissues. **b** In a 25-year-old woman: Severe deformation of medial part of foot. The first metatarsal seems to be absent. Synostosis between the enlarged second and third metatarsals and severely deformed digits are the most distinctive abnormalities. The soft tissues are enlarged and show mottled translucencies

2.2.17 Poland's Syndrome

Synonym: pectoral aplasia-syndactyly syndrome

Poland's syndrome is a nonhereditary disorder characterized by absence of the pectoralis major muscle associated with ipsilateral defects of the upper limb. The majority of the victims are men (78%), and the right upper limb is the one mostly affected (75%) [1]. Soft tissue syndactyly and brachydactyly of the second to fifth fingers are present. The metacarpals may also be shortened. The thumb is usually not affected.

Radiographic Findings [2–4]

Hand

Unilateral brachydactyly, especially of middle phalanges of second to fifth fingers
Soft tissue syndactyly
Unilateral brachymetacarpia
Hypoplasia of whole hand

Other Sites

Upper limb: hypoplasia of (fore)arm
Thorax: translucent hemithorax due to absence of pectoralis major muscle
rib anomalies
elevated scapula
Spine: scoliosis

Differential Diagnosis

Malformation syndromes with: brachydactyly and brachymetacarpia (Sect. 2.2.11)
Syndactyly (Sect. 2.2.14)
Sprengel's deformity

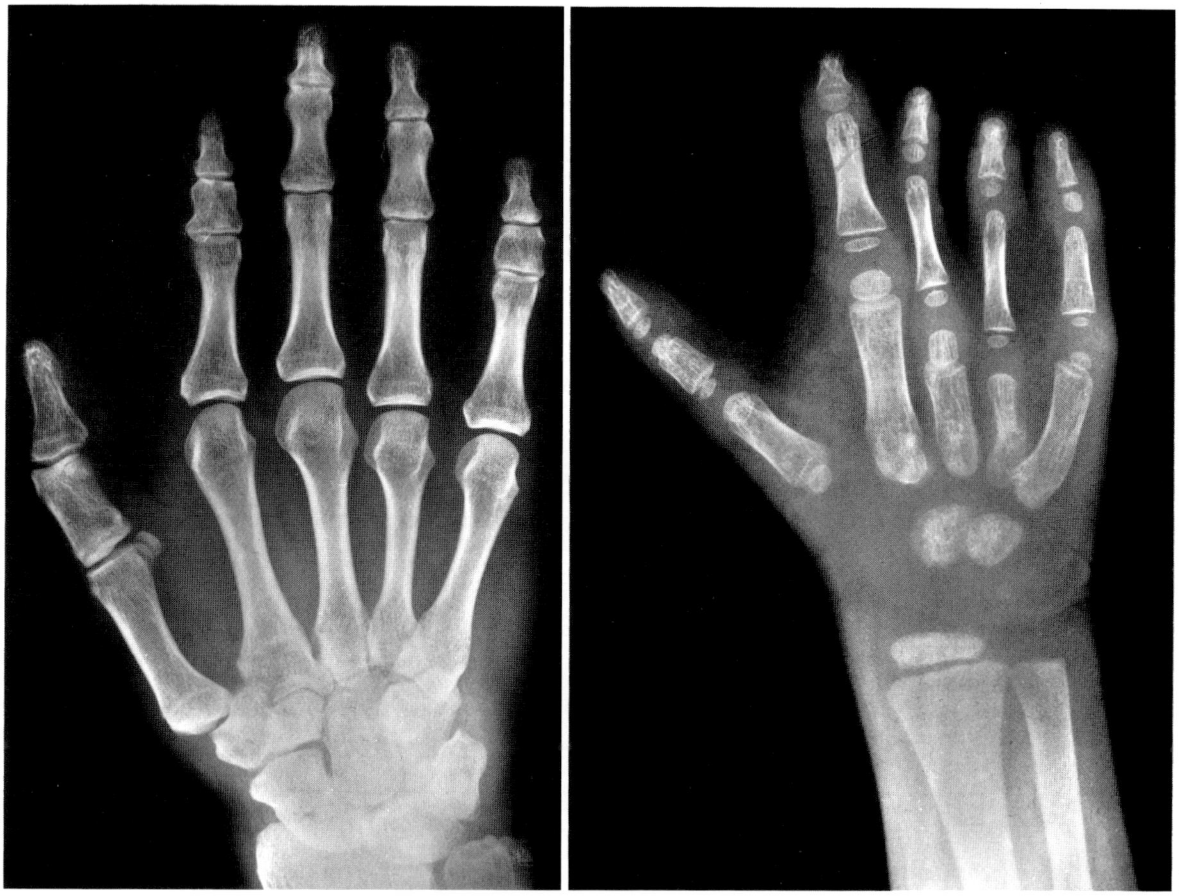

a b

Fig. 1 a, b. Poland's syndrome. **a** In a 24-year-old man: Right hand. Bell type A-1 brachydactyly: all middle phalanges shortened. **b** In a 5-year-old girl: Right hand. Severe hypoplasia of whole hand, syndactyly, short metacarpals and phalanges. Possible fusion between middle and distal phalanges

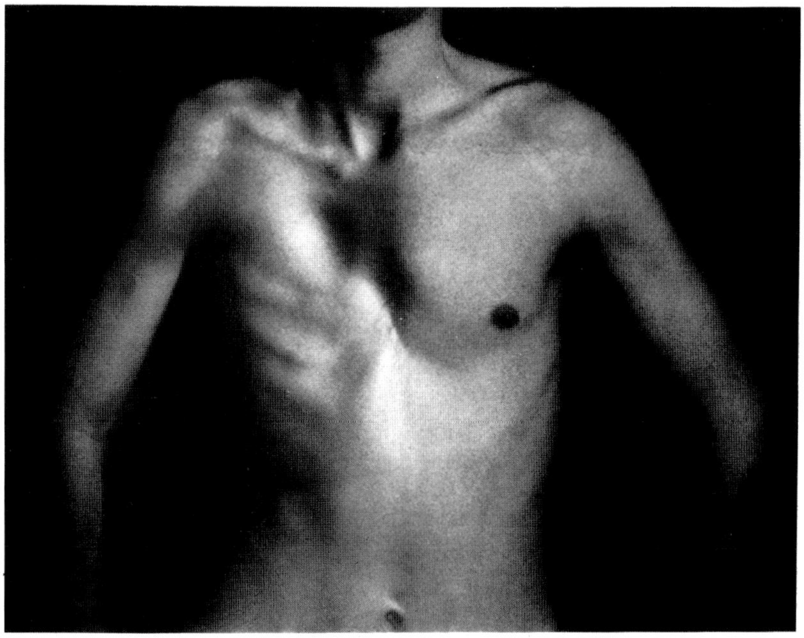

Fig. 2. Poland's syndrome. Absence of right pectoralis major muscle

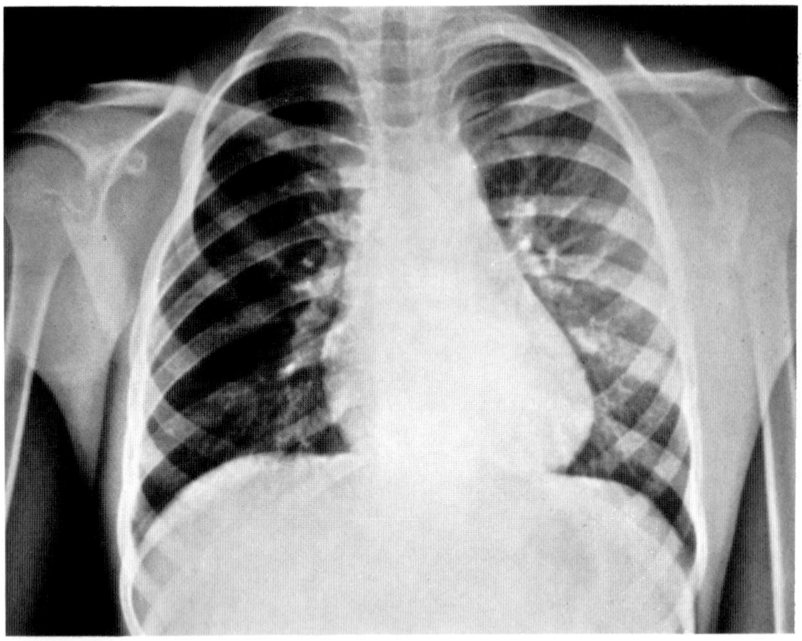

Fig. 3. Poland's syndrome. Translucent right hemithorax, asymmetry of clavicles, rib anomalies

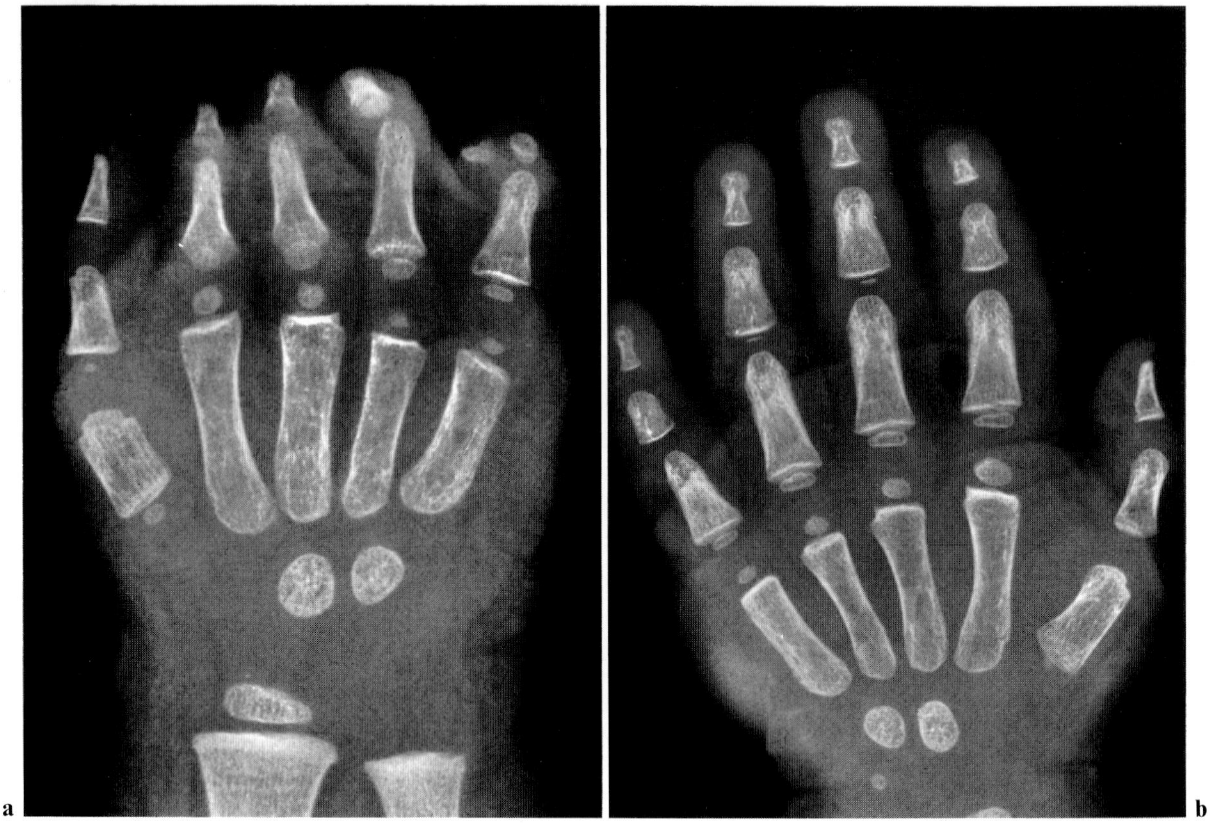

Fig. 4a, b. Poland's syndrome in a 2-year-old boy. **a** Brachydactyly of fingers of right hand associated with syndactyly. **b** Left hand normal

References

1 Mace JW, Kaplan JM, Schauberger JE, Gotlin RW (1972) Poland's syndrome. Report of seven cases and review of the literature. Clin Pediatr 11:98–102

2 Pearl M, Chow TF, Friedman E (1971) Poland's syndrome. Radiology 101:619–623

3 Ireland DCR, Takayama N, Flatt AE (1976) Poland's syndrome. A review of forty-three cases. J Bone Joint Surg 58-A:52–58

4 Steinbach HL, Gold RH, Preger L (1975) Roentgen appearance of the hand in diffuse disease. Year Book, Medical Publishers, Chicago

2.2.18 Rubinstein-Taybi Syndrome

Most cases of Rubinstein-Taybi syndrome are sporadic, and mental retardation is always present. The thumbs and great toes are broad and short. Short stature and a small skull are additional findings. The facies is characteristic with hypertelorism and a prominent beaked or straight nose. Other abnormalities include a high arched palate, low-set ears, high eyebrows, strabismus, ptosis of the upper eyelids, antimongoloid slant of the palpebral fissures, and cryptorchism.

Radiographic Findings [1, 2]

Hand

Thumb: short and broad distal phalanx
comma- or triangle-shaped proximal phalanx (in 35 of 91 patients [1])
abnormal angulation of interphalangeal joint causing radial deviation of thumb
Broad distal phalanges of fingers (in 63 of 114 patients [1])
Brachymesophalangy
Clinodactyly (common)
Delayed skeletal maturation
Syndactyly
Polydactyly

Other Sites

Foot: great toe broad and possibly duplicated
Pelvis: flat acetabular angle
flaring of ilia (small iliac index)
Spine: spina bifida
kyphoscoliosis
lordosis
Skull: high arched palate
wormian bones
Thorax: fusion of ribs
congenital heart defects
sternal anomalies
Urogenital tract: congenital anomalies

Differential Diagnosis

Broad thumbs: acrocephalosyndactyly and acrocephalopolysyndactyly (Sect. 2.1.1)
Leri's pleonosteosis [3]

References

1 Rubinstein JH, Taybi H (1963) Broad thumbs and toes and facial abnormalities. A possible mental retardation syndrome. Am J Dis Child 105:588–608
2 Taybi H, Rubinstein JH (1965) Broad thumbs and toes and unusual facial features. A probable mental retardation syndrome. AJR 92:362–366
3 Rukavinia JG, Falls HF, Holt JF, Block WD (1959) Leri's pleonosteosis. A study of a family with a review of the literature. J Bone Joint Surg 41-A:397–402

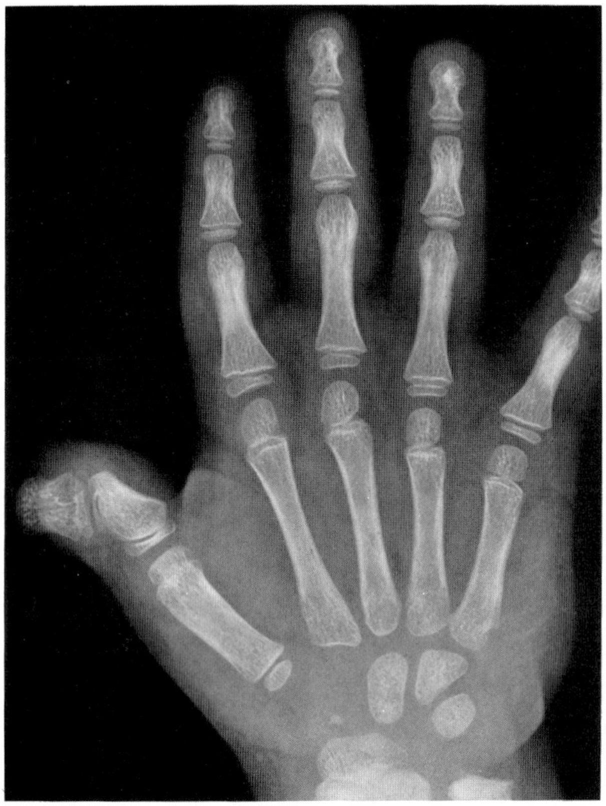

Fig. 1. Rubinstein-Taybi syndrome in a 6-year-old girl. Typical appearance of proximal phalanx of thumb, short and broad distal phalanx. Other distal phalanges also somewhat broadened. Delayed skeletal maturation (corresponding approximately to a normal 4-year-old)

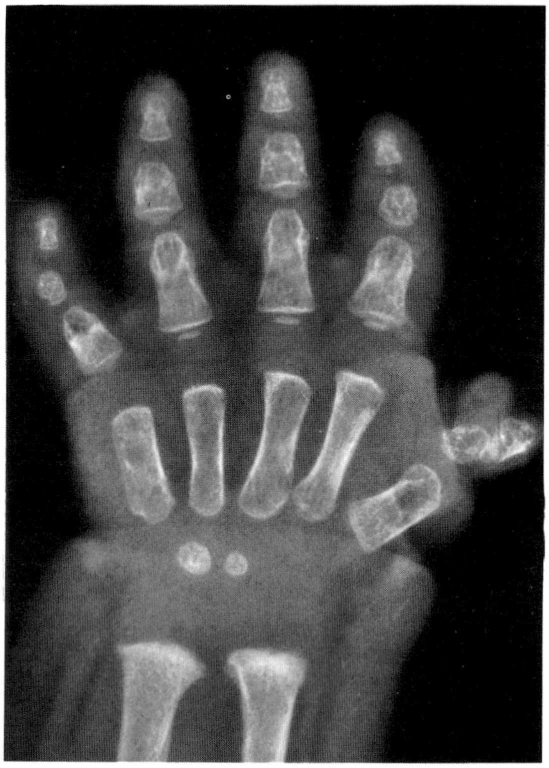

Fig. 2. Rubinstein-Taybi syndrome in a $1\frac{1}{2}$-year-old girl. Both phalanges of the thumb are broad and short. The other digits present brachymesophalangy, including clinodactyly of the fifth finger

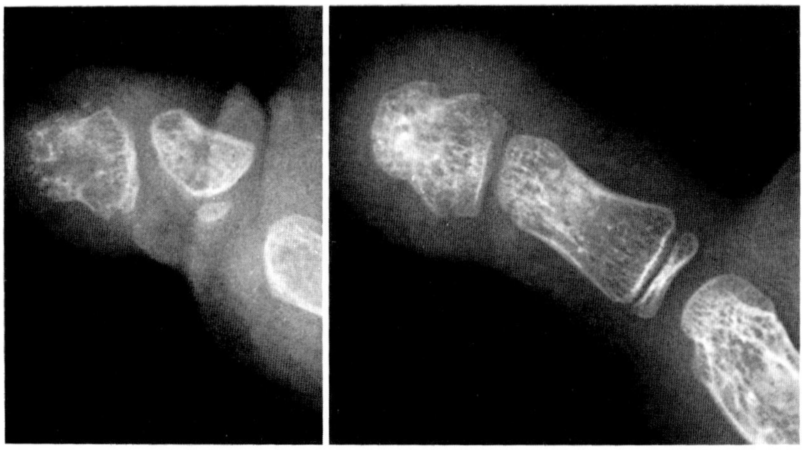

a **b**

Fig. 3a, b. Rubinstein-Taybi syndrome. **a** In a 1-year-old girl: Triangular proximal phalanx, short and broad distal phalanx, radial deviation. **b** In a 4-year-old girl: Proximal phalanx of thumb only slightly abnormal, distal phalanx short and broad

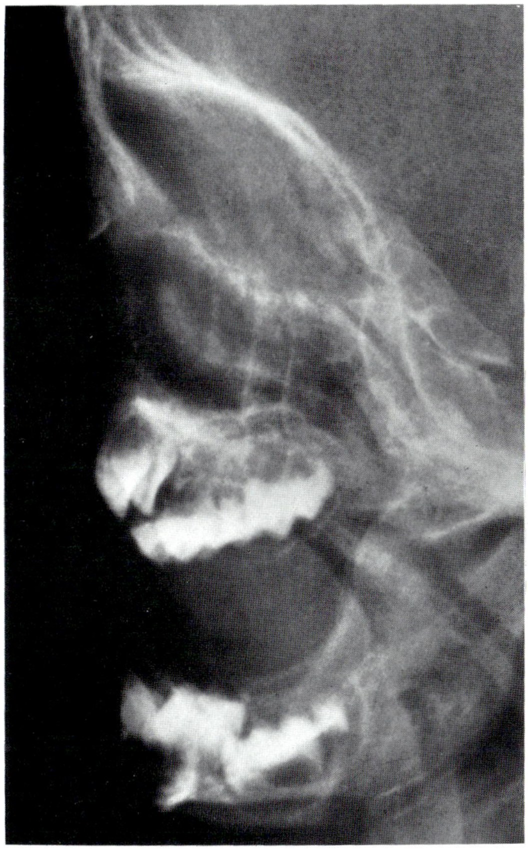

Fig. 4. Same patient as Fig. 2. High arched palate

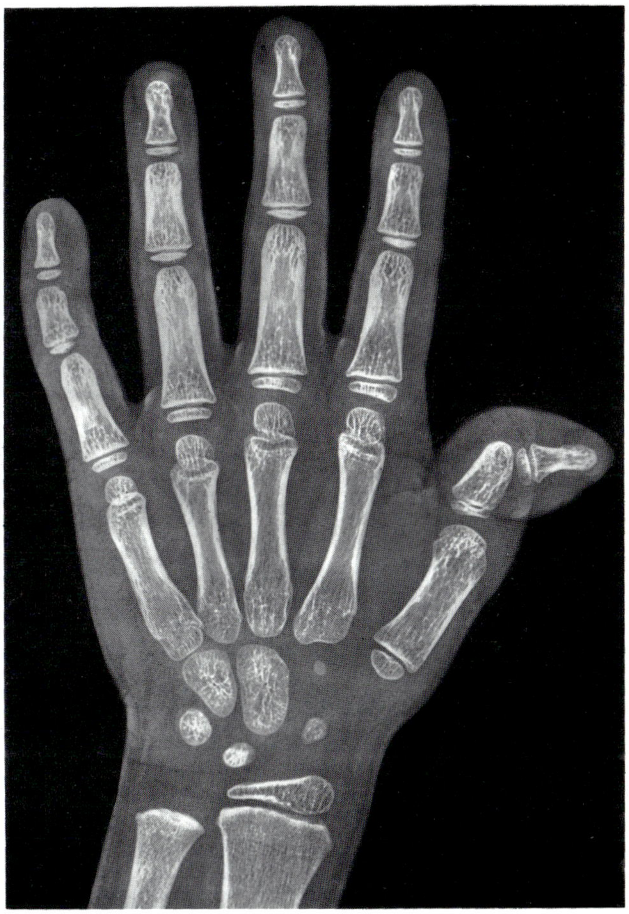

Fig. 5. Thumb abnormality resembling the abnormality found in Rubinstein-Taybi syndrome. In this patient polydactyly of the thumb was the initial finding and one of the distal phalanges was removed

2.2.19 Holt-Oram Syndrome

The Holt-Oram syndrome is a hereditary autosomal dominant disorder with variable expressivity, consisting of upper limb abnormalities, varying from slight to severe radial hypoplasia, and congenital heart defects (mainly atrial and ventricular septal defects and transposition of the great vessels). The abnormalities may be confined to the upper limbs. Besides the hereditary Holt-Oram syndrome, other cardiomelic syndromes can be encountered, such as ventriculoradial dysplasia and congenital radial club hand syndrome with congenital heart disease, in which the association of radial dysplasia and congenital heart disease is characteristic [1–3]. Most cases of these latter syndromes reveal no apparent familial tendency.

Radiographic Findings [1–5]

Hand and Forearm
Radial dysplasia
Carpals: abnormal scaphoid
  carpal fusion
  accessory carpals (os centrale carpi)
Thumb: aplasia or hypoplasia
  triphalangism
Long and slender first metacarpal
Clinodactyly
Brachymesophalangy

Other Sites
Shoulder: rotation of scapula
  short and angulated clavicles

Differential Diagnosis

Radial dysplasia (Sect. 2.2.1)
Abnormalities of carpals (Sect. 2.2.6)
Abnormalities of thumb (Sect. 2.2.11)
Brachydactyly (Sect. 2.2.11)

References

1 Poznanski AK, Stern AM, Gall JC Jr (1971) Skeletal anomalies in genetically determined congenital heart disease. Radiol Clin North Am 9:435–458
2 Holmes LB (1965) Congenital heart disease and upper extremity deformities: a report of two families. N Engl J Med 272:437–444
3 Poznanski AK, Gall JC Jr, Stern AM (1970) Skeletal manifestations of the Holt-Oram syndrome. Radiology 94:45–53
4 Chang CH (1967) Holt-Oram syndrome. Radiology 88:479–483
5 Poznanski AK, Holt JF (1971) The carpals in congenital malformation syndromes. AJR 112:443–448

Fig. 1a, b. Holt-Oram syndrome. **a** In a 6-year-old girl: Atrial septal defect, long and slender first metacarpal, triphalangeal thumb, clinodactyly of fifth finger. **b** In a 13-year-old boy: Ventricular septal defect, os centrale carpi, abnormally shaped scaphoid and trapezium, brachymesophalangy of second and fifth fingers, rather slender first metacarpal ▷

Fig. 2a, b. Holt-Oram syndrome or ventriculoradial dysplasia in a 9-year-old girl. Atrial and ventricular septal defects. **a** The left hand presents severe radial dysplasia with aplasia of the thumb and the radius. A "new thumb" has been made by transplantation of the second finger. **b** In the right hand a hypoplastic thumb is associated with an abnormal arrangement of the carpals ▷

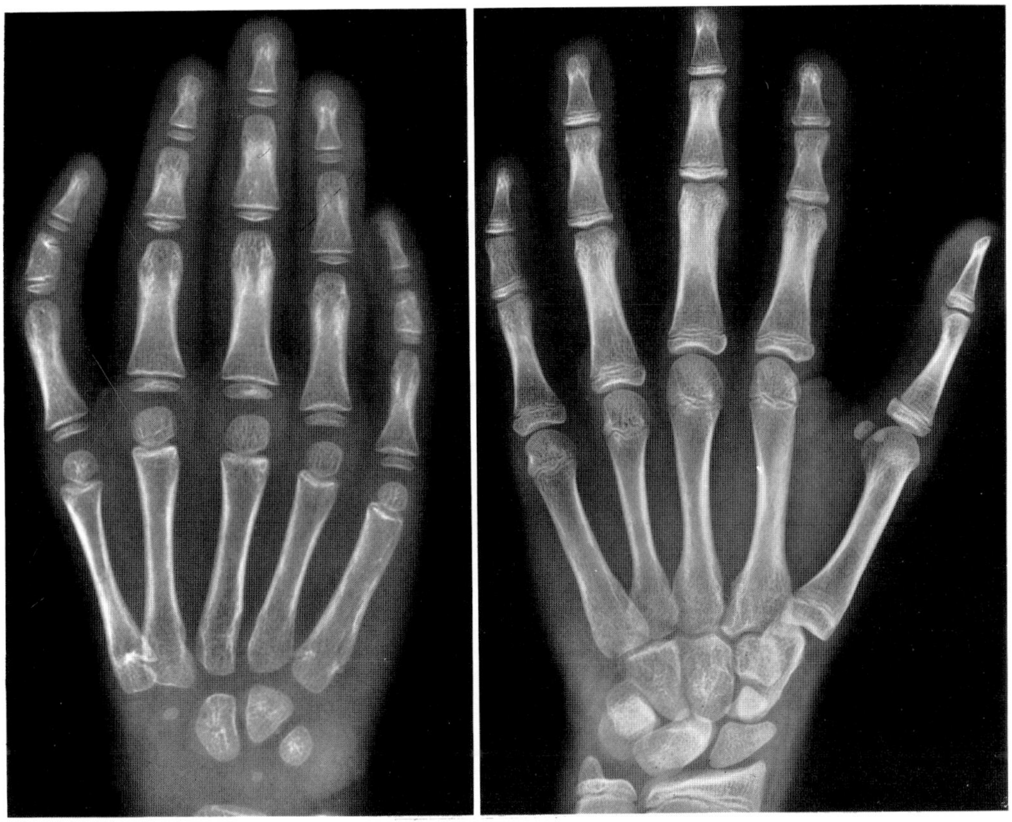

1a b

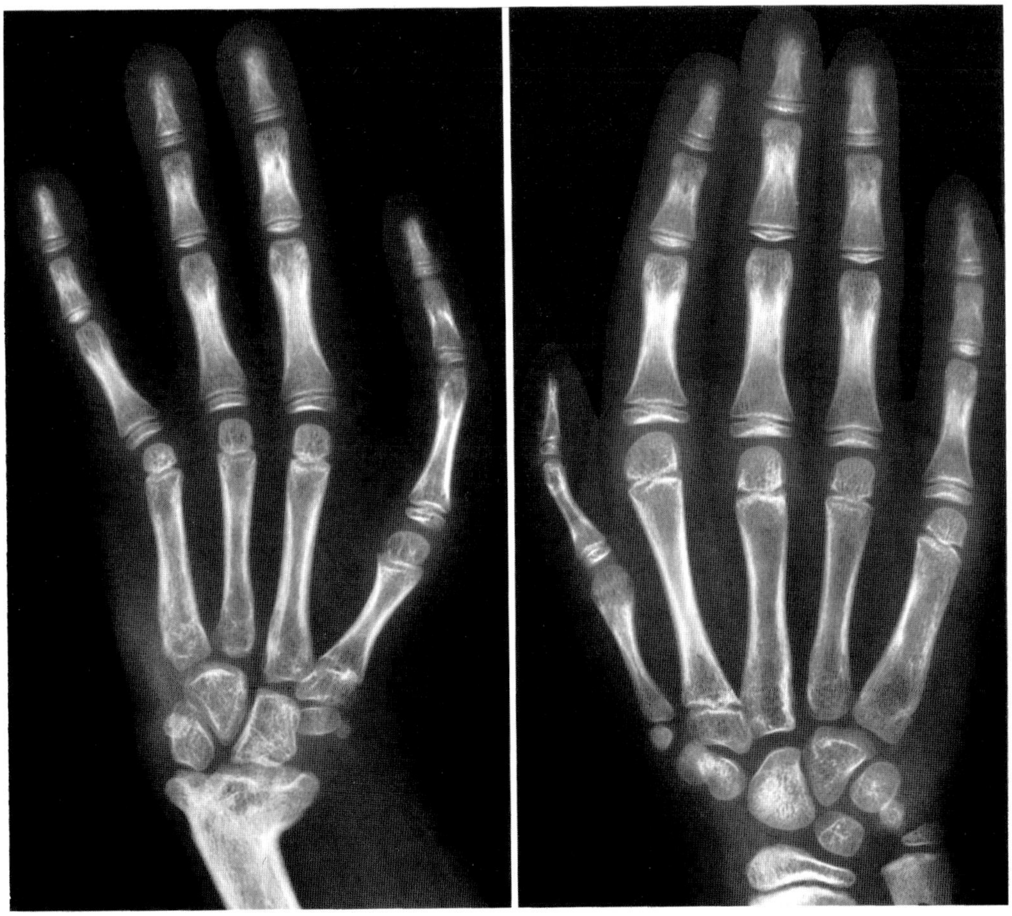

2a b

3 Idiopathic Osteolyses

3.1 Phalangeal Acro-Osteolysis

3.1.1 Hadju-Cheney Syndrome

Hadju-Cheney syndrome is a rare and autosomal dominant disorder with clinical manifestation in the second decade of life. Progressive clubbing of the fingers and toes and resorption of the terminal phalanges are associated with a number of abnormalities in other parts of the skeleton. In some cases, the middle and proximal phalanges and even the distal ends of the metacarpals and metatarsals may also be involved [1, 2].

Radiographic Findings [1, 2]

Hand
Soft tissue swelling (clubbing of fingers)
Osteoporosis
Osteolysis (resorption)
  tufts
  occasional involvement of middle and proximal phalanges, distal ends of metacarpals

Other Sites
Foot: abnormalities similar to those in hand
Skull: wormian bones
  basilar impression
  premature loss of permanent dentition
Spine: osteoporosis
  compression fractures
  kyphosis
Long tubular bones: osteoporosis
  increased tendency to fractures
  hypermobile joints

Differential Diagnosis

Pyknodysostosis [3] (Sect. 1.2.3)
Other conditions involving acro-osteolysis (Sect. 3.1.2 below)

3.1.2 Other Conditions Involving Acro-Osteolysis

One Digit

Osteomyelitis (Sect. 7.3.3)
Bone tumors
  epidermoid cyst (Sect. 7.4.3.2)
  chondroma (Sect. 7.4.1.3)
  glomus tumor
Traumatic amputation

Multiple Digits

Hyperparathyroidism (Sect. 6.2.3)
Scleroderma (Sect. 7.6.3)
Cleidocranial dysplasia (Sect. 1.1.8)
Raynaud's phenomenon (Sect. 7.6.3)
Psoriatic arthritis (Sect. 7.3.6)
Rheumatoid arthritis (Sect. 7.3.4)
Gout (Sect. 7.3.8)
Leprosy (Sect. 7.3.10)
Chemical damage
Pachydermoperiostitis (Sect. 1.2.8) [4]
Syringomyelia (Sect. 7.6.5)
Amniotic bands (Sect. 2.2.4) [5]
Sarcoidosis (Sect. 7.3.12)
Idiopathic multicentric osteolysis [6]
Sjögren's syndrome
Frostbite (Sect. 7.6.2)
Insensitivity to pain [7]
Rothmund's syndrome [8]
Pseudoxanthoma elasticum [9]
Osteopetrosis (Sect. 1.2.2) [10]
Epidermolysis bullosa [11]
Progeria [12]
Pyknodysostosis (Sect. 1.2.3) [3]
Polyvinylchloride exposure
Congenital porphyria [13]
Keratosis palmaris [14]
Guitar player's acro-osteolysis [15]

References

1 Cheney WD (1965) Acroosteolysis. AJR 94:595–607
2 Vanék TJ (1978) Idiopathische Osteolyse von Hadju-Cheney. Fortschr Geb Röntgenstr Nuklearmed Ergänzungsband 128:75–79
3 Muthukrishnan N, Shetty MVK (1972) Pycnodysostosis. AJR 114:247–252
4 Harbison JB, Nice CM (1971) Familial pachydermoperiostosis presenting as an acromegalylike syndrome. AJR 112:532–536
5 Baker CJ, Rudolph AJ (1971) Congenital ring constrictions and intrauterine amputations. Am J Dis Child 121:393–400
6 De Smet AA (1980) Acroosteolysis occurring in a patient with idiopathic multicentric osteolysis. Skeletal Radiol 5:29–34
7 Siegelman SS, Heimann WG, Manin MC (1966) Congenital indifference to pain. AJR 97:242–247
8 Maurer RM, Langford OL (1967) Rothmund's syndrome. A cause of resorption of phalangeal tufts and dystrophic calcification. Radiology 89:706–708
9 James AE Jr, Eaton SB, Blazek JV, Donner MW, Reeves RJ (1969) Roentgen findings in pseudoxanthoma elasticum (PXE). AJR 106:642–647
10 Moss AA, Mainzer F (1970) Osteopetrosis: an unusual cause of terminal-tuft erosion. Radiology 97:631–632
11 Brinn LB, Khilnani MT (1967) Epidermolysis bullosa with characteristic hand deformities. Radiology 89:272–274
12 Margolin FR, Steinbach HL (1968) Progeria, Hutchinson-Gilford syndrome. AJR 103:173–178
13 Small P, Dickson R (1970) The radiological features of congenital porphyria. Br J Radiol 43:732–734
14 Schlansky R, Kucer KA, De Horatius RJ, Abruzzo JL, Schmukler NM (1981) Arthritis and distal tuft resorption associated with keratosis palmaris et plantaris. Arthritis Rheum 24:726–728
15 Destouet JM, Murphy WA (1981) Guitar player acroosteolysis. Skeletal Radiol 6:275–277

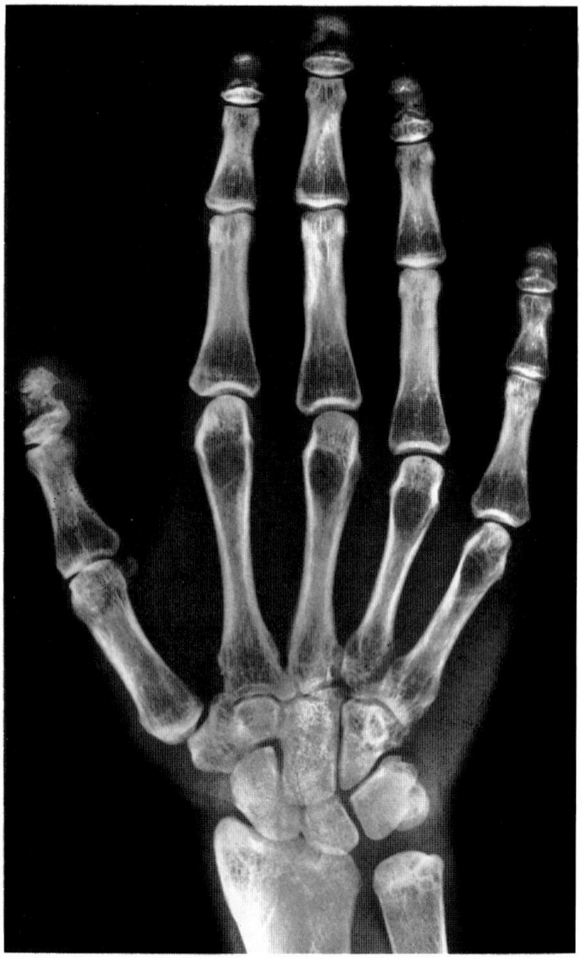

Fig. 1. Hadju-Cheney syndrome in a 26-year-old woman. Typical osteolysis of tufts, diminished number of trabeculae in metaphyses of tubular bones

Fig. 2a–c. Same patient as Fig. 1. **a** Osteolysis of distal phalanx of great toe, fractured fourth metatarsal, osteoporosis of tubular bones in foot. **b** Osteoporosis at knee joint. **c** Compression fractures in vertebral bodies ▷

Fig. 3a–j. Phalangeal acro-osteolysis. **a** Pyknodysostosis; **b** pachydermoperiostosis; **c** traumatic amputation; **d** epidermoid cyst; **e** Raynaud's phenomenon; **f** scleroderma; **g** secondary hyperparathyroidism; **h** after meningococcal sepsis; **i** leprosy; **j** after burning with hydrochloric acid

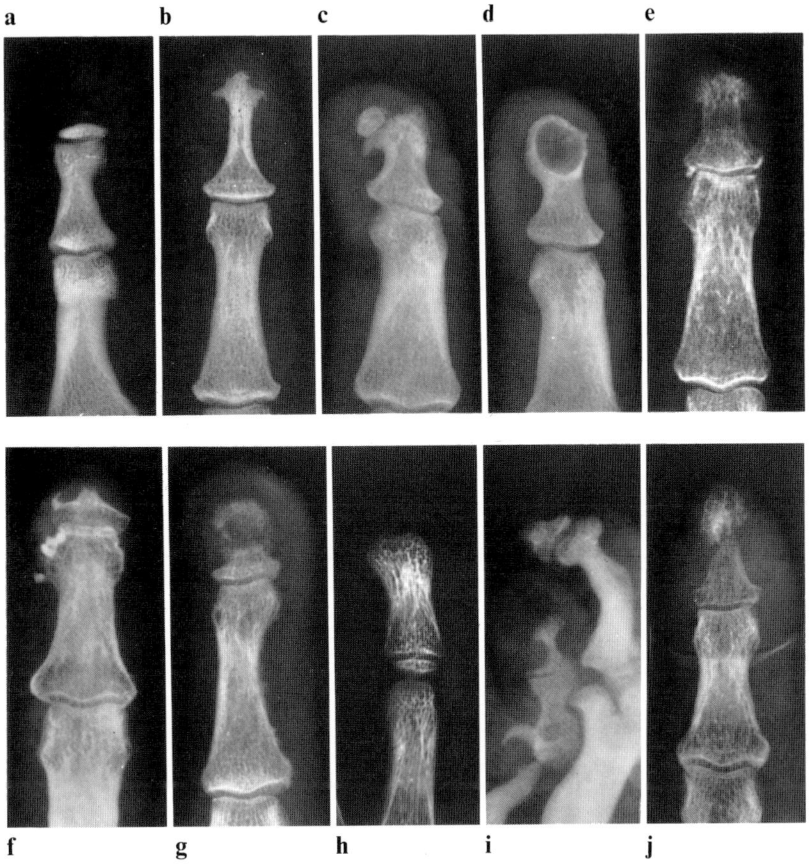

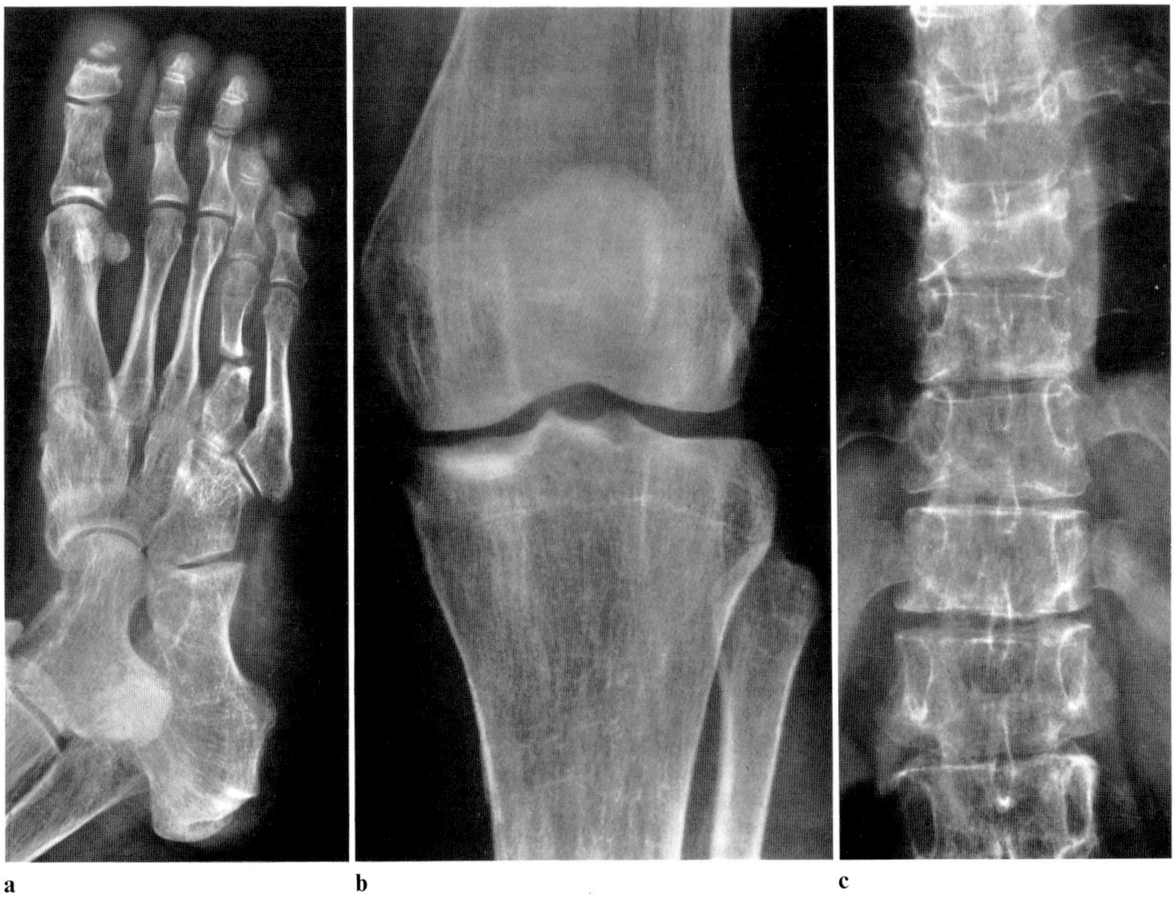

3.2 Carpotarsal Osteolysis

Osteolysis of both the carpals and tarsals may be:

1. Associated with nephropathy, without a family history [1]
2. A hereditary disorder (autosomal dominant or autosomal recessive) [2–5]
3. Caused by miscellaneous disorders [6, 7]

Carpotarsal osteolysis is probably a result of a disturbed metabolism of the connective tissue which generates a highly inflammatory state with hyperemia. An arthritic period in early childhood is usually the first clinical manifestation. Progressive painless osteolysis of the carpals and tarsals follows. The osteolysis is usually bilateral and stops in the third decade of life [1–3].

Radiographic Findings

Hand

Osteolysis of carpals
Partial osteolysis of metacarpals, radius, and ulna
Demineralization
Advanced skeletal maturation prior to osteolysis (caused by hyperemia)
Long and slender phalanges

Other Sites

Foot: findings similar to those in hand
pes cavus, hammer toes, overlapping toes
plantar cysts
Skull: oval shape
micrognathia
frontal bossing
Miscellaneous: bone destruction of large joints
osteoporosis
scoliosis
Marfan-like habitus

References

1 Torg JS, Steel HH (1968) Essential osteolysis with nephropathy. A review of the literature and case report of an unusual syndrome. J Bone Joint Surg 50-A:1629–1634
2 Amin PH, Evans ANW (1978) Essential osteolysis of carpal and tarsal bones. Br J Radiol 51:539–543
3 Tyler T, Rosenbaum HD (1976) Idiopathic multicentric osteolysis. AJR 126:23–27
4 Gluck J, Miller JJ (1972) Familial osteolysis of the carpal and tarsal bones. J Pediatr 81:506–510
5 Kohler E, Babbitt D, Huizenga B, Good TA (1973) Hereditary osteolysis. A clinical, radiological and chemical study. Radiology 108:99–105
6 Winchester P, Grossman H, Wan Ngo Lim, Shannon DB (1969) A new acid mucopolysaccharidosis with skeletal deformities simulating rheumatoid arthritis. AJR 106:121–128
7 Mathias K, Ludwig U (1977) Idiopathische multizentrische Osteolyse mit Kranio-Dysplasie und Schwachsinn: ein neues Syndrom? Fortschr Geb Röntgenstr Nuklearmed Ergänzungsband 127:255–261

Fig. 1a, b. Carpotarsal osteolysis in an 8-year-old boy: both hands. **a** Left hand: The carpals are all absent. Distinct osteolysis of second to fifth metacarpals, osteolysis of ulna, probably some osteolysis of radius. **b** Right hand: Same radiographic findings ▷

Fig. 2. Same patient as Fig. 1 at 11 years of age. Left hand: Progressive osteolysis at proximal ends of metacarpals, deformation of proximal interphalangeal joint and cyst-like translucency in proximal epiphysis of second finger, long and slender phalanges, demineralization of skeleton ▷

Fig. 3a, b. Same patient as Fig. 1 at 8 years of age. Destruction of the tarsals. The metatarsals are not affected

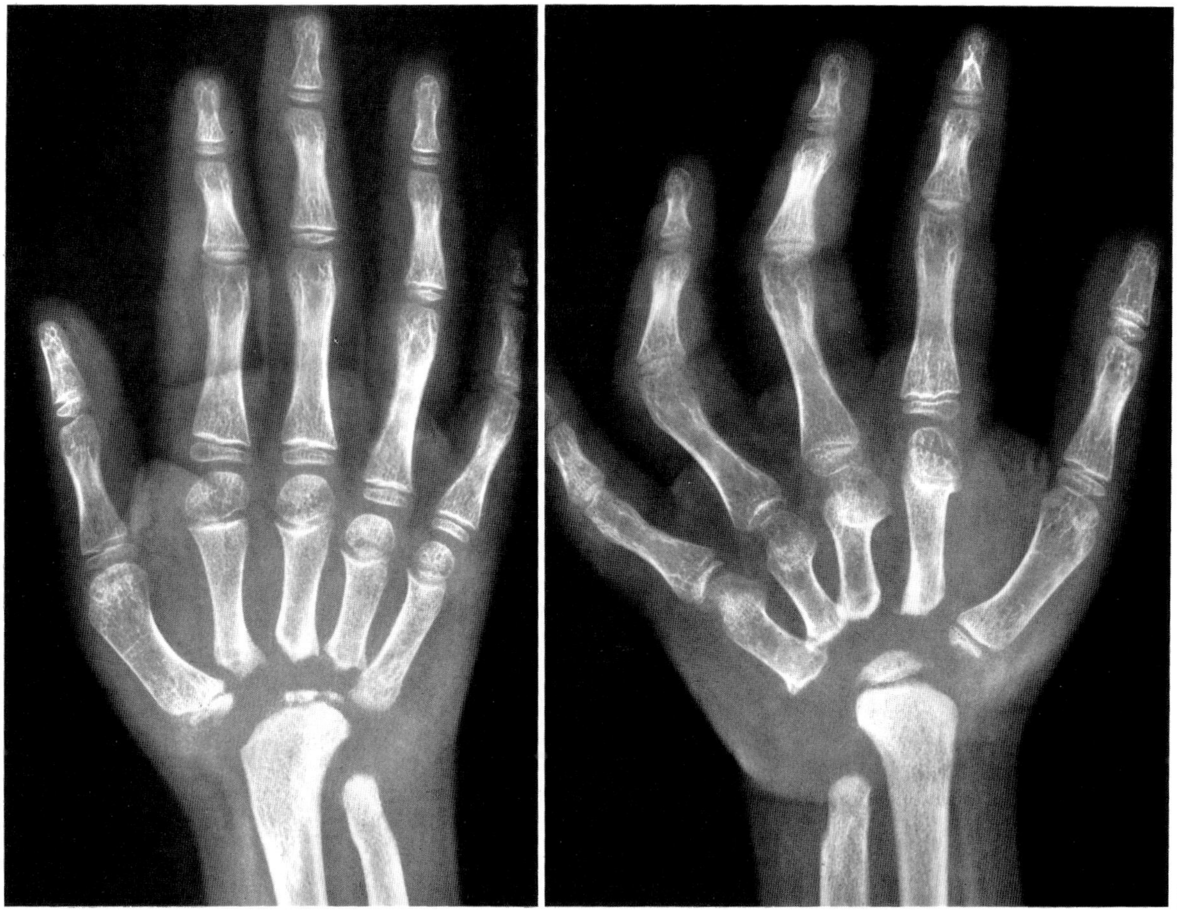

1a b

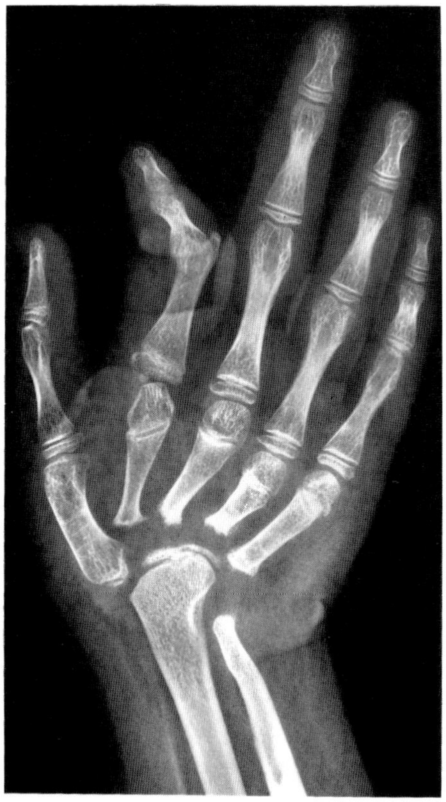

2

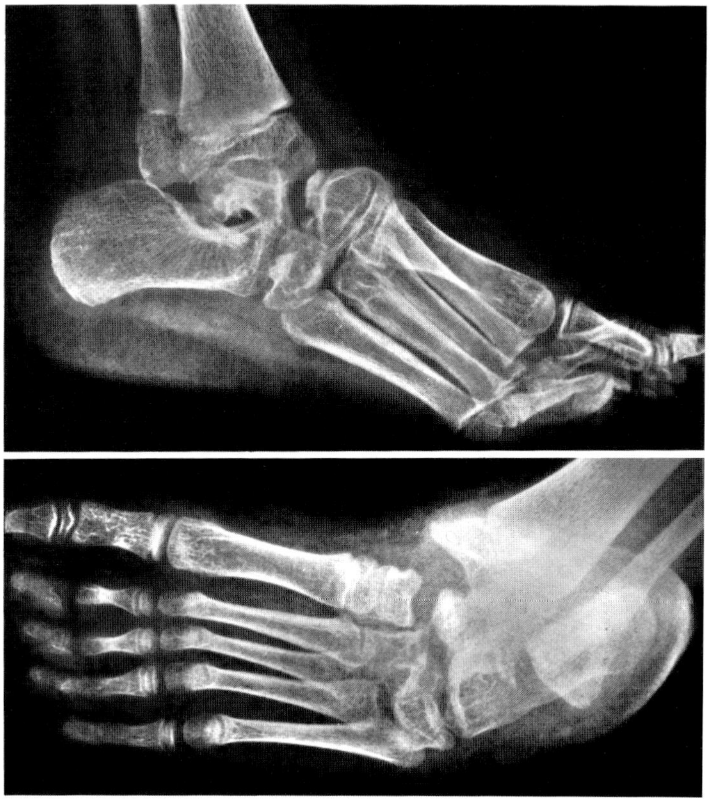

a b

3

4 Chromosomal Aberrations

4.1 Trisomy 18 Syndrome

Synonym: Edwards' syndrome

After mongolism, trisomy 18 is the second most common syndrome of multiple abnormalities [1]. It is usually caused by a full trisomy of the number 18 chromosome. A large variety of abnormalities may be found [1–3]:

Head: psychomotor retardation
  micrognathia
  high arched palate
  low-set ears
  prominent occiput
Thorax: short sternum
  congenital heart disease (ventricular septal disease, patent ductus arteriosis)
  diaphragmatic hernia
Gastrointestinal tract: intestinal malrotation
  heterotopia of pancreatic tissue
Urogenital tract: renal anomalies
Pelvis: congenital dislocation of hips
Hand: flexion deformities of fingers
  specific dermatoglyphic patterns
Foot: rocker-bottom deformity
  short and dorsally flexed big toe

Radiographic Findings [1, 3–6]

Hand

Ulnar deviation of some or all fingers
Gap between second and third fingers
Flexion of fingers, with second and fifth overlapping third and fourth
Short and high-set thumb with ulnar deviation
Hypoplasia of first metacarpal
Delayed skeletal maturation
Small distal phalanges
Radial dysplasia
Clinodactyly of fifth finger
Syndactyly of third and fourth fingers (rare)

Other Sites

Foot: rocker-bottom deformity
  short big toe
  deviation of toes
  hypoplasia of distal phalanges
Skull: prominent occiput
  hypoplasia of facial bones
  high arched palate
Thorax: thin and hypoplastic ribs
  congenital heart disease
Pelvis: congenital dislocation of hips

Differential Diagnosis

Other disorders with radial dysplasia (Sect. 2.2.1)
Arthrogryposis multiplex congenita (Sect. 7.1.1)

References

1 Steinbach HL, Gold RH, Preger L (1975) Roentgen appearance of the hand in diffuse disease. Year Book, Medical Publishers, Chicago
2 Temtamy SA, McKusick VA (1978) The genetics of hand malformations. Liss, New York
3 Poznanski AK (1984) The hand in radiologic diagnosis. Saunders, Philadelphia
4 James AE Jr, Belcourt CL, Atkins L, Janower ML (1969) Trisomy 18. Radiology 92:37–43
5 Robinson AE, Parry WH, Blizard EB (1971) Mosaic trisomy 18. A case report with some unusual radiographic features. Radiology 100:379–380
6 Ozonoff MB, Steinbach HL, Manunes P (1964) The trisomy 18 syndrome. AJR 91:618–628

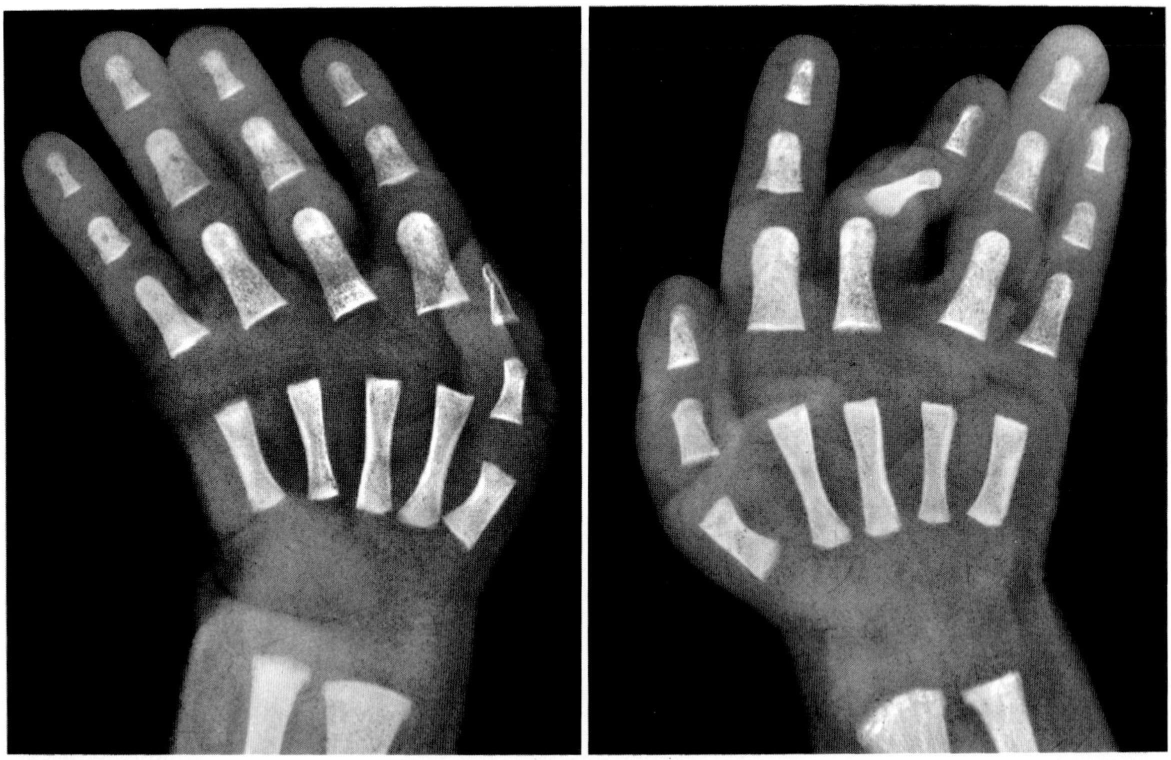

1a b

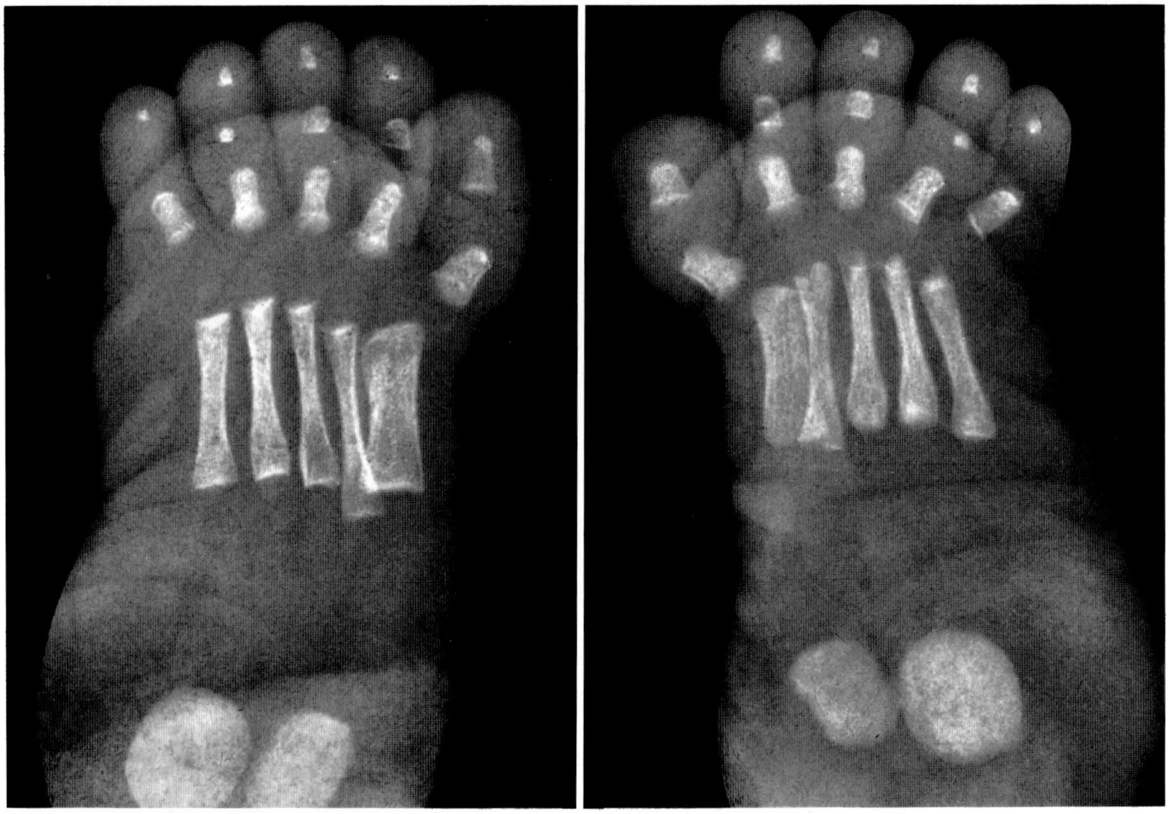

2a b

Fig. 1a, b. Trisomy 18 syndrome in a 2-day-old boy. Short first metacarpals in both hands with ulnar deviation of fingers, particularly in left hand (**a**). In right hand (**b**) third finger is abnormally flexed and overlies fourth finger

Fig. 2a, b. Same patient as Fig. 1. Soft tissue thickening of both feet, big toes short and dorsally flexed. Deviation of other toes most obviously present in right foot (**b**)

4.2 Trisomy 21

Synonyms: mongolism, Down's syndrome, G trisomy

In the great majority of patients with trisomy 21 an extra 21st chromosome is present, but in some patients a translocation or a mosaic chromosomal pattern may be found. The clinical severity is variable. Facial appearance is characteristic, mental retardation is present, and congenital heart disease is encountered in about 50% of sufferers.

Radiographic Findings [1–6]

Hand

Some shortening of tubular bones
Short middle phalanx of fifth finger
Clinodactyly in approximately 50% of cases
Delayed skeletal maturation (disharmonic maturation of carpals)
Small scaphoid
Increased carpal angle

Other Sites

Skull: thin calvarium
 hypoplasia of facial bones
 hypotelorism
 hypoplasia of frontal sinuses
 persistent metopic suture
 high arched palate
 abnormal dentition
Spine: atlantoaxial instability
 cuboid vertebral bodies
 relative increase in height of lumbar vertebral bodies
Pelvis: flattened acetabular roofs
 flared iliac wings
 reduction of iliac index
Thorax: 11 pair of ribs

Differential Diagnosis

Other conditions with: clinodactyly (Sect. 2.2.11)
 brachydactyly (Sect. 2.2.11)
 delayed skeletal maturation

References

1 Hefke HW (1940) Roentgenologic study of anomalies of the hands in one hundred cases of mongolism. Am J Dis Child 60:1319–1323
2 Roche AF (1964) Skeletal maturation rates in mongolism. AJR 91:979–987
3 Caffey J, Ross S (1958) Pelvic bones in infantile mongoloidism. Roentgenographic features. AJR 80:458–467
4 Martel W, Tischler JM (1966) Observations on the spine in mongoloidism. AJR 97:630–638
5 Poznanski AK (1984) The hand in radiologic diagnosis. Saunders Philadelphia
6 Willich E, Fuhr U, Kroll W (1977) Die Skeletveränderungen beim Down-Syndrom. Korrelation röntgenologischer und zytogenetischer Befunde. Fortschr Geb Röntgenstr Nuklearmed Ergänzungsband 127:135–142

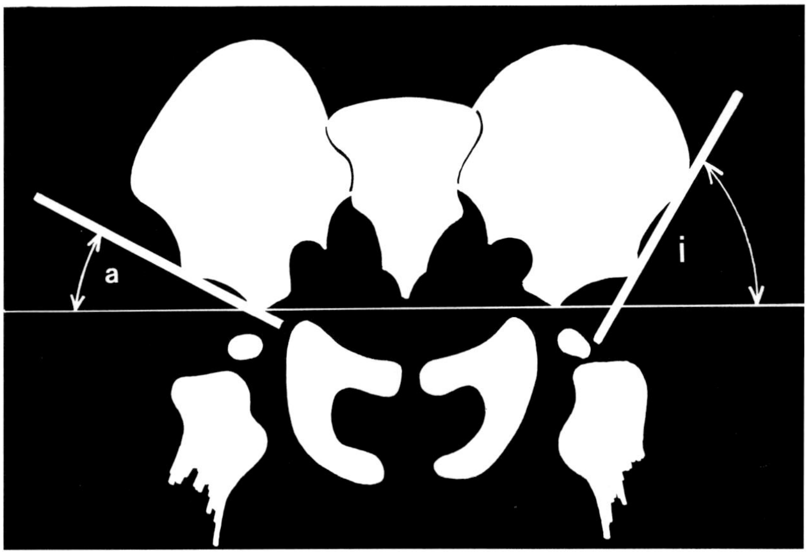

Fig. 1. Iliac index in young mongoloid infants and in normal infants. Iliac index = both acetabular angles (a) + both iliac angles (i)/2. Mongolism: 49°–80° (average 60°); normal: 65°–97° (average 81°) Modified from Caffey and Ross [3]

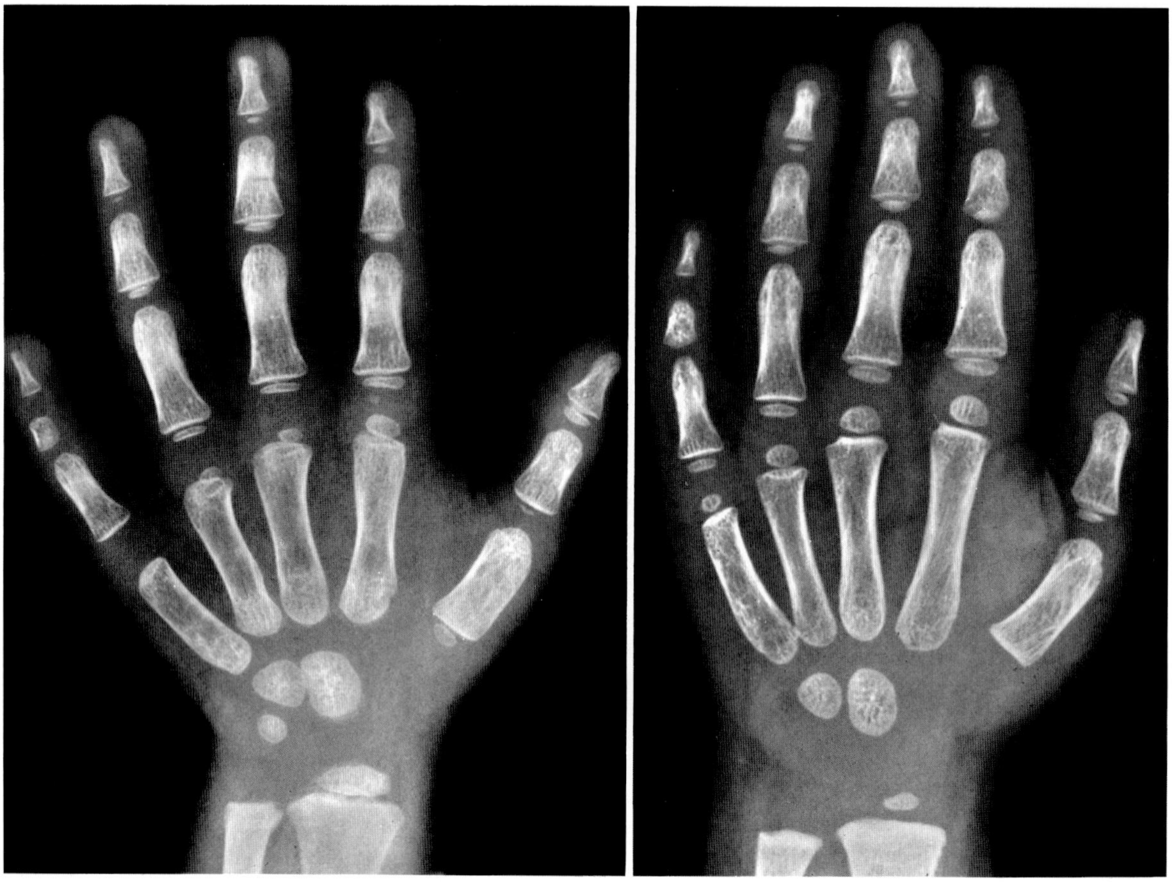

a b

Fig. 2a, b. Trisomy 21. a In **a** 4-year-old boy: Distinct shortening of middle phalanx of fifth finger, delayed skeletal maturation (corresponding to a normal 3-year-old), shortening of all other tubular bones. **b** In another 4-year-old boy: Tubular bones only slightly shortened, except middle phalanx of fifth finger. Delayed skeletal maturation (corresponding to a normal 2-year-old)

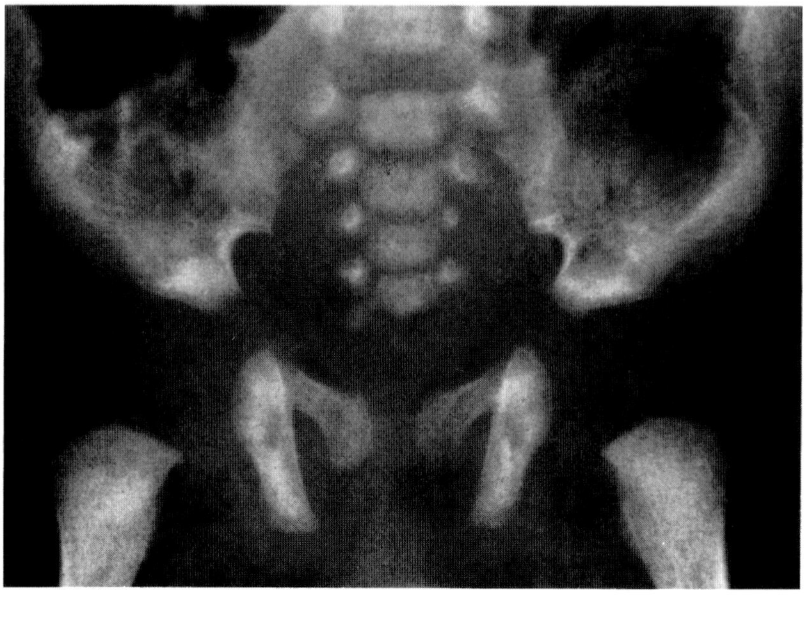

Fig. 3. Trisomy 21 in a 2-week-old boy. Flat acetabular roofs. Iliac index 51° (average in normal individuals 81°)

4.3 Turner's Syndrome

Turner's syndrome is a malformation syndrome characterized by complete or partial absence of a second X chromosome. In the classic syndrome a 45 XO chromosomal pattern is found, but in many patients mosaic types of chromosomal patterns are present. The clinical expression of Turner's syndrome shows great variability. There is agenesis or dysgenesis of the ovaries and the uterus remains in an infantile stage of development. Webbing of the neck, cubitus valgus, and short stature are other classic findings. Renal tract anomalies and congenital heart defects are also commonly encountered.

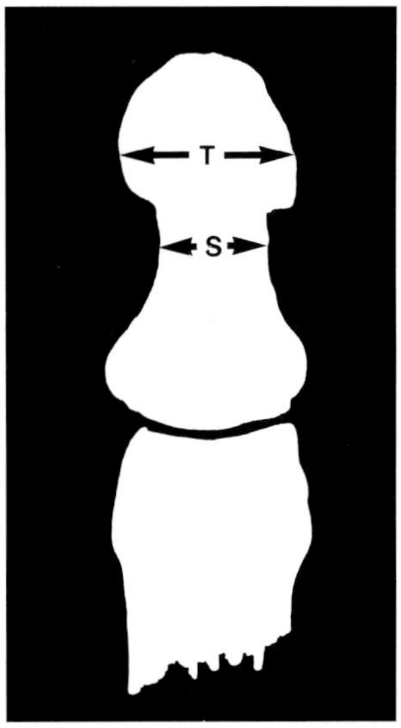

Fig. 1. Tuft-to-shaft ratio. Normal 1.3:1 (SD 0.17); Turner's syndrome > 1.7:1. *T*, tuft; *S* shaft. Modified from Kosowicz [12]

Radiographic Findings [1–5]

Hand

Short fourth metacarpal (metacarpal sign)
Osteoporosis
Delayed skeletal maturation, especially delayed epiphyseal fusion
Drumstick appearance of distal phalanges (tuft-to-shaft ratio > 1.7:1 [1])
Carpal fusion
Reduced carpal angle
Madelung's deformity
Occasionally: short fifth metacarpal
clinodactyly of fifth finger

Other Sites

Foot: short fourth metatarsal
Major joints: deformities of the medial femoral and tibial condyles of knee
cubitus valgus
Spine: developmental anomalies of cervical spine (odontoid, atlas)
kyphosis
scoliosis
Heart: coarctation
aortic stenosis
anomalous pulmonary venous return
dextrocardia
atrial septal defect
aortic aneurysm
Kidneys: horseshoe kidney
duplication

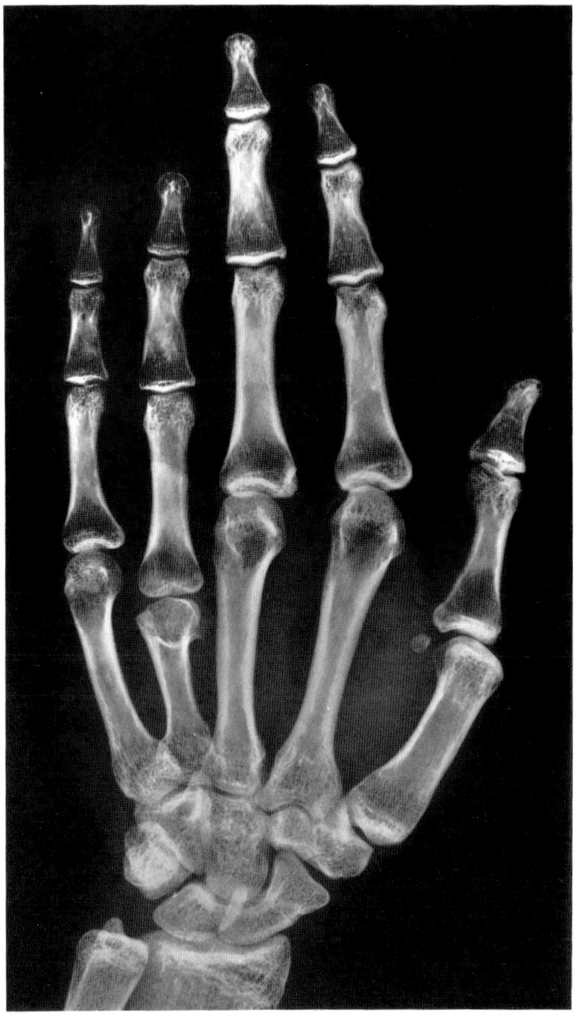

Fig. 2. Turner's syndrome in a 19-year-old woman. Severe shortening of fourth metacarpal. Carpal angle 120° (normal 129.6° ± 8.7°). The tuft-to-shaft ratio of the third and fourth distal phalanges is 1.6:1

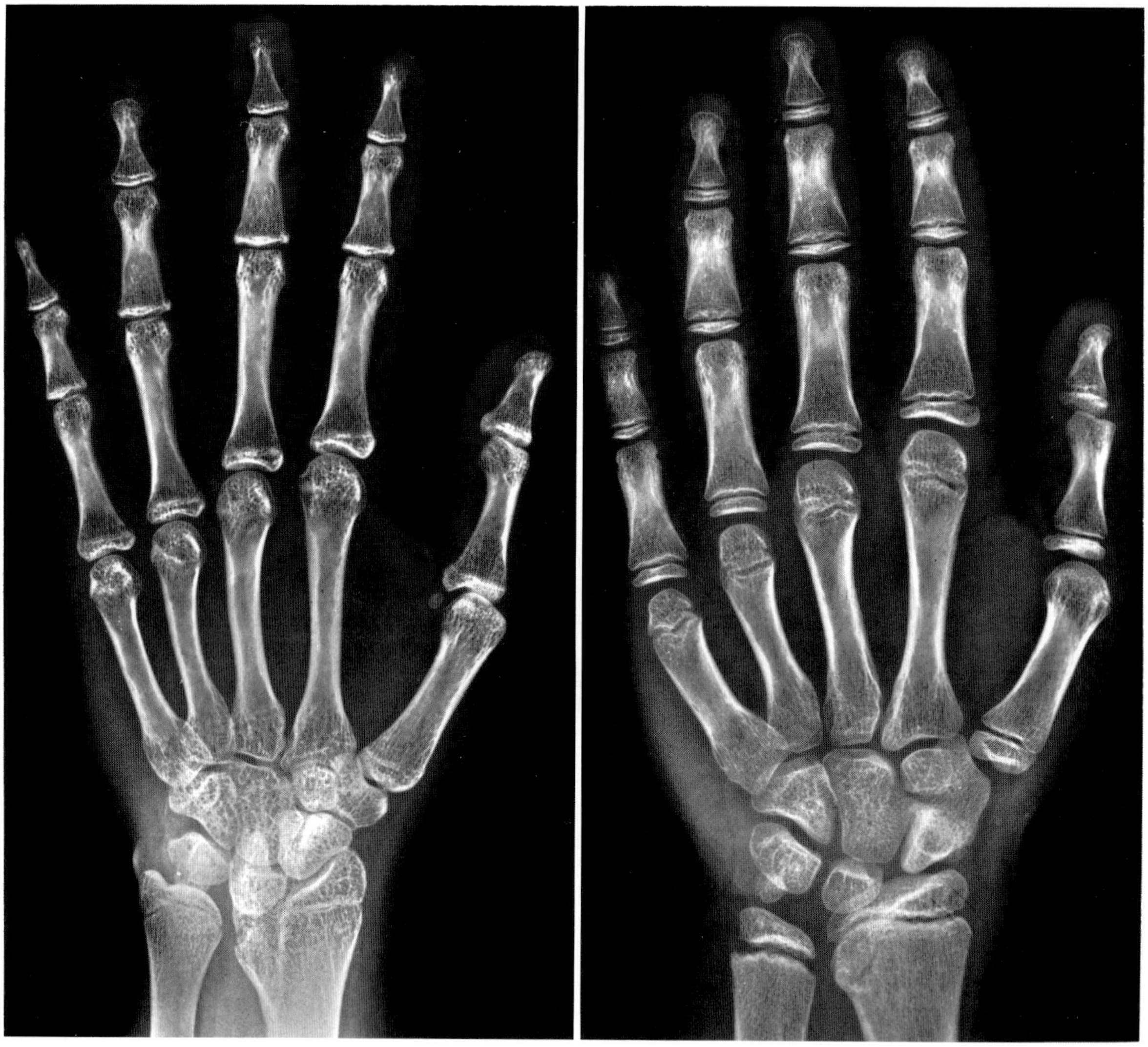

a b

Fig. 3a, b. Turner's syndrome. **a** In an 18-year-old woman: Madelung's deformity, somewhat shortened fourth metacarpal bone, abnormal arrangement of carpals in proximal row. Carpal angle 112°. **b** In a 13-year-old girl. Abnormal bone structure in radial metaphysis associated with scaphoid-trapezium fusion. Carpal angle 130°. Delayed skeletal maturation (corresponding approximately to a normal 10-year-old child)

Differential Diagnosis

Noonan's syndrome [6, 7]
Carpal fusion (Sect. 2.2.7)
Short fourth metacarpal (Sect. 2.2.11)
Madelung's deformity (Sect. 2.2.8)

References

1 Kosowicz J (1965) The roentgen appearance of the hand and wrist in gonadal dysgenesis. AJR 93:354–361
2 Steinbach HL, Gold RH, Preger L (1975) Roentgen appearance of the hand in diffuse disease. Year Book Medical Publishers Chicago
3 Baker DK, Berdon WE, Morishima A, Conte F (1967) Turner's syndrome and pseudo-Turner's syndrome. AJR 100:40–47
4 Finby N, Archibald RM (1963) Skeletal abnormalities associated with gonadal dysgenesis. AJR 89:1222–1235
5 Poznanski AK, Garn SM, Shaw HA (1976) The carpal angle in the congenital malformation syndromes. Ann Radiol (Paris) 19:141–150
6 Riggs W Jr (1970) Roentgen findings in Noonan's syndrome. Radiology 96:393–396
7 Summitt RL (1969) Turner's syndrome and Noonan's syndrome. J Pediatr 74:155–156

5 Primary Growth Disturbances

5.1 Cornelia de Lange's Syndrome

Synonym: Brachmann-de Lange syndrome

Cornelia de Lange's syndrome is an occasional familial syndrome characterized by severe mental retardation, peculiar facies (low hairline, heavy confluent eyebrows, small upturned nose, micrognathia, wide and downturned upper lip), delayed skeletal maturation, and small hands and feet. Cutaneous syndactyly of the feet, proximal insertion of the thumbs, and clinodactyly are often present. In severe cases, any of the upper extremity bones can be absent. The elbows present flexion deformities or contractures with or without luxation. Hiatus hernia, intestinal malrotation, eye anomalies, cryptorchism, hypospadias, congenital heart disease, hirsutism, and cutis marmorata are other features which have been mentioned.

Radiographic Findings [1–6]

Hand

Radial dysplasia (hypoplasia of first metacarpal, possible complete absence of thumb)
Ulnar dysplasia (hypoplasia or aplasia of fifth finger, clinodactyly very common)
Delayed skeletal maturation
Cone-shaped epiphyses (especially in metacarpals)
Brachymetacarpia
Brachymesophalangy of second finger
Syndactyly
Monodactyly (uncommon)

Other Sites

Foot: small
cutaneous syndactyly of second and third toes
Elbow: hypoplasia and posterior luxation of radial head
bowing of radius and ulna
Skull: microcephaly
brachycephaly
hypoplasia of mandible
high arched palate
Pelvis: small acetabular angles
increased iliac angles
coxa valga
Thorax: rounded thoracic outlet
short sternum
congenital heart disease
Abdomen: hiatus hernia
intestinal duplication
malrotation
pyloric stenosis
inguinal hernia

Differential Diagnosis

Luxation of radial head:
chondroectodermal dysplasia (Sect. 1.1.6)
acrocephalosyndactyly (Apert; Sect. 2.1.1)
Turner's syndrome (Sect. 4.3)
arthrogryposis multiplex congenita (Sect. 7.1.1) [10]
Klinefelter's syndrome [7]
Fanconi's anemia
nail-patella syndrome [8]
Nievergelt's syndrome
Ehlers-Danlos syndrome [9]
Radial dysplasia (Sect. 2.2.1)
Ulnar dysplasia (Sect. 2.2.2)
Clinodactyly (Sect. 2.2.11)

References

1 Steinbach HL, Gold RH, Preger L (1975) Roentgen appearance of the hand in diffuse disease. Year Book Medical Publishers, Chicago
2 Kurlander GJ, Demyer W (1967) Roentgenology of the Brachmann-de Lange syndrome. Radiology 88:101–110
3 Silver HK (1964) The de Lange syndrome. Am J Dis Child 108:523–529
4 Taybi H (1973) Cornelia de Lange syndrome. Semin Roentgenol 8:198–199

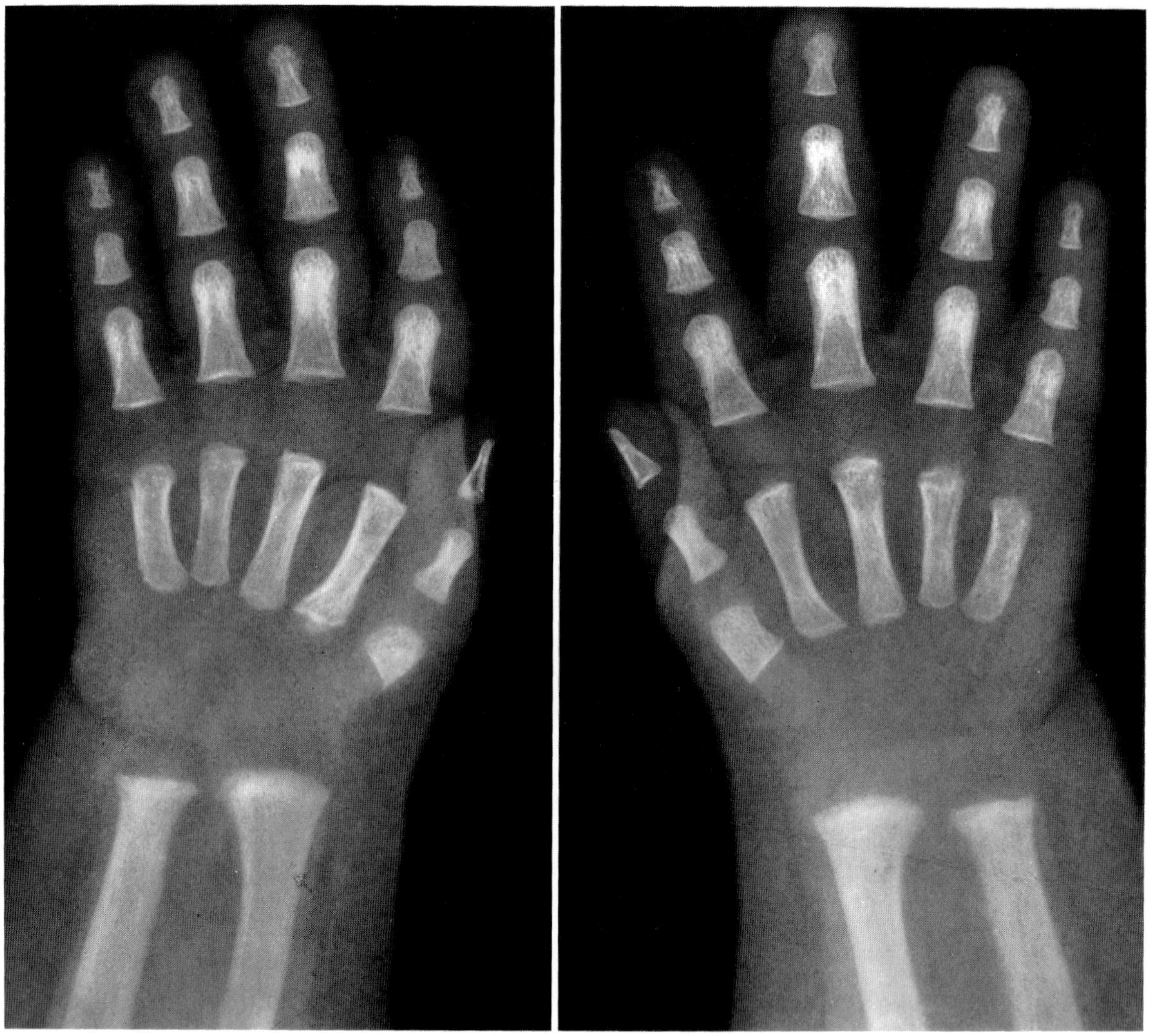

a b

Fig. 1a, b. Cornelia de Lange's syndrome in a 1-year-old boy. Shortening of tubular bones, marked hypoplasia of first metacarpal and some hypoplasia of proximal phalanx of thumb. Delayed skeletal maturation. Brachymesophalangy of second and fifth fingers

5 Lee FA, Kenny FM (1967) Skeletal changes in the Cornelia de Lange syndrome. AJR 100:27–39
6 Gerald B, Udamsky R (1967) The Cornelia de Lange syndrome, radiographic findings. Radiology 88:96–100
7 Almquist EA, Gordon LH, Blue AI (1959) Congenital dislocation of the head of the radius. J Bone Joint Surg 51-A:1118–1127
8 Mino RA, Mino VH, Livingstone RG (1948) Osseous dysplasia and dystrophy of the nails. Review of the literature and report of a case. AJR 60:633–641
9 Hass J, Hass R (1958) Arthrochalasis multiplex congenita. Congenital flaccidity of the joints. J Bone Joint Surg 40-A:663–674
10 Cockshott WP, Omolulu A (1958) Familial congenital posterior dislocation of both radial heads. J Bone Joint Surg 40-A:483–492

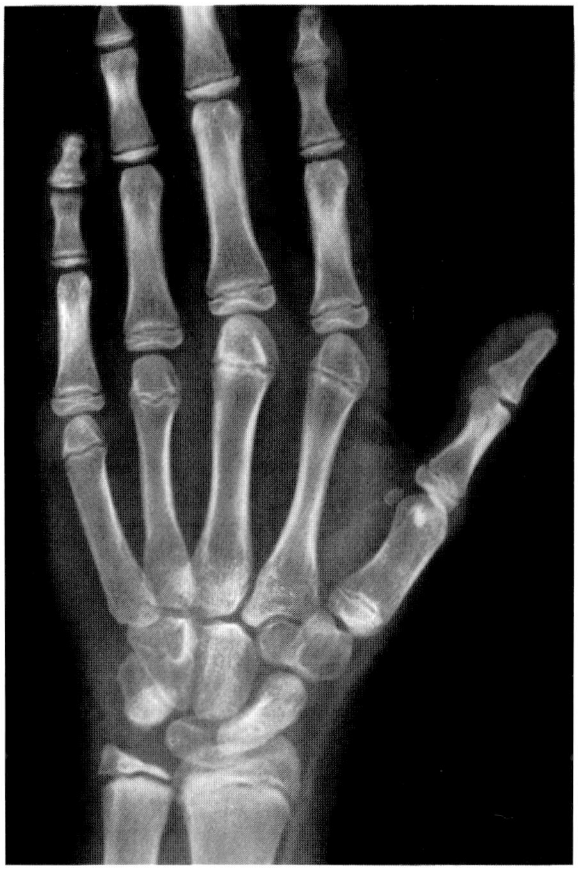

Fig. 2. Cornelia de Lange's syndrome in a 17-year-old male. Brachymesophalangy of second finger and brachytelephalangy of second and fifth fingers, some shortening of first metacarpal. Delayed skeletal maturation

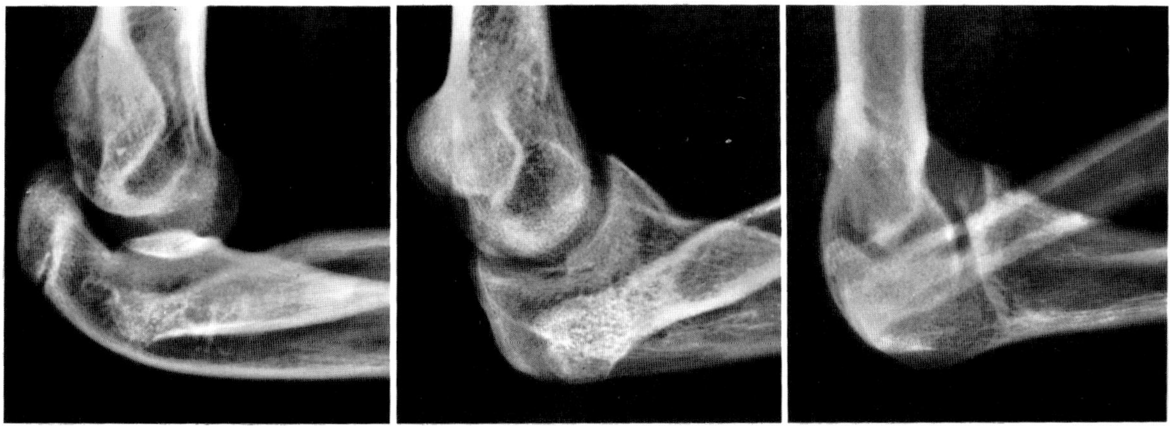

a b c

Fig. 3a–c. Hypoplastic radial head and posterior luxation. **a** Cornelia de Lange's syndrome; **b** nail-patella syndrome; **c** Klinefelter's syndrome

5.2 Marfan's Syndrome

Marfan's syndrome is an autosomal dominant hereditary disorder of the connective tissue. The skeleton, the eyes, and the cardiovascular system are involved. Sufferers may present slender long tubular bones, joint laxity, diminution of the soft tissue, scoliosis, dislocation of the ocular lens, and insufficiency of the aortic valve due to dilatation of the thoracic aorta.

Radiographic Findings [1–3]

Hand

Arachnodactyly without accompanying increase in width
Increased metacarpal index
Flexion deformity of fifth digit

Other Sites

Long tubular bones: slender
premature osteoarthrosis
subluxation
Spine: posterior scalloping (widened neural canal)
thoracolumbar kyphoscoliosis
occasionally: Scheuermann's disease
spondylolysis
Thorax: pectus excavatum
pectus carinatum
dilatation of thoracic aorta
dissecting aneurysm
other congenital heart disease

Differential Diagnosis

Homocystinuria [3, 4], autosomal recessive disease characterized by:
high arched palate
dental abnormalities
protrusion of incisors
large paranasal sinuses
increased metacarpal index
osteoporosis
scoliosis
Ehlers-Danlos syndrome [5]
Multiple endocrine neoplasia syndrome (type II b)

References

1 Parish JG (1960) Heritable disorders of connective tissue. Proc R Soc Med 53:515–518
2 Parish JG (1966) Radiographic measurements of the skeletal structure of the normal hand. Br J Radiol 39:52–62
3 Brenton DP, Dow CJ (1972) Homocystinuria and Marfan's syndrome. A comparison. J Bone Joint Surg 54-B:277–284
4 Hunter KR (1969) Homocystinuria or Marfan's syndrome. Lancet 1:842–849
5 Beighton P, Thomas ML (1969) The radiology of Ehlers-Danlos syndrome. Clin Radiol 20:354–359

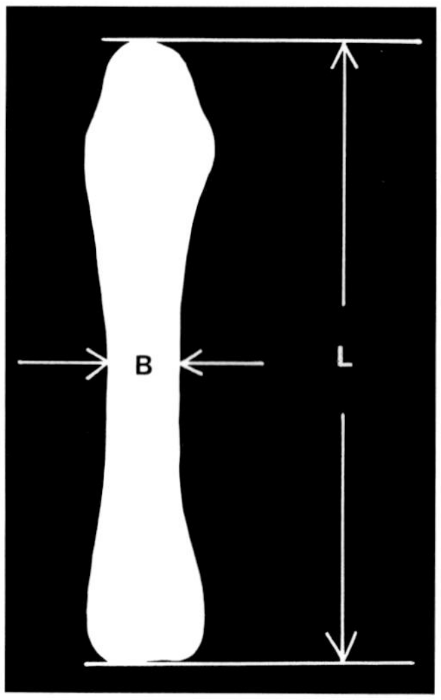

Fig. 1. Relative slenderness (RS).

$$\text{RS} = \frac{\text{length } (L)}{\text{breadth at midpoint } (B)}$$

$$\text{metacarpal index} = \frac{\text{RS2} + \text{RS3} + \text{RS4} + \text{RS5}}{4}$$

Normal values	Men		Women	
	Mean	Range	Mean	Range
Right	6.8	5.9–7.6	7.7	6.3–8.9
Left	7.0	6.0–8.0	7.8	6.8–9.0

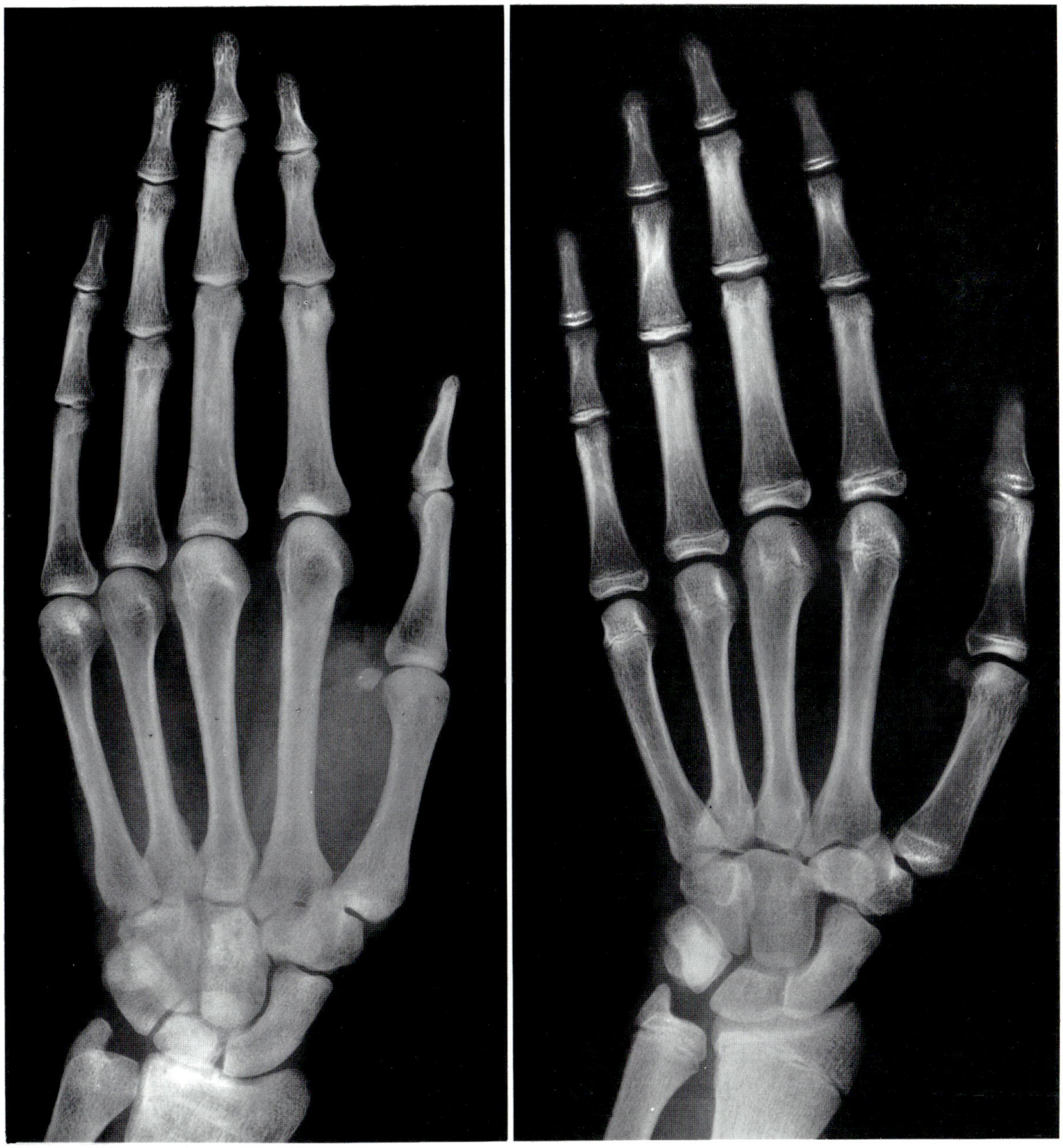

a b

Fig. 2a, b. Marfan's syndrome. **a** In a 20-year-old man: Arachnodactyly (metacarpal index 10.1). This patient presented the additional findings of dislocation of the eye lenses, high arched palate, joint laxity, thoracolumbar scoliosis, and insufficiency of the aortic valve due to dilatation of the thoracic aorta. **b** In a 17-year-old male: Arachnodactyly (metacarpal index 9.0). Some shortening of fourth metacarpal. Additional findings: high arched palate, joint laxity, scoliosis

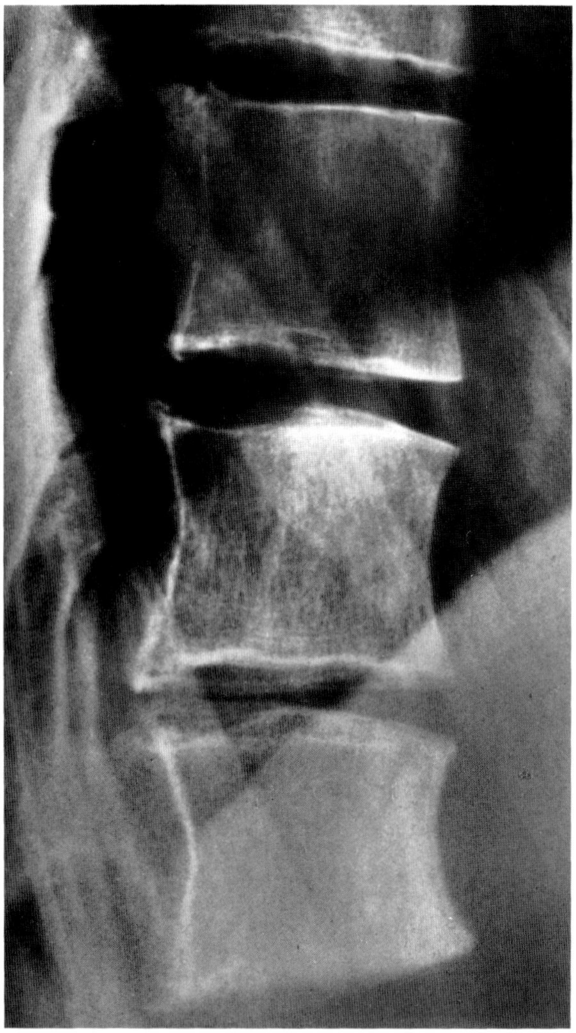

Fig. 3. Same patient as Fig. 2a. Posterior scalloping of lumbar vertebral bodies (dural ectasia)

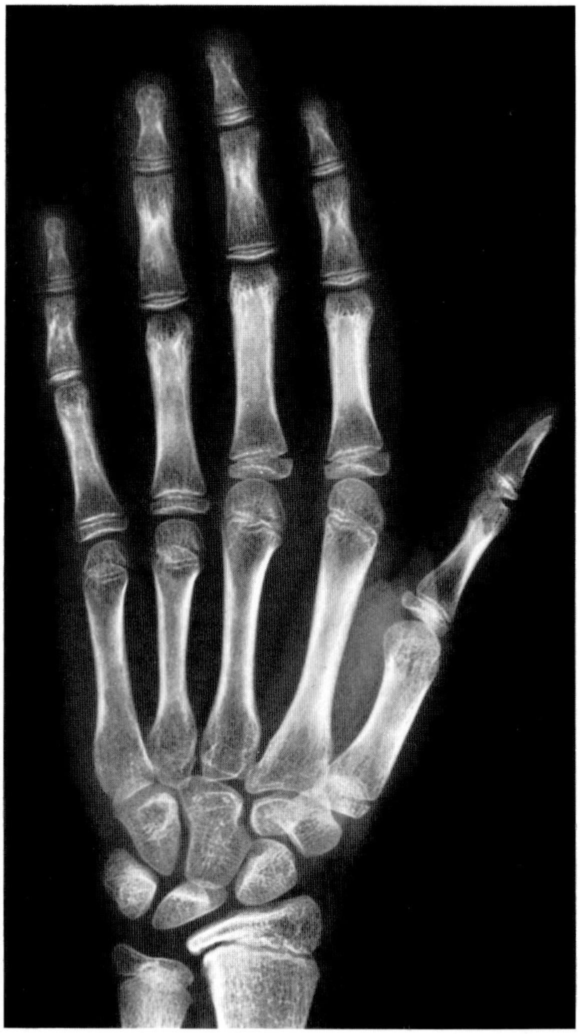

Fig. 4. Homocystinuria in a 14-year-old girl: Elongated and slender tubular bones, metacarpal index 9.1. Relative shortening of fourth metacarpal. Demineralization of skeleton and delayed skeletal maturation (corresponding approximately to a normal 9-year-old child)

6 Metabolic Bone Diseases

6.1 Primary Diseases

6.1.1 Mucopolysaccharidosis

Mucopolysaccharidosis (MPS) is divided into the following types [1]:

MPS I Alpha-L-iduronidase deficiency
- a) Hurler
- b) Scheie
- c) other forms

MPS II Hunter (sulfoiduronate sulfatase deficiency)

MPS III San Filippo
- a) heparin sulfomidase deficiency
- b) *N*-acetyl-alpha-glucosaminidase deficiency

MPS IV Morquio (*N*-acetylgalactosamine-6-sulfate-sulfatase deficiency)

MPS VI Maroteaux-Lamy (arylsulfatase B deficiency)

MPS VII Aspartylglucosaminuria (aspartylglucosaminidase deficiency)

Differential Diagnosis

Achondroplasia (Sect. 1.1.3)
Metaphyseal chondrodysplasia (Sect. 1.1.10)
Multiple epiphyseal dysplasia (Sect. 1.1.11)
Spondyloepiphyseal dysplasia
Mucolipidosis I, II, and III [5, 6]

References

1 "Special report" (1978) AJR 131:352–354
2 McKusick VA (1969) The nosology of the mucopolysaccharidoses. AJR 47:730–747
3 Spranger JW (1972) The systemic mucopolysaccharidoses. Ergeb Inn Med Kinderheilkd 32:165–173
4 Grossman HL, Dorst JP (1973) The mucopolysaccharidoses. Prog Pediatr Radiol 4:495–544
5 Melhem R, Dorst JP, Scott CI Jr, McKusick VA (1973) Roentgen findings in mucolipidosis III (pseudo Hurler polydystrophy). Radiology 106:153–160
6 Staalman CR, Bakker HD (1984) Mucolipidosis I. Roentgenographic follow-up. Skeletal Radiol 12:153–161
7 Murray RO, Jacobson HG (1977) The radiology of skeletal disorders. Churchill Livingstone, Edinburgh

Radiographic Findings [2–4, 7]

Findings	MPS Ia 1–2 years	MPS Ib First decade	MPS II 2–5 years	MPS III 4–5 years	MPS IV 1–1½ years	MPS VI 0–1 year	MPS VII
Hand							
Metacarpals							
Shaft constriction					+		
Proximal tapering	++	±	+		++	++	+
Wide/short	++	±	+		++	++	
Thin cortex	++	±	±		+	+	
Phalanges							
Wide/short	++		±		++	++	
Shaft constriction					+		
Thin cortex	++				+	++	
Carpals							
Small	+	±	±		+	+	
Irregular	+		±		+	+	
Delayed maturation	+	±	±		+	+	
Decreased carpal angle	+				+		
Claw hand		+		±			
Spine							
Thoracolumbar anterior beaking	+		±	±	++	+	+
Flat vertebral bodies		±	±		+		
Concave anterior and posterior surfaces of the vertebral bodies	+		±			±	
AP diameter							
increased				±			
decreased	+				±		
Caudo/cranial surfaces convex		±	+	+		±	
Wide intervertebral spaces					+		
Hypoplasia of odontoid process					+	+	+
Skull							
Frontal bossing	+		±				
Thickening	+		±	+			
Deep optic chiasm	+		±			+	+
Sutures: premature fusion	+		±			+	+
Mastoids: nonpneumatized				+			
Low nasal bridge	+		±				
Dental abnormalities	+		±		+		
Long tubular bones							
Metaphyses: splayed	+				+		
Metaphyses: constricted						+	
Shaft widening		±	+		±	+	
Cortical thickening	+		±		+		
Bowing			±		+	+	
Pelvis							
Flared iliac wings	+		±			±	
Steep acetabular roof	+				+	+	
Abnormal femoral epiphyses	+				+	+	
Coxa vara	+		±				
Coxa valga	+		±		+	+	
Dislocation of the hip	+				+		
Thorax							
Ribs:							
Thickening	+				+		
Anterior widening	+	±	±		+	+	+
Small scapula						+	+

a 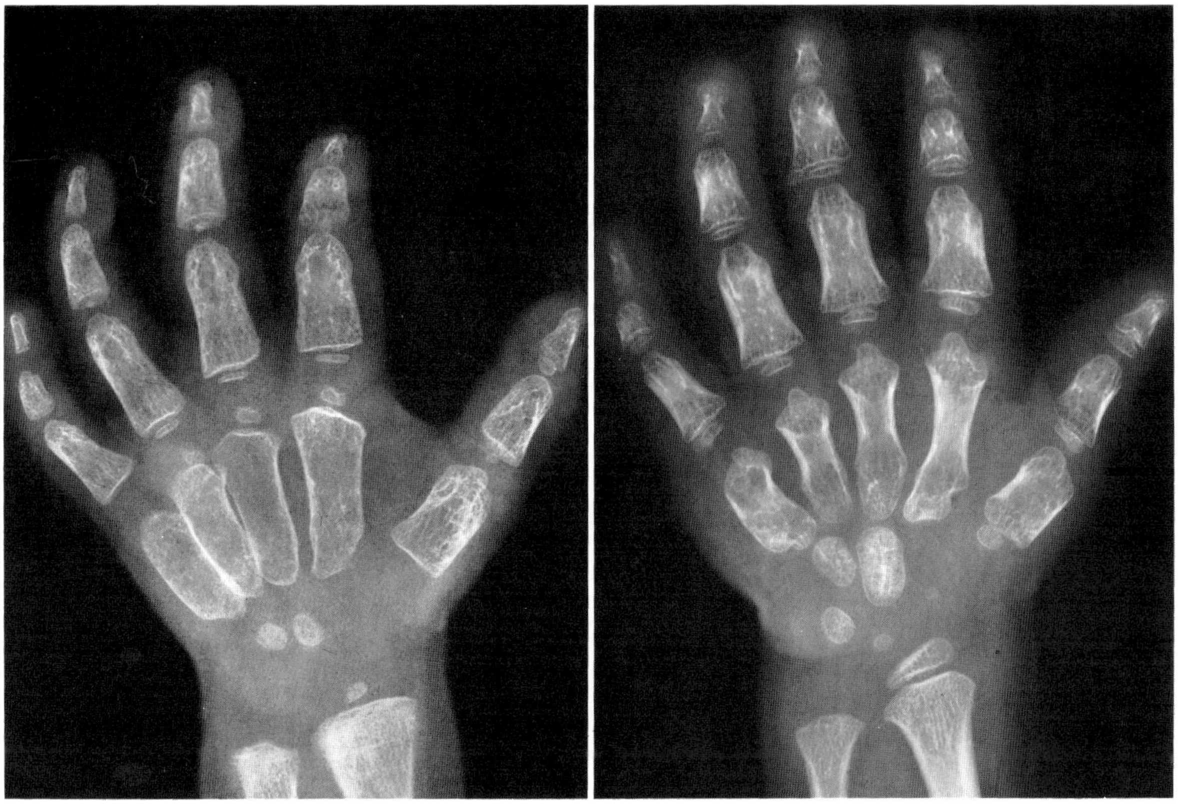 b

Fig. 1a, b. Mucopolysaccharidosis. **a** MPS Ia, HURLER in a 2-year-old boy: Tapering of metacarpals, short and wide tubular bones, thin cortex, small carpals, delayed skeletal maturation. **b** MPS Ia, HURLER in an 8-year-old girl: Tapering of metacarpals, short and wide tubular bones, thin cortex, delayed skeletal maturation

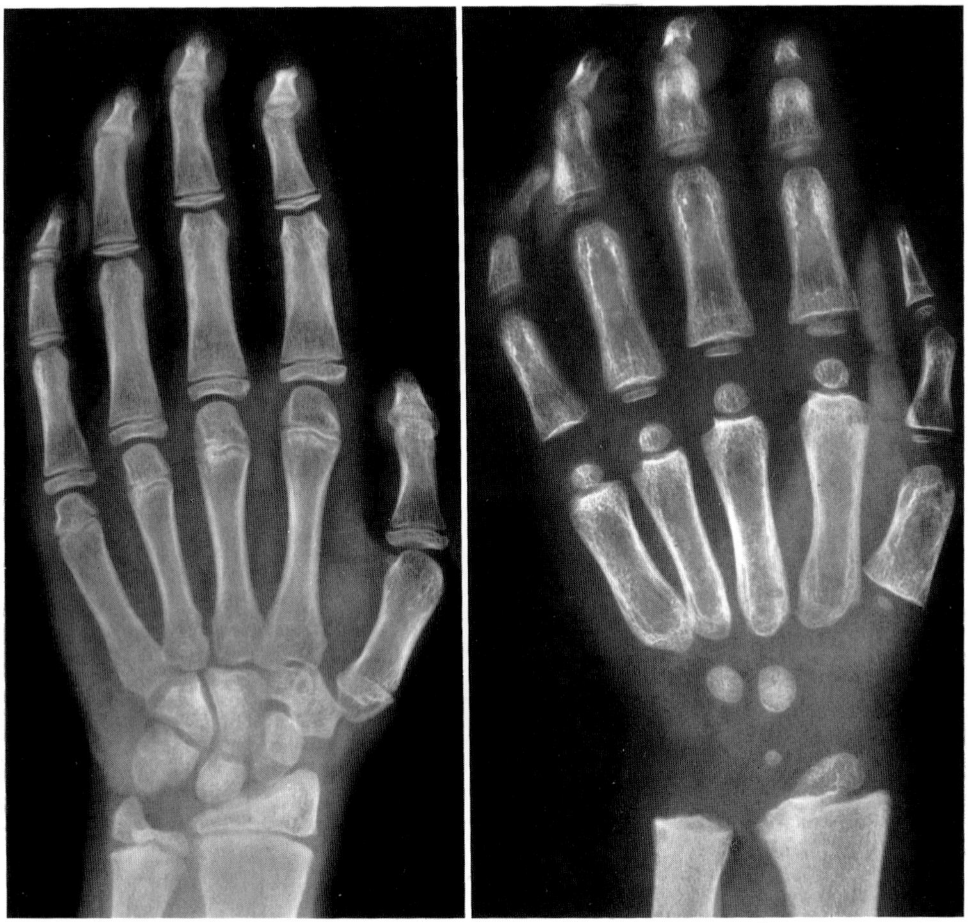

2a b

Fig. 2a, b. Mucopolysaccharidosis. **a** MPS I b, Scheie in a 13-year-old boy: Rather well developed tubular bones, normal skeletal maturation, claw hand. **b** MPS II, Hunter. 4-year-old boy: Some tapering of metacarpals, short and wide tubular bones, widened shafts of distal radius and ulna, small carpals, delayed skeletal maturation

Fig. 3a, b. Mucopolysaccharidosis. **a** MPS III, San Filippo (type III a) in a 10-year-old girl: No significant abnormalities of tubular bones. Delayed skeletal maturation, small carpals, scaphoid still absent. **b** MPS IV, Morquio in a 5-year-old girl: Very short and wide tubular bones with thin cortex, irregular and small carpal bones with delayed skeletal maturation. Radial and ulnar metaphyses splayed and irregularly bordered ▷

Fig. 4a–d. Mucopolysaccharidosis. **a** MPS I a, Hurler in a 2-year-old boy: Hypoplasia of anterior-upper border of L2, somewhat concave anterior surfaces of lumbar vertebral bodies, thoracolumbar kyphosis, anterior beaking of L2. **b** MPS II, Hunter in a 4-year-old boy: Only somewhat concave anterior and posterior surfaces of lumbar vertebral bodies. Same aspect higher in vertebral column. Cranial and caudal surfaces of the vertebral bodies slightly convex. **c** MPS III, San Filippo (type III a) in a 10-year-old girl: Concave anterior surface of T12, convex cranial and caudal surfaces of vertebral bodies. **d** MPS IV, Morquio in a 5-year-old girl: Thoracolumbar kyphosis, flat vertebral bodies and wide intervertebral discs, anterior beaking, concave posterior surfaces of vertebral bodies ▷

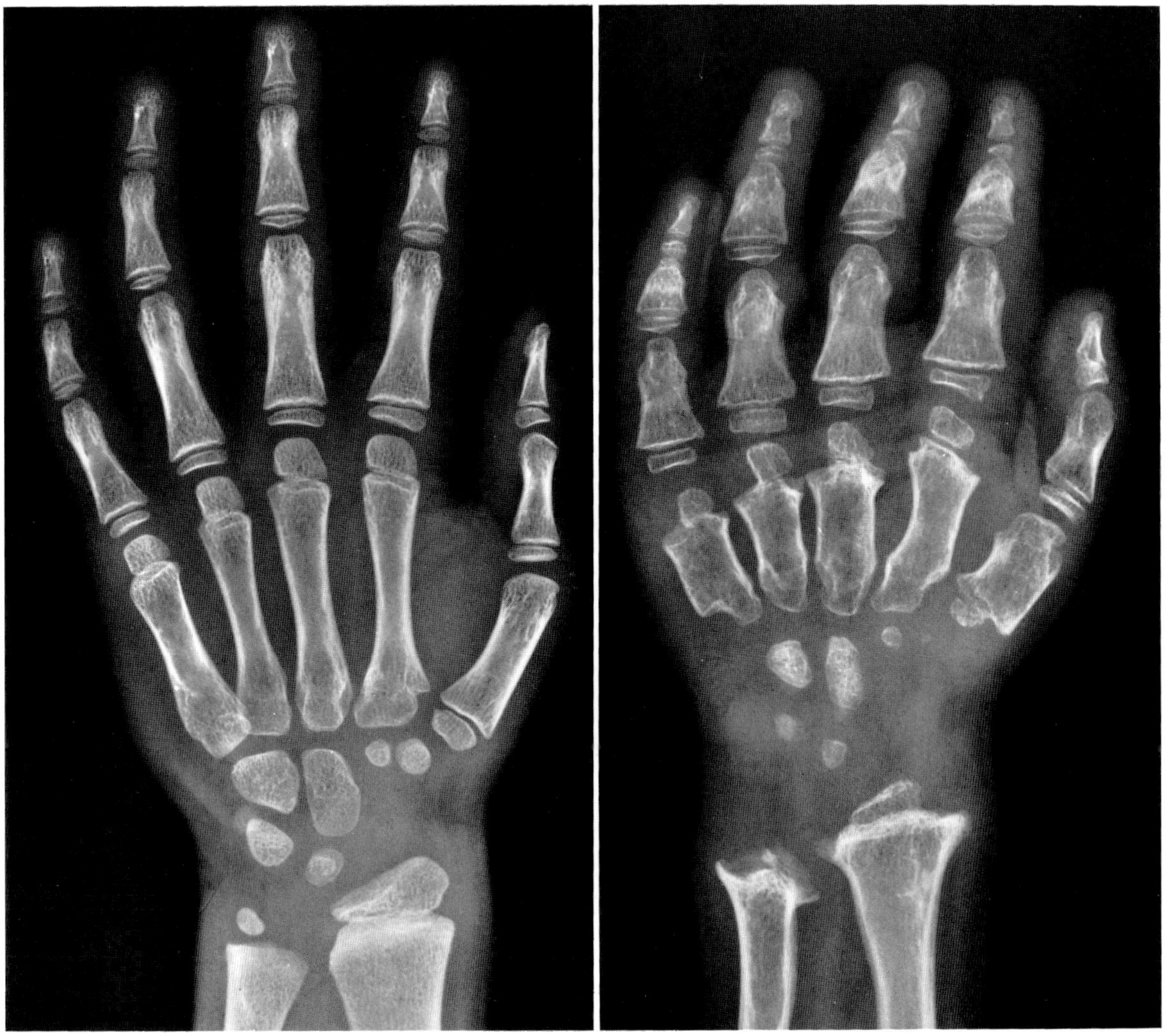

3a b

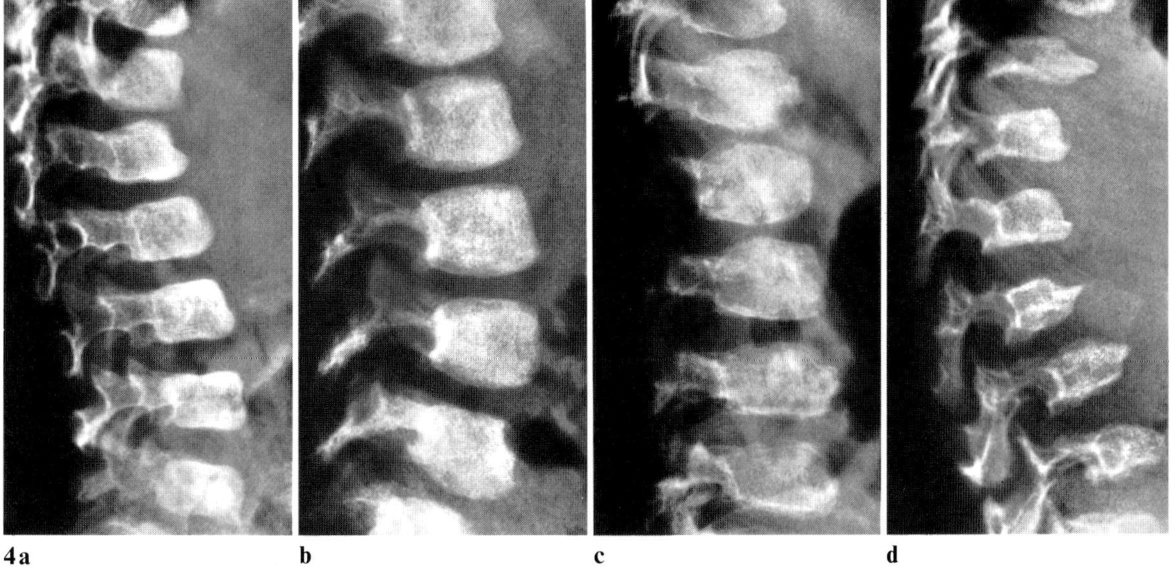

4a b c d

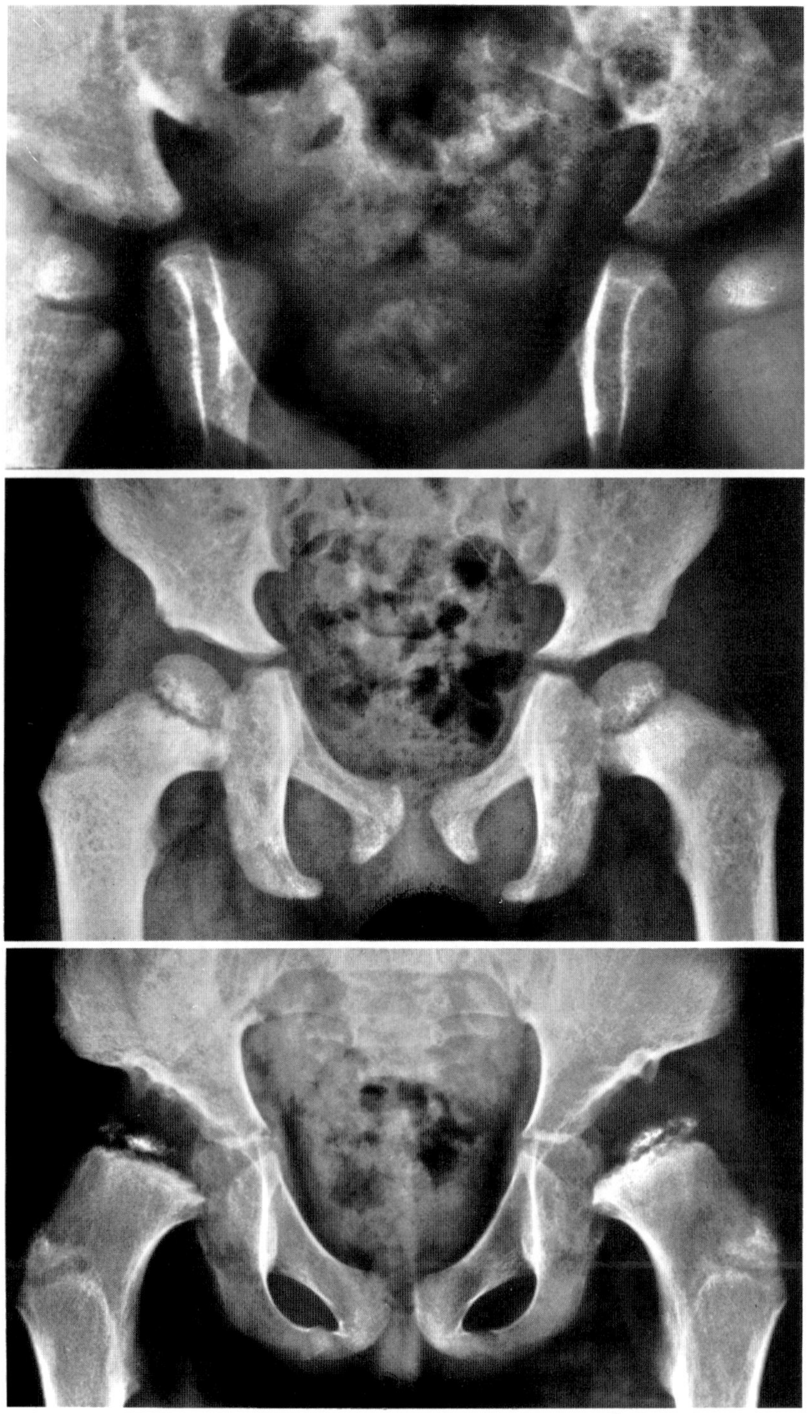

a

b

c

Fig. 5a–c. Mucopolysaccharidosis. **a** MPS Ia, HURLER in a 2-year-old boy: Steep acetabular roof and subluxation of both femoral heads. **b** MPS II, HUNTER in a 4-year-old boy: Well-developed acetabular roofs, wide femoral shafts, cortical thickening, coxa vara. **c** MPS IV, MORQUIO in a 6-year-old boy: Steep and irregular acetabular roofs, fragmentation of femoral heads, coxa valga

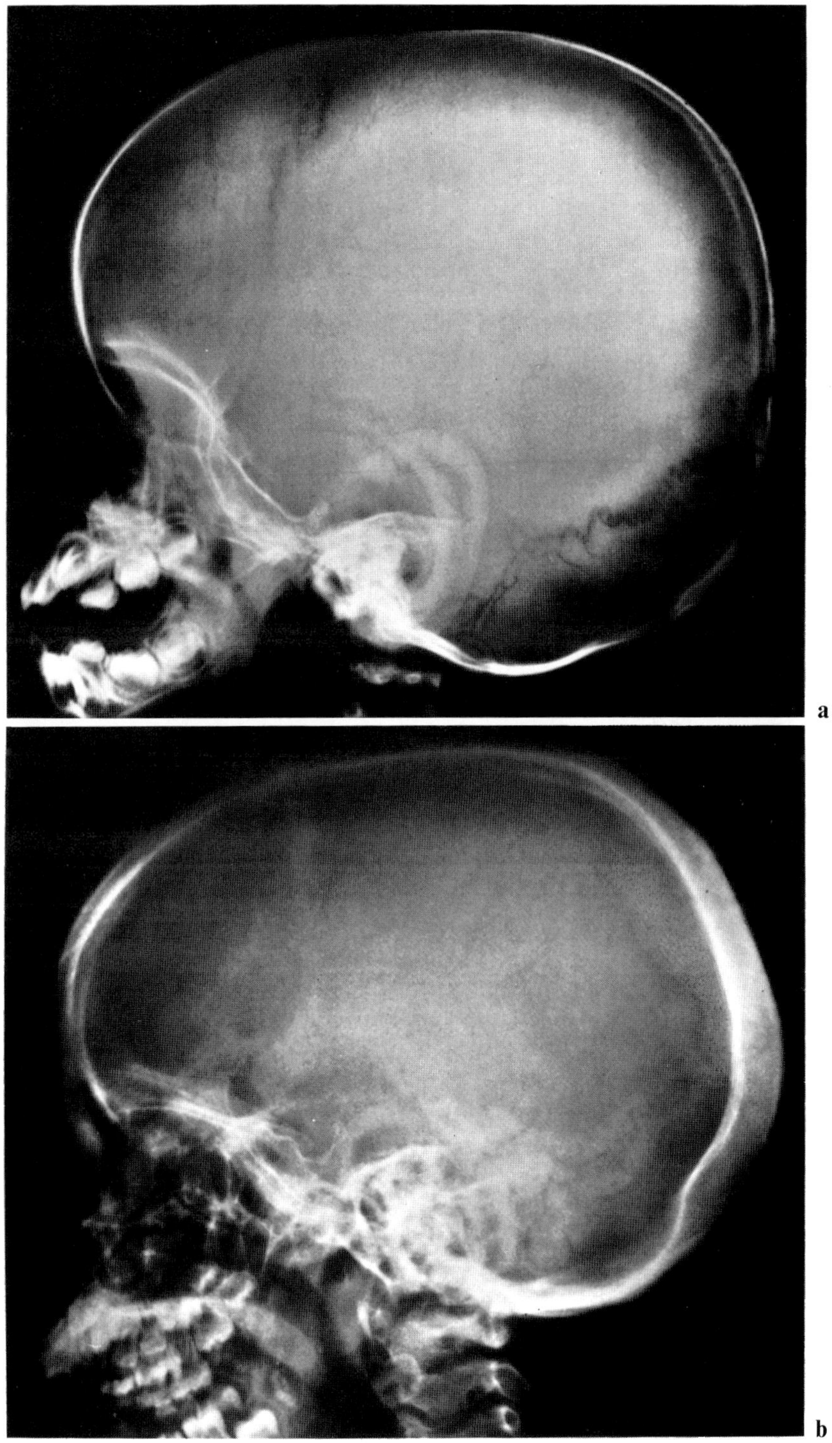

Fig. 6 a, b. Mucopolysaccharidosis. **a** MPS I a, HURLER in a 1-year-old girl: Deepening of optic chiasm and elongated sella, frontal bossing, low nasal bridge. **b** MPS III, SAN FILIPPO (type III a) in an 8-year-old girl: Thickening of parietal and occipital bones, a characteristic finding in MPS III

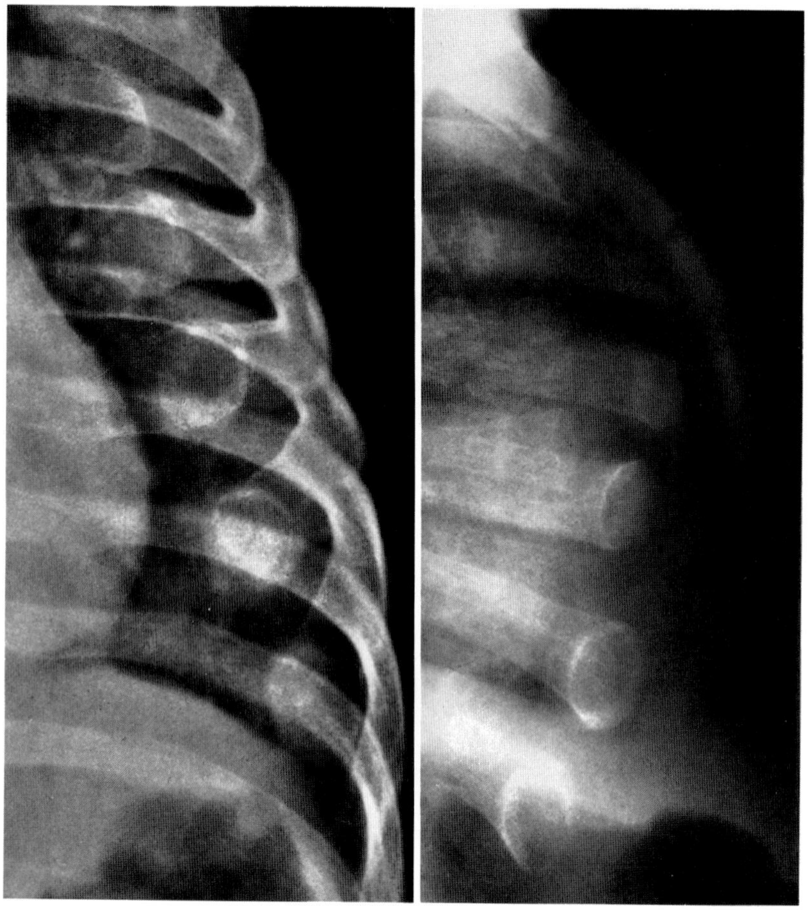

a b

Fig. 7a, b. Mucopolysaccharidosis. **a** MPS Ia, HURLER in a 2-month-old boy: Widened anterior rib ends. **b** MPS IV, MORQUIO in a 5-year-old girl: Widened ribs with cupped anterior ends

6.1.2 Hypoparathyroidism, Pseudohypoparathyroidism, and Pseudo-pseudohypoparathyroidism

Synonym: Albright's hereditary osteodystrophy

In hypoparathyroidism (H) a deficiency in the production of parathyroid hormone leads to hypocalcemia. The cause of H is either congenital hypoplasia of the parathyroid glands or an inadequate supply of parathyroid hormone due to reduced function (disease, surgical removal). In (pseudo)pseudohypoparathyroidism the end-organ system is unresponsive to parathyroid hormone. Pseudohypoparathyroidism (PH) and pseudopseudohypoparathyroidism (PPH) have been found in members of the same family. The two conditions represent different manifestations of the same autosomal dominant disorder. In PH an inadequate end-organ response to endogenous parathyroid hormone causes signs of hypoparathyroidism. The parathyroid glands are often hyperplastic, and hypocalcemia and hyperphosphatemia are present. In PPH the blood chemistry is normal (normal calcium level). The victims are usually short and obese and are mentally retarded (1, 4, 5).

Radiographic Findings [1–3, 5]

Hand

Short metacarpals: PH 75%; PPH 90% (fourth and fifth fingers)

Short phalanges (especially distal phalanges)

Premature fusion of phalangeal and metacarpal epiphyseal plates

Soft tissue calcifications (usually periarticular)

Cone-shaped epiphyses

Small carpal angle
Occasionally: osteoporosis and subperiosteal bone resorption by secondary hyperparathyroidism
Bone density normal, increased, or decreased

Other Sites
Foot: short metatarsals [1] PH 40%–70% (third and fourth toes); PPH nearly 100% (all five toes)
short phalanges
exostoses
Skull: calvarial thickening [1]: PH 20%–37%; PPH 25%
calcification of basal ganglia [1]: PH 33%–50%; PPH 4.8%; H frequently abnormal dentition (especially PH)
Long tubular bones: exostoses (short, broad-based, and diaphyseal)
metaphyseal bands of increased density
bowing
Miscellaneous findings: coxa vara/valga
fractures
osteoporosis

Differential Diagnosis

Renal osteodystrophy (Sect. 6.2.4)
Other disorders with soft tissue calcifications (Sect. 6.2.7)
Paget's disease (Sect. 6.2.9)
Fluorosis (Sect. 7.5.1)
Mastocytosis (Sect. 7.6.7)
Myelosclerosis
Osteoblastic metastases
Sickle cell anemia

Differences Between PH and PPH [1]

	PH (%)	PPH (%)
Short metacarpals	69–75	86–90
Short metatarsals	40–70	97
Soft tissue calcifications	42–60	27–40
Calcifications in basal ganglia	33–50	4.8
Abnormal dentition	37	–
Calvarial thickening	20–37	25
Increased bone density	5–15	–
Diminished bone density	15–22	5
Hyperparathyroidism	5–10	–

References

1 Murray RO, Jacobson HG (1977) The radiology of skeletal disorders. Churchill Livingstone, Edinburgh
2 Steinbach HL, Young DA (1966) The roentgen appearance of pseudohypoparathyroidism (PH) and pseudo-pseudohypoparathyroidism (PPH). Differentiation from other syndromes associated with short metacarpals, metatarsals and phalanges. AJR 97:49–66
3 Steinbach HL, Rudhe U, Jonsson M, Young DA (1965) Evolution of skeletal lesions in pseudohypoparathyroidism. Radiology 85:670–676
4 Mann JB, Alterman S, Hills AG (1962) Albright's hereditary osteodystrophy comprising pseudohypoparathyroidism and pseudohypoparathyroidism with a report of two cases representing the complete syndrome occurring in successive generations. Ann Intern Med 56:315–322
5 Taybi H, Keele D (1962) Hypoparathyroidism: a review of the literature and report of two cases in sisters, one with steatorrhea and intestinal pseudo-obstruction. AJR 88:432–442

a b c

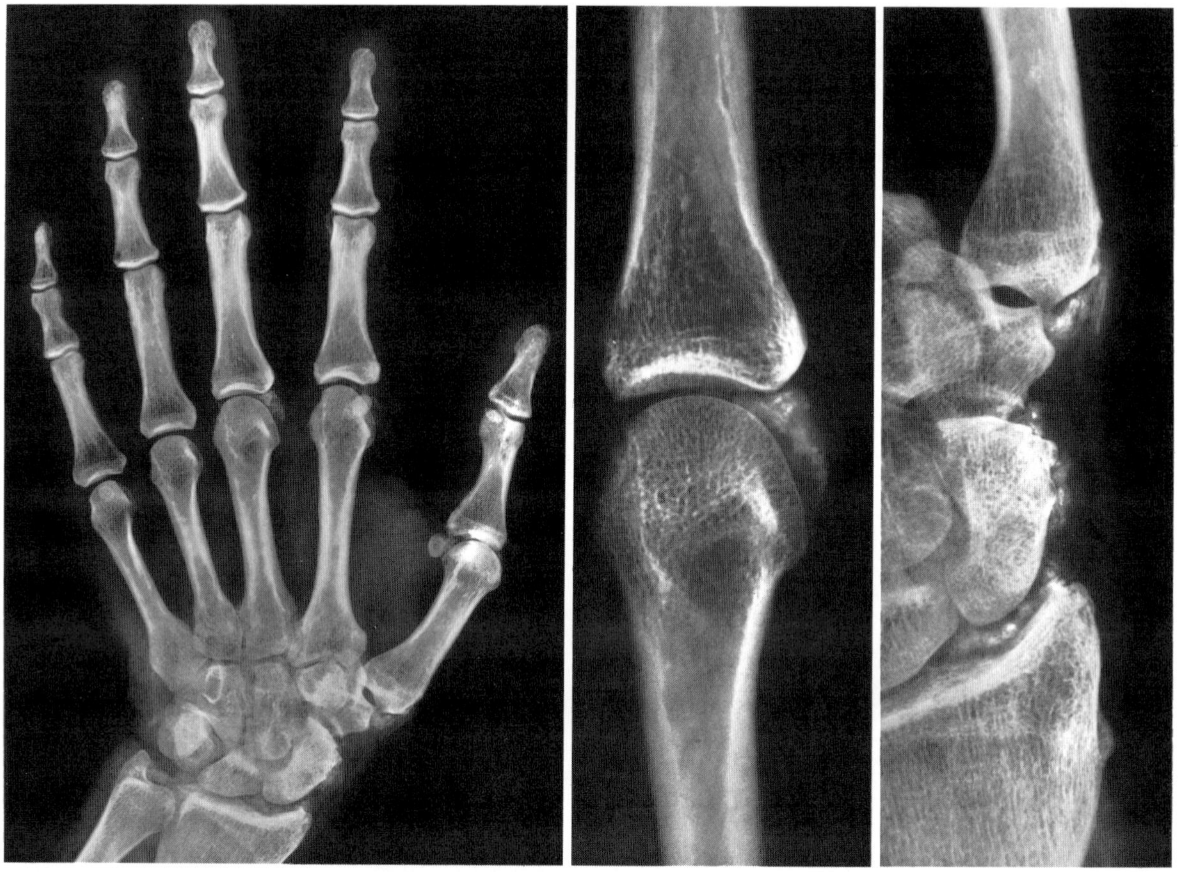

1

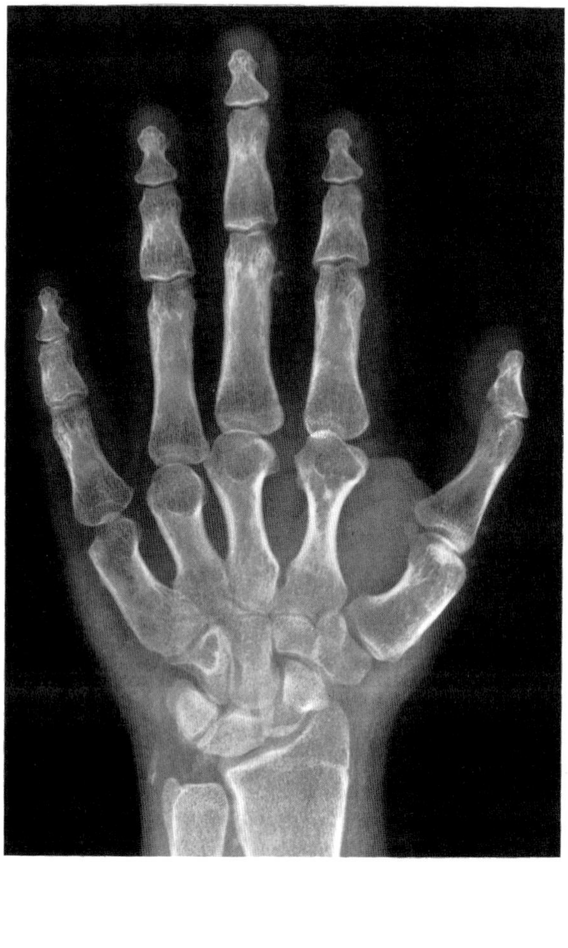

2

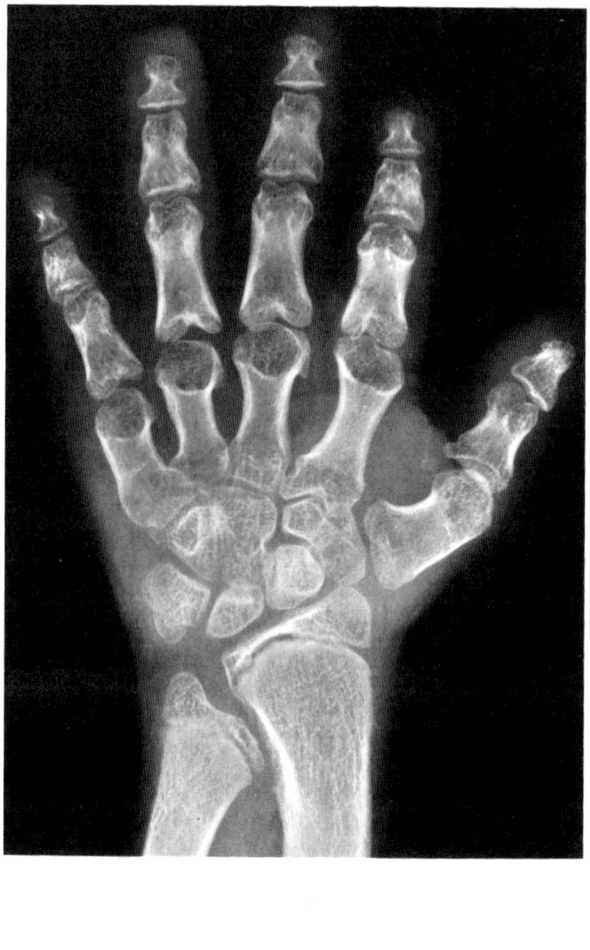

3

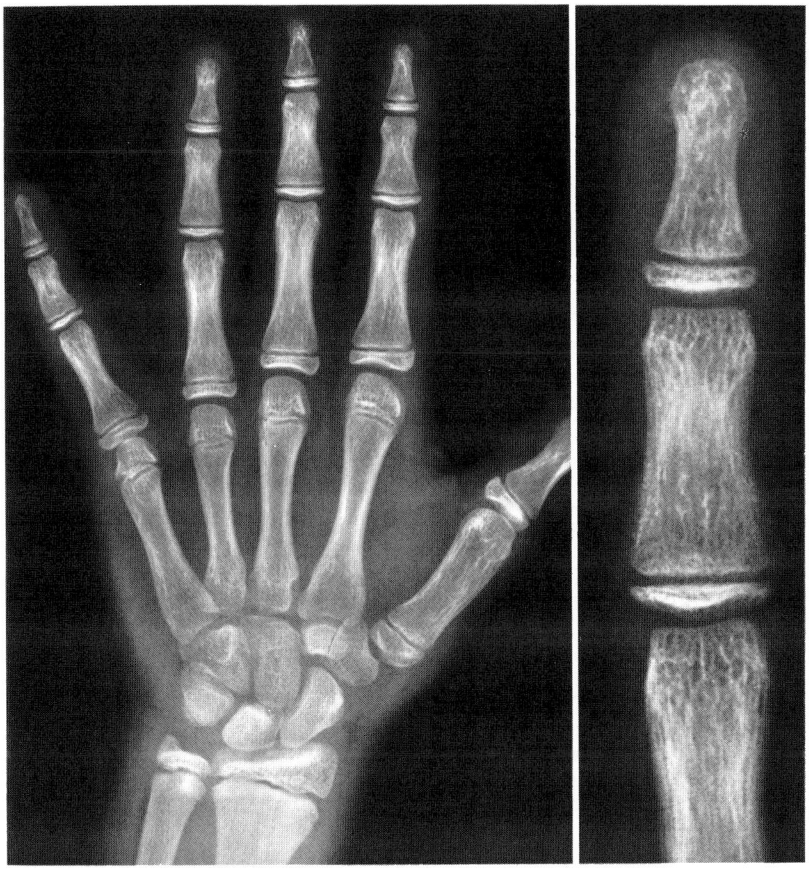

Fig. 4. PH in a 10-year-old girl. Mild shortening of third, fourth, and fifth metacarpals, subperiosteal bone resorption by secondary hyperparathyroidism (*detail*)

◁ **Fig. 1a–c.** H in a 63-year-old woman after removal of parathyroid glands. Chondrocalcinosis and extensive periarticular calcifications, particularly around wrist and adjacent to several metacarpophalangeal joints (**b, c**)

Fig. 2. PH in a 14-year-old girl. All metacarpals and majority of phalanges short, advanced epiphyseal fusions, soft tissue calcifications especially around wrist and in third digit

Fig. 3. PPH in a 13-year-old boy. Severe shortening of all tubular bones in hand, cone-shaped epiphyses at bases of proximal phalanges, short ulna. Hand findings are similar to those in acrodysostosis

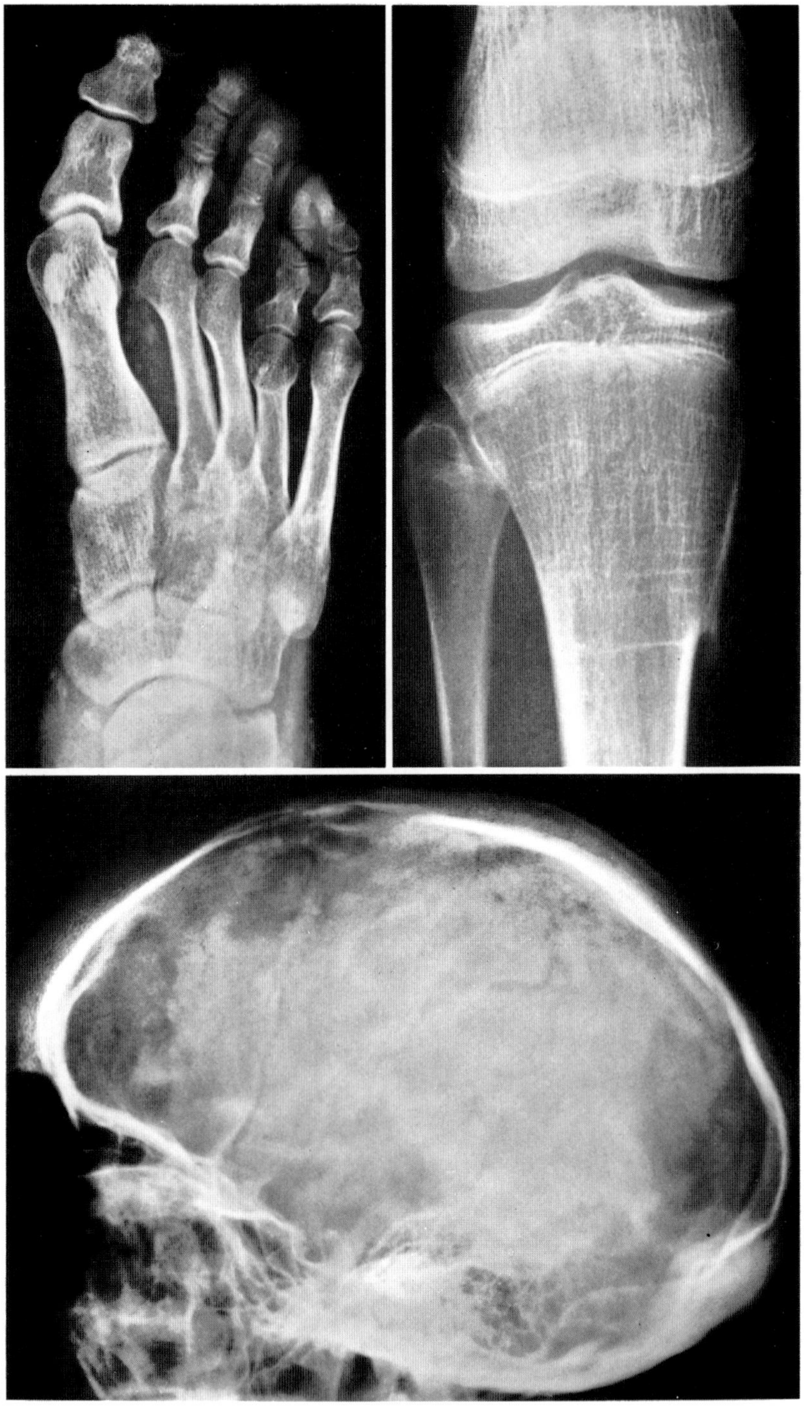

a b c

Fig. 5. a PH (same patient as Fig. 2). Right foot: soft tissue calcifications, shortening of third and fourth metatarsals and most phalanges. **b** PPH (same patient as Fig. 3). Widening of both femoral and tibial metaphyses, small metadiaphyseal exostosis with broad base. **c** PH (same patient as Fig. 2). Thickening of calvarium by hyperplasia of tabula interna

6.2 Acquired Diseases

6.2.1 Rickets and Osteomalacia

Ordinary rickets in early infancy is mostly caused by poor intake of vitamin D or deficient absorption of vitamin D and calcium in the intestinal tract.

Vitamin D Metabolism [1, 2]

1. Vitamin D2 (ergocalciferol): intestinal absorption of this vitamin derived from plant sterols
2. Vitamin D3 (cholecalciferol): (a) intestinal absorption; (b) skin: ultraviolet irradiation of 7-dehydrocholecalciferol
3. In the liver: hydrolysis of cholecalciferol and ergocalciferol in 25-hydroxycholecalciferol (25-OH-D3 and 25-OH-D2)
4. In the blood: especially 25-OH-D3 circulates conjugated with alpha globulin
5. In the kidneys: hydrolysis of 25-OH-D3 into 1,25 dihydroxycholecalciferol ($1,25(OH)_2$ D3)

$1,25(OH)_2D3$ has the following functions:

1. It is very active in the intestinal absorption of calcium and phosphate.
2. It controls calcium transport to and from the skeleton.
3. It controls phosphate excretion.

Causes of Rickets and Osteomalacia [3]

1. Deficiency states:
   vitamin D deficiency
   calcium deficiency
2. Intestinal tract:
   partial gastrectomy
   biliary obstruction
   celiac disease
   sprue
   gluten-sensitive enteropathy
3. Organic renal disease:
   polycystic disease
   ureteropelvic obstruction
   acquired renal disease (renal osteodystrophy)
4. Tubular resorption defects:
   hypophosphatemia (vit D resistant rickets) [4]
   congenital cystinuria
   aminoaciduria
   hepatolenticular degeneration
   idiopathic Fanconi-De Toni-Debré syndrome (loss of phosphate, glucose, and amino acids)
   acquired Fanconi-De Toni-Debré syndrome
   glucosuric rickets
5. Hypophosphatasia
6. Miscellaneous [5]

Laboratory Findings

Blood: calcium low or normal (secondary hyperparathyroidism)
phosphate low
alkaline phosphatase normal

Radiographic Findings [3–7]

The radiographic findings depend on the patient's age. In infants, they are often very typical, and there are no differences between those findings in rickets due to vitamin D deficiency and those in so-called renal rickets. Mostly, the clinical differential diagnosis will not be difficult.

Children

Abundant masses of noncalcified osteoid
Wide epiphyseal plates
Metaphyses: irregular, splayed, and cupped
Severe demineralization
Pseudofractures and fractures
Retardation of skeletal maturation
In healing rickets: recalcification of epiphyseal and periosteal osteoid, provisional zones first
In long-standing vitamin D deficiency and in familial hypophosphatemia (vitamin-D-resistant rickets): short stature, bowing of legs, pelvic abnormalities, thoracic kyphosis

Adults

Hand: In many cases the hand bones do not present significant abnormalities
Typical findings at other sites in osteomalacia: demineralization
Looser's zones
fish vertebrae
coxa vara
gross fractures
basilar impression of skull

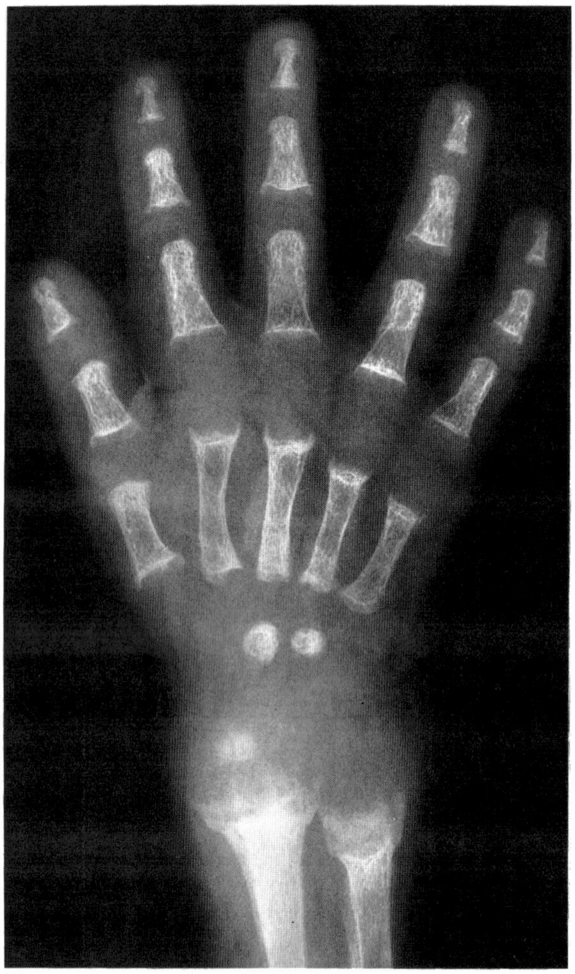

1

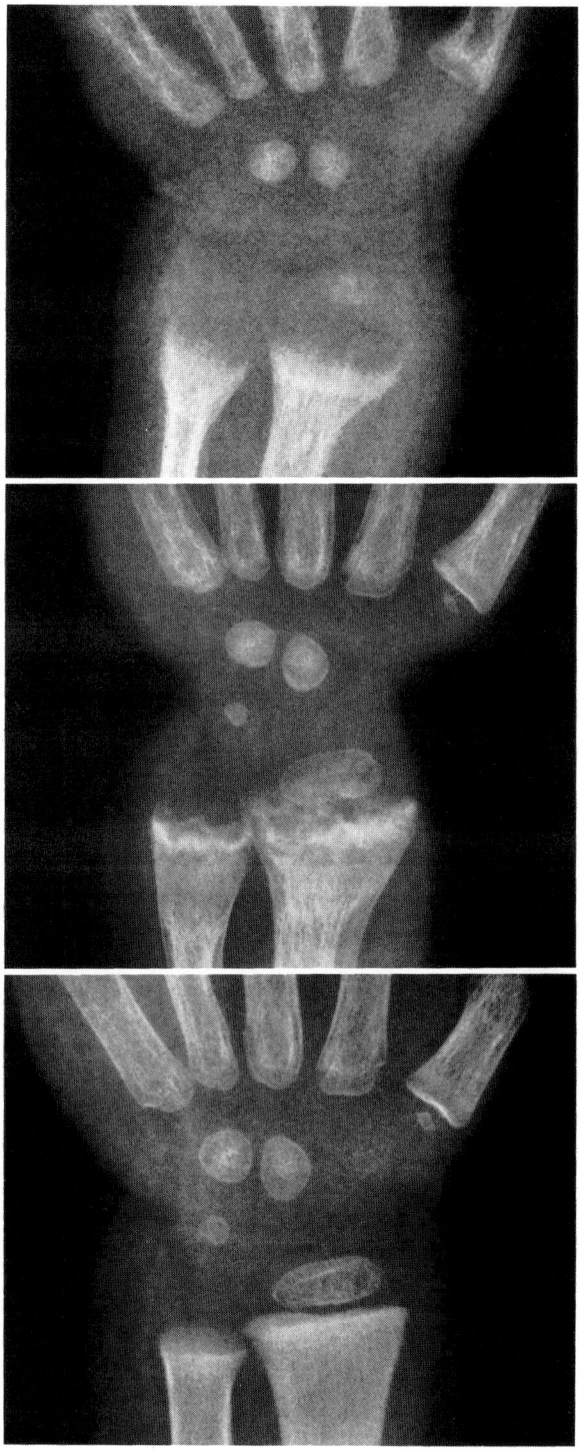

a

b

c

2

Fig. 1. Vitamin D deficiency rickets in a 2-year-old boy. Differential diagnosis: hypophosphatasia

Fig. 2a–c. Vitamin D deficiency rickets. **a** Before treatment; **b** after 6 weeks of treatment; **c** after 3 months of treatment

Fig. 3a–d. Vitamin D deficiency rickets. **a** Demineralization, wide growth plate, irregular demarcation of metaphysis (splaying and cupping). **b** After 1 month of treatment: some calcification of osteoid. **c** After 4 months of treatment: provisional zones of ossification, translucent areas between these zones and remainder of metaphyses. **d** After 9 months of treatment: remarkable improvement. Normal aspect of tubular bones

Fig. 4a–d. Renal rickets (Fanconi-De Toni-Debré syndrome). **a** 1966: distinct radiographic features of rickets. **b** 1974: normal hand bones. **c** April 1981: abnormalities of radial and ulnar metaphyses. **d** November 1981: regression of metaphyseal abnormalities

a b c d

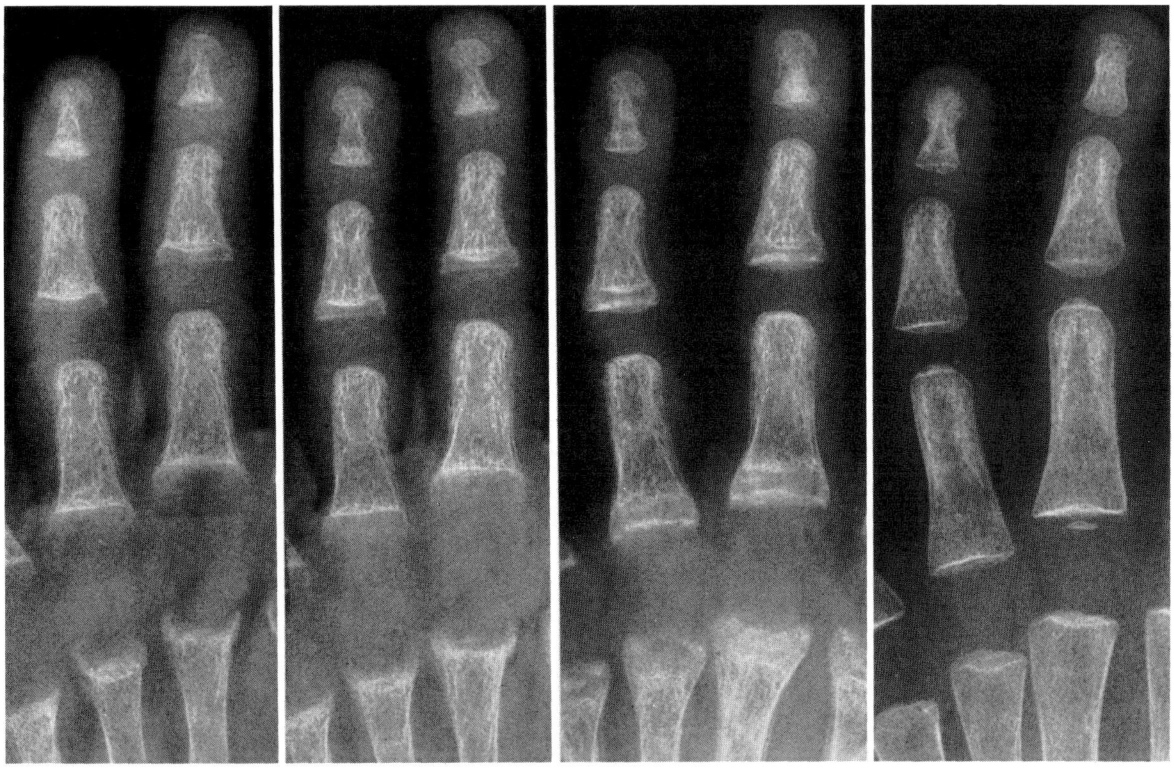

3

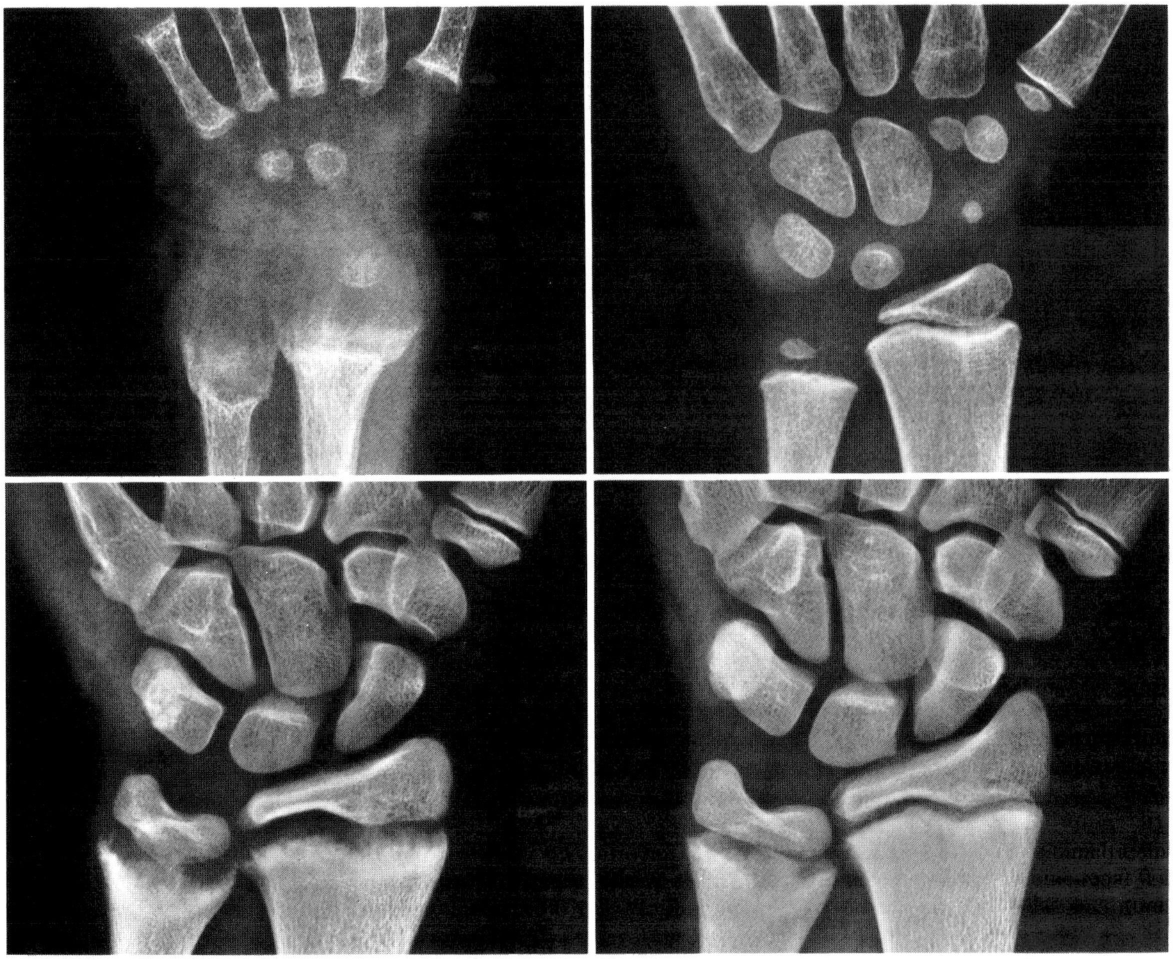

a b

4 c d

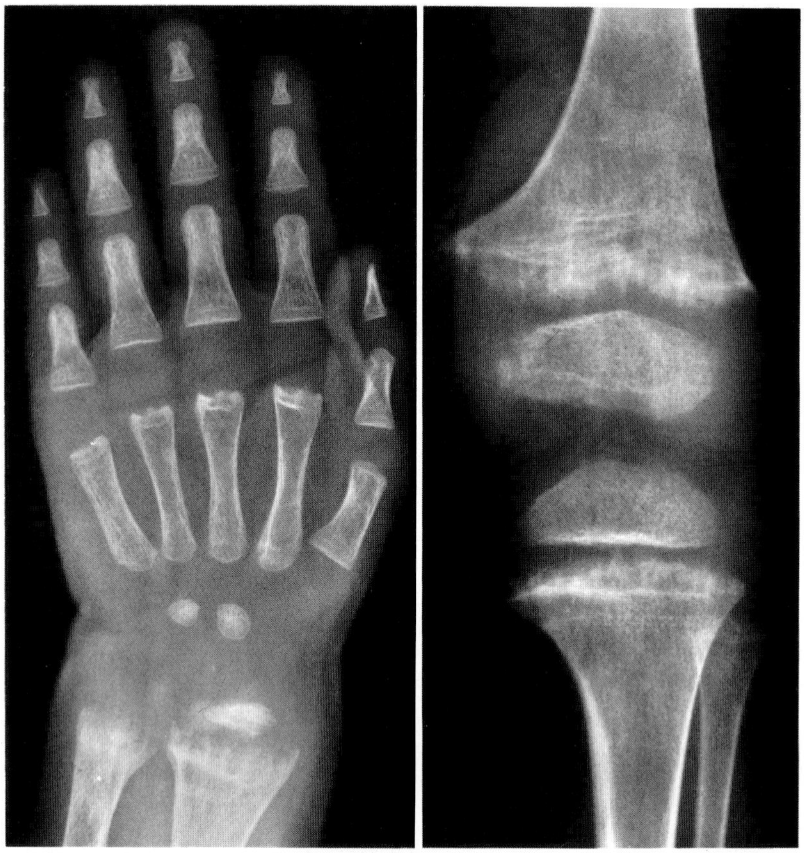

a b

Fig. 5a, b. Renal rickets (Fanconi-De Toni-Debré syndrome) in a 3-year-old boy. **a** Left hand: findings of rickets. **b** Right knee: wide epiphyseal plates with irregular demarcation of metaphyses. Differential diagnosis: metaphyseal chondrodysplasia (Schmid)

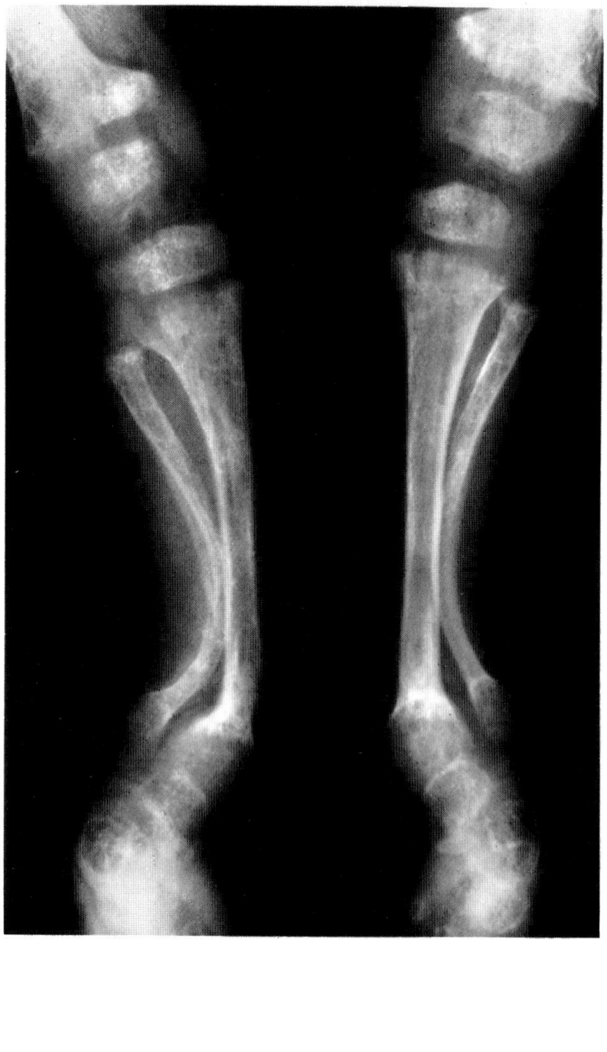

6

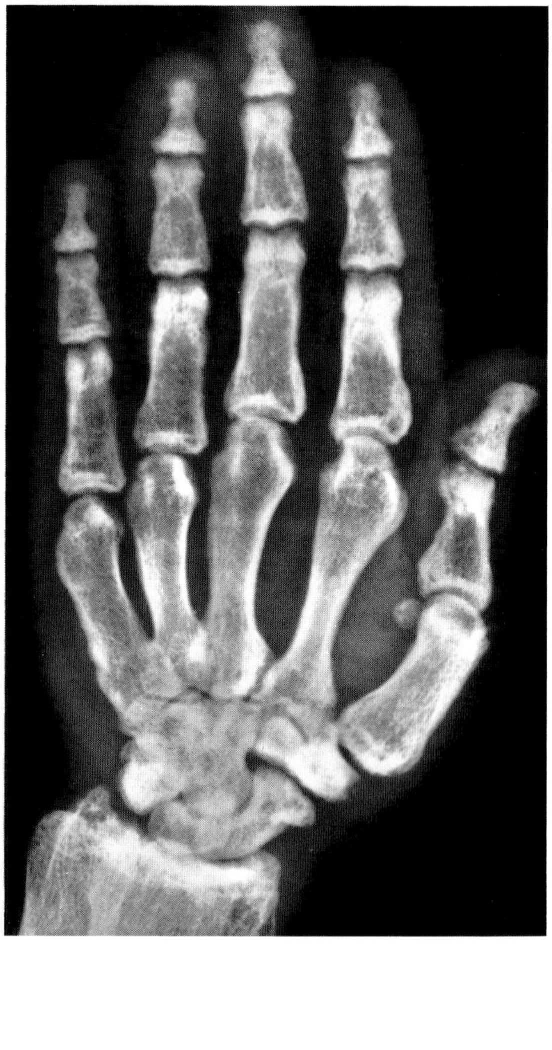

7

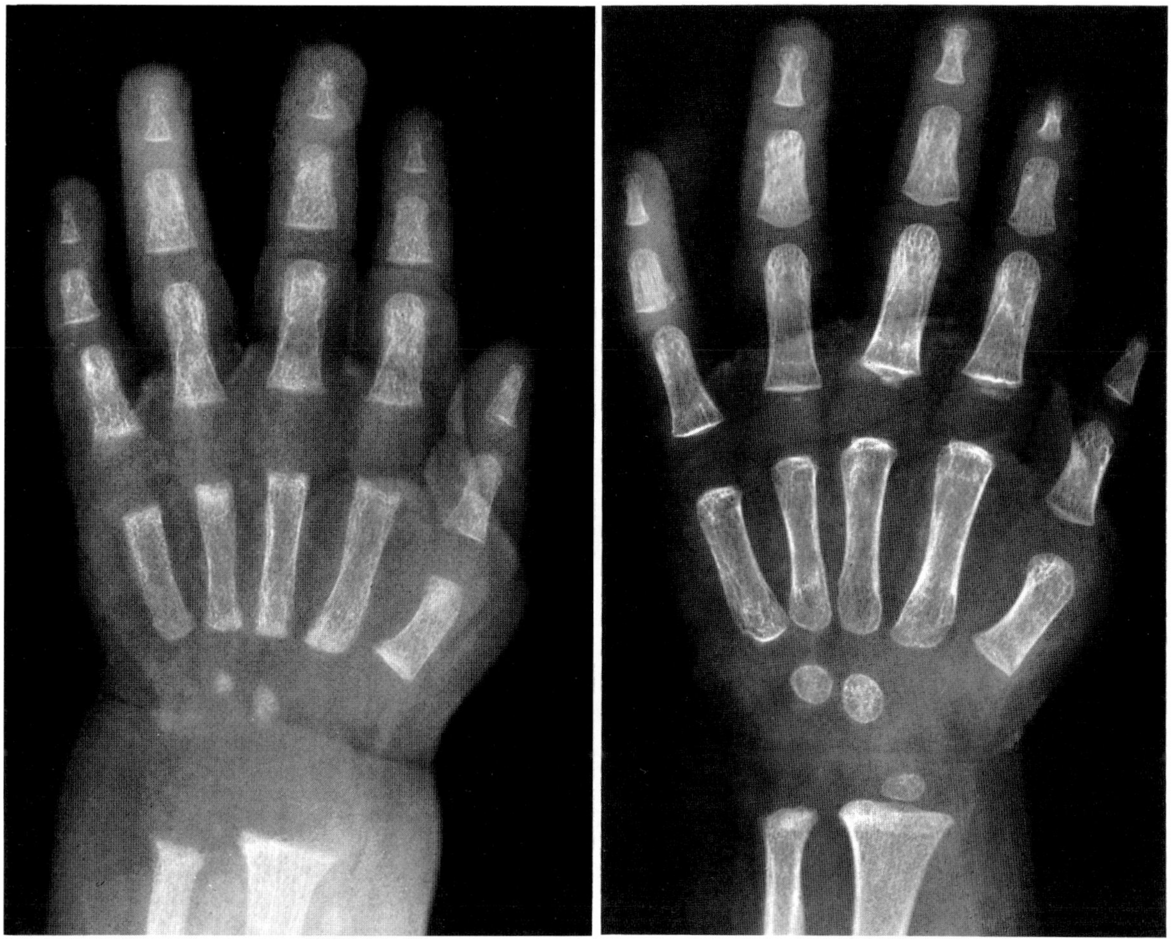

a b

Fig. 8a, b. Familial hypophosphatasia (excretion of phosphoethanolamine, a constituent of alkaline phosphatase, in the urine). **a** In a 1-month-old boy. Radiographic findings similar to those in rickets. **b** After 7 months of treatment: normal hand bones

◁ **Fig. 6.** Vitamin D deficiency rickets. Characteristic and severe affection of lower legs with bowing of tibia and fibula on both sides

Fig. 7. Familial hypophosphatemia (phosphate diabetes) with secondary hyperparathyroidism in a 22-year-old man. Short, wide, and dense bones in hand. Osteosclerosis probably due to secondary hyperparathyroidism

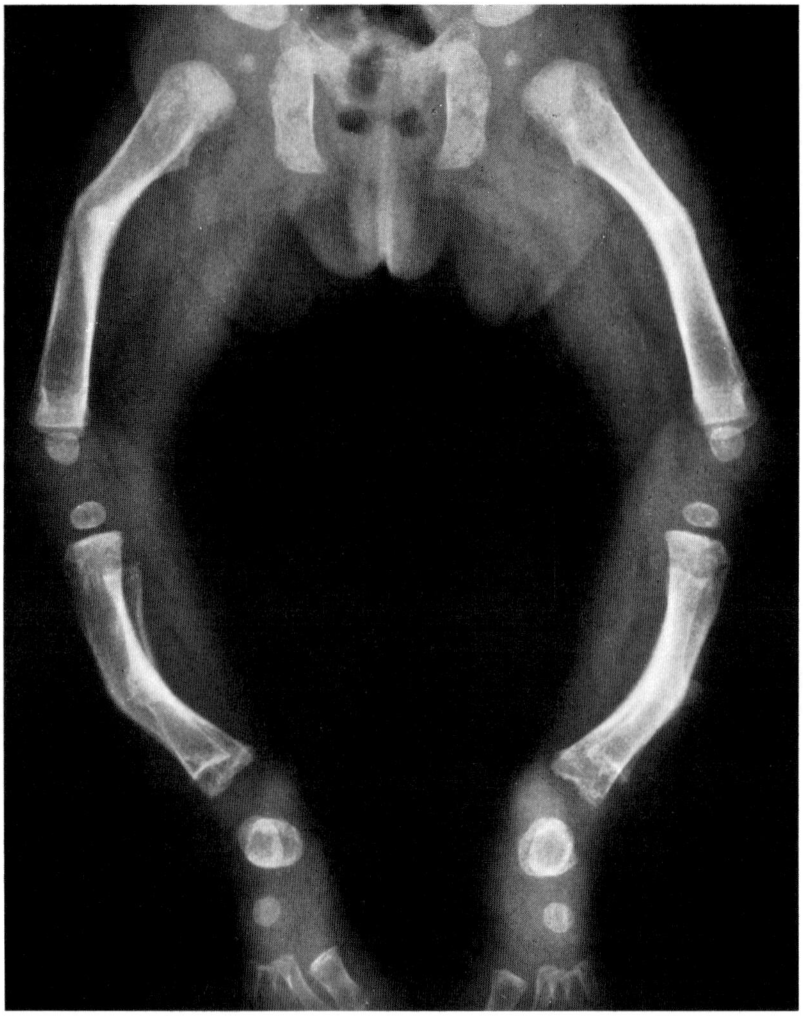

Fig. 9. Familial hypophosphatasia. Bowing of legs, severe demineralization, stress fractures in long tubular bones

Differential Diagnosis in Children

Metaphyseal chondrodysplasia (Sect. 1.1.10)
Hypophosphatasia

References

1 Kanis JA (1982) Vitamin D metabolism and its clinical application. J Bone Joint Surg [Br] 64-B:542–560
2 Pitt MJ, Haussler MR (1977) Vitamin D: biochemistry and clinical applications. Skeletal Radiol 1:191–208
3 Murray RO, Jacobson HG (1977) The radiology of skeletal disorders. Churchill Livingstone, Edinburgh
4 Schmidberger H, Grubbauer HM, Holzer H (1974) Die familiäre primäre Vitamin-D-resistente Rachitis (Phosphatdiabetes). Fortschr Geb Röntgenstr Nuklearmed Ergänzungsband 120:200–209
5 Wendenburg HH, Baldauf G, Barwich D (1976) Vitamin-D-Mangel-Osteopathie nach antikonvulsiver Langzeitbehandlung. Fortschr Geb Röntgenstr Nuklearmed Ergänzungsband 124:7–11
6 Steinbach HL, Noetzli M (1964) Roentgen appearance of the skeleton in osteomalacia and rickets. AJR 91:955–972
7 Griffin CN Jr (1982) Symmetric ilial pseudofractures: a complication of chronic renal failure. A case report with a review of the literature. Skeletal Radiol 8:295–298

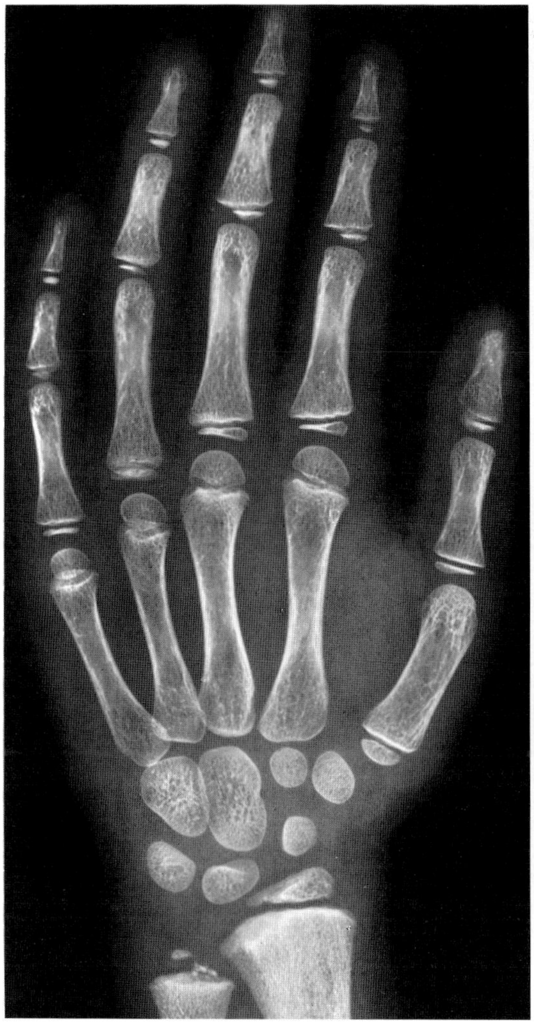
a

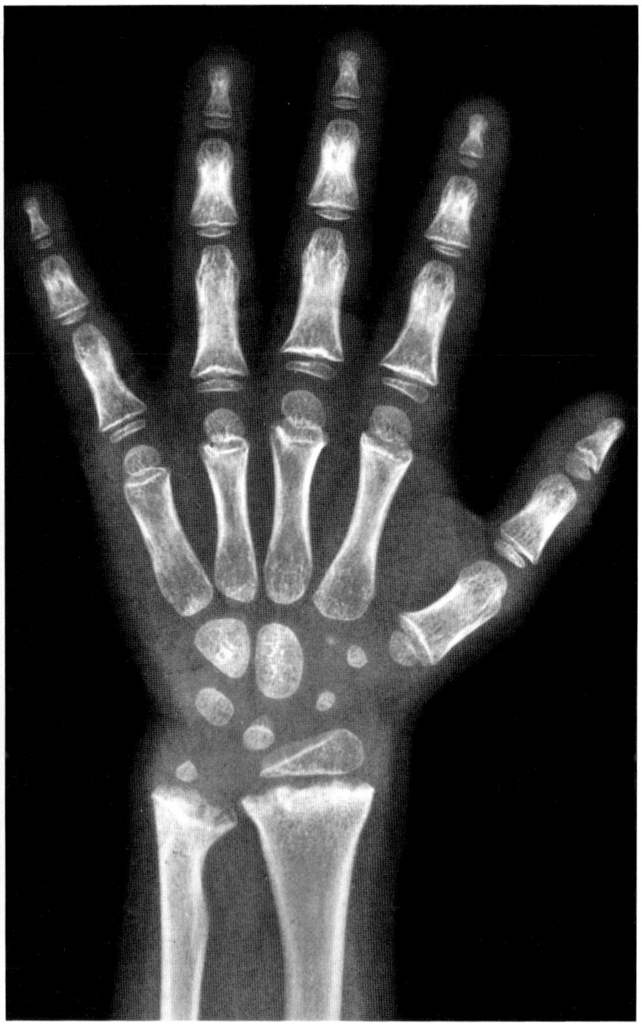
b

Fig. 10. a Renal rickets in a 6-year-old-boy. Multiple ivory and dense epiphyses, irregular distal radial and ulnar metaphyses. Signs of secondary hyperparathyroidism. **b** Metaphyseal dysplasia (Schmid) in a 5-year-old girl. Irregular metaphyses in radius and ulna, mimicking findings in rickets

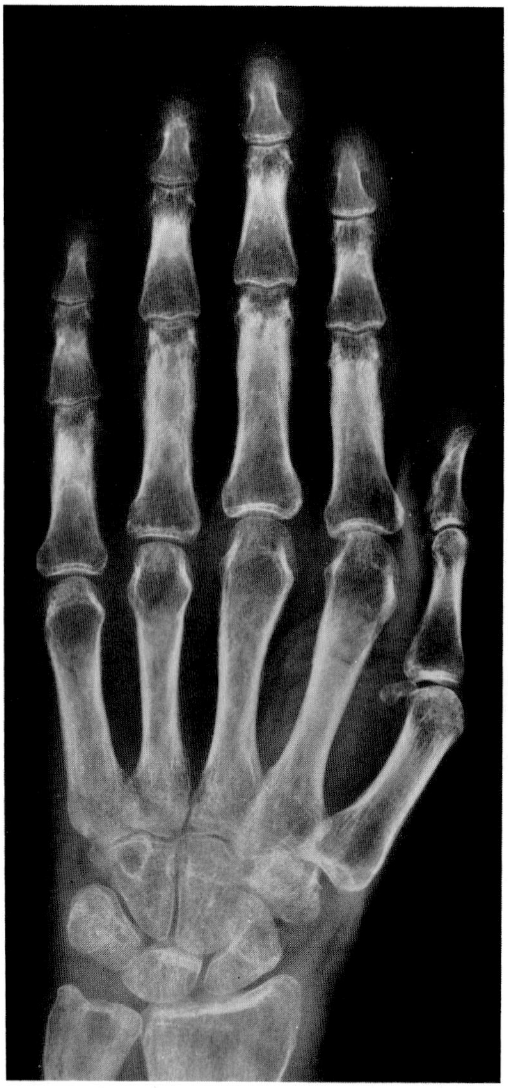

Fig. 11. Osteomalacia caused by biliary cirrhosis in a 46-year-old woman. Demineralization of tubular bones, signs of periostitis (hypertrophic osteoarthropathy) in first and third metacarpals

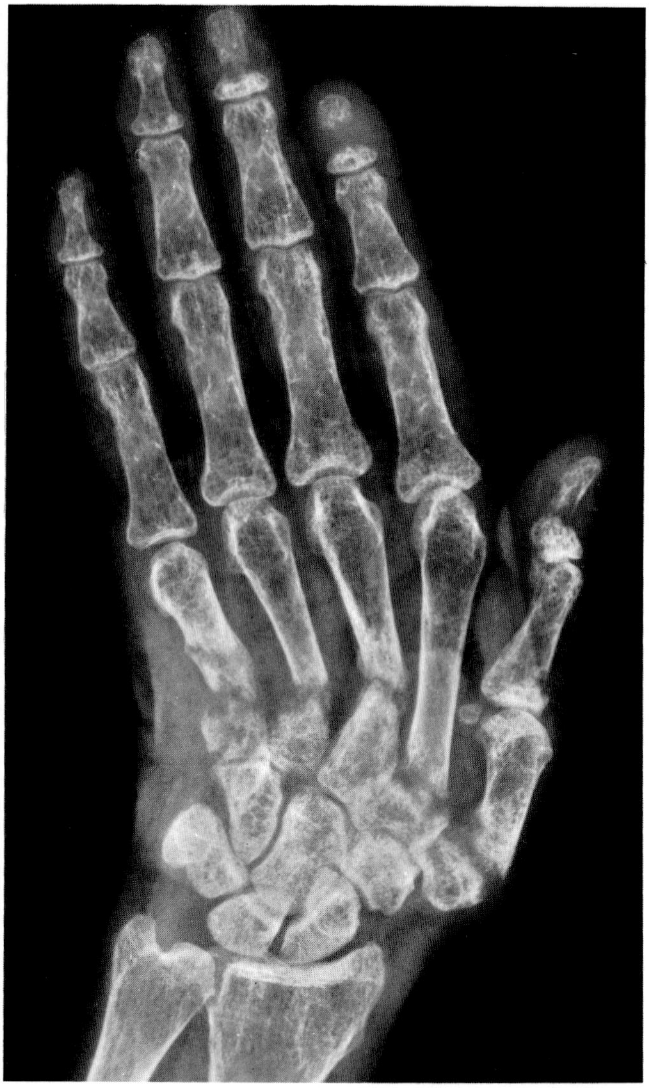

Fig. 12. Osteomalacia caused by hypophosphatemia in a 43-year-old man. Left hand: severe demineralization with fractures in all metacarpals

a b c

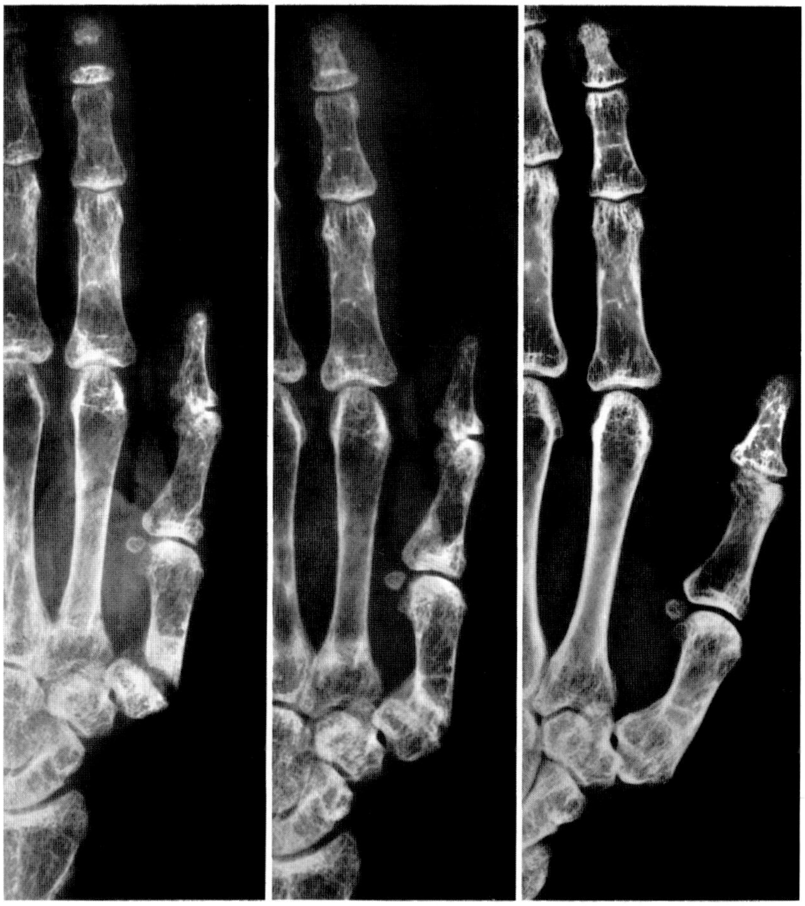

Fig. 13a–c. Same patient as Fig. 12. Right hand. **a** March 1969: severe osteomalacia with fractures and acro-osteolysis at distal phalanx of second finger. **b** May 1969: during therapy, reossification of skeleton with healing of fractures. **c** 1981: during therapy, tolerable mineralization of hand bones

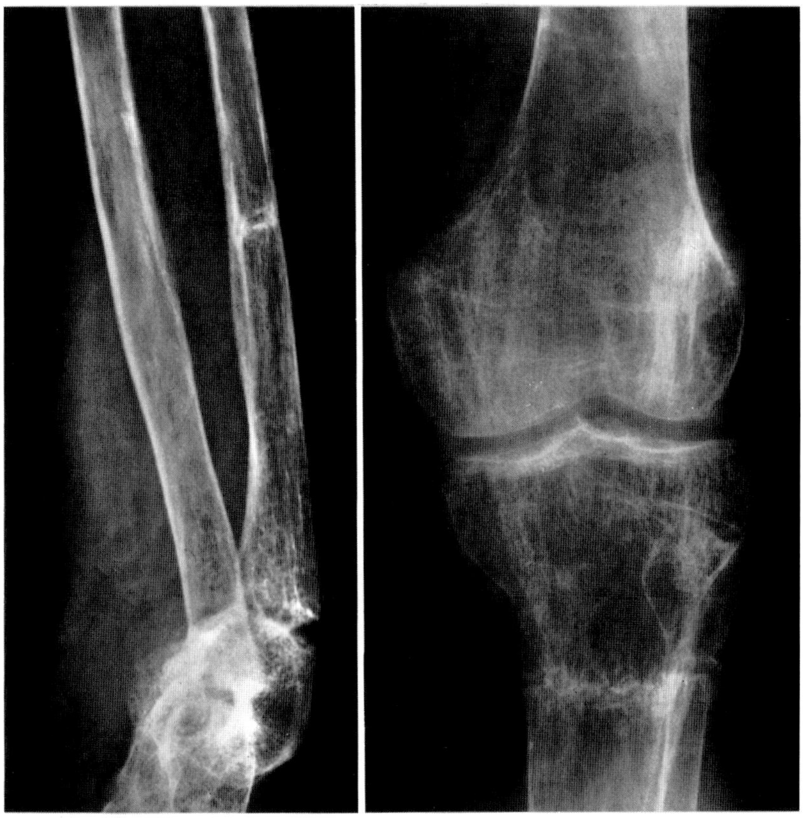

a b

Fig. 14a, b. Same patient as Fig. 12. Stress fractures: **a** ulna and radius; **b** tibia and fibula

6.2.2 Hypervitaminosis D

High vitamin D intake is more dangerous in young children than in adults: In childhood, intake of 50000 units vitamin D per day over a period of weeks or months is toxic [1]. Hypervitaminosis D promotes calcium and phosphate absorption in the intestinal tract and reduces phosphate excretion by the kidneys. Metatastic accretions (usually of hydroxyapatite) are deposited in the soft tissues and kidneys, causing renal insufficiency and secondary hyperparathyroidism. Increased plasma protein binding (early pregnancy) and ectopic hormone production (sarcoidosis) can also cause increased hormone levels of vitamin D.

Laboratory Findings

Blood: calcium high
phosphate high

Radiographic Findings [2–4]

Children

Metaphyseal bands of increased density
Osteoporosis and osteosclerosis
Periosteal bone formation and cortical thickening
Metastatic calcifications (viscera, blood vessels, and periarticular structures)
Delayed skeletal maturation

Adults

Massive calcium deposits in periarticular tissues
Focal or generalized osteoporosis
Osteosclerosis
Calcifications in arterial vessels, kidneys, stomach, heart, lungs, and adrenals
Other signs of secondary hyperparathyroidism (see also renal osteodystrophy, Sect. 6.2.4)

Differential Diagnosis for Periarticular Calcifications

Hyperparathyroidism (Sect. 6.2.3)
Renal osteodystrophy (Sect. 6.2.4)
Collagen vascular disorders (Sect. 7.6.3)
Tumoral calcinosis [5]
Milk-alkali syndrome

References

1 Haddad JG, Stamp TCB (1974) Circulating 25-hydroxyvitamin D in man. Am J Med 57:57–64
2 Christensen WR, Liebman C, Sosmar MC (1951) Skeletal and periarticular manifestations of hypervitaminosis D. AJR 65:27–41
3 Swoboda W (1952) Die Röntgensymptomatik der vit-D-Intoxikation im Kindesalter. Fortschr Geb Röntgenstr Nuklearmed Ergänzungsband 77:534–545
4 Holman CB (1952) Roentgenologic manifestations of vitamine D intoxication. Radiology 59:805–816
5 Bishop AF, Destouet JM, Murphy WA, Gilula LA (1982) Tumoral calcinosis: case report and review. Skeletal Radiol 8:269–274

Fig. 1. Hypervitaminosis D. Thin bands of sclerosis in metaphyses of tubular bones and in carpals. Dense metaphyses of radius and ulna ▷

Fig. 2a, b. Same patient as Fig. 1. **a** 1938: Very dense bone structure in metaphyses as well as in epiphyses. Several growth-arrest lines in femur and tibia. No cortical thickening and normal modeling of metaphyses. **b** 1939: Parallel dense bands in epiphyses, alternating bands of sclerosis and translucency in metaphyses

Fig. 3. Same patient as Fig. 1. Multiple parallel dense bands in pelvic bones and femoral epiphyses ▷

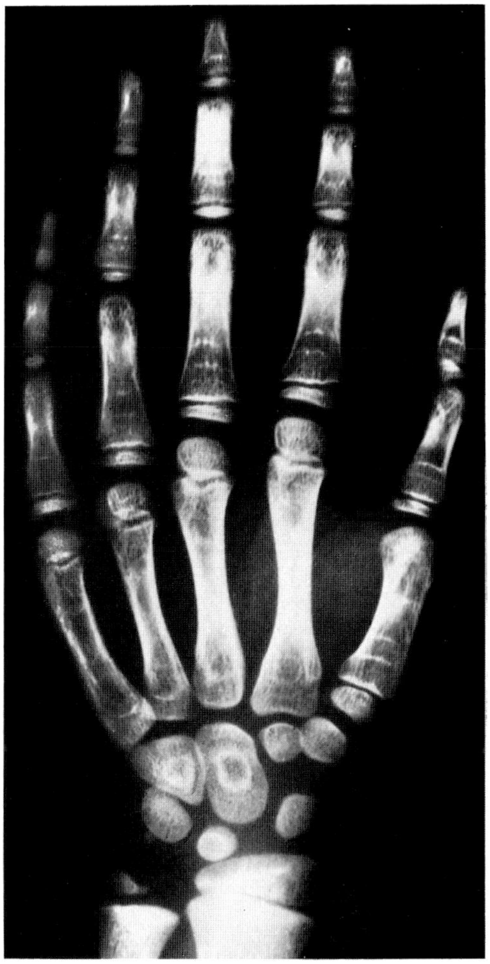

1

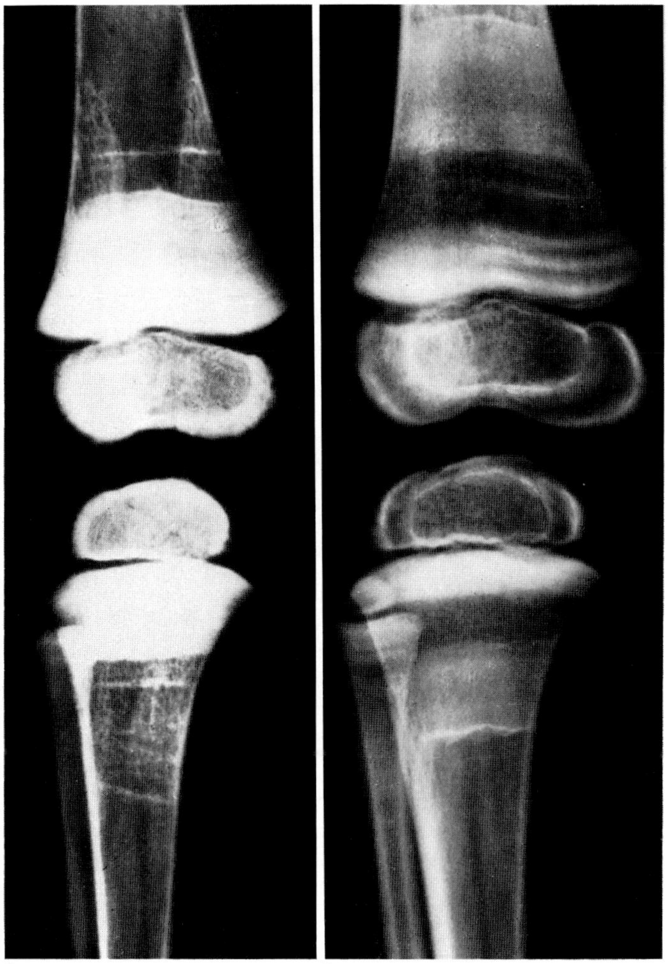

2a b

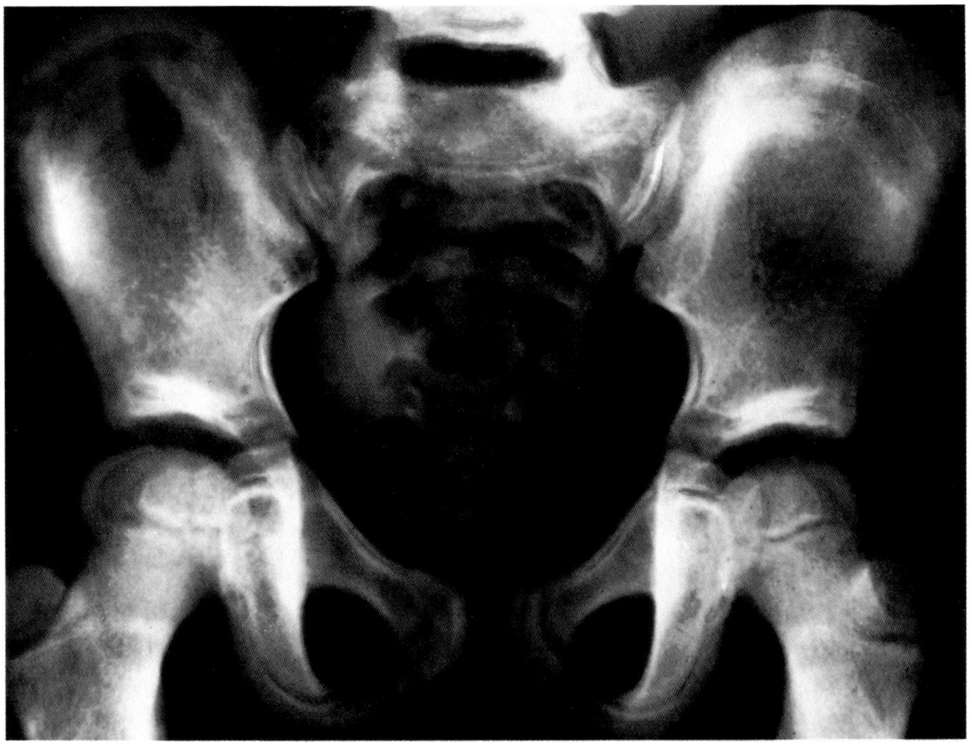

3

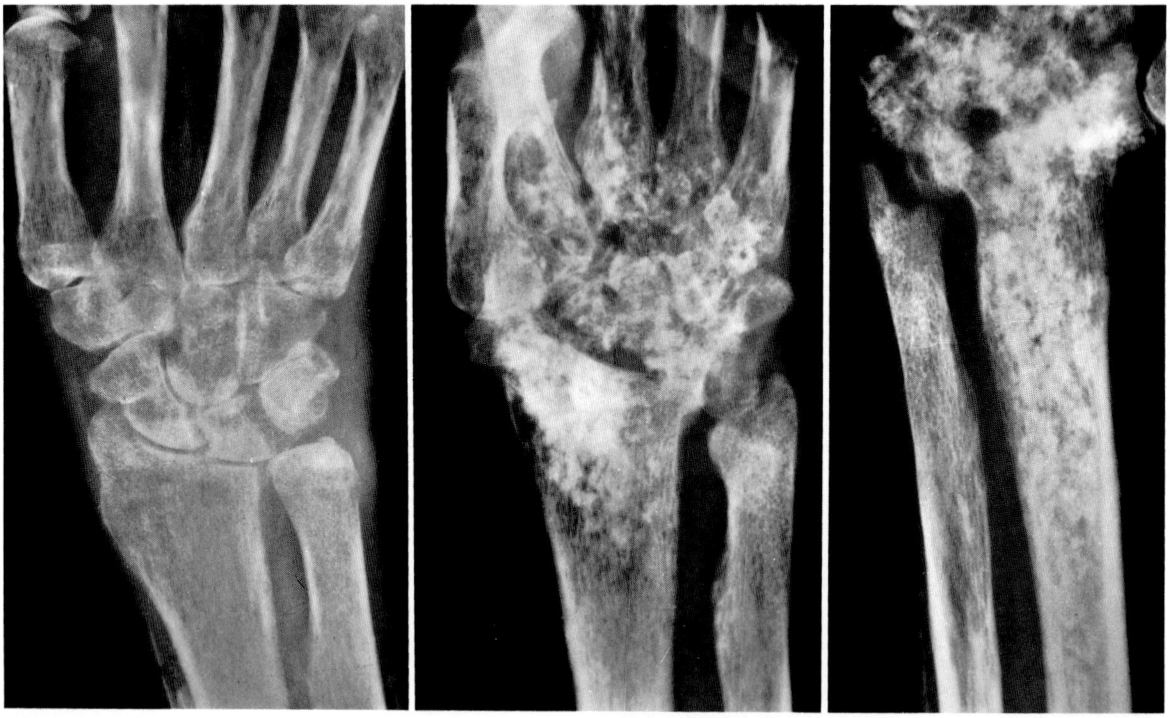

a, b c

Fig. 4a–c. Lupus erythematosus, hypervitaminosis D, and terminal renal insufficiency in a 28-year-old woman: **a** 1980: Calcifications in soft tissues and demineralization of skeleton in left wrist. **b** 1982: Increased demineralization, soft tissue calcifications, carpal destruction with spotted osteosclerosis. **c** 1983: Destruction of carpals with ankylosis. Extensive number of rosette-like osteosclerotic foci in carpals and, especially, in metaphysis of radius. These abnormalities can be explained by renal osteodystrophy

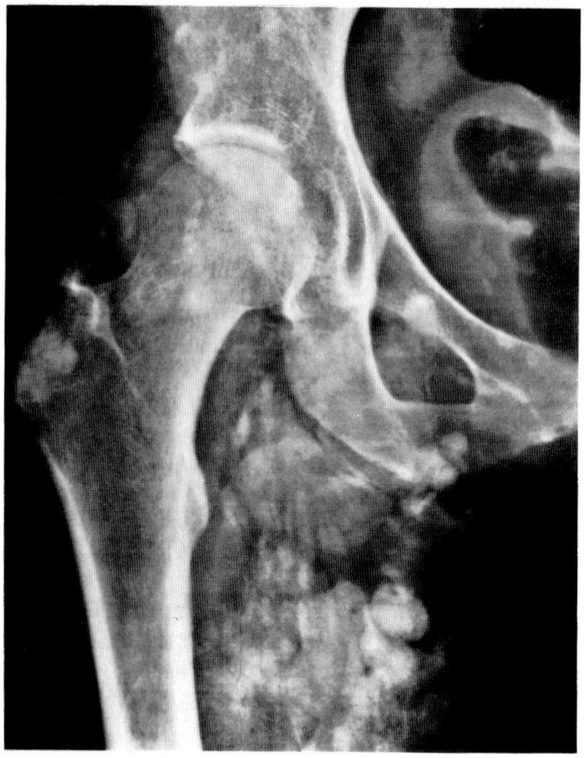

Fig. 5. Same patient as Fig. 4. Right hip: extensive soft tissue calcifications around the hip joint and intramuscularly

6.2.3 Hyperparathyroidism

Primary Hyperparathyroidism

Increased secretion of parathormone due to hyperplasia (10%–20%), adenoma (80%–90%), or carcinoma (2%) of the parathyroid glands. The raised level of parathormone causes an increase in excretion of phosphate and calcium, resulting in demineralization of the skeleton. Radiological features of primary hyperparathyroidism are described in about 20%–30% of sufferers. Many cases are diagnosed clinically before the radiographs are conclusive [1–3, 5].

Laboratory Findings
Blood: calcium high
phosphate low/normal
alkaline phosphatase normal/high
Urine: calcium high
phosphate high

Secondary Hyperparathyroidism [3, 4]

Etiology
Vitamin D deficiency (Sect. 6.2.1)
Malabsorption syndrome (deficient resorption of calcium in intestinal tract) (Sect. 6.2.1)
Chronic renal failure (Sect. 6.2.4)

Laboratory Findings
Blood: phosphate high
calcium low

Radiographic Findings [1–4]

Demineralization
Bone resorption: subperiosteal (phalanges and tuft erosions)
endosteal
intracortical (around haversian canals)
subchondral
subligamentous
trabecular bone
Cystic lesions (brown tumors)
Osteosclerosis
Chondrocalcinosis (18%–40% in primary hyperparathyroidism)
Periostitis
Soft tissue and vascular calcifications

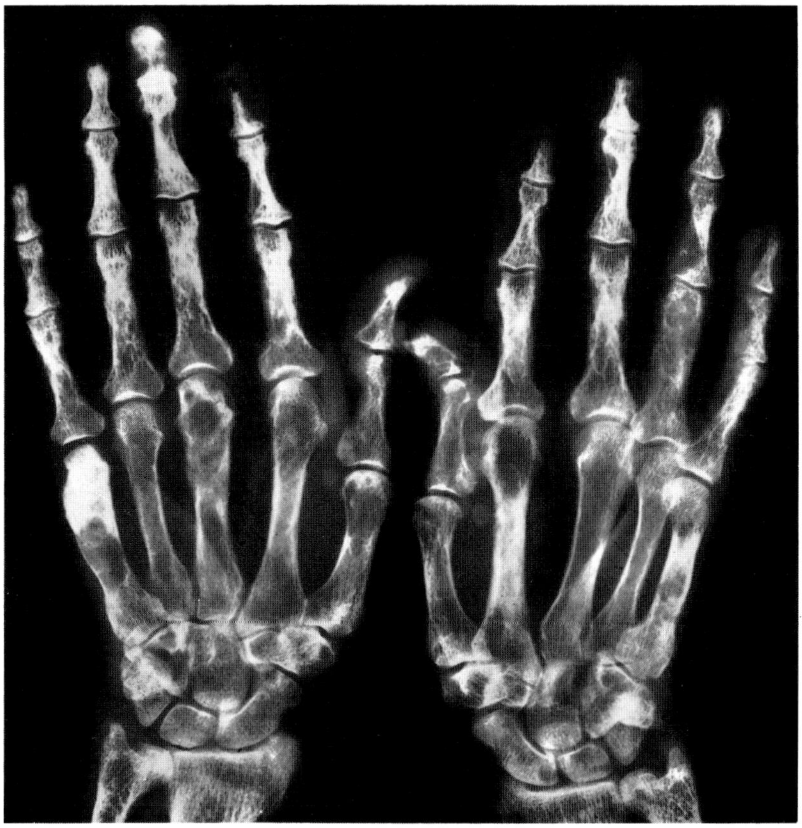

Fig. 1. Primary hyperparathyroidism in a 65-year-old woman. Extensive bone resorption, demineralization, cystic lesions

a b c d

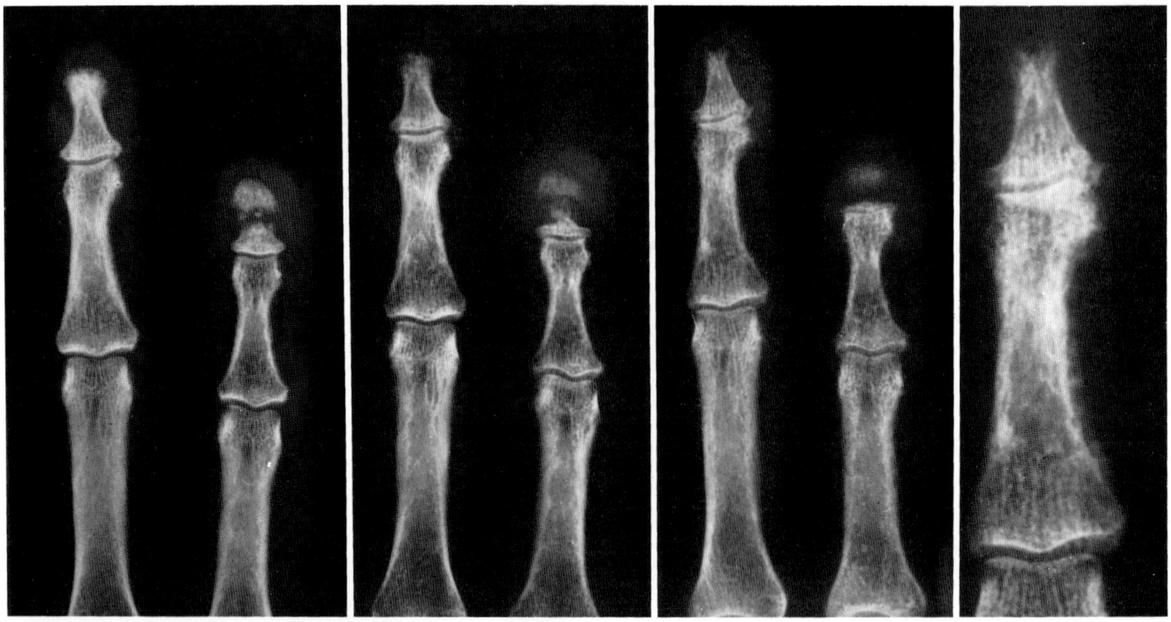

Fig. 3a–d. Renal osteodystrophy in a 44-year-old woman. **a** Subperiosteal and intracortical bone resorption associated with tuft erosions. **b** After 1 year: Progressive radiographic findings. **c** After a further 2 years: Progressive bone resorption and demineralization. **d** Detail: Significant bone resorption and tuft erosion

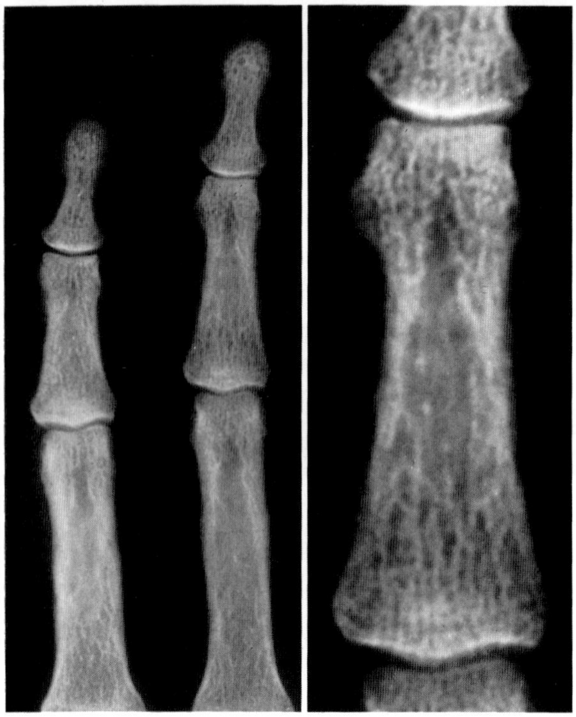

a b

◁**Fig. 2a, b.** Primary hyperparathyroidism in a 30-year-old woman. Typical subperiosteal bone resorption, slight erosion of tufts

Osteomalacia (see also renal osteodystrophy, (Sect. 6.2.4)

In primary hyperparathyroidism, brown tumors and chondrocalcinosis are regularly seen, whereas in secondary hyperparathyroidism, osteosclerosis and periostitis are more frequent. Parathormone activates bone resorption as well as bone formation. Osteosclerosis is probably due to this osteoblastic action as well as the action of calcitonin.

In renal osteodystrophy, additional findings are observed in association with secondary hyperparathyroidism: rickets/osteomalacia, soft tissue calcifications, vascular calcifications [3].

References

1 Genant HK, Heck LL, Lanzl LH, Rossman K, Horst JV, Paloyan JE (1973) Primary hyperparathyroidism. A comprehensive study of clinical, biochemical and radiographic manifestations. Radiology 109:513–524

2 Teng CT, Nathan MH (1960) Primary hyperparathyroidism. AJR 83:716–731

3 Resnick D, Niwayama G (1981) Diagnosis of bone and joint diseases. Saunders, Philadelphia

4 Jensen PS, Kliger AS (1977) Early radiographic manifestations of secondary hyperparathyroidism associated with chronic renal disease. Radiology 125:645–652

5 Juttmann JR, Bruining HA, Birkenhäger JC (1980) Diagnostic aspects of primary hyperparathyroidism (in Dutch). Ned Tijdschr Geneeskd 124:1002–1007

6.2.4 Renal Osteodystrophy

In chronic renal failure the changes in the osseous structures are caused by secondary hyperparathyroidism and osteomalacia. Radiographic abnormalities are found in approximately 50% of patients with renal osteodystrophy [1]. Long-term hemodialysis diminishes the radiographic findings.

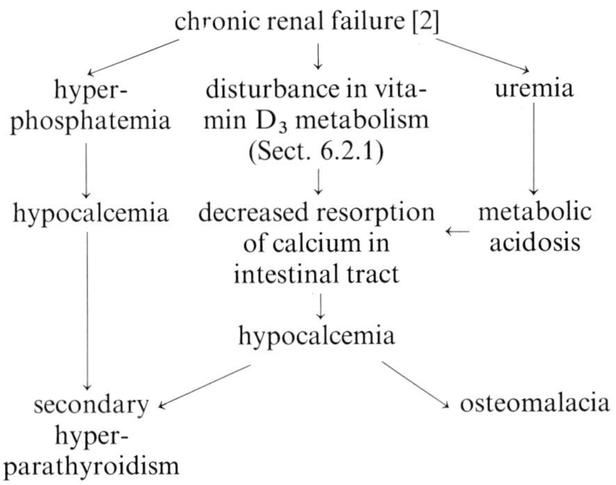

Bone Histology

From the histological findings in renal osteodystrophy one can conclude that the turnover of bone is high and that increased destruction of bone predominates over the mass of well-mineralized bone osteoid. Sometimes osteosclerosis can also be found in the biopsy specimens (actions of parathormone and calcitonin [3]).

Laboratory Findings

Blood: calcium low
  phosphate high
  alkaline phosphatase normal/high

Radiographic Findings [2–6]

Demineralization
Bone resorption: subperiosteal (phalanges and tuft)
  endosteal
  intracortical
  subchondral (periarticular, especially distal interphalangeal joints of fourth and fifth fingers)
  subligamentous
  trabecular bone
Metastatic calcifications of soft tissue (periarticular) and arterial walls
Osteosclerosis: rugger-jersey spine
  metaphyseal areas of tubular bones (especially long bones)
  skull base
(Pseudo)fractures
Chondrocalcinosis (uncommon)
Cystic lesions (uncommon)
(See also secondary hyperparathyroidism, Sect. 6.2.3)

Differential Diagnosis

Tuft erosions: Acro-osteolysis (Sect. 3.1)
Multiple soft tissue calcifications in hand:
  Hypoparathyroidism (Sect. 6.1.2) and Pseudohypoparathyroidism (Sect. 6.1.2) [7]
  Hypervitaminosis D (Sect. 6.2.2)
  Werner's syndrome (Fig. 5 in Sect. 6.2.7)
  Gout (Sect. 7.3.8)
  Sarcoidosis (Sect. 7.3.12)
  Scleroderma (Sect. 7.6.3)
  Dermatomyositis [8]

References

1 Graaf P de (1980) Renal bone disease and extraskeletal calcifications during dialysis and after transplantation. Thesis, Pasmans, Leyden
2 Raber-Durlacher JE, Schächter MEJ, Abraham-Inpijn L, Bras J, Ooy CP van, Wilmink JM (1983) Renal osteodystrophy II. Pathology and roentgenologic diagnosis (in Dutch). Ned Tijdschr v Geneesk 127:1578–1584
3 Resnick D, Niwayama G (1981) Diagnosis of bone and joint diseases. Saunders Philadelphia
4 Meema HE, Oreopoulous DG, Meema S (1978) A roentgenologic study of cortical bone resorption in chronic renal failure. Radiology 126:67–74
5 Lewis VL, Keats TE (1982) Bone and sclerosis in renal osteodystrophy simulating osteonecrosis. Skeletal Radiol 8:275–278
6 Sundaram M, Joyce PF, Shields JB, Riaz MA, Sagar S (1979) Terminal tufts of the hands-site for earliest changes of renal osteodystrophy in patients on maintenance hemodialysis. AJR 133:25–29
7 Hall FM, Segall-Blank M, Genant HK, Kolb FO (1981) Pseudohypoparathyroidism presenting as renal osteodystrophy. Skeletal Radiol 6:43–46
8 Sewell JR, Liyanage B, Ansell BM (1978) Calcinosis in juvenile dermatomyositis. Skeletal Radiol 3:137–143

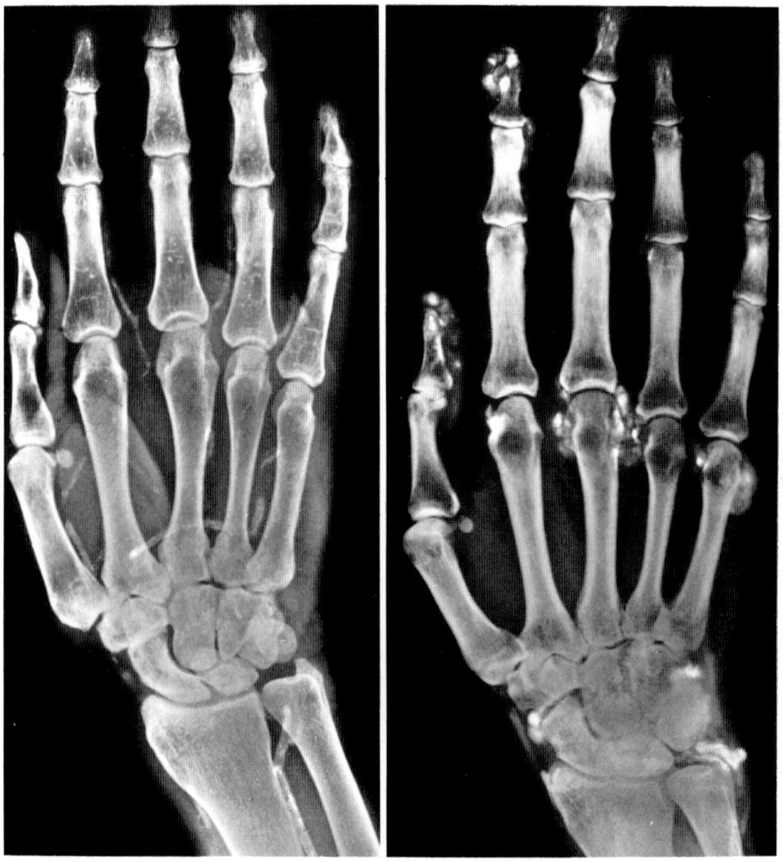

a b

Fig. 1a, b. Renal osteodystrophy. **a** In a 65-year-old man: Metastatic calcifications in arterial walls, slight, rather diffuse osteosclerosis. **b** In a 37-year-old woman: Metastatic calcifications in periarticular soft tissues, probable chondrocalcinosis in wrist, osteosclerosis in distal ulna and radius

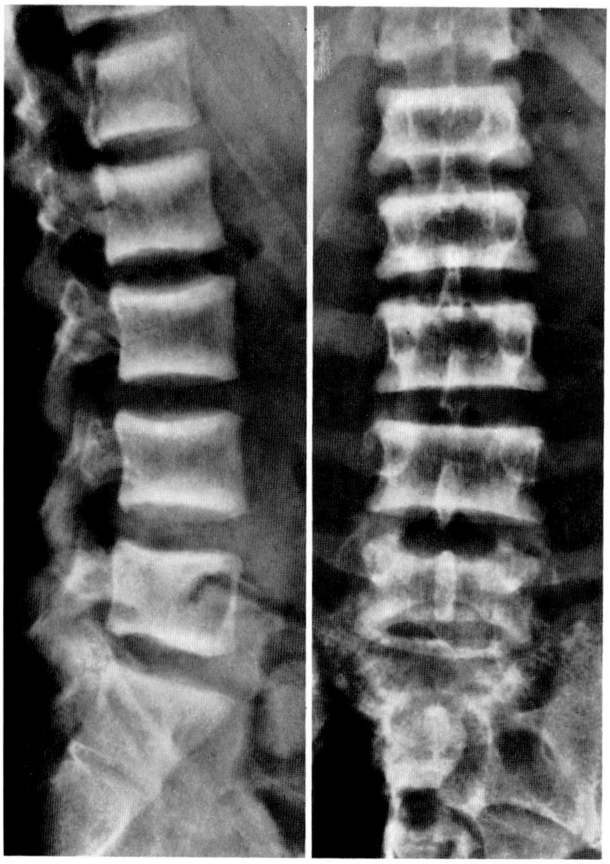

2a **b**

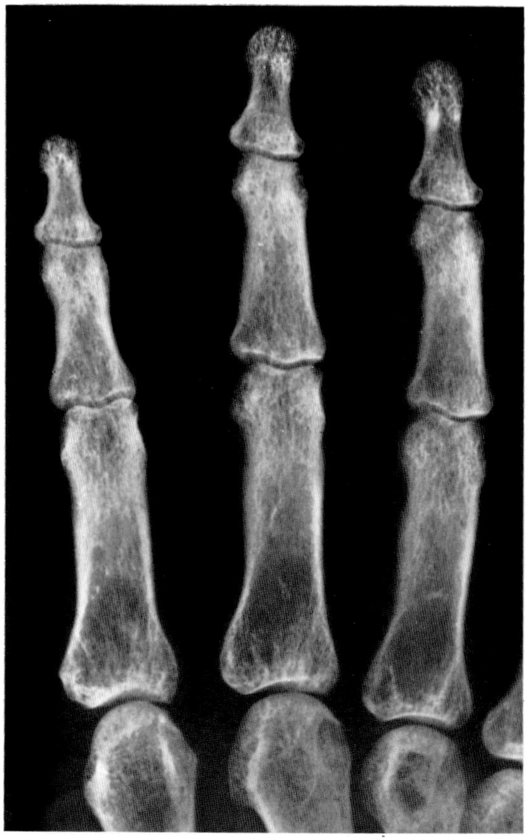

4

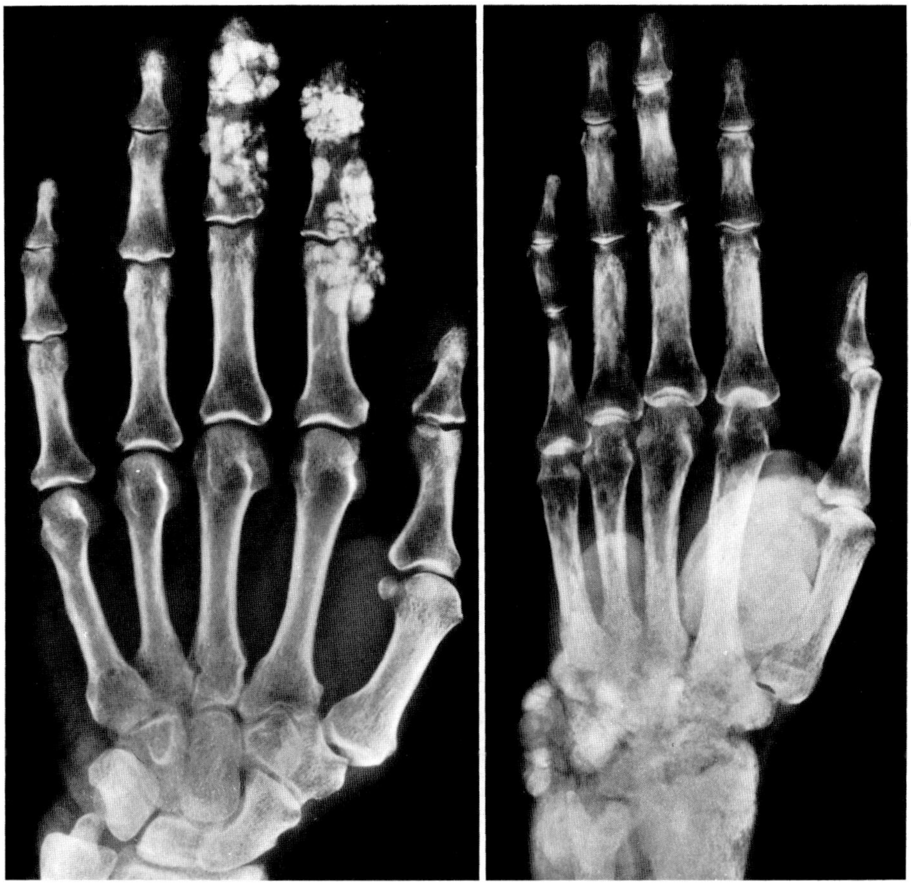

a b

Fig. 3a, b. Multiple soft tissue calcifications. **a** In a 55-year-old woman with scleroderma. **b** In a 29-year-old woman with hypervitaminosis D: Huge calcifications around wrist, osteosclerosis of carpals and distal ends of radius and ulna

◁ **Fig. 2.** Renal osteodystrophy in a 43-year-old man. Rugger-jersey spine

Fig. 4. Renal osteodystrophy in a 41-year-old man with chronic renal failure. Increased bone density, predominantly in metaphyseal areas of phalanges. Spine displayed characteristic rugger-jersey appearance

6.2.5 Scurvy

Synonym: hypovitaminosis C

Sufficient vitamin C in the diet is necessary for normal formation of osteoid tissue. Deficiency of vitamin C impairs osteoblastic activity and osteoid formation. On radiographs, a dense zone of provisional calcification lies adjacent to the growth plate (Wimberger's white line). This zone is brittle and commonly the site of microfractures. Lateral extension of the zone of provisional calcification leads to elevation of the periosteal membrane and spurs. On the diaphyseal side of the provisional zone, the formation of bony matrix is decreased and calcification is replaced by fibrous tissue. Hemorrhages usually begin in this radiolucent zone (Trümmerfeld's zone) and may produce periosteal hemorrhages. Clear radiographic signs of scurvy are found in the skeleton of children, particularly around the knees. In adults, usually only nonspecific osteoporosis is present [1–4].

Radiographic Findings [1–4]

Hand/forearm:

Osteoporosis of formed bone (more osteoclastic than osteoblastic activity)
Metaphyseal bands of increased bone density adjacent to growth plates (Wimberger's white lines)
Metaphyseal bands of radiolucency (Trümmerfeld's zone)
Metaphyseal fractures
Periosteal new bone formation (remote hemorrhages)
Thin cortex
Delayed skeletal maturation
Radiodense shell around epiphyseal centers and carpals

Differential Diagnosis

Congenital syphilis (Sect. 7.3.1)
Leukemia
Metastases of neuroblastoma (Sect. 7.4.2.5)

References

1 McCann P (1962) The incidence and value of radiological signs of scurvy. Br J Radiol 35:683–686
2 Bromer RS (1973) A critical analysis of the roentgen signs of infantile scurvy. AJR 49:575–579
3 Resnick D, Niwayama G (1981) Diagnosis of bone and joint disorders. Saunders, Philadelphia
4 Steinbach HL, Gold RH, Preger L (1975) Roentgen appearance of the hand in diffuse disease. Year Book Medical Publishers, Chicago

Fig. 1a–d. Scurvy in three patients. **a, b** Significant metaphyseal bands of radiolucency in distal radius and ulna (Trümmerfeld's zones), some periosteal new bone formation, some fragmentation of dense provisional zones. **c** Wimberger's white line and Trümmerfeld's zone both present, scalloping of radial and ulnar cortices due to periosteal new bone formation. **d** Distinct Wimberger's white lines, incipient ossification of carpals ▷

Fig. 2. Scurvy. Severe osteoporosis, dense and radiolucent bands in metaphyses, spurs at metaphyseal margins, microfractures and periosteal new bone formation at many sites. The fibulae are bowed ▷

Fig. 3. Congenital syphilis. Metaphyseal affection of radius and ulna with cortical erosions and fracture of ulna. Neither Wimberger's white line nor Trümmerfeld's zone present

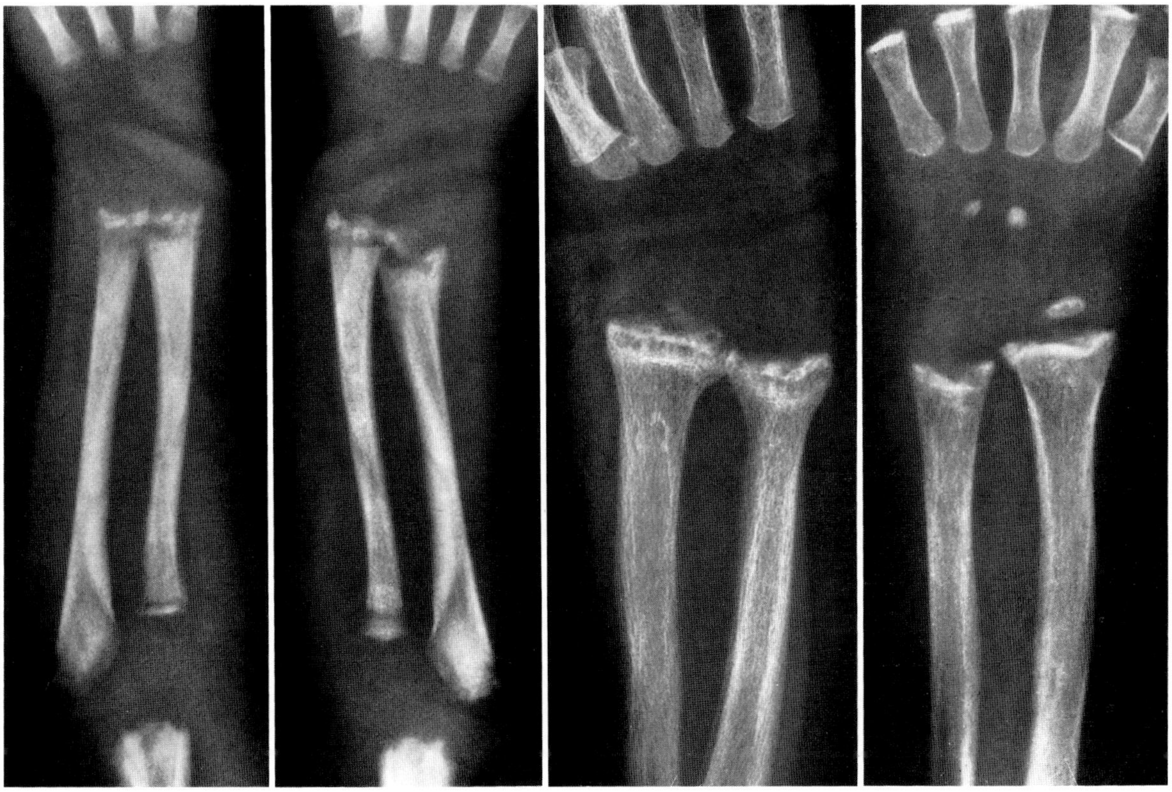

1a **b** **c** **d**

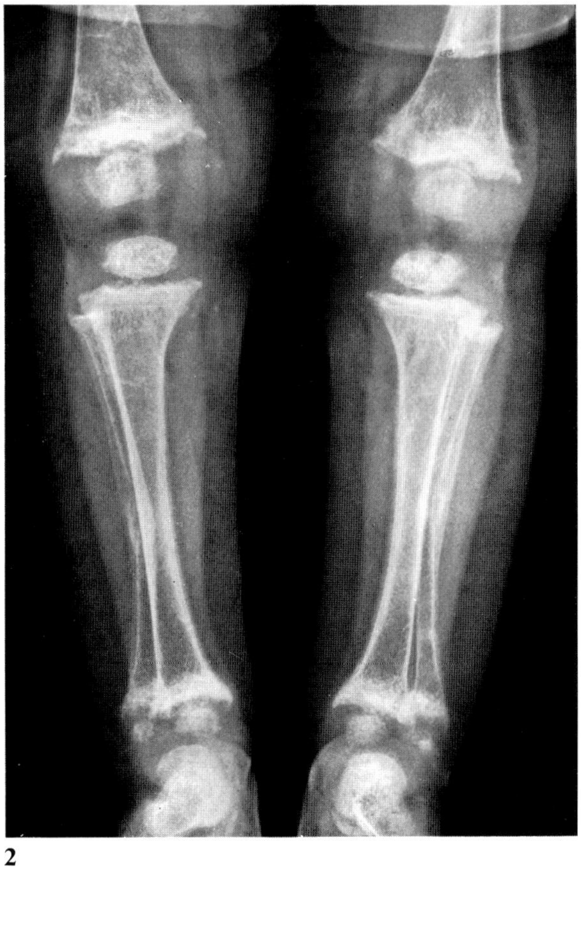

2

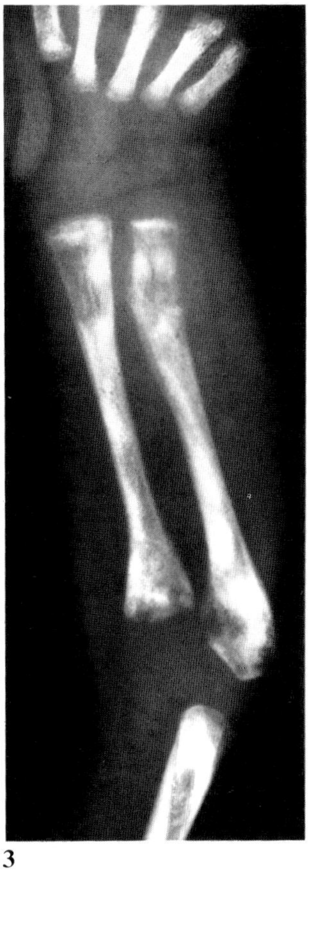

3

6.2.6 Chondrocalcinosis

Chondrocalcinosis probably originates from abnormal excretion of calcium pyrophosphate dihydrate (CPPD) crystals by the chondrocytes as a result of changes in the chondrocytic metabolism. Reduced activity of pyrophosphatase (pyrophosphatase hydrolyses calcium pyrophosphate to the more soluble orthophosphate) in the aging patient or suppression of pyrophosphatase activity by calcium, ferrous, and cupric ions are thought to be the inducing etiologic factors in chondrocalcinosis [1]. This inhibition of the pyrophosphatase action causes an increase in the amount of calcium pyrophosphate in the joint cartilage. Acute synovitis may be related to "crystal shedding": cartilaginous deposits are cast into the articular cavity. The association between CPPD chondrocalcinosis and the articular calcifications in hemochromatosis, hyperparathyroidism, and Wilson's disease can be explained in this way [2].

Clinical Findings

The following CPPD syndromes can be encountered [3]:

1. Asymptomatic CPPD deposition, especially in older people (25% over the age of 75 years)
2. Acute inflammatory joint attacks (pseudogout), mainly in one of the larger joints
3. Pseudorheumatoid arthritis, which may simulate seronegative rheumatoid arthritis, mainly in the larger joints
4. Severe osteoarthrosis
5. Recurrent joint hemorrhage (knee joint)

Classification [3, 4]

1. Primary or idiopathic CPPD: a sometimes familial disease based on autosomal dominant inheritance
2. Secondary CPPD:
   a) hemochromatosis (41% CPPD)
   b) hyperparathyroidism (18%–40% CPPD)
   c) Wilson's disease
   d) gout (5%–32% CPPD)
   e) osteoarthrosis
   f) diabetes mellitus
   g) neuropathic arthropathy
   h) ochronosis
   i) hypophosphatasia
   j) miscellaneous conditions

Radiographic Findings [3–5]

Hand

Chondrocalcinosis in hyaline cartilage and fibrocartilage
Joint effusion
Small or larger (more than 1 cm) subchondral pseudocysts
Degenerative joint destruction (severe destruction mimics neuropathic arthropathy or ischemic necrosis)
Synovial calcifications, large tophaceous CPPD deposits (uncommon)
Linear calcifications in tendons
Osteochondral intra-articular bodies

Other Sites

Involvement of hips, knees, shoulders, elbows, symphysis pubis, sacroiliac joints, and lumbar spine
Linear calcifications in Achilles tendon and quadriceps femoris tendon

Hemochromatosis [6–9]

Primary hemochromatosis is a congenital defect involving the absorption of excessive amounts of iron in the gastrointestinal tract. The iron ions disturb the cartilage metabolism by suppressing pyrophosphatase activity. A second defect seems to be the inability of the reticuloendothelial cells to store this iron. *Secondary* hemochromatosis can result from increased oral intake of iron, repeated blood transfusions, prolonged or repeated iron therapy, or cirrhosis of the liver.

Radiographic Findings

Hand

Signs of arthritis caused by crystal-induced synovitis
Osteoarthrosis of small joints (especially second to fourth metacarpophalangeal joints) with joint space narrowing, subchondral cysts, osteophytes, subchondral sclerosis, and erosions
Chondrocalcinosis
Osteoarthrosis of carpal joints
Focal osteoporosis of wrist

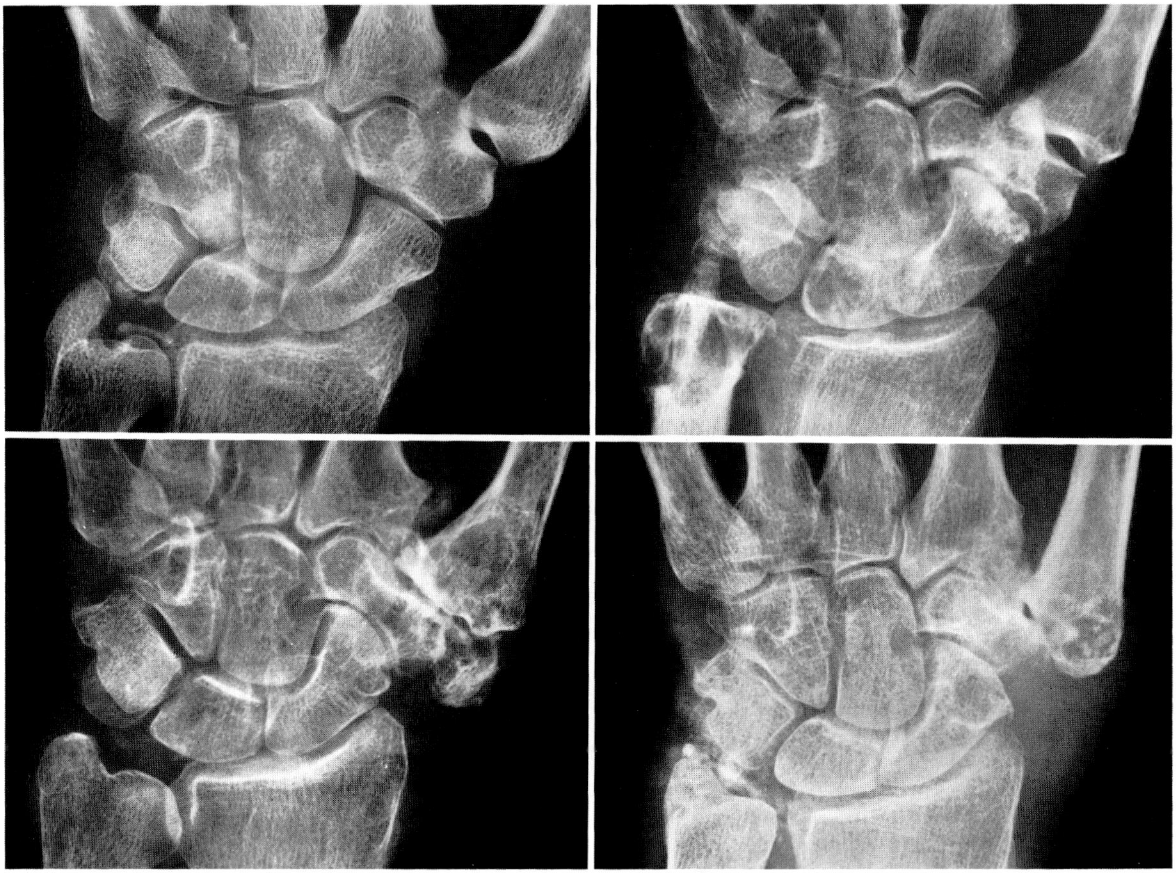

Fig. 1 a–d. CPPD chondrocalcinosis. **a** In a 60-year-old woman: Calcifications in triangular and intercarpal cartilages of wrist, no significant osseous changes. **b** In a 71-year-old woman: Chondrocalcinosis and some tendon calcifications. Degenerative joint diseases with large cavities in ulna and lunate. **c** In a 69-year-old woman: Small calcifications in triangular cartilage of wrist, severe osteoarthrosis of first carpometacarpal joint, soft tissue calcifications on radial side of wrist (probably hydroxyapatite). **d** In a 65-year-old woman: Acute inflammatory attack of chondrocalcinosis in first carpometacarpal joint (pseudogout attack). Joint presents severe osteoarthrosis and large pseudocysts in first metacarpal. Triangular cartilage calcified

Other Sites

Osteoarthrosis of small and large joints

Calcifications of intervertebral discs

Uncommon: periostitis and osteonecrosis of femoral head

References

1 McCarty DJ (1979) Calcium pyrophosphate dihydrate crystal deposition disease: pseudo-gout: articular chondrocalcinosis. In: McCarty DJ (ed) Arthritis and allied conditions, 9th edn. Lea and Febiger. Philadelphia

2 McCarty DJ (1976) Calcium pyrophosphate dihydrate crystal deposition disease. Arthritis Rheum 19[suppl]: 275–282

3 Resnick D, Niwayama G, Goergen TG, Utsinger PD, Shapiro RF, Haselwood DH, Wiesner KB (1977) Clinical, radiographic and pathologic abnormalities in calcium pyrophosphate dihydrate deposition disease (CPPD): pseudo-gout. Radiology 122:1–16

4 Resnick D, Niwayama G (1981) Diagnosis of bone and joint disorders. Saunders Philadelphia

5 Martel W, McCarter DK, Solsky MA, Good AE, Hart WR, Braunstein EM, Brady TM (1981) Further observations on arthropathy of calcium pyrophosphate crystal deposition disease. Radiology 141:1–15

6 Twersky J (1975) Joint changes in idiopathic haemochromatosis. AJR 124:139–144

7 Weber J (1982) Haemochromatosis. Boerhaave course: metabolic joint disease. PAO, Leyden, pp 59–61

8 Sella EJ, Goodman AH (1973) Arthropathy secondary to transfusion haemochromatosis. J Bone Joint Surg [Am] 55:1077–1081

9 Mall K, Zander W (1980) Arthropathie bei Hämochromatose. Fortschr Geb Röntgenstr Nuklearmed Ergänzungsband 132:442–446

a b

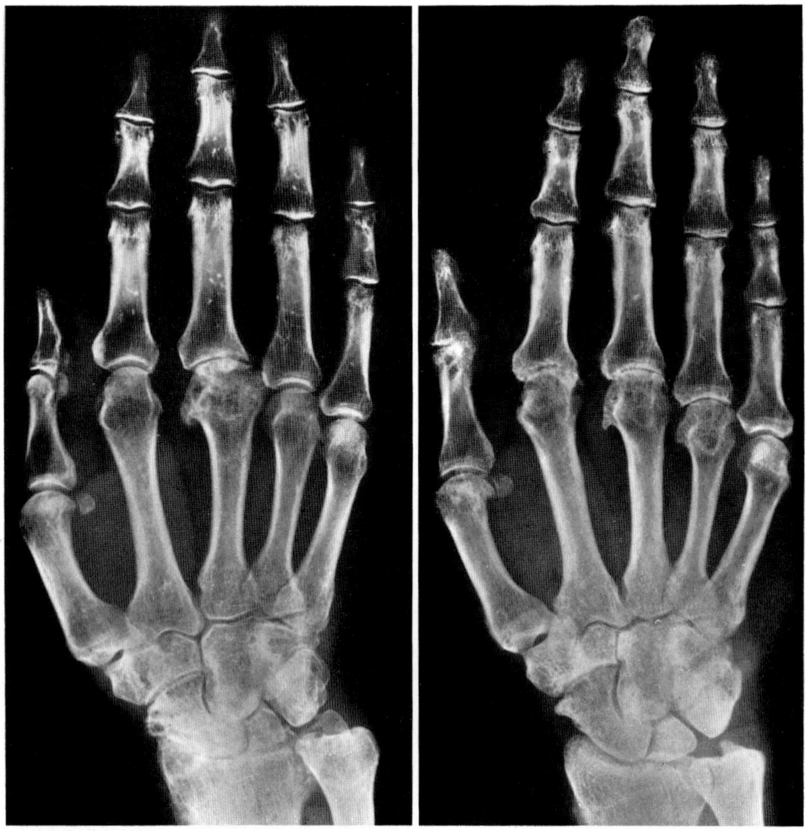

Fig. 2a, b. Primary hemochromatosis. **a** In a 58-year-old man: Chondrocalcinosis of triangular cartilage of wrist, severe osteoarthrosis of radiocarpal joint and third metacarpophalangeal joint. **b** In a 62-year-old man: Severe osteoarthrosis of second to fourth metacarpophalangeal joints. These are the predominantly affected hand joints in hemochromatosis

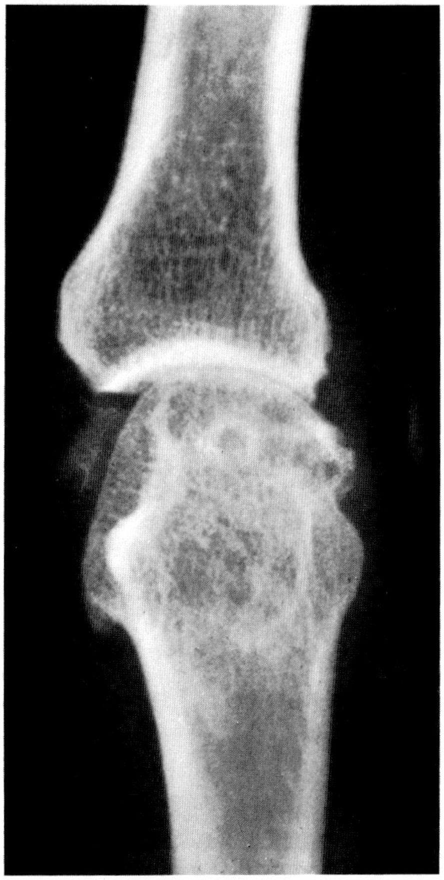

Fig. 3. Chondrocalcinosis and osteoarthrosis. Faint calcifications of joint cartilage, joint space narrowing, sclerosis, small exophytes

6.2.7 Other Crystal-Induced Diseases

Deposition of crystals may be facilitated by alterations in the structure and metabolism of cartilage. Joint damage can cause crystal shedding, and free crystals in the synovial fluid can activate mechanisms which will accelerate joint destruction. These particles are therefore a potential amplification mechanism in the pathogenesis of chronic destructive arthritis, as well as a cause of acute synovitis [1–3].

Hydroxyapatite Deposition Disease

Hydroxyapatite is the main constituent of most ectopic calcifications. It has been suggested that the crystals are formed in chondrocytic matrix vesicles. Especially in the more severe destructive forms of osteoarthritis, these crystals have been found in the articular cartilage, synovial membrane, and synovial fluid. They can induce the generation of prostaglandins and destructive enzymes from the synovial cells [1, 2]. Hydroxyapatite deposition disease (HADD) has sometimes proved to be a familial disorder [4].

Clinical Findings

HADD presents with clinical features of acute monoarticular periarthritis, polyarticular disease, or joint destruction.

Radiographic Findings [4, 5]

Solitary or multiple calcifications in vicinity of joints (tendons, bursae, joint capsules), initially thin and poorly defined, later more homogeneous and dense
Diffuse amorphous pattern of intra-articular calcifications
Well-defined deposits of HADD: (a) in fibrocartilage (for instance within menisci); (b) sometimes accompanying CPPD deposits in hyaline cartilage
Osseous lesions (osteoporosis, cysts, reactive sclerosis, contour irregularities)
Osteoarthrosis
Ankylosis

Differential Diagnosis of Soft Tissue Calcifications

Osteoarthrosis (Sect. 7.3.13)
Renal osteodystrophy (Sect. 6.2.4)
CPPD crystal deposition disease (Sect. 6.2.6)
Scleroderma (Sect. 7.6.3)
Dermatomyositis
Vascular disease (arteriosclerosis)
Hyperparathyroidism (Sect. 6.2.3)
Hypervitaminosis D (Sect. 6.2.2)
Sarcoidosis (Sect. 7.3.12)
Hypoparathyroidism and pseudohypoparathyroidism (Sect. 6.1.2)
Gout (Sect. 7.3.8)
Tuberculosis (Sect. 7.3.9)
Werner's syndrome (progeria adultorum) (Fig. 5)
Sequelae of trauma
Chondromatosis capsulae (Fig. 4)
Tumoral calcinosis [6]
Calcinosis universalis
Soft tissue tumors (hemangiomas, synovial sarcoma, chondromas) (Sect. 7.4.1.3, 7.4.2.4)

Other Crystals

The role of other crystals in joint disease remains unclear. The following crystals can be found [47]:
Calcium orthophosphate
Octacalcium phosphate
Brushite
Cholesterol and other lipid crystals
Calcium oxalate crystals in patients with renal diseases

References

1 Dieppe PA (1982) Other crystal-induced arthropathies. Boerhaave course: metabolic joint diseases. PAO, Leyden
2 Dieppe PA, Crocker P, Huskisson EC, Willoughby DA (1976) Apatite deposition disease (a new arthropathy). Lancet 1:266–269
3 Halverson PB, McCarty DJ (1978) Identification of hydroxyapatite crystals in synovial fluid. Arthritis Rheum 21:563–569 (abstr)
4 Marcos JC, de Benyacar MA, Garcia-Morteo O, Arturi AS, Maldonado-Cocco JA, Morales VH, Laguens R (1981) Idiopathic familial chondrocalcinosis due to apatite crystal deposition. Am J Med 71:557–564
5 Bonavista JA, Dalinka MK, Schumacher HR (1980) Hydroxyapatite deposition disease. Radiology 134:621–625
6 Bishop AF, Destouet JM, Murphy WA, Gilula LA (1982) Tumoral calcinosis: case report and review. Skeletal Radiol 8:269–274

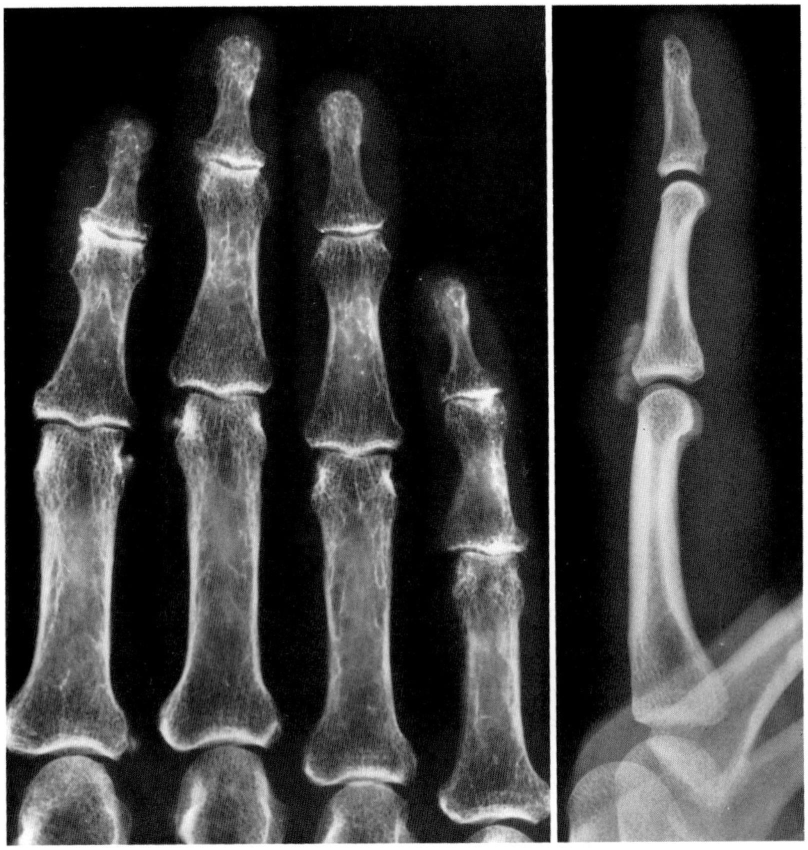

a b

Fig. 1 a, b. Periarticular calcifications, probably hydroxyapatite. **a** In an 80-year-old woman: Multiple periarticular soft tissue calcifications. **b** In a 41-year-old woman: Painful proximal interphalangeal joint, periarticular calcifications, normal joint space

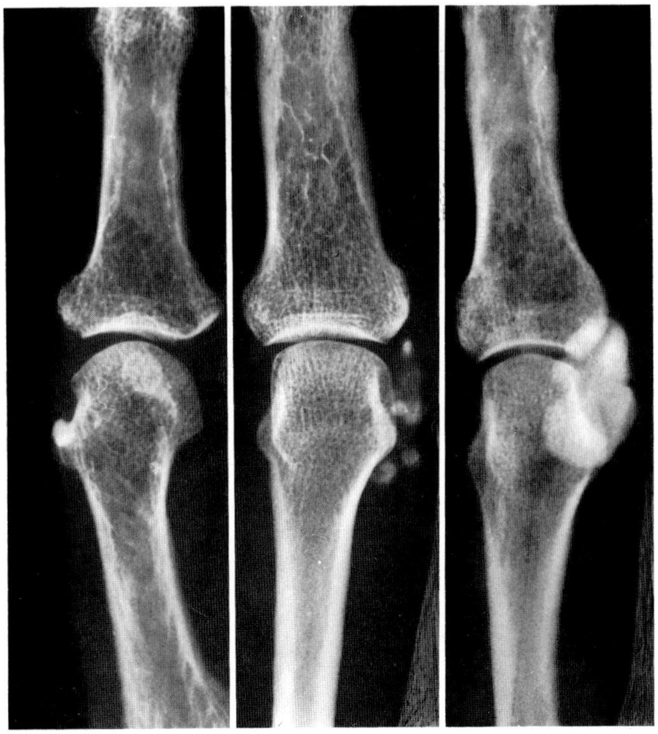

a b c

Fig. 2 a–c. Periarticular calcifications, probably hydroxyapatite. **a** In a 78-year-old woman: Amorphous circumscribed calcification in vicinity of fifth metacarpophalangeal joint. **b** In a 74-year-old man: Painful fourth metacarpophalangeal joint, multiple calcifications adjacent to this normal joint. Possibly tendinitis calcarea. **c** In a 57-year-old woman: Painful fourth metacarpophalangeal joint, probably well-defined hydroxyapatite deposition. Complaints and deposit disappeared after a period of 6 months

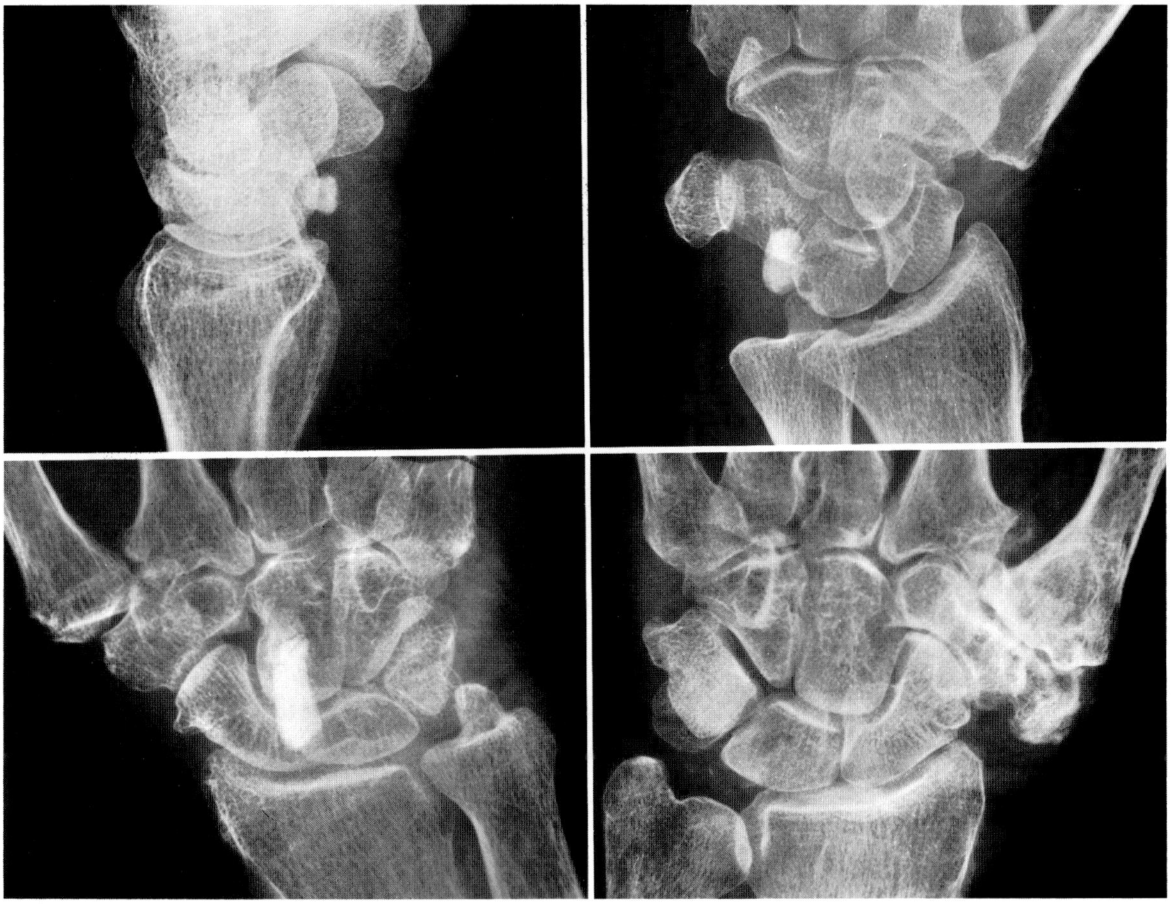

a b c d

Fig. 3a–d. Periarticular calcifications, probably hydroxyapatite. **a** In a 49-year-old man: Painful wrist, circumscribed calcification volar to the wrist (tendinitis?). **b** 69-year-old woman: Painful wrist, circumscribed calcification near ulnar styloid (tendinitis?). **c** 72-year-old woman: Painful wrist, large soft tissue calcification. Probably tendinitis. **d** 69-year-old woman: Faint calcification by CPPD crystals in triangular cartilage, amorphous calcification, probably hydroxyapatite deposition, near first carpometacarpal joint, severe osteoarthrosis of this joint

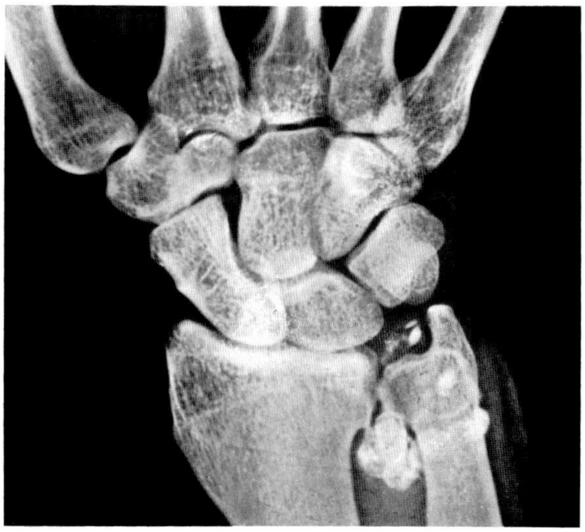

Fig. 4. Chondromatosis capsulae of distal radioulnar joint. A number of dense deposits of calcium salts in chondromatous tissue are present

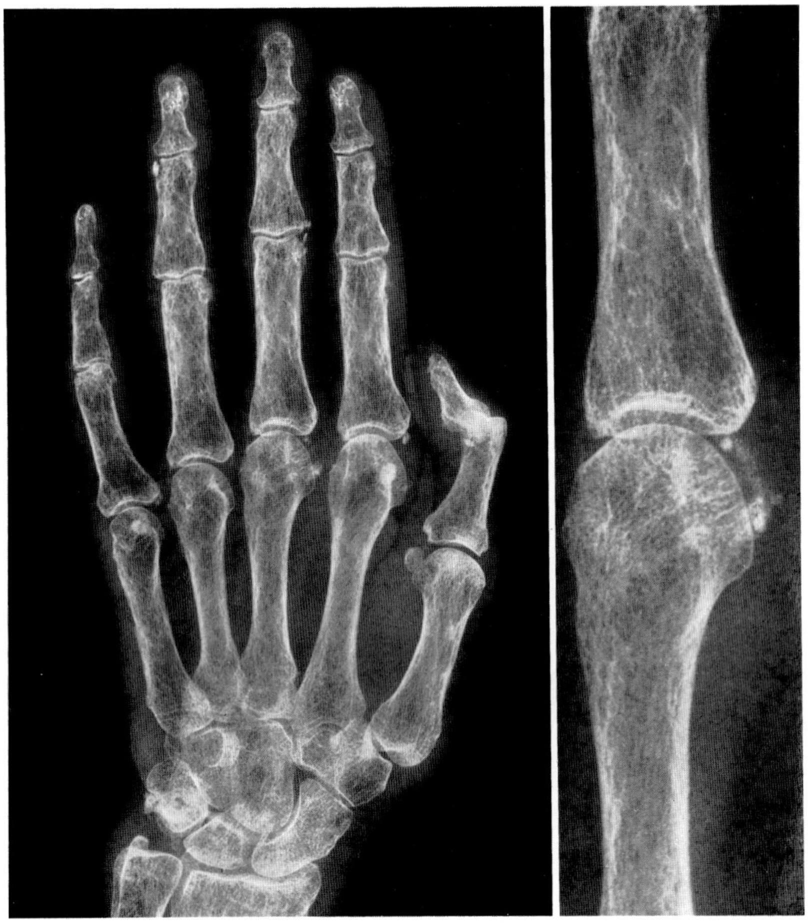

a b

Fig. 5a, b. Werner's syndrome (progeria adultorum) in an adult female. Severe osteoporosis, multiple calcifications. Most of the calcifications are periarticular, and some chondrocalcinosis also seems to be present (**b**)

6.2.8 Oxalosis

Oxalosis involves widespread deposition of calcium oxalate crystals in renal and several extrarenal tissues. It may be an acquired disorder, or may represent one aspect of primary hyperoxaluria, a rare autosomal recessive disease. There are two types of primary hyperoxaluria:

Type I absence of alpha-ketoglutarate-glyoxylate-carboxylase activity

Type II lack of D-glyceric-dehydrogenase activity

In both types, excessive production of oxalate leads to deposition in the body tissues, and increased excretion, of calcium oxalate. Nephrolithiasis and nephrocalcinosis are usually followed by uremia. Progressive renal failure causes renal osteodystrophy (secondary hyperparathyroidism and osteomalacia). Thanks to long-term renal dialysis, these patients can survive into adult life. In biopsy specimens, extensive destruction of cortical bone trabeculae and deposition of rosette-like arrangement of oxalate crystals may be found. These deposits of calcium oxalate are surrounded by giant cell granulomas and an abundance of unmineralized osteoid tissue [1, 2].

Radiographic Findings [1–5]

Hand

Osteosclerosis: metaphyseal bands
  spotty metaphyseal osteosclerosis

Signs of renal osteodystrophy (secondary hyperparathyroidism and osteomalacia)

Coarse trabeculae

Acro-osteolysis

Soft tissue and vascular calcifications

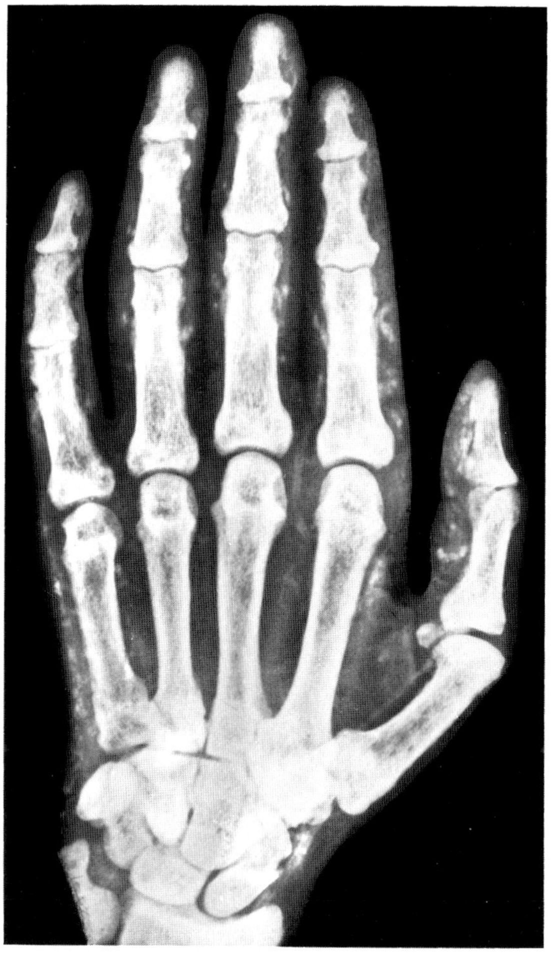

Fig. 1. Oxalosis in a 44-year-old man. Primary hyperoxaluria, chronic hemodialysis. Osteosclerosis, predominantly in the metaphyseal areas, coarsening of trabeculae, subperiosteal bone resorption by secondary hyperparathyroidism, excessive calcification of soft tissues

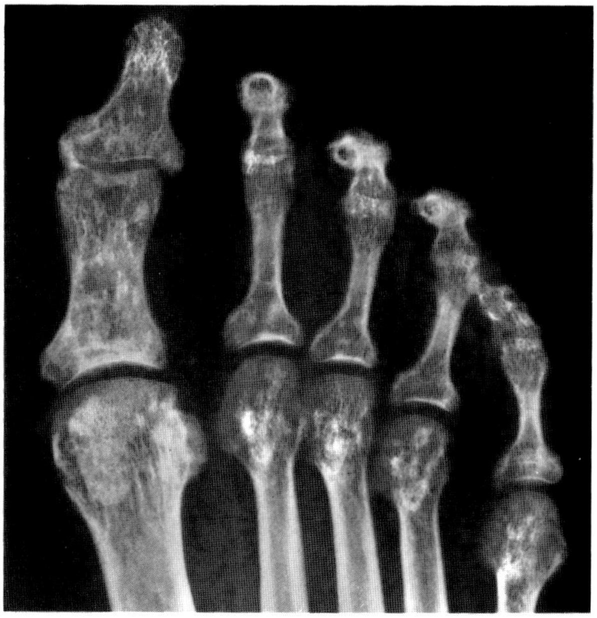

Fig. 2. Oxalosis in a 49-year-old man. Foci of osteosclerosis in metaphyseal regions (differential diagnosis osteopoikilosis; Sect. 1.2.4). Some subperiosteal bone resorption and faint soft tissue calcifications

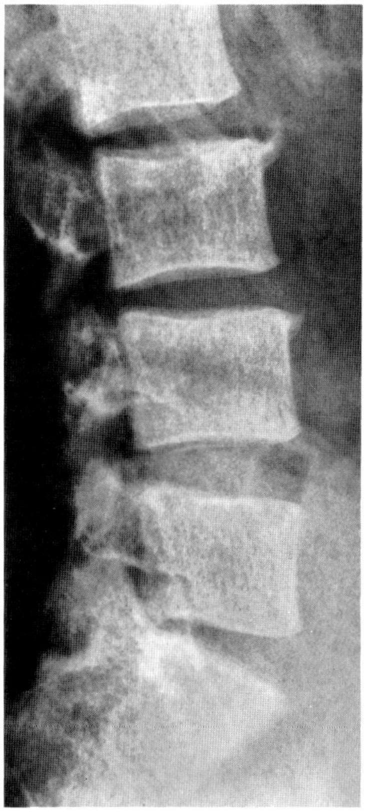

Fig. 3. Same patient as Fig. 2. Woolly osteosclerosis of vertebral bodies due to deposition of calcium oxlate and secondary hyperparathyroidism (rugger-jersey spine)

Other Sites
Foot: findings similar to those in hand
Long tubular bones: metaphyseal bands of osteosclerosis and rosettes
soft tissue calcifications
Spine: osteosclerosis and coarsening of trabeculae in vertebral bodies

Differential Diagnosis

Hypervitaminosis D (Sect. 6.2.2)
Fluorosis (Sect. 7.5.1)
Mastocytosis (Sect. 7.6.7)

References

1 Breed A, Chesney R, Friedman A, Gilbert E, Langer L, Lattoraca R (1981) Oxalosis-induced bone disease: a complication of transplantation and prolonged survival in primary hyperoxaluria. J Bone Joint Surg [Am] 63-A:310–316
2 Brancaccio D, Poggi AM, Ciccarelli C, Bellini F, Galmozzi C, Poletti I, Maggiore Q (1981) Bone changes in end-stage oxalosis. AJR 136:935–939
3 Martijn A, Thijn CJP (1982) Radiologic findings in primary hyperoxaluria. Skeletal Radiol 8:21–24
4 Kalifa G, Dossans B, Gagnadoux MF, Sauvegrin J (1979) Aspects radiologiques de l'oxalose. J Radiol 60:45–49
5 Hug I, Mihatsch JM (1975) Die primäre Oxalosis. Fortschr Geb Röntgenstr Nuklearmed Ergänzungsband 123:153–162

6.2.9 Paget's Disease

Synonym: osteitis deformans

Paget's disease is probably caused by a slow viral infection of the osteoblasts. Both the affected hyperactive osteoclasts and a large number of osteoblasts are responsible for the changes in size, shape, and structure of the affected bones [1]. The abnormalities usually start in the proximal end of the bone and spread in a distal direction. A predilection for the pelvis, skull, spine, and long tubular bones is obvious.

Radiographic Findings [2–4]

Osteolysis, occasionally as numerous small resorption clefts of cortex [2]
Osteosclerosis (increases after treatment with calcitonin)
Coarse trabecular bone structure
Enlargement and deformation of bones
Widening of shaft by cortical thickening

Differential Diagnosis

Chronic osteomyelitis (Sect. 7.3.3)
Fibrous dysplasia (Sect. 7.4.3.1)
Osteoblastic metastasis

References

1 Bijvoet OLM, Frijlink WB, Vellenga CJLR (1982) Paget's disease. Boerhaave course: metabolic joint diseases. PAO, Leyden, pp 95–103
2 Doyle FH, Banks LM, Pennock JM (1980) Radiologic observations on bone resorption in Paget's disease. Arthritis Rheum 23:1205–1210
3 Haverbush TJ, Wilde AH, Phalen GS (1972) The hand in Paget's disease of bone. Report of two cases. J Bone Joint Surg [Am] 54-A:173–175
4 Wilner D, Sherman RS (1966) Roentgen diagnosis of Paget's disease (osteitis deformans). Med Radiogr Photogr 42:35–41

a 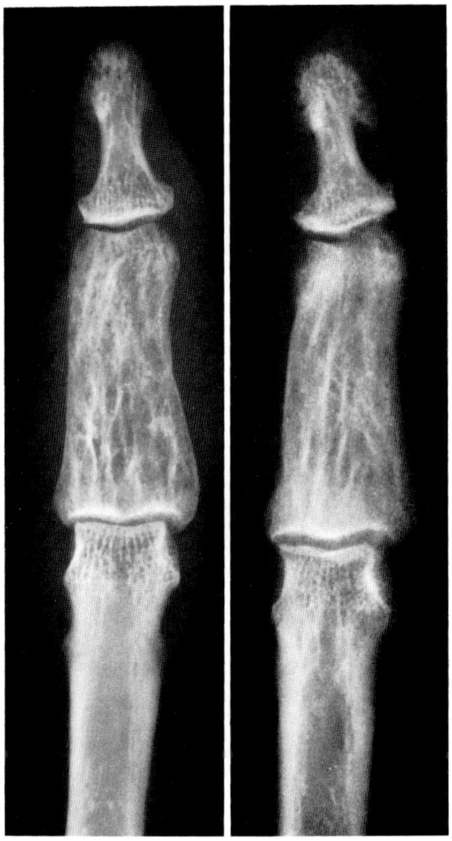 b

Fig. 1a, b. Paget's disease. a In a 39-year-old woman: Middle phalanx of right third finger enlarged, with widening of shaft, coarse trabecular bone structure, and predominant osteolytic appearance. b In a 77-year-old woman: Middle phalanx of left third finger enlarged and widened with coarse trabecular bone structure and some osteosclerosis

a 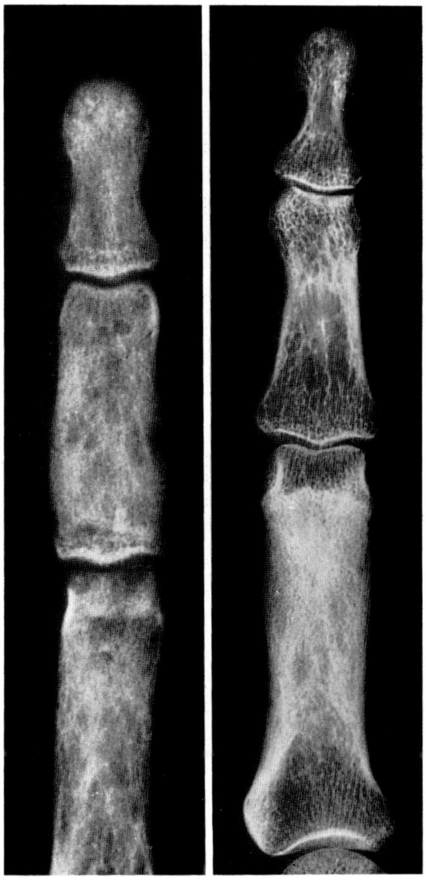 b

Fig. 2a, b. Fibrous dysplasia. a In a 17-year-old boy: Polyostotic fibrous dysplasia. Bone changes resemble Paget's disease, but patient's age makes Paget's disease impossible. b In a 60-year-old woman: Dense bone structure in diaphysis with slight widening of phalanx. Distal and proximal ends of bone display normal structures. Sparing of the bone ends is very rare in Paget's disease

7 Other Disorders of Bones and Joints

7.1 Constitutional Diseases

7.1.1 Arthrogryposis Multiplex Congenita

Synonym: amyoplasia congenita

Arthrogryposis multiplex congenita is probably a primary neurogenic abnormality. Decreased motion leads to deformity, muscle atrophy, musculoligamentous contractures, and joint ankylosis. On autopsy, a decrease in the size of the spinal cord, a decreased number of anterior horn cells, and signs of motor demyelinization are found [1]. In some cases autosomal recessive inheritance is likely, but most cases are sporadic. The clinical picture is characterized by: limitation of active and passive motility, symmetrical joint contractures (usually flexion contractures), pes equinovarus, hip dislocation (mostly bilateral), and scoliosis (15%–40% of cases). Congenital heart anomalies, microcephaly, esophageal atresia, and genitourinary malformations have also been described [2].

Radiographic Findings [1–4]

Hand

Contractures (clawhand)
Carpal fusion in second decade of life
Carpometacarpal fusion
Increased carpal angle (for normal values, see Sect. 2.2.8)
Syndactyly
Symphalangism
Ulnar deviation of wrist
Delayed skeletal maturation
Congenital amputation
Hypoplasia of distal phalanges

Other Sites

Pelvis: dislocation of hips (bilateral in two-thirds of cases)
coxa vara/valga
Soft tissue: decreased size of muscular structures
increased amount of subcutaneous and intermuscular fat
Long tubular bones: thinness and fragility
osteoporosis
bowing
radio-ulnar synostosis
Patella: hypoplasia
Foot: clubfoot
tarsal fusion
Spine: Klippel-Feil deformity
scoliosis

Differential-Diagnosis

Osteogenesis imperfecta (Sect. 1.2.1)
Amyotonia congenita

References

1 Ozonoff MB (1971) Pediatric orthopedic radiology. Saunders, Philadelphia
2 Christ F, Anders G (1981) Die Röntgenmorphologie der Arthrogryposis multiplex congenita. Fortschr Geb Röntgenstr Nuklearmed Ergänzungsband 135:592–596
3 Friedlander HL, Westin GW, Wood L Jr (1968) Arthrogryposis multiplex congenita. A review of forty-five cases. J Bone Joint Surg [Am] 50:89–112
4 Poznanski AK, La Rowe PC (1970) Radiographic manifestations of the arthrogryposis syndrome. Radiology 95:353–358

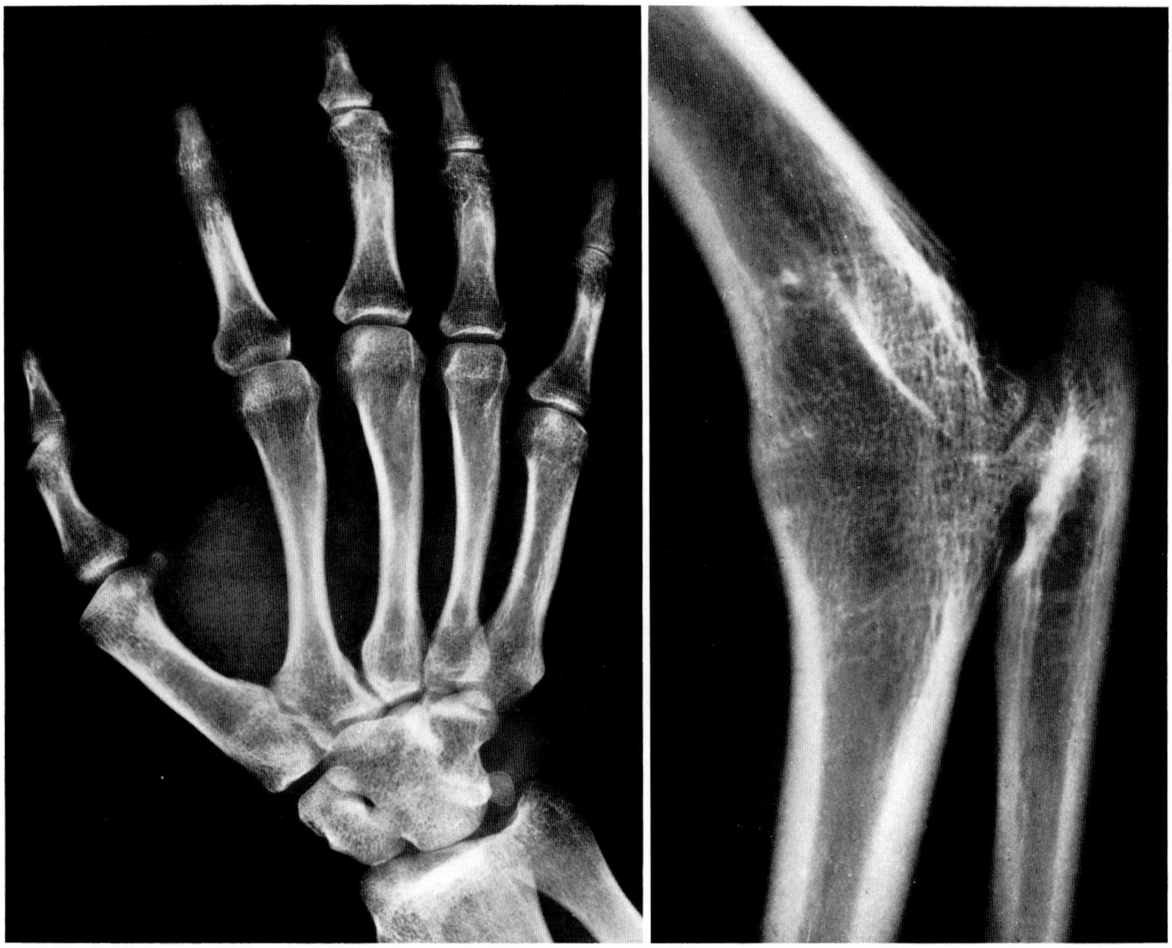

a b

Fig. 1a, b. Arthrogryposis multiplex congenita in a 28-year-old man. **a** Right hand: Carpal fusion and fusion between trapezoid and first metacarpal, short fingers with rather normal distal phalanges, middle phalanges absent, symphalangism between phalanges of second digit. Same type of abnormalities in left hand and in feet. **b** Right elbow: Ankylosis between radius and humerus

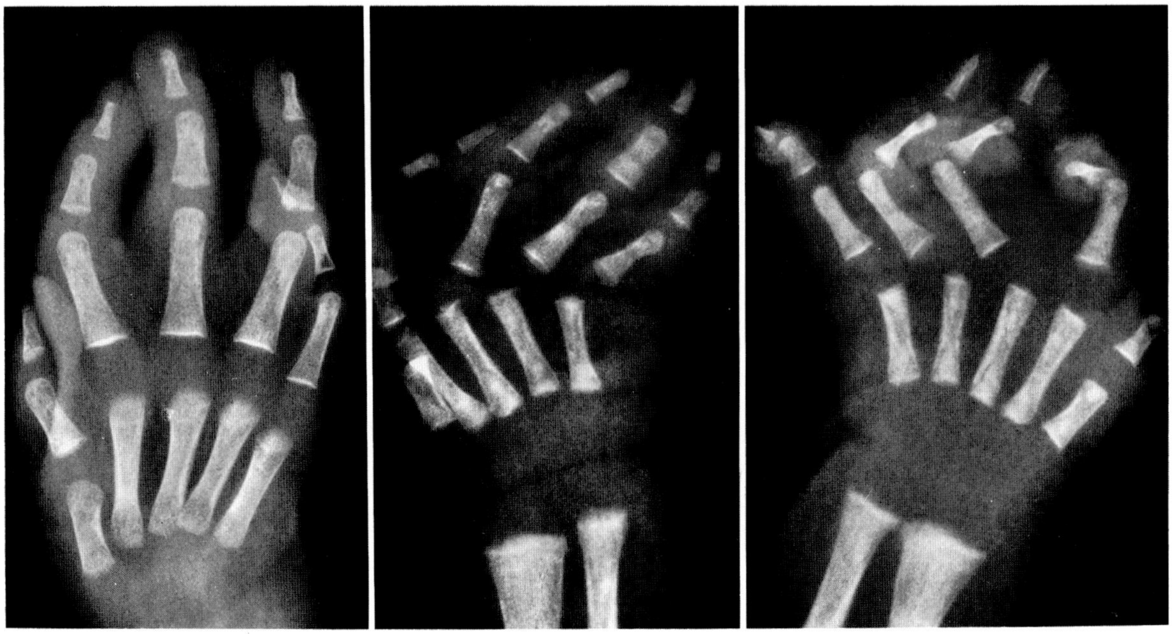

a b c

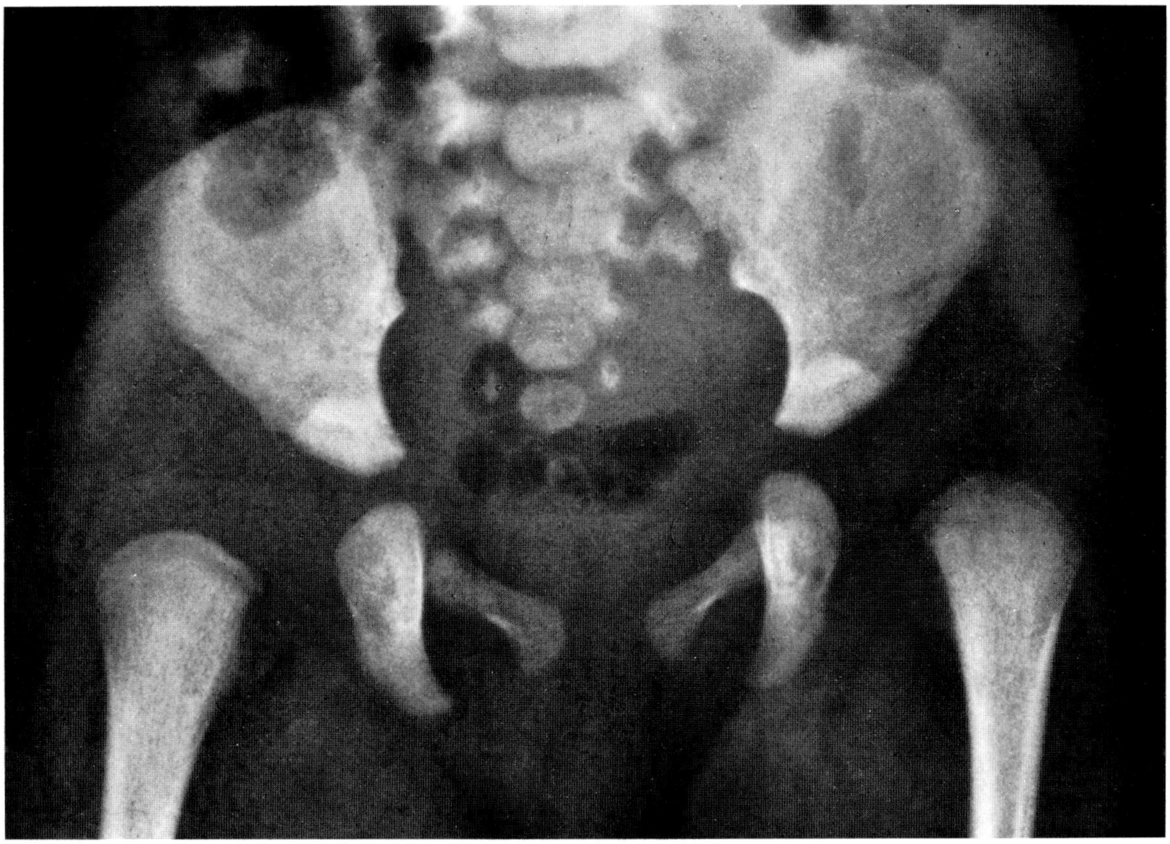

Fig. 3. Same patient as Fig. 2b. Bilateral luxation of hips

◁ **Fig. 2a–c.** Arthrogryposis multiplex congenita. **a** In a 2-month-old boy: Bowing of fingers and clawhand deformity. **b, c** In a 9-day-old boy: Severe contractures in both hands

7.1.2 Tuberous Sclerosis and Neurofibromatosis

Various types of neuroectodermatoses (phakomatoses) are known:

1. Tuberous sclerosis (Bourneville-Pringle syndrome)
2. Neurofibromatosis (Recklinghausen's disease)
3. Cephalotrigeminal hemangiomatosis (Sturge-Weber syndrome)
4. Cerebelloretinal hemangiomatosis (Hippel-Lindau syndrome)

7.1.2.1 Tuberous Sclerosis

Tuberous sclerosis is an autosomal dominant hereditary disease characterized by convulsions, mental retardation and skin lesions (adenoma sebaceum) [1–3]. In patients with tuberous sclerosis, multiple hamartomas may be found in almost all organs:

Skin: adenoma sebaceum (80%–90%)
  shagreen patches (20%–50%)
  periungual fibromas
  café-au-lait and white macules
Brain: nodular lesions with extensive gliosis
Eyes: retinal tumors (phakomas)
Heart: rhabdomyo(sarco)mas
Lungs: myofibrosis
Kidneys: angiomyolipomas
Liver, adrenals: hamartomas

Radiographic Findings [1–6]

Hand

Periosteal new bone formation
Subperiosteal bony nodules (periosteal warts)
Thickening of cortex (undulating contour)
Endosteal sclerosis

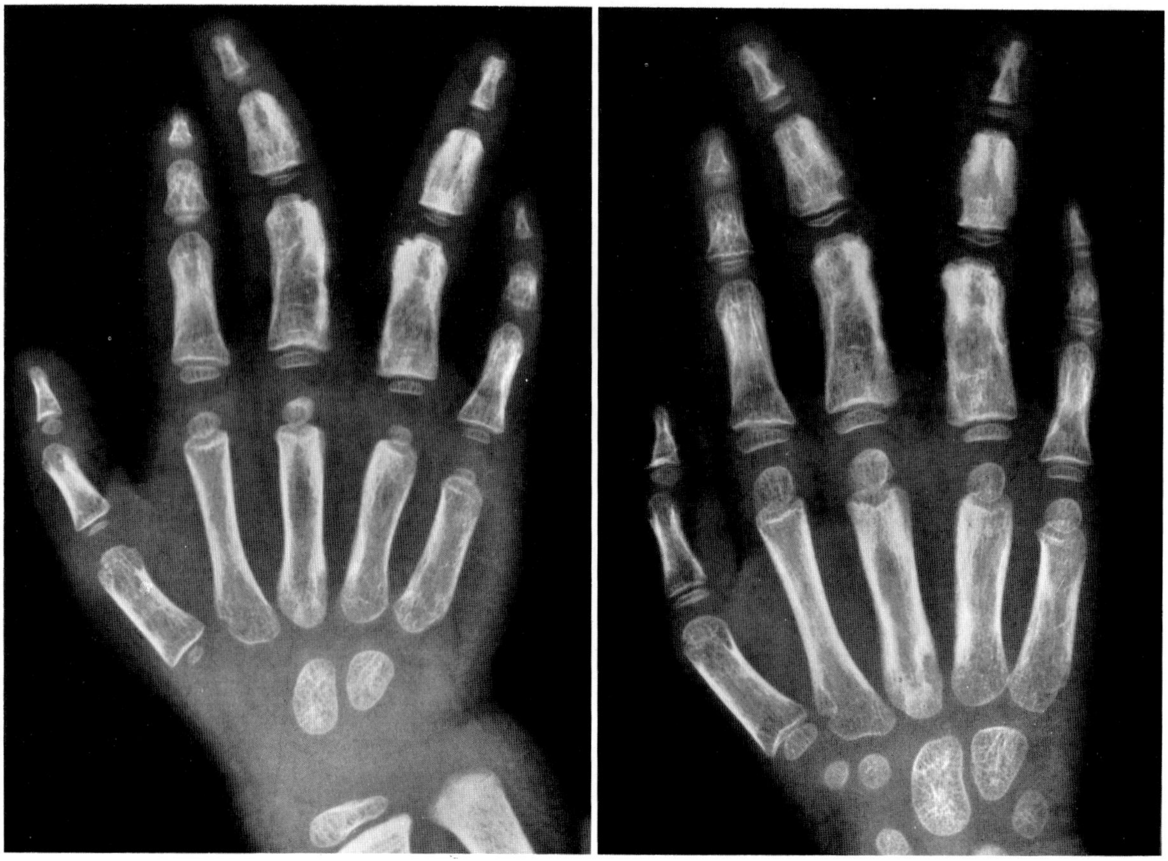

a b

Fig. 1 a, b. Tuberous sclerosis. **a** In a 3-year-old girl: Bowing of third and fourth digits with phalangeal thickening and irregular cortical margins due to periosteal new bone formation. **b** Same patient at age of 6 years: The radiographic findings are more distinct. Endosteal sclerosis of third and fourth metacarpals, cyst-like defects of phalanges, small tuft defects

Cyst-like cortical defects, particularly in distal phalanges (cortical pitting)
Tuft erosions by subungual fibromas

Other Sites
Foot: periosteal new bone formation along metatarsals
Long tubular bones: irregular cortical thickening
subperiosteal bony nodules
cyst-like areas of fibrosis
coarsened trabecular pattern
Pelvis: patchy ovoid, round, or flame-shaped areas of increased bone density
Spine: osteoblastic deposits i vertebral bodies
Viscera: hamartomas in kidney (40%–80%), heart, lungs (1%), and endocrine glands

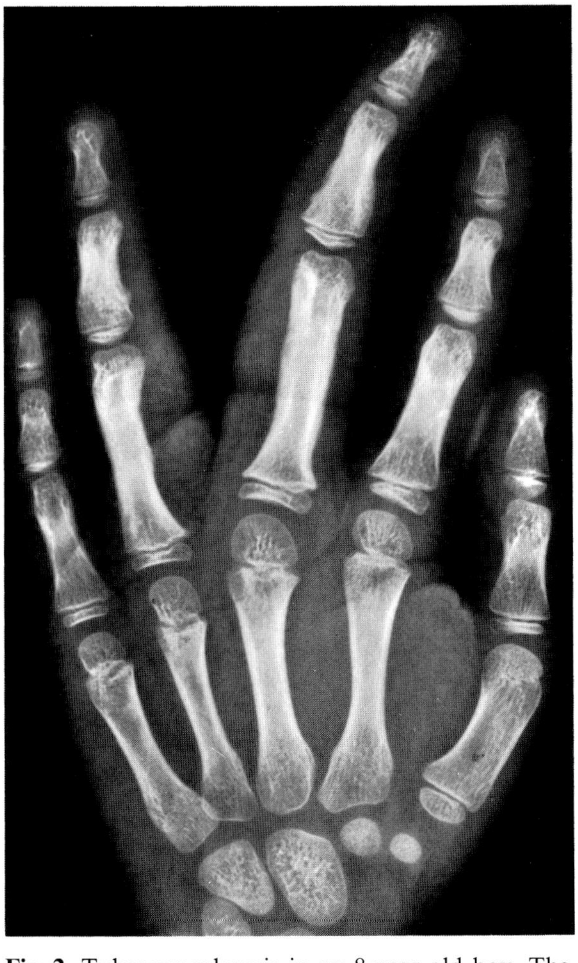

Fig. 2. Tuberous sclerosis in an 8-year-old boy. The third and fourth digits are thickened and the phalanges present undulating surfaces due to periosteal new bone formation. Several small subperiosteal bony nodules (periosteal warts) are present. The metacarpals are normal

Differential Diagnosis of Small Cyst-Like Bone Defects in Phalanges

Basal cell nevus syndrome (Sect. 2.1.2)
Hyperlipoproteinemia (Sect. 7.1.5)
Sarcoidosis (Sect. 7.3.12)

7.1.2.2 Neurofibromatosis

Neurofibromas develop from nerve sheath elements. In neurofibromatosis the following triad may be found: (a) café-au-lait spots on the skin, (b) multiple neurofibromas, and (c) multiple bone lesions (in 50% of patients).

Radiographic Findings [7, 8]

Hand
Localized hypertrophy of bone and soft tissue
Small erosions of outer bone contour (rarely intraosseous defects)
Bone hypoplasia
Diaphyseal slenderness (sometimes caused by adjacent soft tissue hypertrophy)

Other Sites
Skull: hypoplasia of posterior orbital wall
deformation of clinoid processi
cranium bifidum
enlargement of middle cranial fossa
shoe-shaped sella
Spine: widening of intervertebral foramina
pressure defects of pedicles
concave posterior surface of vertebral bodies
kyphosis
Thorax: intercostal neurofibromas
GI tract: neurofibromas
Limbs: overgrowth of bone, or hypoplasia of bone due to adjacent hypertrophy of soft tissue

Differential Diagnosis

Macrodystrophia lipomatosa (Sect. 2.2.16)
Angiodysplasia (Sect. 7.1.4)

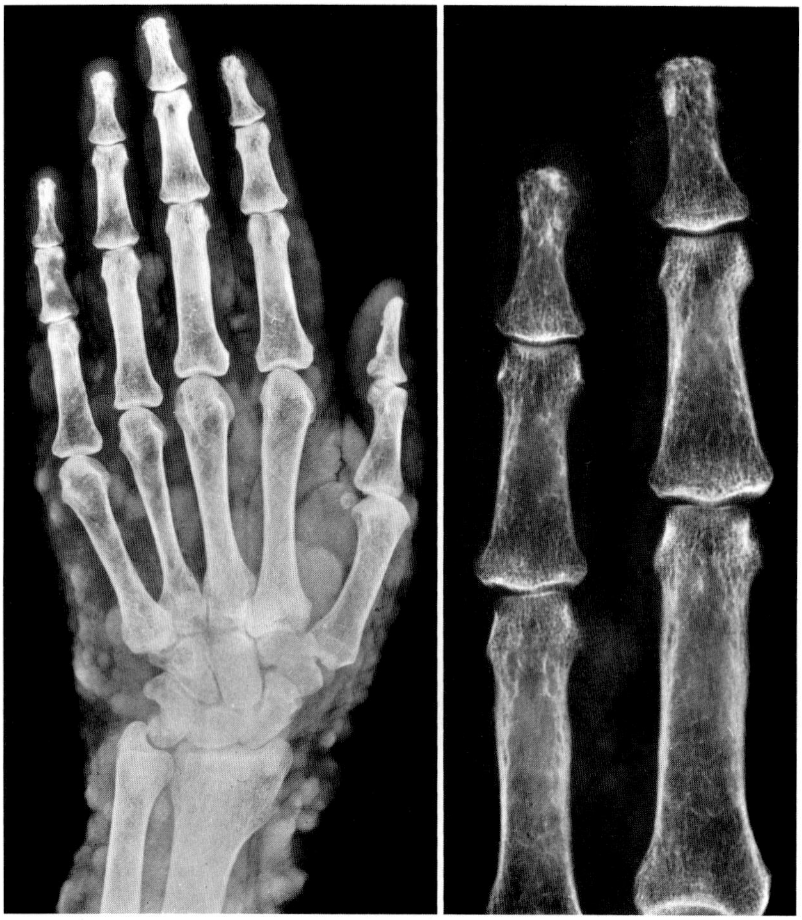

a b

Fig. 1 a, b. Neurofibromatosis in a 66-year-old woman. Multiple neurofibromas of skin. The tufts present irregular distal margins with small defects and some focal sclerosis (**b**)

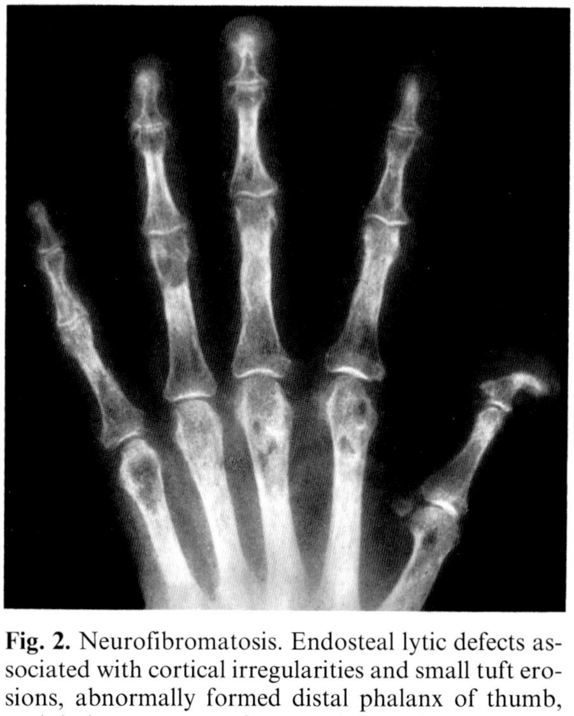

Fig. 2. Neurofibromatosis. Endosteal lytic defects associated with cortical irregularities and small tuft erosions, abnormally formed distal phalanx of thumb, undulating contour of cortex in proximal phalanx of third finger

References

1 Resnick D, Niwayama G (1981) Diagnosis of bone and joint disorders. Saunders, Philadelphia
2 Steinbach HL, Gold R, Preger L (1975) Roentgen appearance of the hand in diffuse disease. Year Book Medical Publishers, Chicago
3 Teske HJ, Heckemann R, Mayer HJ, Odenwälder H, Krautzun K (1978) Zum Stellenwert der Röntgendiagnostik bei der tuberösen Sklerose (Morbus Bourneville). Fortschr Geb Röntgenstr Nuklearmed Ergänzungsband 129:770–777
4 Whitaker PH (1959) Radiological manifestations in tuberous sclerosis. Br J Radiol 32:152–156
5 Green GJ (1968) The radiology of tuberous sclerosis. Clin Radiol 19:135–147
6 Holt JF, Dickerson WW (1952) The osseous lesions of tuberous sclerosis. Radiology 58:1–8
7 Pitt MJ, Mosher JF, Edeiken J (1972) Abnormal periosteum and bone in neurofibromatosis. Radiology 103:143–146
8 Steinbach HL, Gold RH, Preger L (1975) The hand in diffuse disease. Year Book Medical Publishers, Chicago

7.1.3 Fibrodysplasia Ossificans Progressiva

Synonym: myositis ossificans progressiva

Fibrodysplasia ossificans progressiva is a rare hereditary disease involving progressive ossification of striated muscles, tendons, fascia, ligaments, and aponeuroses. Ectopic periosteal tissue may be responsible for the development of the abnormal bone structures through a process of intramembranous bone formation. Local trauma is an exacerbating factor. Large ossifications and ankylosis lead to immobility of the patient. Death from pulmonary complications and inanition is typical [1–3].

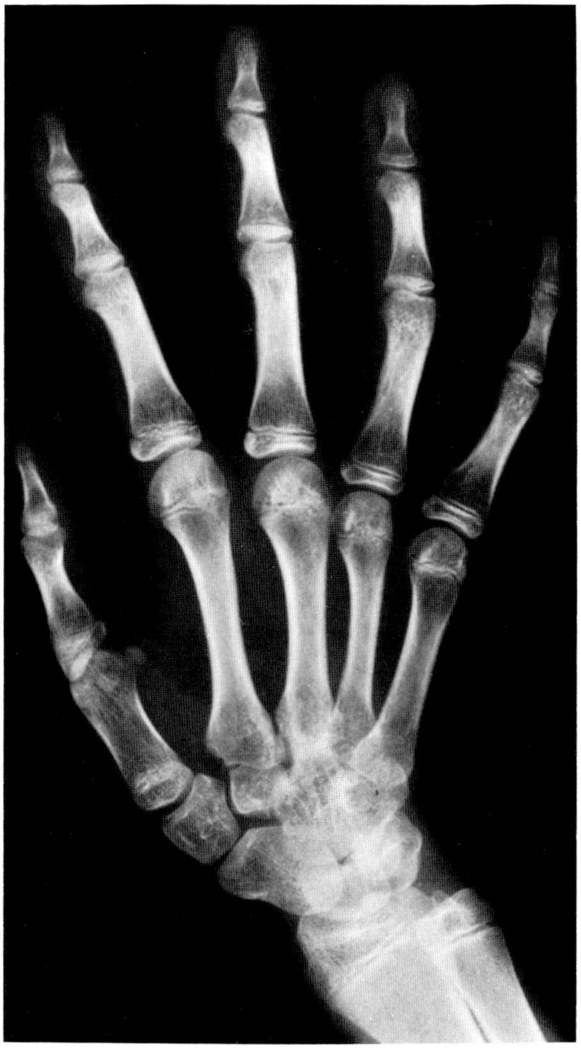

Fig. 1. Fibrodysplasia ossificans progressiva in a 15-year-old girl. Right hand: Short first metacarpal, peculiar epiphysis of proximal phalanx of thumb, small exostosis on proximal phalanx of fifth finger

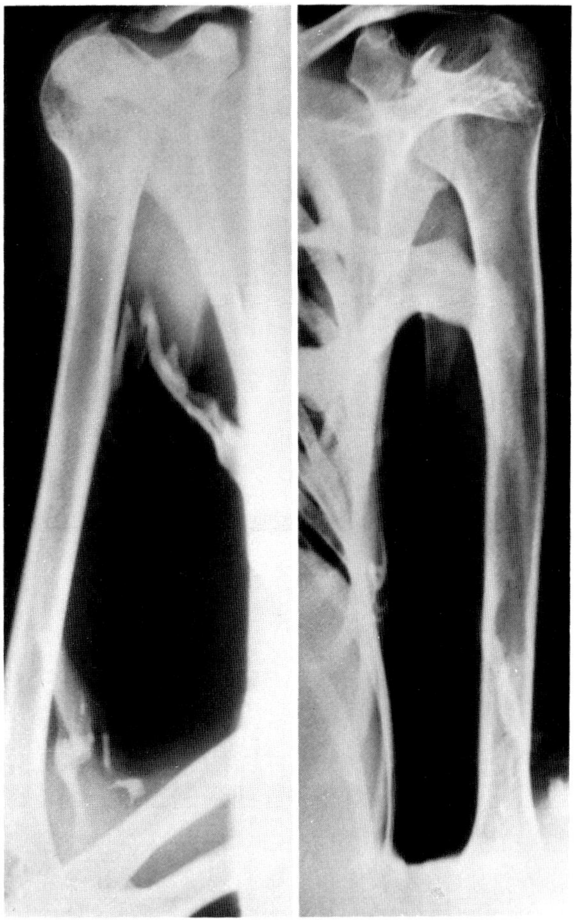

Fig. 2. Fibrodysplasia ossificans progressiva in same patient as Fig. 1: Both upper arms: Extensive ossified masses in soft tissues

Radiographic Findings [1–4]

Hand
Hypoplasia of proximal phalanx of thumb
Hypoplasia of first metacarpal
Clinodactyly
Exostoses

Other Sites
Foot: short first toe
Spine: ankylosis of cervical vertebral arches
hypoplasia of vertebral bodies
ossification of intervertebral ligaments
Soft tissues: ossified masses

Differential Diagnosis

Juvenile rheumatoid arthritis (Sect. 7.3.5)
Ankylosing spondylitis

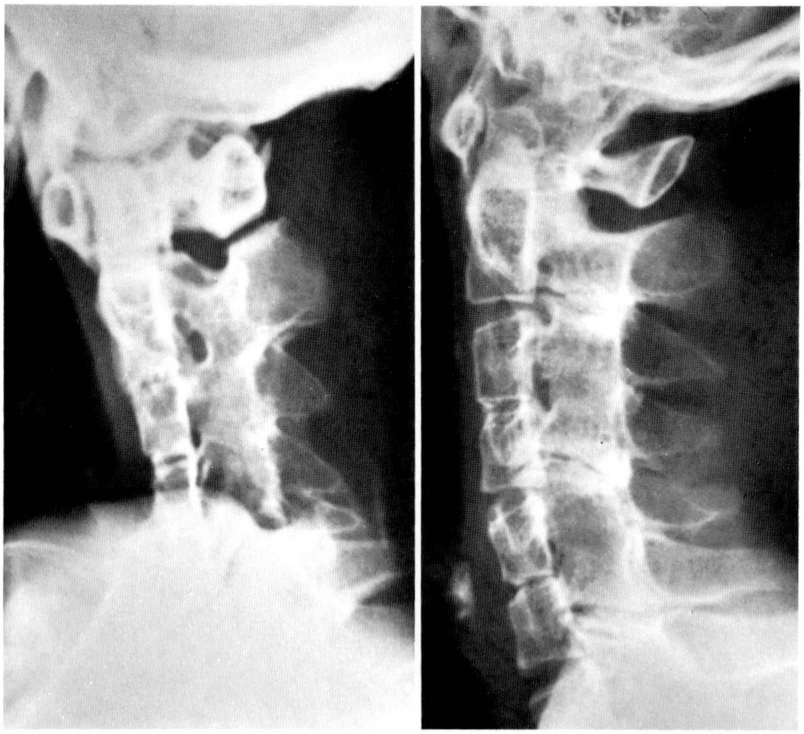

Fig. 3. a Fibrodysplasia ossificans progressiva in same patient as Fig. 1: Hypoplasia of vertebral bodies, ankylosis of vertebral arches. **b** Juvenile rheumatoid arthritis in a 19-year-old woman: Hypoplasia of vertebral bodies and ankylosis of some vertebral arches

References

1 Resnick D (1983) Case report 240. Skeletal Radiol 10:131–136
2 Rogers JG, Geho WB (1979) Fibrodysplasia ossificans progressiva. A survey of forty-two cases. J Bone Joint Surg [Br] 58:48–57
3 Connor JM, Evans DAP (1982) Fibrodysplasia ossificans progressiva. The clinical features and natural history of 34 patients. J Bone Joint Surg [Br] 64:76–83
4 Smith R, Russell RGG, Woods CG (1976) Myositis ossificans progressiva. J Bone Joint Surg [Br] 58:48–57

7.1.4 Angiodysplasia

Synonyms: angio-osteohypertrophy syndrome, nevus varicosis osteohypertrophicus, Klippel-Trénaunay-Weber syndrome

The syndrome of congenital vascular abnormalities associated with increased bone length in an extremity is infrequent. The cause of these embryonic disturbances of vascular development is probably abnormal development of the vessels, in which nevi, vascular growths, lymphangiomas, arteriovenous fistulas, and absence of the deep venous system may occur. Five groups of abnormalities are found [1–6]:

I Nevi, venectasias, and increased bone length (Klippel-Trénaunay syndrome)
II Arteriovenous fistulas, venectasias, and increased bone length (Parkes Weber's syndrome)
III Nevi, venectasias through lack or compression of deep veins and some increased bone length (Servelle's syndrome)
IV Cavernous angiomas with hypertrophy of the soft tissues (venectasia) and decreased bone length (Servelle-Trinquecoste-Martorell syndrome)
V Nevi, lymphedema and some increased bone length

Radiographic Findings [1–9]

Soft tissue swelling
Increased bone length
Decreased bone length
Phleboliths
Abnormal bone structure
Osteoporosis
On angiography: arteriovenous fistulas
venectasias
lymphvessel abnormalities

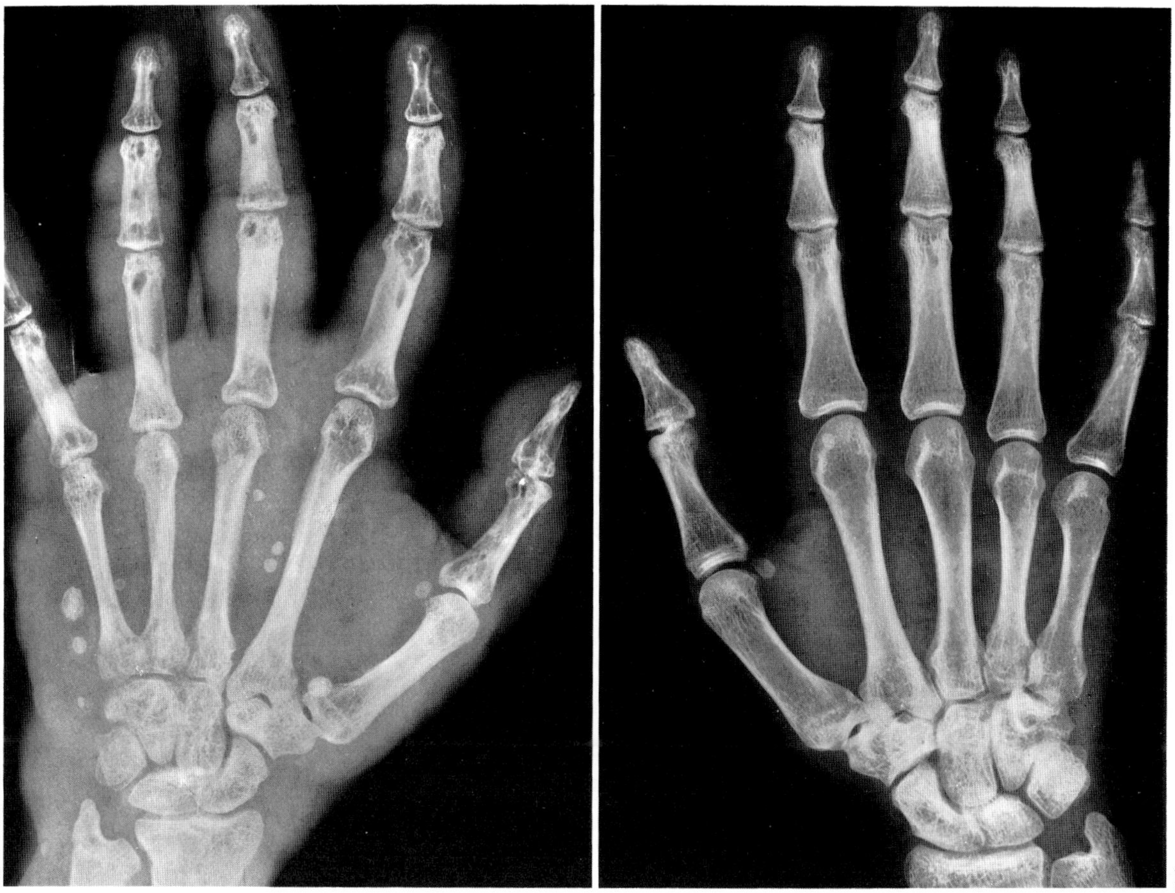

a b

Fig. 1a, b. Angiodysplasia (groups II and IV) in a 21-year-old man. Both hands: Decreased bone length and abnormal bone structure (**a**), multiple phleboliths, soft tissue swelling (cavernous angiomas). Several souffles were audible along the affected extremity due to arteriovenous fistulas (group II)

Finding	Group				
	I	II	III	IV	V
Extremity predominantly affected	lower	upper	lower	upper	lower
Soft tissue swelling				+	+
Increased bone length	+	+	±		±
Decreased bone length				+	
Phleboliths				+	
Abnormal bone structure		+		+	
Arteriovenous fistulas		+			
Venectasias	+	+	+	±	±
Cavernous angiomas				+	
Lymphvessel abnormalities					+

References

1 Bourde C (1974) The Klippel-Trénaunay-Weber syndromes; a practical and therapeutic classification based on angiographic findings. Ann Radiol (Paris) 17:101–106

2 May R, Nissl R (1959) Die angeborenen venösen Mißbildungen und Anomalien. Die Phlebographie der unteren Extremität. Thieme, Stuttgart

3 Hoogendam IJ (1974) Aangeboren vaatmisvormingen in de extremiteiten. Congenital vascular malformations in the extremities. Thesis, Van der Loeff BV, Enschede

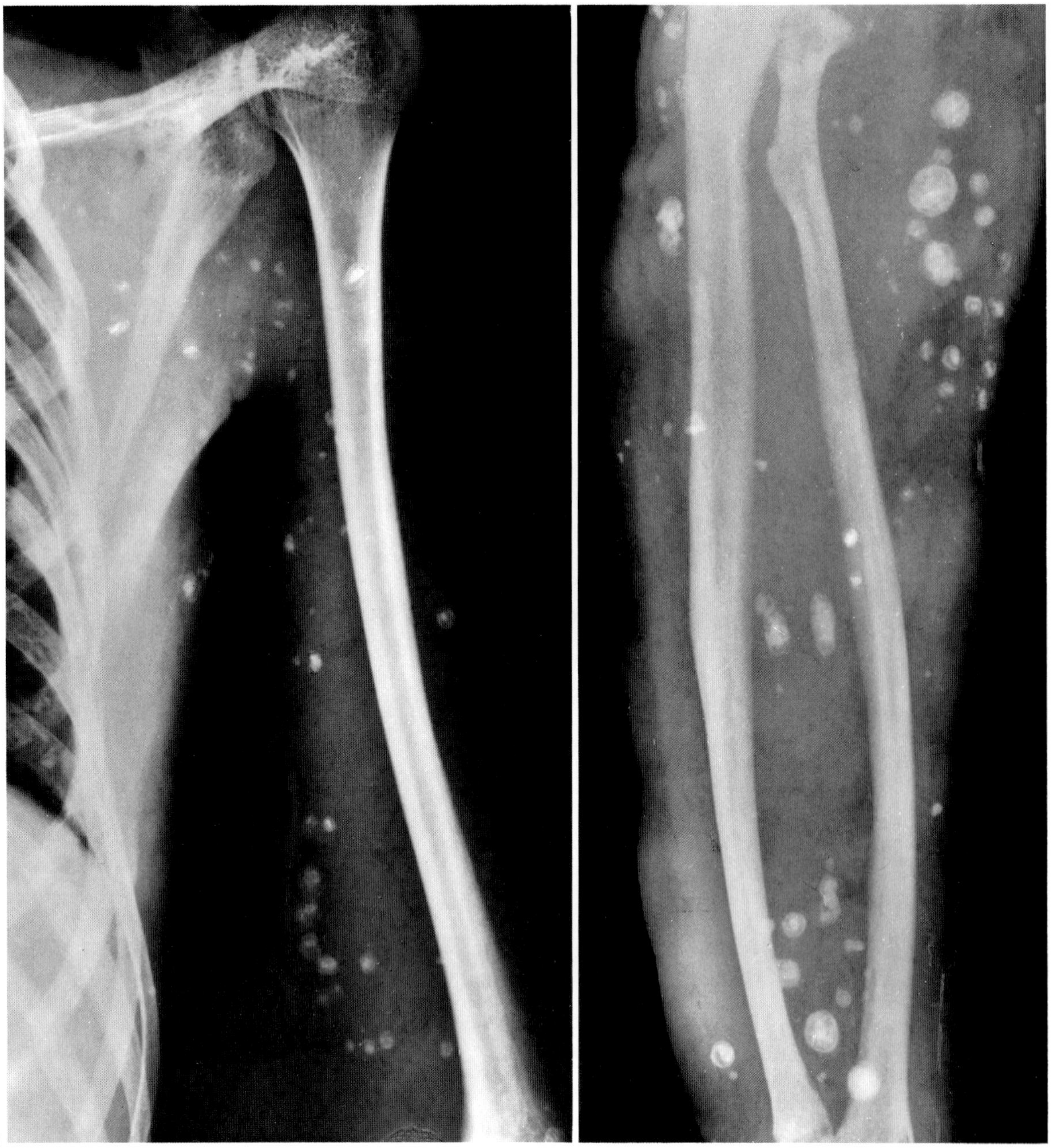

a b

Fig. 2a, b. Same patient as Fig. 1. Multiple phleboliths in soft tissues of arm, abnormal bone structure of radius, ulna, humerus, and ribs

4 Schönenberg H, Redemann M (1972) Klippel-Trénaunay-Weber Syndrom. Klin Pädiatr 184:449–460
5 Brooksaler F (1966) The angioosteohypertrophy syndrome. Klippel-Trénaunay-Weber syndrome. Am J Dis Child 112:161–164
6 Becker C, Becker HW (1967) Beitrag zur vasculo-ossalen Dysembryoplasie nach Klippel-Trénaunay mit Fehlen der tiefen Venen. Fortschr Geb Röntgenstr Nuklearmed Ergänzungsband 107:258–264
7 Langer M, Langer R (1982) Radiologisch erfaßbare Veränderungen der Angiodysplasien Typ Klippel-Trénaunay und Typ Servelle-Martorell. Fortschr Geb Röntgenstr Nuklearmed Ergänzungsband 136:557–582
8 Langer M, Langer R (1981) Radiologic analysis of bone structure in congenital angiodysplasia. Eur J Radiol 1:195–199
9 Leipner N, Janson R, Kühr J (1982) Angiomatöse Dysplasie (Typ F.P. Weber). Fortschr Geb Röntgenstr Nuklearmed Ergänzungsband 137:73–77

7.1.5 Hyperlipoproteinemia

Synonym: hyperlipemia

Hyperlipoproteinemia may be found as a primary familial disease or secondary to a variety of disorders. The plasma concentrations of triglycerides and/or cholesterol are increased. Five types can be distinguished [1–3]:

Type I (hypertriglyceridemia):
  Primary, autosomal recessive
  Secondary

Cystic skeletal lesions are sometimes encountered.

Type II (hypertriglyceridemia):
  Primary, autosomal dominant
  Secondary

This type is characterized by an autosomal dominant hereditary pattern and may be associated with hypercholesterolemia. Particularly in hyperlipoproteinemia type IIa (elevated low-density lipoprotein level), hypercholesterolemia, atherosclerosis, xanthomas, joint complaints, and radiographic findings are frequently present.

Type III (hypertriglyceridemia, elevated intermediate-density lipoprotein level):
  Primary, autosomal recessive
  Secondary

Type IV (hypertriglyceridemia, elevated very-low-density lipoprotein level):
  Primary, autosomal recessive
  Secondary

This type may be associated with primary gout. Polyarthritis and radiographic findings (periarticular osteoporosis, cystic lesions) may be present.

Type V (hypertriglyceridemia, elevated very-low-density lipoprotein level):
  Primary, autosomal dominant?
  Secondary

Radiographic Findings [2–5]

Bony lesions caused by focal collections of cholesterol-laden marrow foam cells, intraosseous xanthomas, as well as extrinsic involvement of bone by tendon xanthomas may be found.

Hand

Periarticular soft tissue swelling by xanthomas
Small lytic intraosseous lesions
Bony erosions
Periarticular osteoporosis

Other Sites

Long tubular bones: soft tissue swelling (tendon xanthomas)
  scalloping of external bony surface (subperiosteal xanthomas)
  intraosseous lytic lesions
  pathologic fractures
  signs of avascular osteonecrosis

Differential-Diagnosis

Rheumatoid arthritis (Sect. 7.3.4)
Gout (Sect. 7.3.8)
Sarcoidosis (Sect. 7.3.12)
Pyogenic arthritis (Sect. 7.3.2)

References

1 Fredrickson DS, Goldstein JL, Brown MS (1978) The familial hyperlipoproteinemias. In: Stanbury JB, Wijngaarden J, Fredrickson DS (eds) The metabolic basis of inherited disease. McGraw Hill, New York
2 Resnick D, Niwayama G (1981) Diagnosis of bone and joint disorders. Saunders, Philadelphia
3 Vermeer BJ (1979) Biochemical and ultrastructural investigations on hyperlipoproteinemia and xanthomatosis. Thesis, Leyden
4 Yaghmai I (1978) Intraosseous and extraosseous xanthomata associated with hyperlipemia. Radiology 128:49–54
5 Bjersand AJ (1979) Bone changes in hypercholesterolemia. Radiology 130:101–102

Differential Diagnosis

Macrodystrophia lipomatosa (Sect. 2.2.16)
Tuberous sclerosis (Sect. 7.1.2.1)
Neurofibromatosis (Sect. 7.1.2.2)
Maffucci's syndrome (Sect. 7.4.1.3)

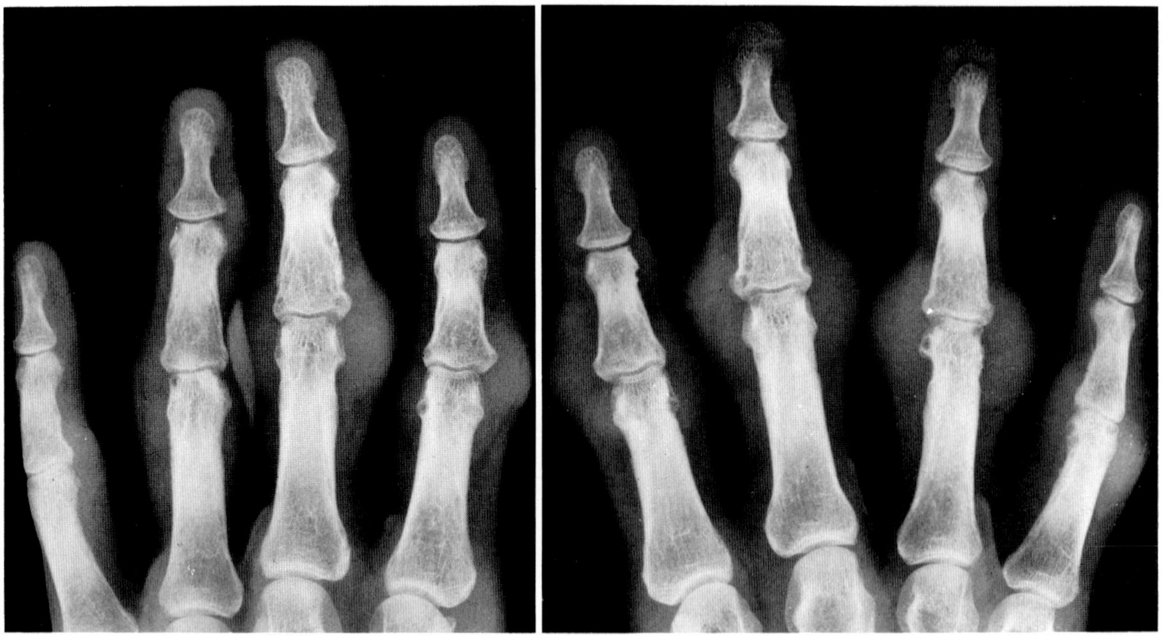

a b

Fig. 1a, b. Hyperlipoproteinemia, type IIa in a 34-year-old man with familial hypercholesterolemia: Xanthomas around joints of fingers, elbows, and ankles, involvement of Achilles tendons. Characteristic radiographic findings in hand, with soft tissue swelling and lytic bony lesions (both intraosseous and extraosseous)

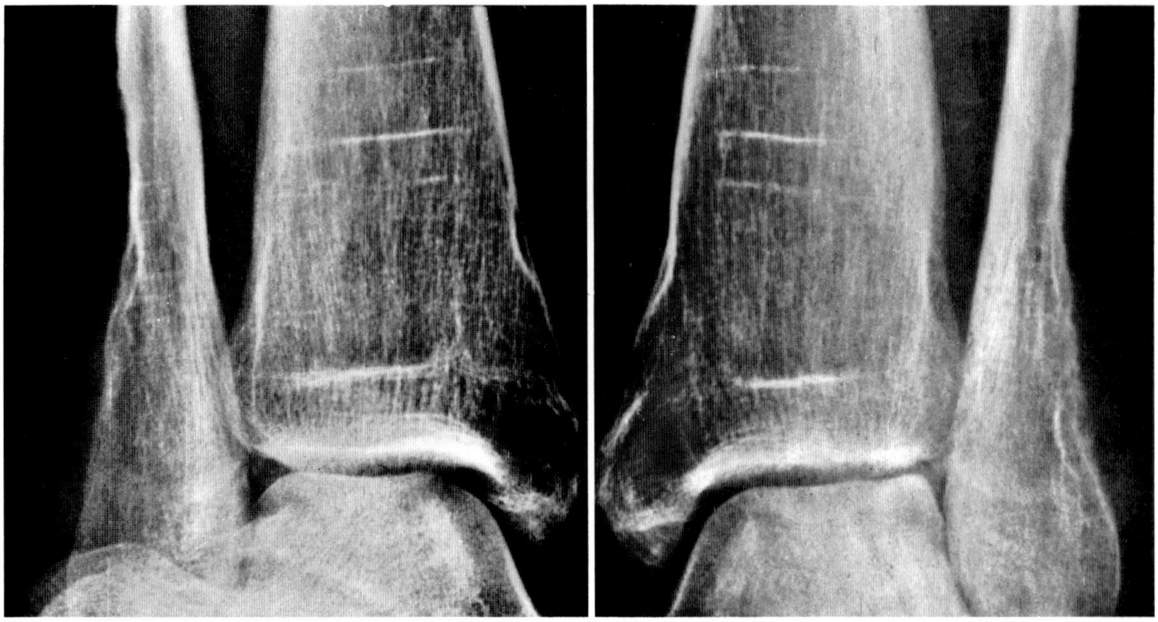

a b

Fig. 2a, b. Same patient as Fig. 1. Both ankle joints: Symmetric subperiosteous xanthomas have resulted in scalloping of external bony surface in metaphyseal areas of tibia and fibula

7.2 Endocrine Diseases

7.2.1 Hypothyroidism

The clinical findings in hypothyroidism depend on the age of onset.

Congenital hypothyroidism: cretinism

Hypothyroidism in growing child: juvenile myxedema

Adult hypothyroidism: only mild bone abnormalities

Delayed maturation of the skeleton is the reason for most of the radiographic abnormalities. Thyroid hormone stimulates the linear growth of the tubular bones, but does not influence the formation of periosteal bone, so the tubular bones become relatively short and wide. Hypercalcemia may be present, caused by an elevated threshold for calcium excretion and hypersensitivity to vitamin D (soft tissue calcifications and nephrocalcinosis).

Radiographic Findings [1–4]

Hand

Delayed skeletal maturation

Short tubular bones (particularly metacarpals)

Value of R $\left(\frac{\text{second metacarpal length}}{\text{skeletal age}}\right) > 1$

Occasionally: multiple epiphyseal centers (epiphyseal dysgenesis)
increased density of epiphyses
increased density of metaphyses
distal phalanges: osseous enlargement of midportion of metaphyses [4]

a 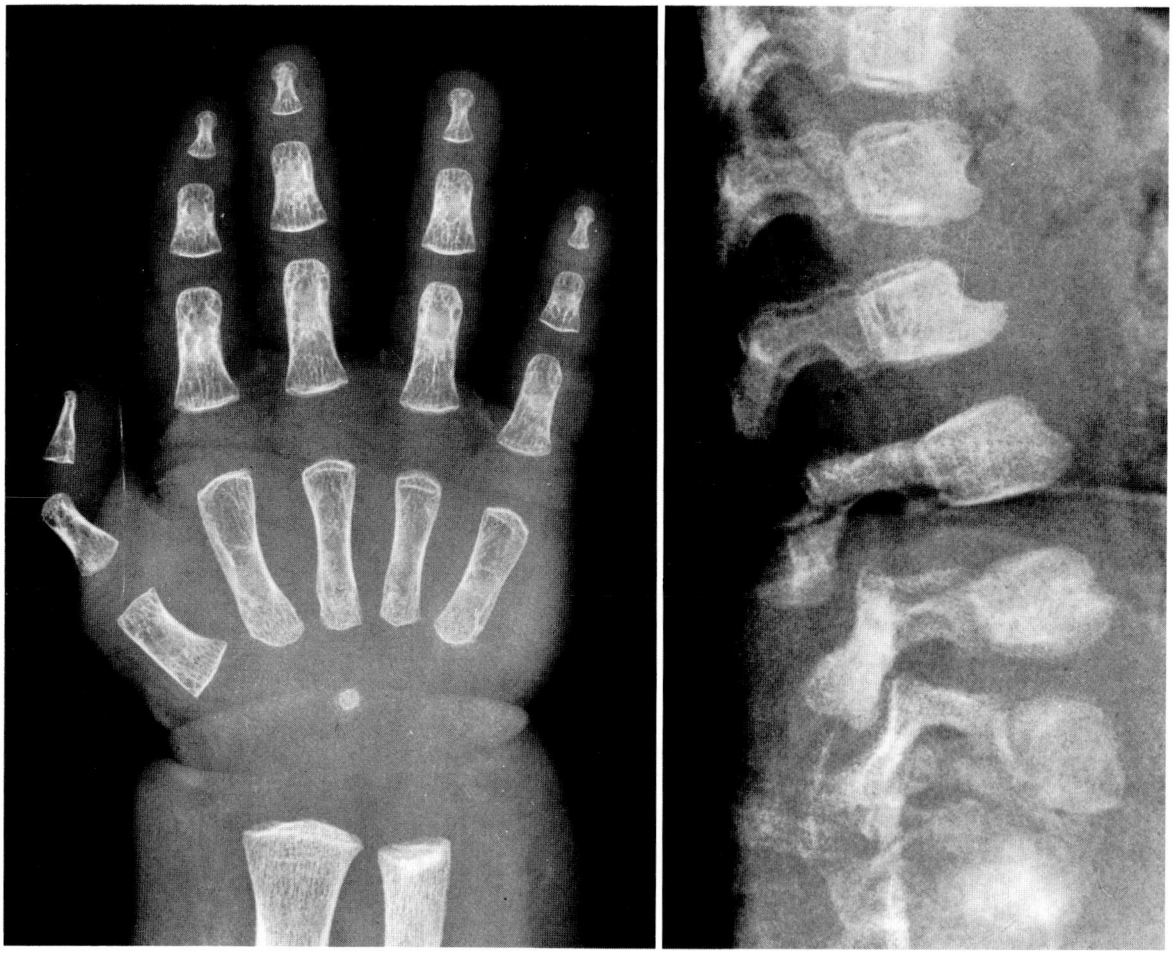 b

Fig. 1a, b. Hypothyroidism (cretinism) in a 3-year-old girl. **a** Strikingly delayed skeletal maturation (equivalent to a normal 3-month-old child). Otherwise no abnormalities. **b** Lumbar spine: Beak-shaped vertebral bodies, particularly L 2

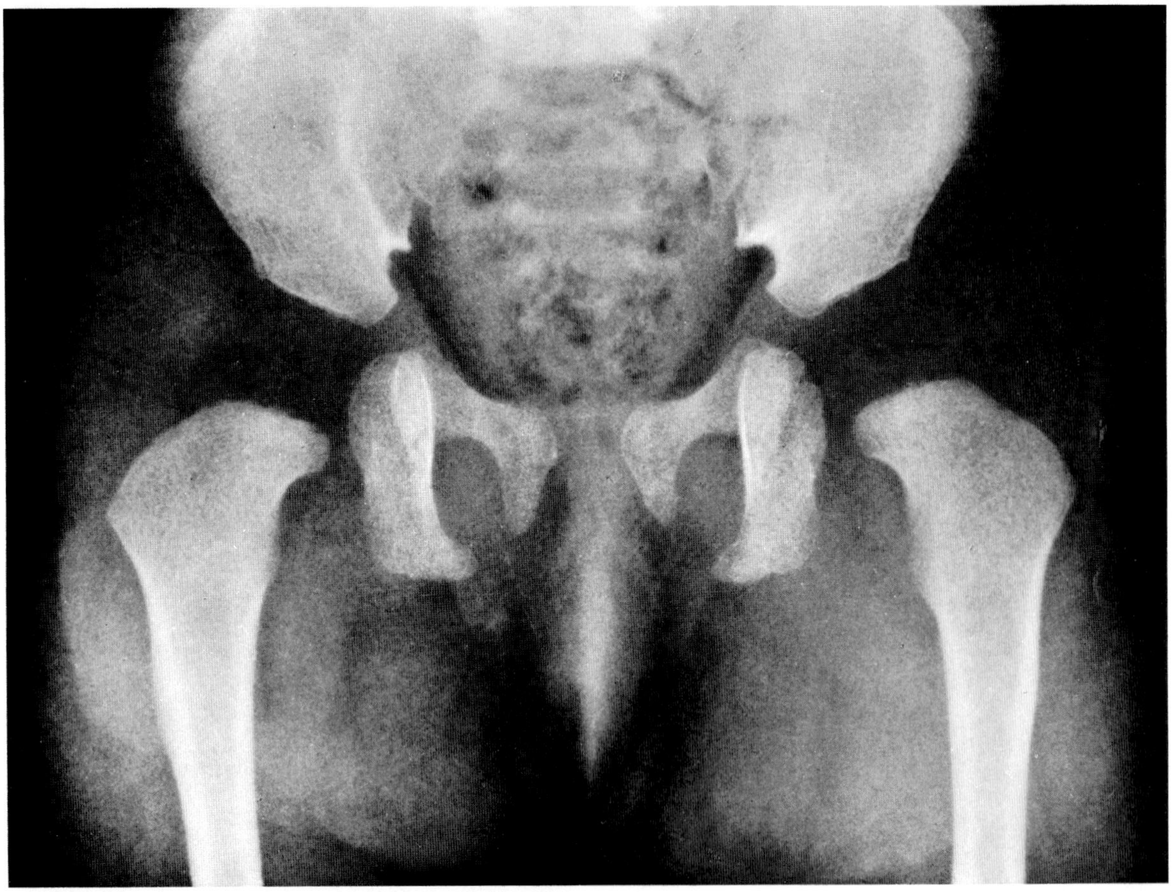

Fig. 2. Same patient as Fig. 1. Delayed skeletal maturation: Proximal epiphyses of femur not yet ossified, slight increase in density of metaphyses

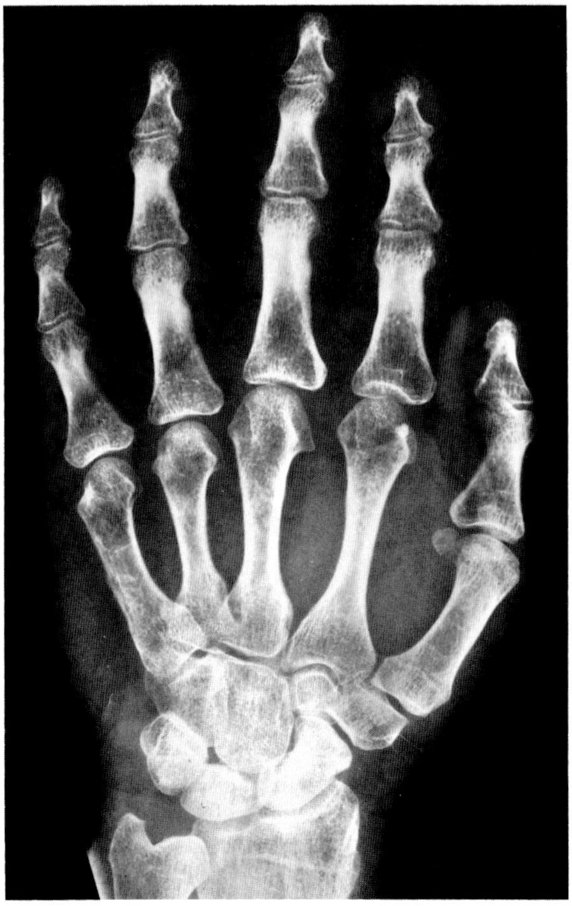

Fig. 3. Hypothyroidism (cretinism) in a 53-year-old woman. Short tubular bones, thin sclerotic band in former radial growth plate

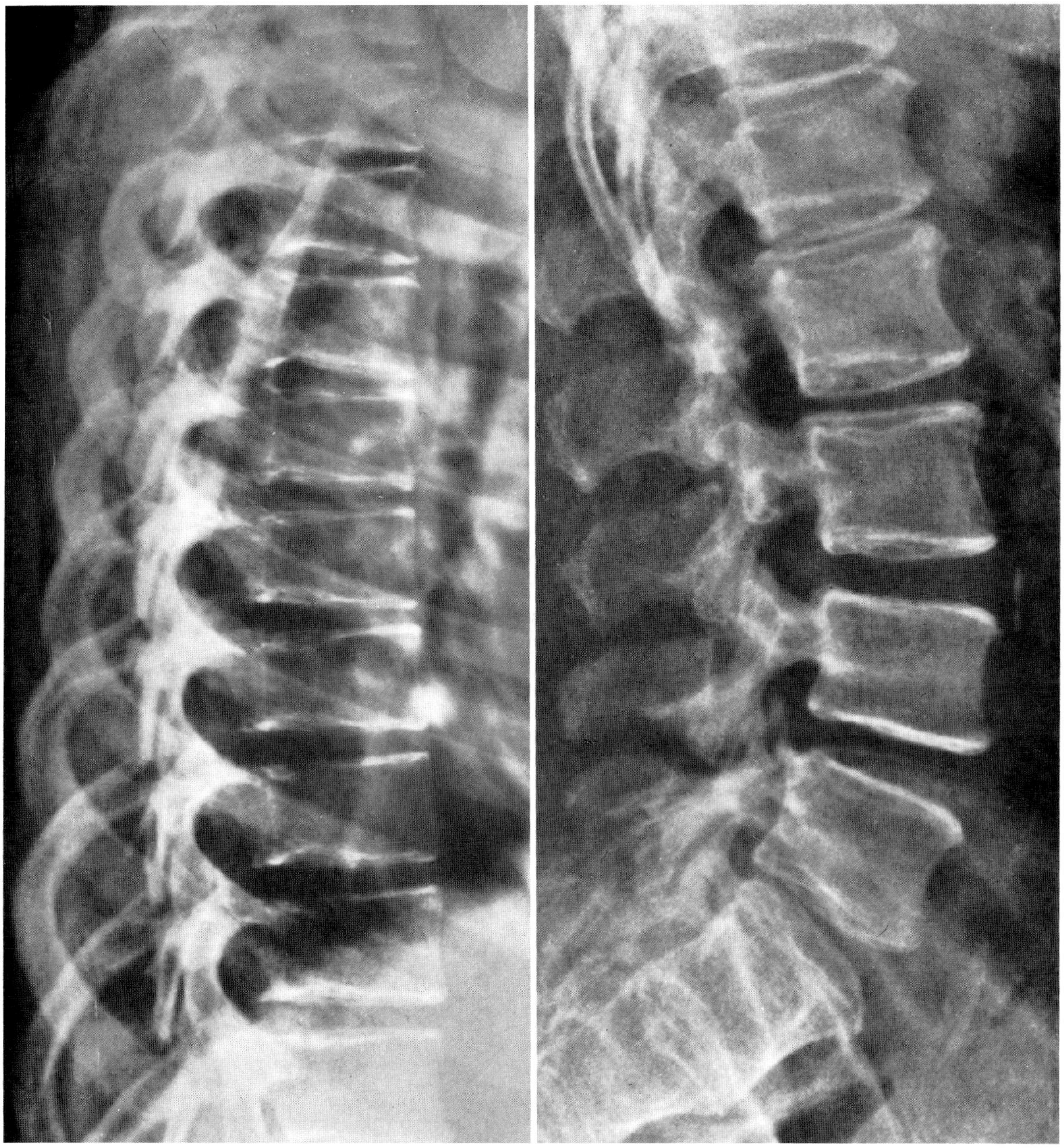

a

Fig. 4a, b. Same patient as Fig. 3. Platyspondylisis and some sclerosis of upper and lower margins of vertebral bodies

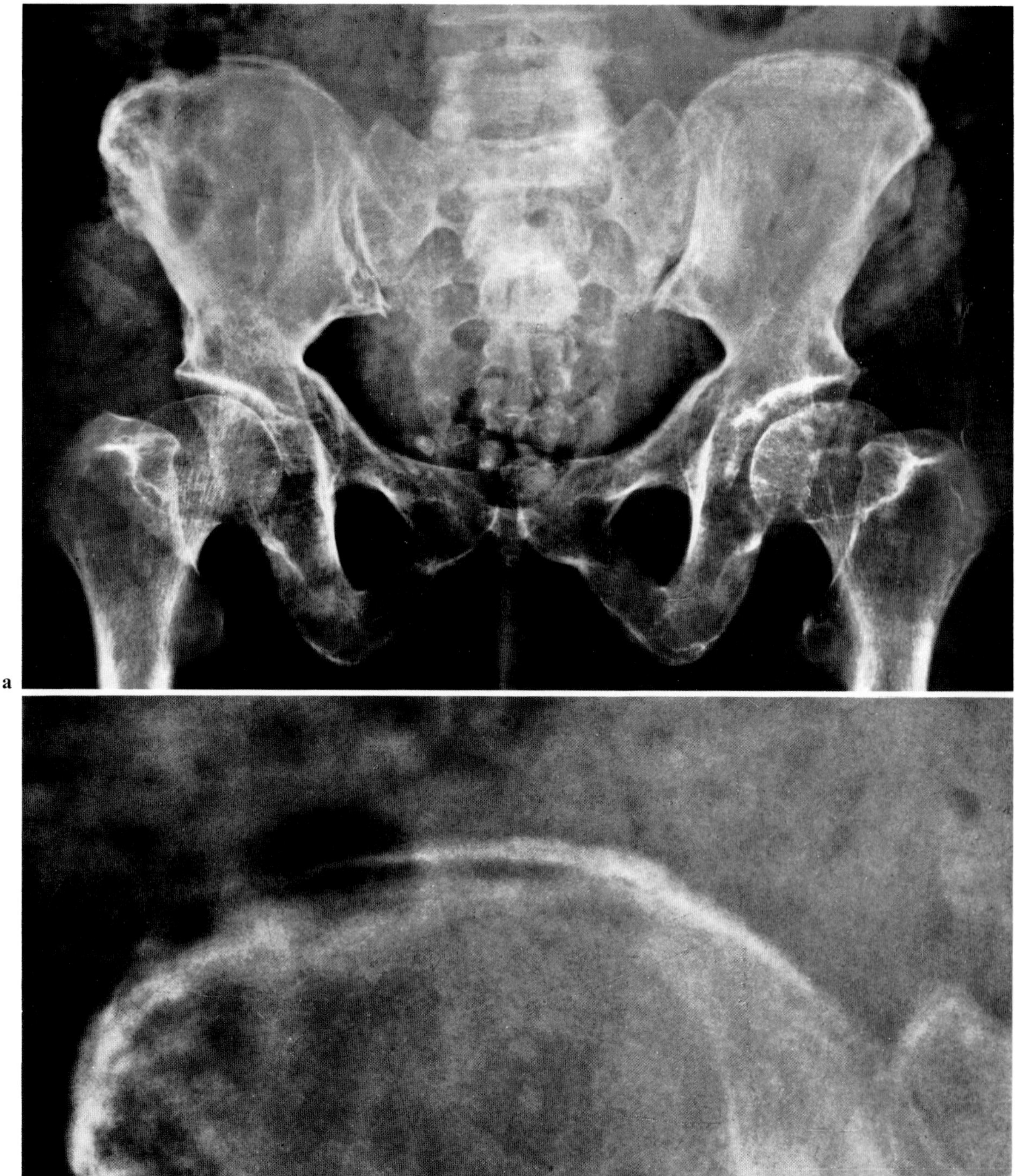

Fig. 5a, b. Same patient as Fig. 3. Unfused iliac apophyses (**b** detail)

Other Sites

Skull: wide sutures
- wormian bones
- hypoplastic paranasal sinuses
- prognathism
- delayed dental development
- enlarged sella turcica

Spine: beak-shaped anterior surface of vertebral bodies (differential diagnosis: mucopolysaccharidosis, Sect. 6.1.1)
- thoracolumbar kyphosis
- poorly ossified and unfused ring apophyses
- platyspondylisis in adults
- sclerosis of upper and lower vertebral margins
- wide intervertebral disc spaces

Long tubular bones: delayed skeletal maturation
- shortening of tubular bones
- irregular metaphyses
- cortical thickening
- multiple epiphyseal ossification centers (hips)
- slipped capital femoral epiphysis
- coxa vara

Miscellaneous: hypercalcemia (CPPD, premature arterial calcification, nephrocalcinosis)
- unfused iliac apophyses

Differential Diagnosis

Achondroplasia (Sect. 1.1.3)
Epiphyseal dysplasia (Sect. 1.1.11)
Mucopolysaccharidosis (Sect. 6.1.1)
Hypopituitarism [3]

References

1 Rybak M (1969) Dysplasie du squelette et maturation osseuse dans l'insuffisance thyroïdienne de l'enfant. Ann. Radiol. 13:243–249

2 Borg SA, Fitzer PM, Young LW (1975) Roentgenologic aspects of adult cretinism. Two case reports and review of the literature. AJR 123:820–828

3 Hernandez RJ, Poznanski AK, Hopwood NJ (1979) Size and skeletal maturation of the hand in children with hypothyroidism and hypopituitarism. AJR 133:405–408

4 Hernandez RJ, Poznanski AK (1979) Distinctive appearance of the distal phalanges in children with primary hypothyroidism. Radiology 132:83–84

7.2.2 Acromegaly

Overproduction of growth hormone caused by an eosinophilic adenoma of the hypophysis (after closure of the growth plates) initiates hypertrophy of bones, cartilage, and soft tissues.

Radiographic Findings [1–5]

Hand

Prominent tufts of fingers (arrowheading)
Widening of joint spaces (cartilage hypertrophy)
Exostoses around metacarpal and proximal phalangeal heads
Soft tissue thickening
Large sesamoid in first metacarpophalangeal joint
Thick bones
Coarse trabecular pattern
Periosteal bone apposition
Periarticular calcifications
Premature osteoarthrosis (especially in metacarpophalangeal joints)

Other Sites

Skull: enlarged sella turcica
enlarged mandible
calvarial hyperostosis
Spine: posterior scalloping of vertebral bodies
thickening of intervertebral discs
Joints: premature degenerative disease (spine, hips, knees)
Soft tissue: heel pad thickening
subligamentous bone formation (patella, calcaneus)

Differential Diagnosis

Pachydermoperiostosis (Sect. 1.2.8)
Osteoarthrosis (Sect. 7.3.13)
Thyroid acropachy (Sect. 7.6.8) [6]
Hypertrophic osteoarthropathy (Sect. 7.6.8)
Diffuse idiopathic skeletal hyperostosis [5]

References

1 Anton HC (1972) Hand measurements in acromegaly. Clin Radiol 23:445–450
2 Lin SR, Lee KF (1971) Relative value of some radiographic measurements of the hand in the diagnosis of acromegaly. Invest Radiol 6:426–431
3 Resnick D, Niwayama G (1981) Diagnosis of bone and joint disorders. Saunders, Philadelphia
4 Erbe W von, Stephan G, Böttcher H (1975) Das Muster der Skelettveränderungen bei der Akromegalie. Fortschr Geb Röntgenstr Nuklearmed Ergänzungsband 122:317–322
5 Littlejohn GO, Urowitz MB, Smythe HA, Keystone EC (1981) Radiographic features of the hand in diffuse idiopathic skeletal hyperostosis (DISH): comparison with normal subjects and acromegalic patients. Radiology 140:623–629
6 Moule B, Grant MC, Boyle IT, May H (1970) Thyroid acropachy. Clin Radiol 21:329–333

Dimensions in normal adulthood and in acromegaly [1–3]

	Normal		Acromegaly		SD
	Men	Women	Men	Women	
Width of index finger at midportion of proximal phalanx (right angles to longitudinal axis; AD in Fig. 1)	23.1 mm	20.4 mm	27.3 mm	25.9 mm	±2.2 mm
Width of proximal phalanx of index finger at midportion (right angles to longitudinal axis; BC in Fig. 1)	10.6 mm	9.1 mm	11.2 mm	10.2 mm	±0.9 mm
Midphalangeal ratio (BC/AD)	0.46	0.45	0.41	0.39	±0.04
Tuft width in third finger	8.5±1.0 mm	7.4±0.95 mm	≧12 mm	≧10 mm	
Sesamoid index	25.1 mm²	20.3 mm²	31.0 mm²	31.2 mm²	±6.0 mm²
Cartilage thickness in second metacarpophalangeal joint	1.7±0.4 mm	1.6±0.4 mm	>2.5 mm	>2.5 mm	
Heel pad thickness	23 mm	21.5 mm	30–35 mm	30–35 mm	

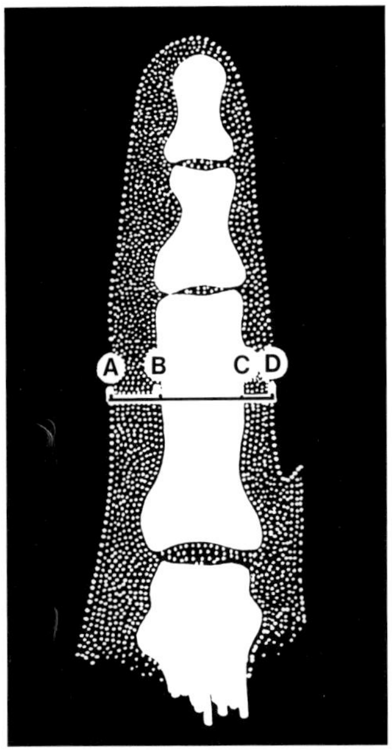

Fig. 1. Proximal phalanx: Midphalangeal ratio = B C/A D. See table for normal and abnormal values. (Modified from LIN and LEE [2])

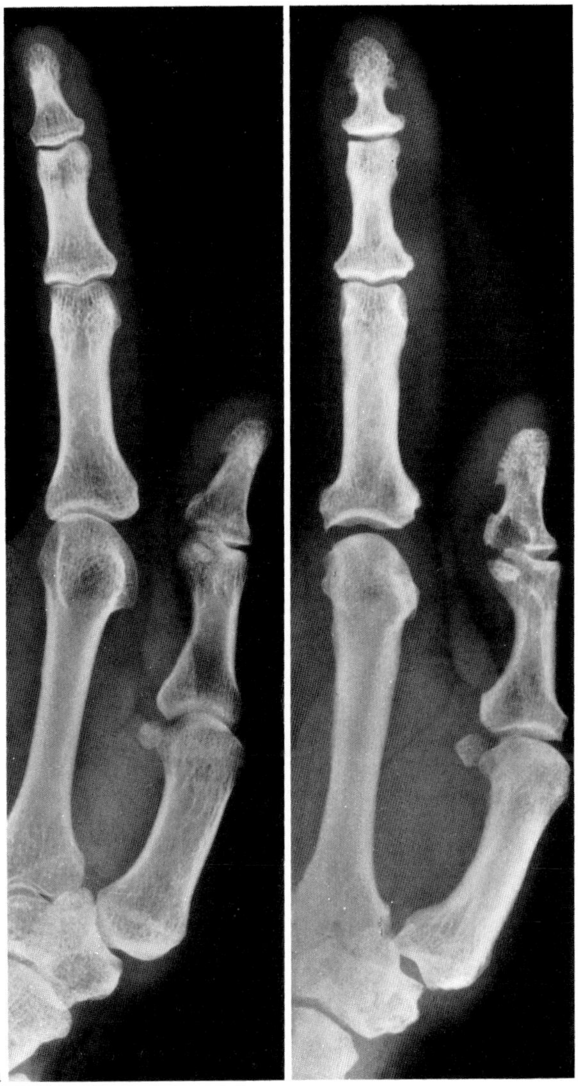

a b

Fig. 3a, b. Normal hand vs acromegaly. **a** Part of a normal female hand. **b** Part of hand of a 47-year-old man with acromegaly: Tuft width in third finger 9 mm (normal 8.5 ± 1.0 mm), cartilage thickening 3 mm (1.7 mm ± 0.4 mm), sesamoid index 30 mm^2 (normal 25.1 ± 6.0 mm^2)

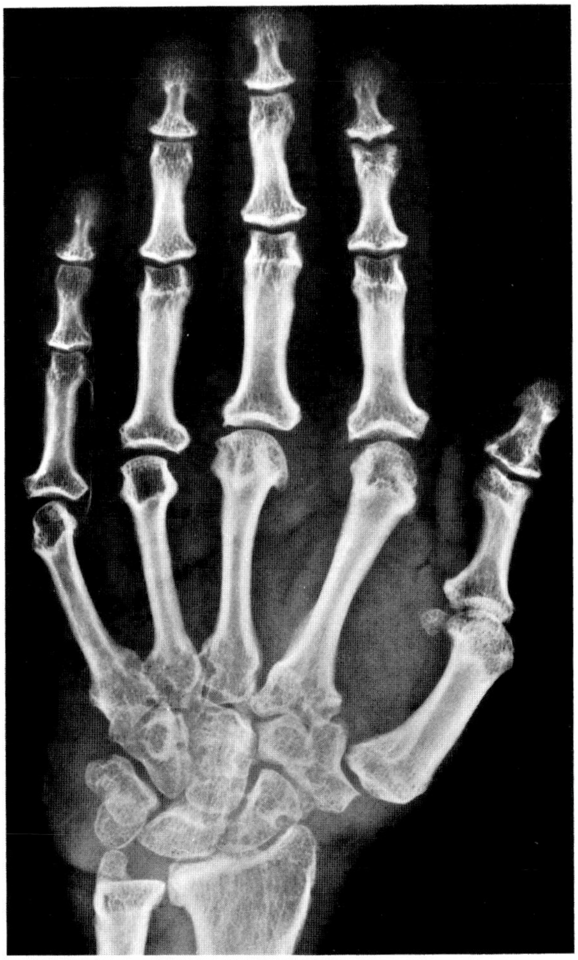

Fig. 2. Acromegaly in a 39-year-old man. Soft tissue thickening, arrowheading of tufts, widening of joint spaces, large sesamoid

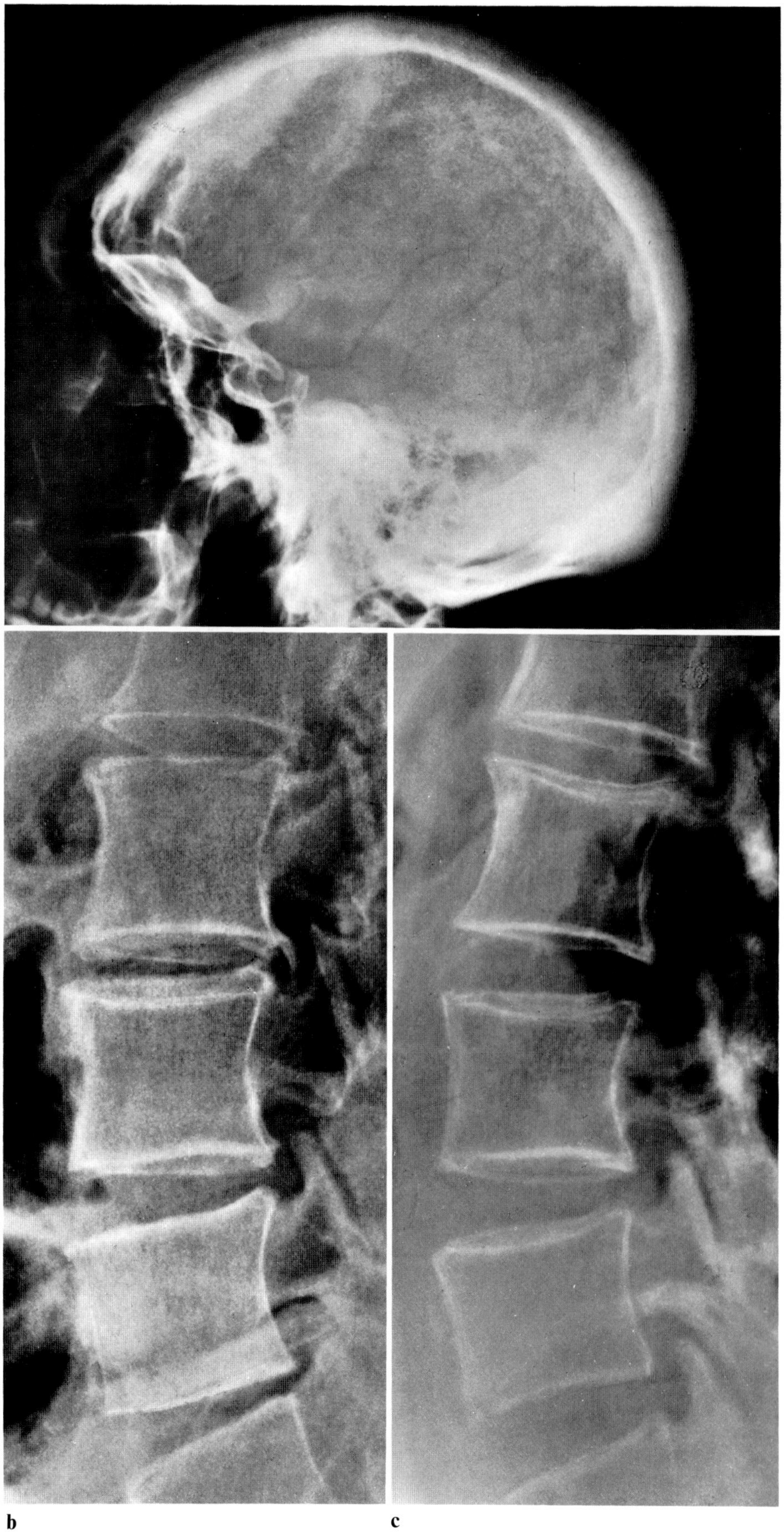

a b c

Fig. 4a–c. Acromegaly.
a Skull thickening with hyperostosis frontalis and enlarged sella turcica.
b, **c** Two different lumbar spines: Marked scalloping of vertebral bodies posteriorly

7.3 Arthritis and Osteomyelitis

7.3.1 Congenital Syphilis

In congenital syphilis, transplacental migration of the spirochete (*Treponema pallidum*) is followed by infection of the fetus. In many cases this infection leads to abortion. Some children born alive present hepatosplenomegaly, skin lesions, and painful extremities. The early osseous lesions of congenital syphilis are usually present in the epiphyseal-metaphyseal areas of the skeleton. The metaphyses of the long tubular bones are often the sites of syphilitic granulation tissue. Dactylitis may be present. In the late first and second decade of life, the radiographic findings are (non)-gummatous osteomyelitis and diffuse periostitis, and destruction of the nasal bones, Hutchinson teeth, saber-shin deformity of the tibiae, and even dactylitis may develop [1–5].

Radiographic Findings in Early Osseous Lesions

Hand/Forearm

Metaphysis: radiolucent bands of granulation tissue
- irregular erosive lesions
- cortex destruction
- fragmentation

Diaphyseal osteomyelitis: osteolysis
- surrounding bony eburnation

Periosteal new bone formation

Dactylitis

Fractures

a

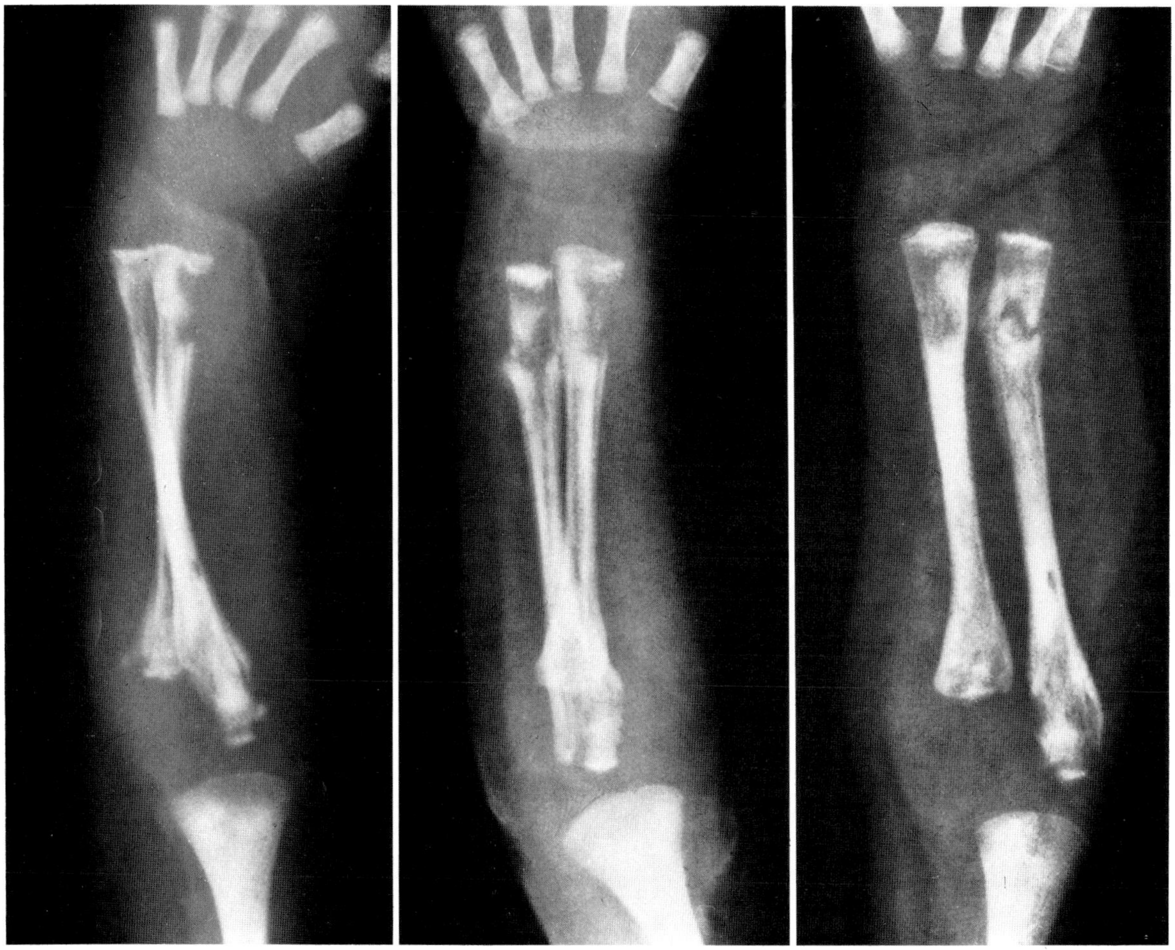

b, c

Fig. 1a–c. Congenital syphilis. **a** Left arm: Severe involvement of radius and ulna with cortical erosions in metaphyseal areas and signs of osteitis and periosteal reaction. **b** Left arm after 2 weeks: Progressive destruction in metaphyses, periosteal reaction and fracture of ulna. Metacarpals not affected. **c** Right arm: Metaphyseal infection of radius and ulna, ulnar fracture and periosteal new formation, cortical erosion in proximal ulna

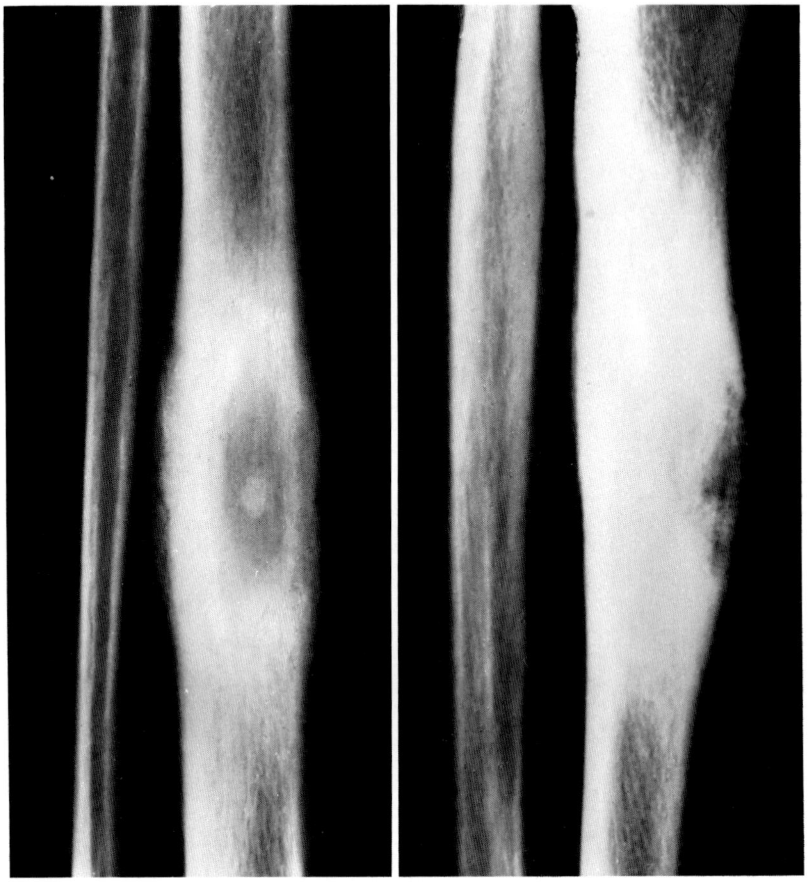

a b

Fig. 3a, b. Acquired syphilis in an adult male. Gummatous osteitis of tibia with bone destruction surrounded by a zone of dense bone. Extensive periosteal new bone formation

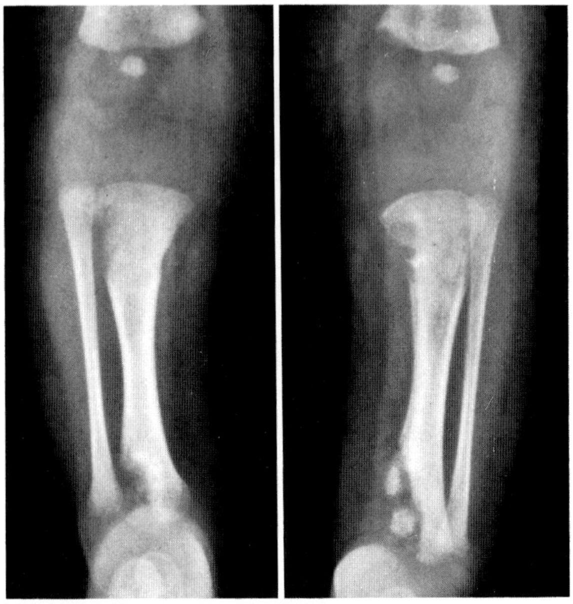

a b

Fig. 2a, b. Same patient as Fig. 1. The tibiae present osteolytic lesions in the proximal ends (Wimberger's sign) as well as in the distal ends. Fragmentation, particularly of left distal metaphysis (**b**), and periosteal new bone formation along tibia

Other Sites

Knees	Costochondral regions
Shoulders	Sternum
Elbows	Vertebral bodies

Differential Diagnosis

Scurvy (Sect. 6.2.5)
Osteomyelitis (Sect. 7.3.3)
Tuberculosis (Sect. 7.3.9)
Yaws (Sect. 7.3.11)

References

1 Cremin BJ, Fisher RM (1970) The lesions of congenital syphilis. Br J Radiol 43:333–341
2 Levin EJ (1970) Healing in congenital osseous syphilis. AJR 110:591–597
3 Murray RO, Jacobson HG (1977) The radiology of skeletal disorders. Churchill Livingstone, Edinburgh
4 Chipps BE, Schwischuk LE, Voelter WW (1976) Single bone involvement in congenital syphilis. Pediatr Radiol 5:30–36
5 Resnick D, Niwayama G (1981) Diagnosis of bone and joint disorders. Saunders, Philadelphia

7.3.2 Pyogenic Arthritis

Many infectious agents can cause pyogenic arthritis, but most cases are staphylococcal in origin [1–6]. The following conditions predispose to pyogenic arthritis [1]:

1. Congenital
   insensitivity to pain
   sickle cell anemia
2. Traumatic
   tissue laceration
   human and animal bites
   frostbite
   burning
   puncture wounds
   fractures
3. Neurological
   syringomyelia
   lepra
   diabetes
4. Hematogenic factors (less common)

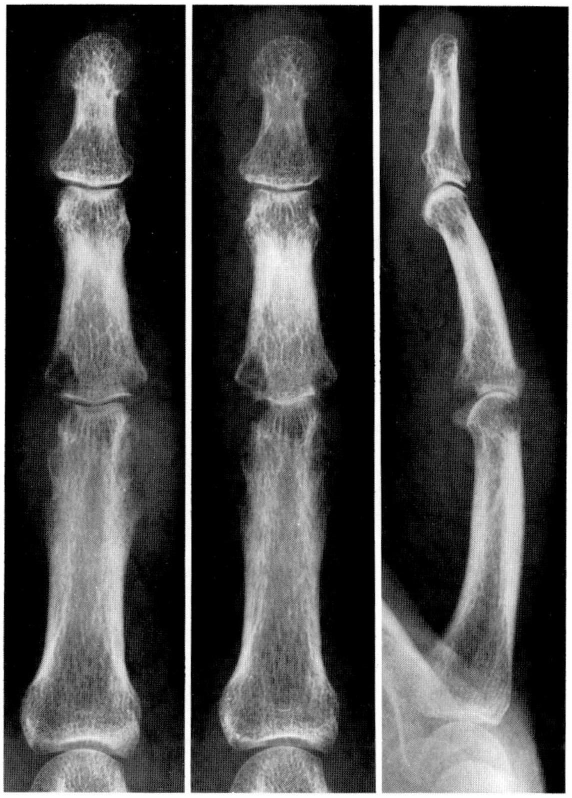

a b c

Fig. 1a–c. Pyogenic arthritis in a 57-year-old man. **a** Soft tissue swelling, some periarticular osteoporosis, joint space still normal, multiple marginal erosions. **b, c** After 2 months: Joint space narrowing, several faint periarticular calcifications, periosteal bone formation

Radiographic Findings [1, 6]

Hand:
Soft tissue swelling
Periarticular osteoporosis
Joint space narrowing
Marginal erosions
Periostitis
Sclerosis
Deformation of the joint
Secondary osteoarthrosis
Periarticular calcifications
Ankylosis

Differential Diagnosis

Hand
Rheumatoid arthritis (Sect. 7.3.4)
Juvenile rheumatoid arthritis (Sect. 7.3.5)
Psoriatic arthritis (Sect. 7.3.6)
Reiter's syndrome (Sect. 7.3.7)
Gout (Sect. 7.3.8)
Osteoarthrosis (Sect. 7.3.13)
Wrist
Carpal fusion (Sect. 2.2.7)
Pseudogout (Sect. 6.2.6)
Rheumatoid arthritis (Sect. 7.3.4)
Juvenile rheumatoid arthritis (Sect.7.3.5)
Gout (Sect. 7.3.8)
Tuberculous arthritis (Sect. 7.3.9)

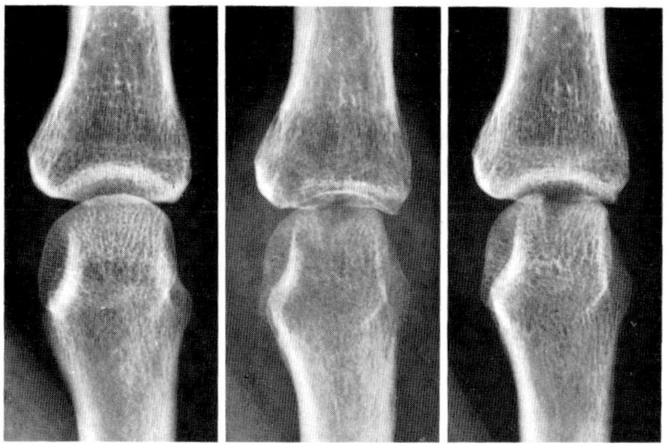

a b c

Fig. 2a–c. Pyogenic arthritis in a 42-year-old man after human bite. **a** Initial radiograph: No abnormalities. **b** After 1 month: Soft tissue swelling, periarticular osteoporosis, joint space narrowing. **c** Four months after treatment: Only slight joint space narrowing, normal bone density, small defect in metacarpal head

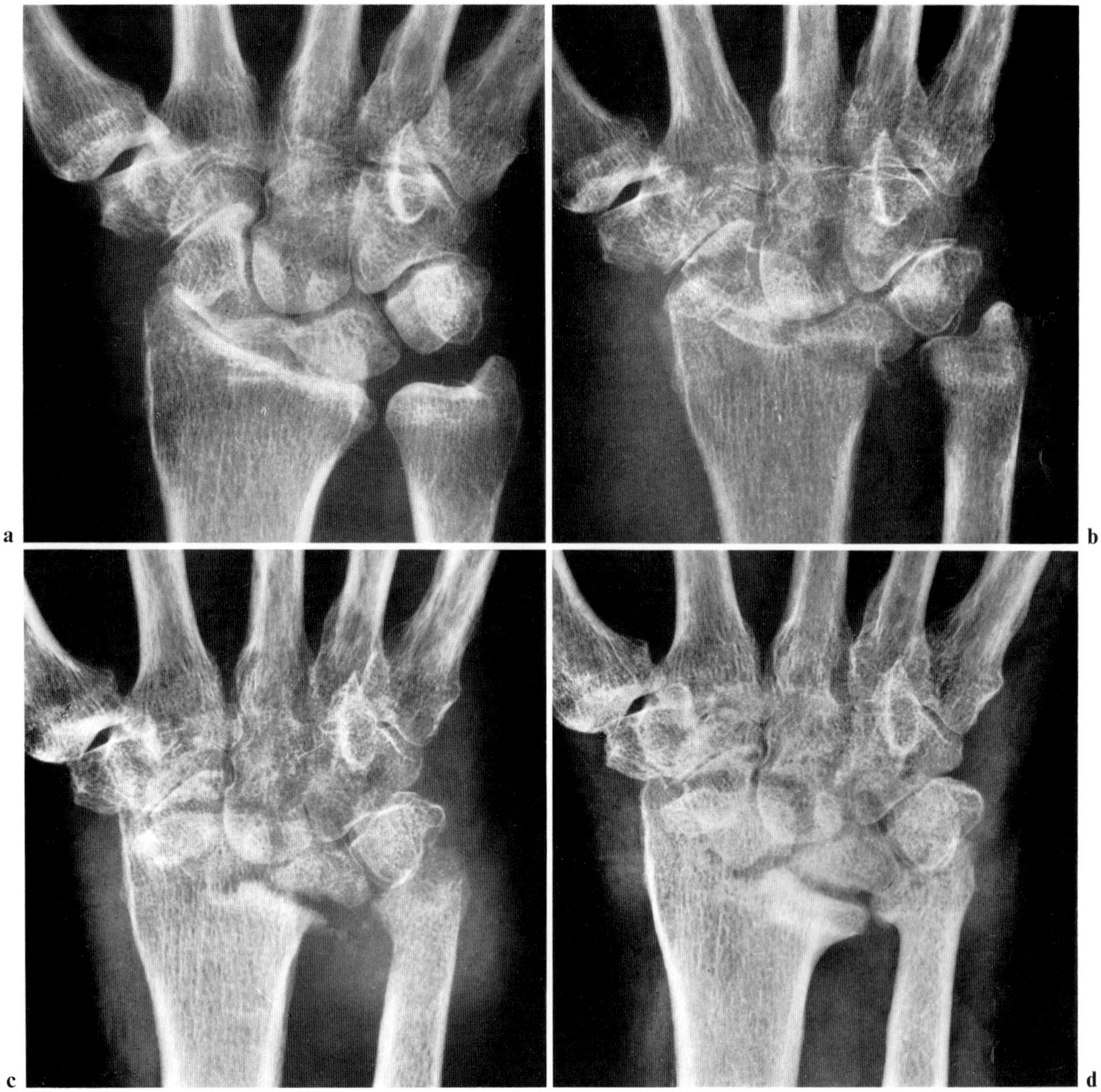

Fig. 3a–d. Pyogenic arthritis (staphylococcus) of the wrist in an 80-year-old woman. **a** Some periarticular osteoporosis and narrowing of radiocarpal joint space. **b** After 7 weeks: Significant periarticular osteoporosis and destruction of radiocarpal joint. **c** After another 4 months: Destruction of radiocarpal and intercarpal joints, improved bone density, several tiny periarticular calcifications in soft tissue. **d** After another year: Increased bone density, bone destruction unchanged in comparison with previous radiograph

References

1 Poznanski AK (1984) The hand in radiologic diagnosis. Saunders, Philadelphia
2 Newman JH (1976) Review of septic arthritis throughout the antibiotic era. Ann Rheum Dis 35:198–201
3 Hutto JH, Ayoub EM (1975) Streptococcal osteomyelitis and arthritis in a neonate. Am J Dis Child 129:1449–1453
4 Kaufmann CA, Watanakunakorn C, Phair JP (1976) Pneumococcal arthritis. J Rheumatol 3:409–412
5 Garcia-Kutzbach, Masi AT (1974) Acute infectious agent arthritis (IAA): a detailed comparison of proved gonococcal and other blood-borne bacterial arthritis. J Rheumatol 1:93–98
6 Resnick D, Niwayama G (1981) Diagnosis of bone and joint disorders. Saunders, Philadelphia

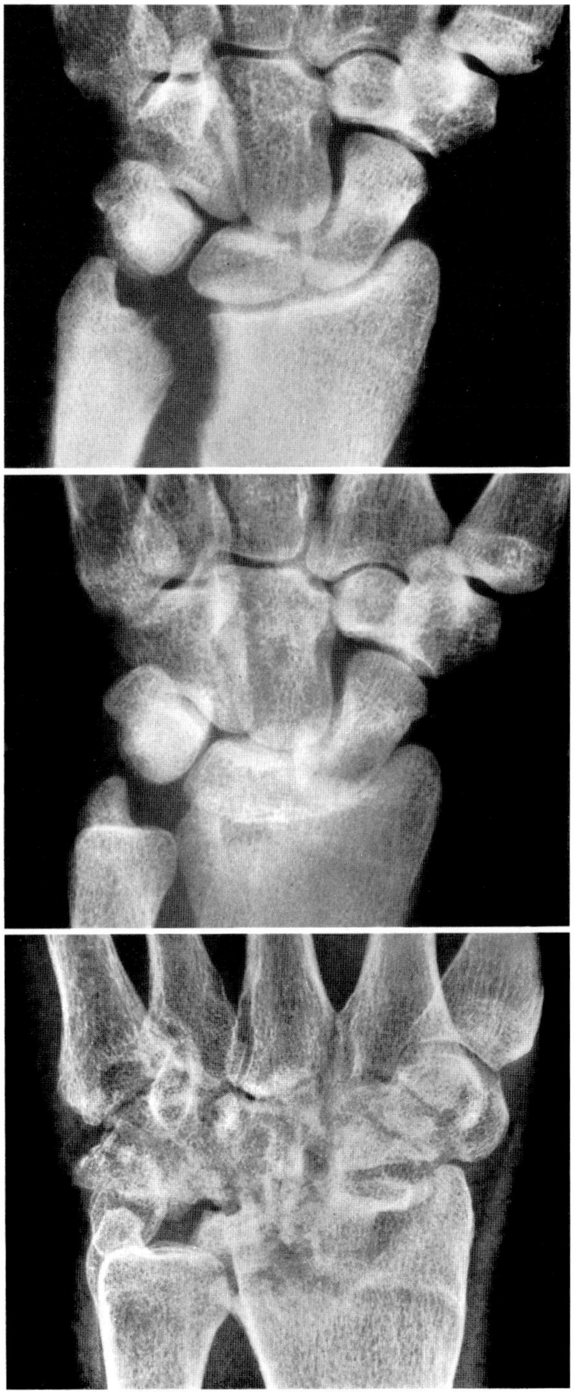

a b c

Fig. 4a–c. Gonococcal arthritis in a 19-year-old woman (a, b). **a** Right wrist: Significant destruction of radioulnar joint, periostitis. **b** Left wrist: Gonococcal arthritis, early ankylosis of radiocarpal joint. **c** Results of tuberculous arthritis in a 22-year-old woman: Severe destruction of wrist with ankylosis

7.3.3 Osteomyelitis

The following disorders predispose to pyogenic infection and subsequent osteomyelitis of the hand:

1. Congenital
   insensitivity to pain
   sickle cell anemia
2. Traumatic
   tissue laceration
   human and animal bites
   burns
   puncture wounds
   fractures
3. Neurological
   syringomyelia
   leprosy
   diabetes

Radiographic Findings [1]

Hand
Soft tissue swelling
Periosteal new bone formation
Bone destruction
Sequestrum

References

1 Capitanio MA, Kirkpatrick JA (1970) Early roentgen observations in acute osteomyelitis. AJR 108:488–496

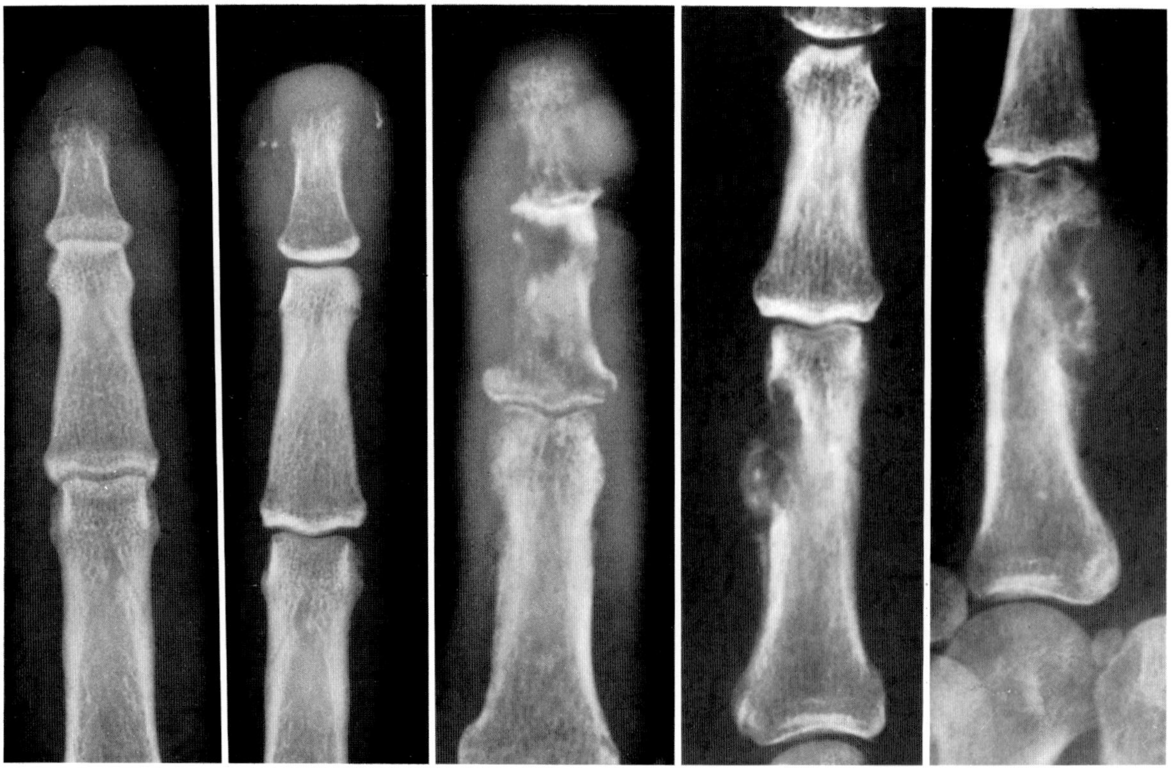

a **b** **c** **d** **e**

Fig. 1a–e. Pyogenic osteomyelitis. **a, b** In a 21-year-old woman. **a** Soft tissue swelling and tuft destruction. **b** After 14 days: Significant demineralization of distal phalanx, distal interphalangeal joint intact. **c** In a 43-year-old man: Osteomyelitis of distal, middle, and proximal phalanges, soft tissue swelling, demineralization, bone destruction. **d, e** In a 40-year-old man: Osteomyelitis of proximal phalanx, bone destruction, only slight demineralization, significant periosteal bone formation. Specific differential diagnosis: osteosarcoma, chondrosarcoma (uncommon)

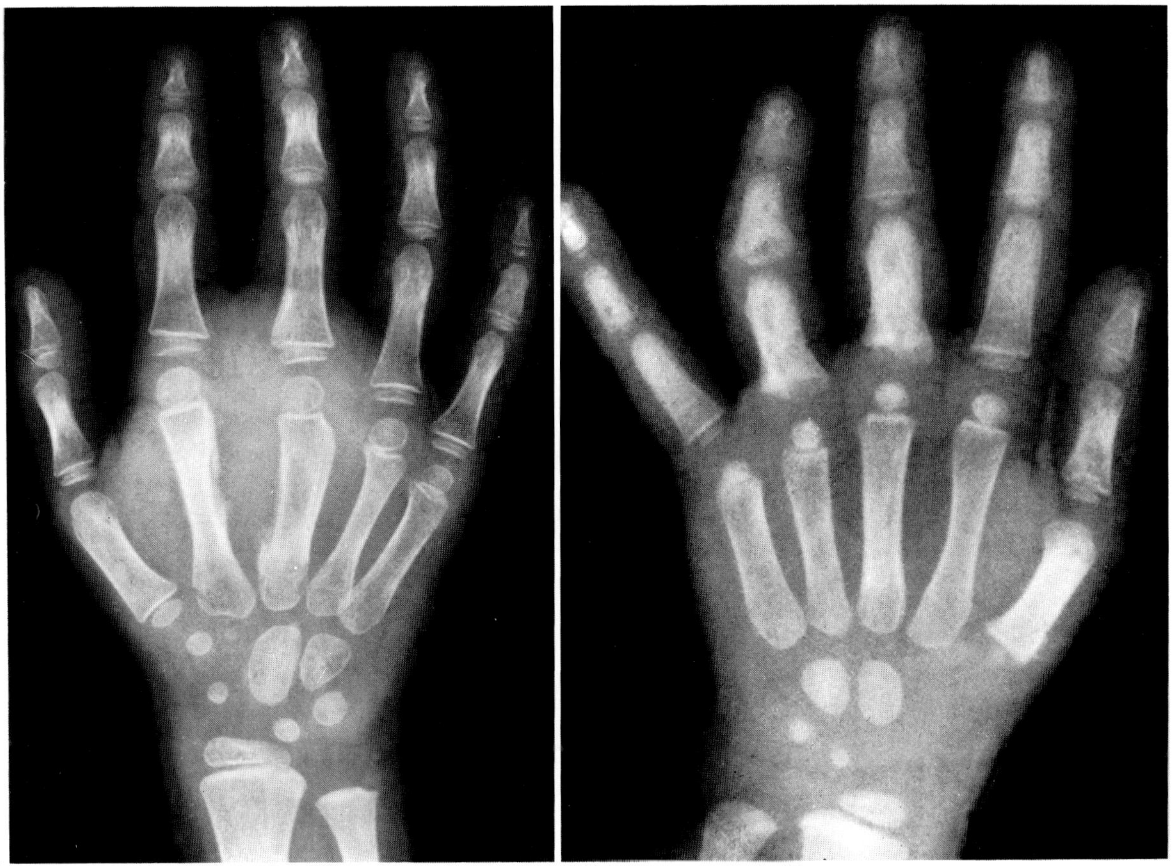

a b

Fig. 2a, b. Osteomyelitis. **a** In a 5-year-old girl: Soft tissue swelling, huge periosteal new bone formation of second and third metacarpals. Specific differential diagnosis: myositis ossificans. **b** In a 4-year-old boy: Sickle cell anemia and salmonella osteomyelitis. Several bones are affected. Significant increased bone density, shaft widening due to periosteal new bone formation

7.3.4 Adult Rheumatoid Arthritis

Rheumatoid arthritis is a chronic systemic and auto-immune disease affecting many organs of the body. Symmetric polyarthritis of the small joints in the hands and feet is often one of the initial features. The affected joints present signs of chronic synovitis, with destruction of joint cartilage, bony structures, and ligaments. The most characteristic findings are the subcutaneous nodules, which are granulomas each consisting of a central necrotic area surrounded by granulomatous tissue. There are similar histologic findings in the synovial membranes, periarticular soft tissues, and tendons, as well as in the heart, lungs, pleura, eyes, spleen, and larynx.

Radiographic Findings [2–8]

Hand

Periarticular soft tissue swelling (synovial thickening and joint distension)
Periarticular demineralization (hyperemia, disuse)
Joint space narrowing
Marginal erosions by rheumatoid pannus (initial erosions of metacarpophalangeal joints usually found on volar side)
Small pseudocysts
Joint destruction (commonly in form of cup and pencil deformity)
Periostitis (rather uncommon)
Subcutaneous nodules
(Sub)luxation
Ulnar deviation of fingers
Ankylosis
Secondary osteoarthrosis

Other Sites
Foot: abnormalities similar to those in hand
Large joints: ankles
knees
elbows
shoulders
hips
Other joints: costovertebral
acromioclavicular
sternoclavicular
craniovertebral

Differential Diagnosis

Chondrocalcinosis (Sect. 6.2.6)
Hyperlipoproteinemia (Sect. 7.1.5)
Juvenile rheumatoid arthritis (Sect. 7.3.5)
Psoriatic arthritis (Sect. 7.3.6)
Reiter's syndrome (Sect. 7.3.7)
Gout (Sect. 7.3.8)
Osteoarthrosis (Sect. 7.3.13)
Systemic lupus erythematosus (Sect. 7.3.14)
Scleroderma (Sect. 7.6.3)
Ankylosing spondylitis
Multicentric reticulohistiocytosis [7, 8]

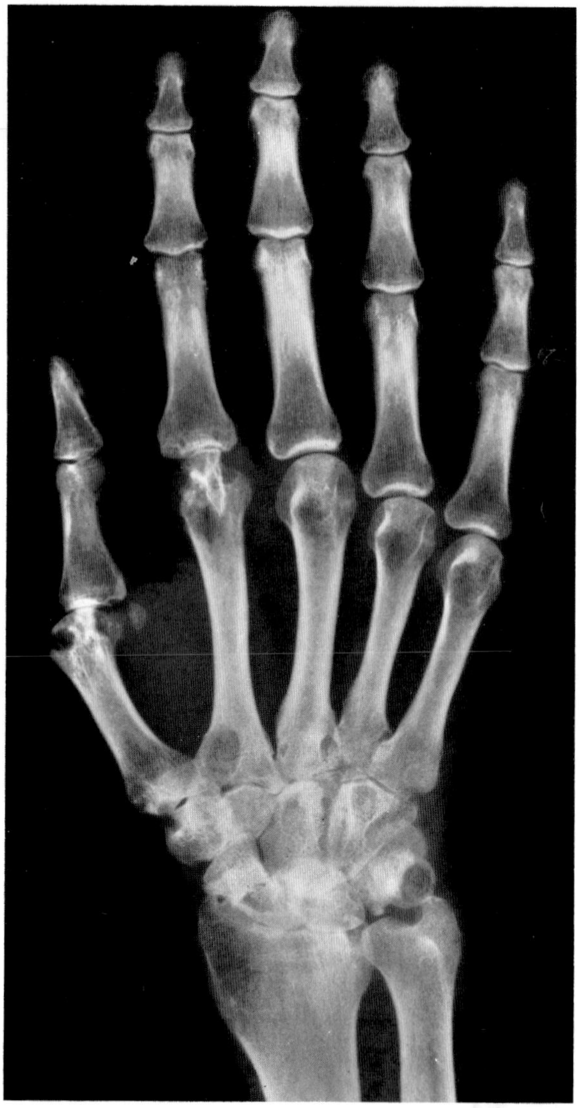

Fig. 1. Rheumatoid arthritis in a 52-year-old woman. Polyarthritis of first and second metacarpophalangeal joints, carpometacarpal joints, intercarpal joints, and radiocarpal joint. The joint spaces of the affected joints are severely narrowed, and multiple pseudocysts are present

The accompanying table shows the comparative laboratory findings for this and other conditions [1]

Condition	Parameter			
	Rheumatoid factor: Rose-Waaler, latex fixation	Antinuclear antibodies	DNA antibodies	Anti-perinuclear factor
Adult rheumatoid arthritis	+70%–80% −20%–30%	+40% −60%	−	+50% −50%
Juvenile rheumatoid arthritis	−	−	−	−
Osteoarthrosis	−	−	−	−
Ankylosing spondylitis	−	−	−	−
Psoriatic arthritis	−	−	−	−
Reiter's syndrome	−	−	−	−
Arthritis in ulcerative colitis	−	−	−	−
Scleroderma	−	+	−	−
Sjögren's syndrome	−	+	−	−
Systemic lupus erythematosus	−	+	±	−
Gout	−	−	−	−

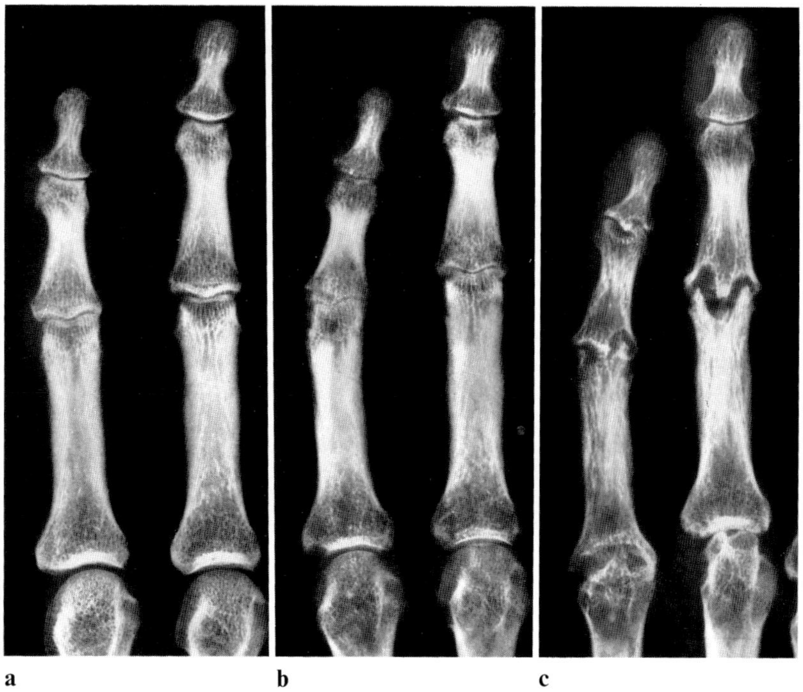

Fig. 2a–c. Rheumatoid arthritis in a woman. **a** August 1978: Normal second and third fingers. **b** December 1978: Periarticular demineralization, joint space narrowing, multiple small marginal erosions. **c** 1980: Severe destruction of affected joints with "seagull" appearance

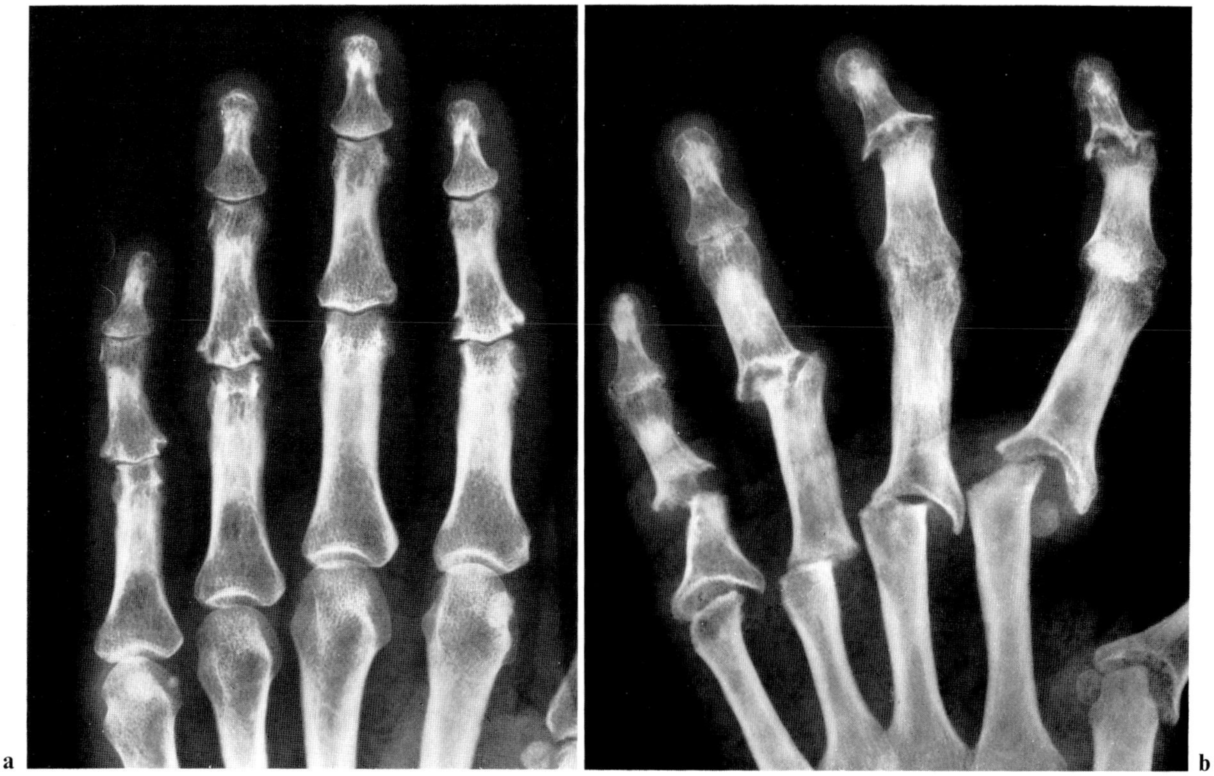

Fig. 3a, b. Rheumatoid arthritis. **a** In a 49-year-old woman: Proximal interphalangeal joints mainly affected, metacarpophalangeal joints normal. **b** In a 40-year-old woman: Severe joint destruction, particularly of metacarpophalangeal joints, cup and pencil deformity

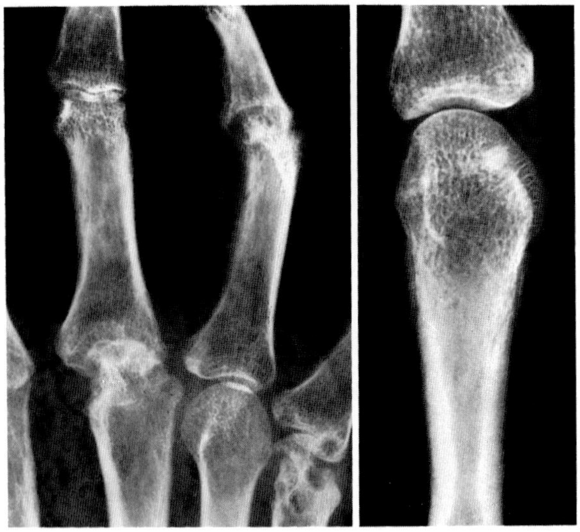

a b

Fig. 4a, b. Rheumatoid arthritis. **a** In a 46-year-old woman: Severe arthritis, periosteal reaction along proximal phalanges. **b** In 25-year-old woman: Periosteal reaction at second metacarpal

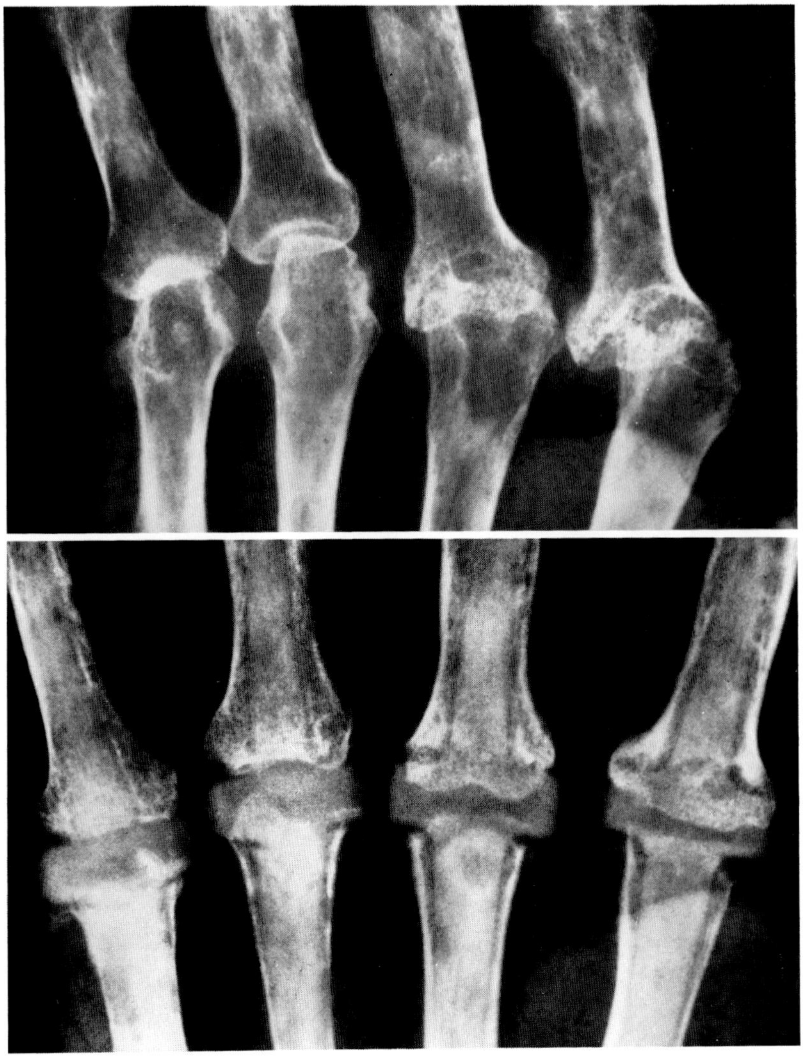

a

b

Fig. 5a, b. Rheumatoid arthritis before and after arthroplasty with silastic Swanson prostheses

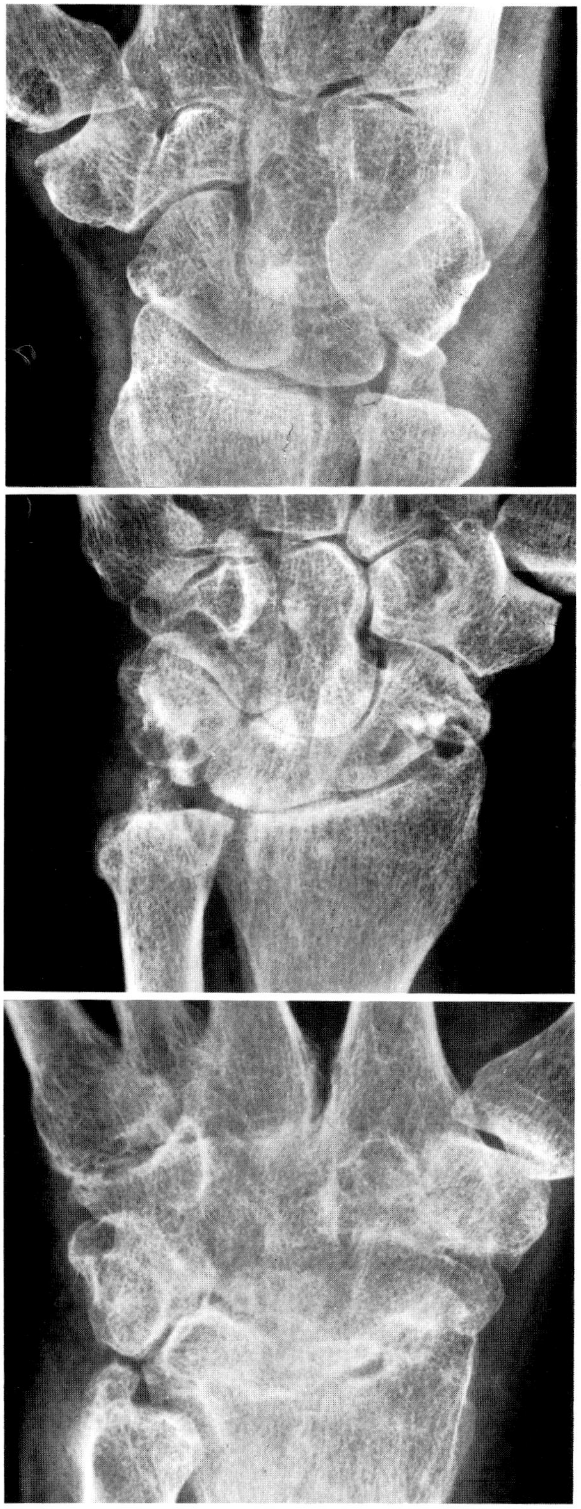

a b c

Fig. 6a–c. Rheumatoid arthritis. **a** In a 47-year-old woman: Significant soft tissue swelling, several small pseudocysts. **b** In a 48-year-old woman: Narrowing of intercarpal and radiocarpal joint spaces, multiple erosions and small cysts. Distal radioulnar joint also affected. **c** In a 46-year-old woman: Ankylosis of wrist

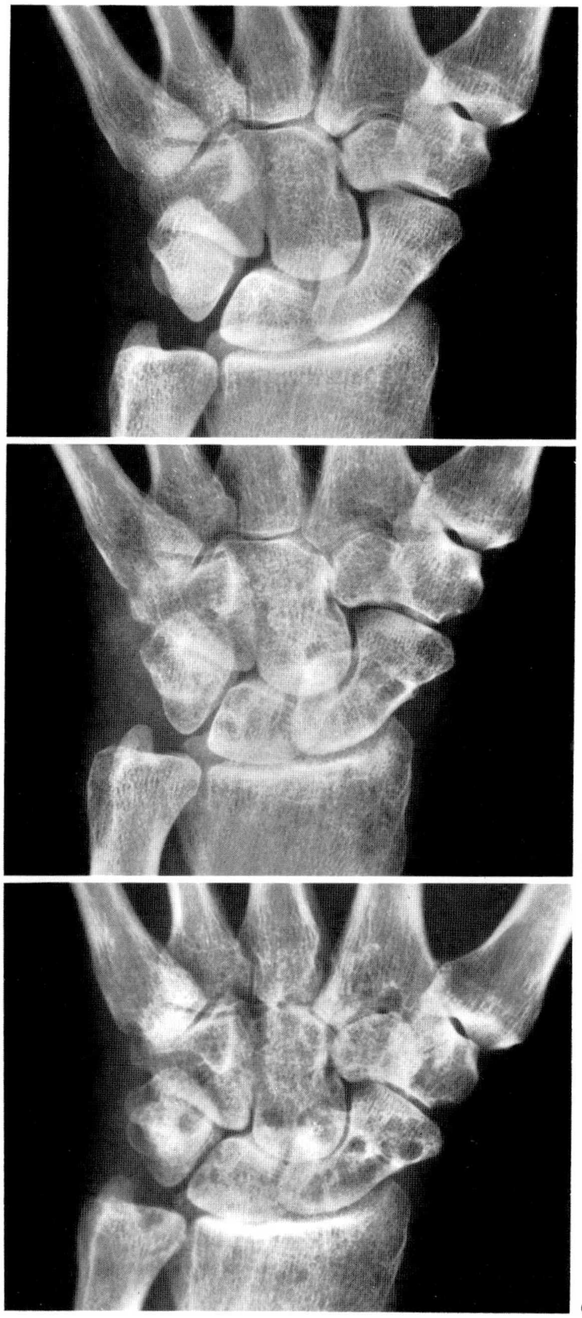

a b c

Fig. 7a–c. Rheumatoid arthritis in a 43-year-old woman. **a** 1981: Normal wrist. **b** 1982: Periarticular demineralization, soft tissue swelling, pseudocysts in scaphoid and lunate. **c** 1984: Progressive joint space narrowing, multiple pseudocysts in carpals

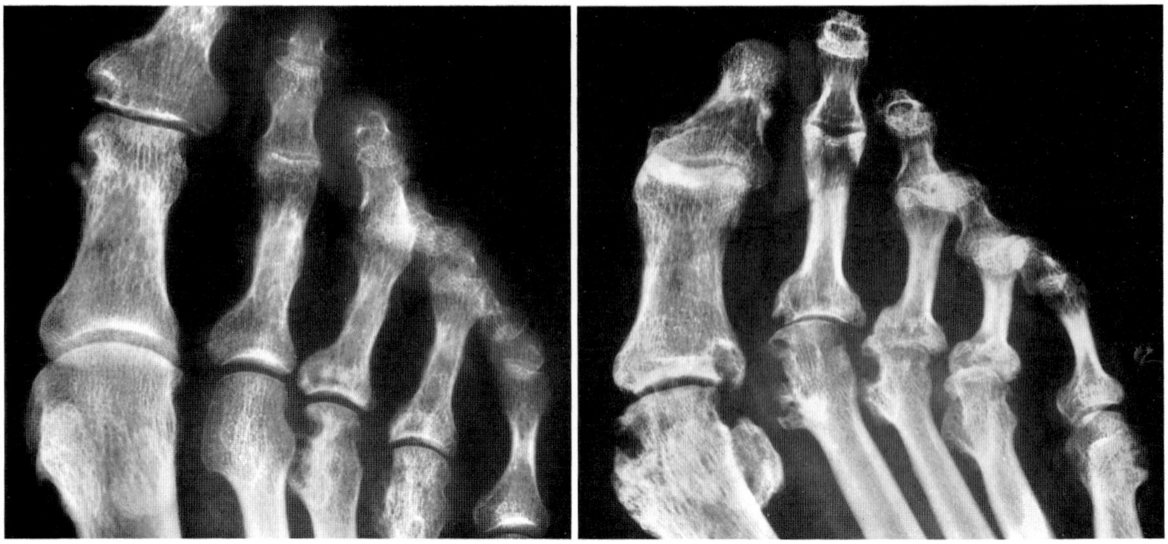

a b

Fig. 8a, b. Rheumatoid arthritis. **a** In a 49-year-old woman: Polyarthritis of metatarsophalangeal joints and first interphalangeal joint. **b** In a 70-year-old man: Severe affection of all metatarsophalangeal joints and deviation of toes

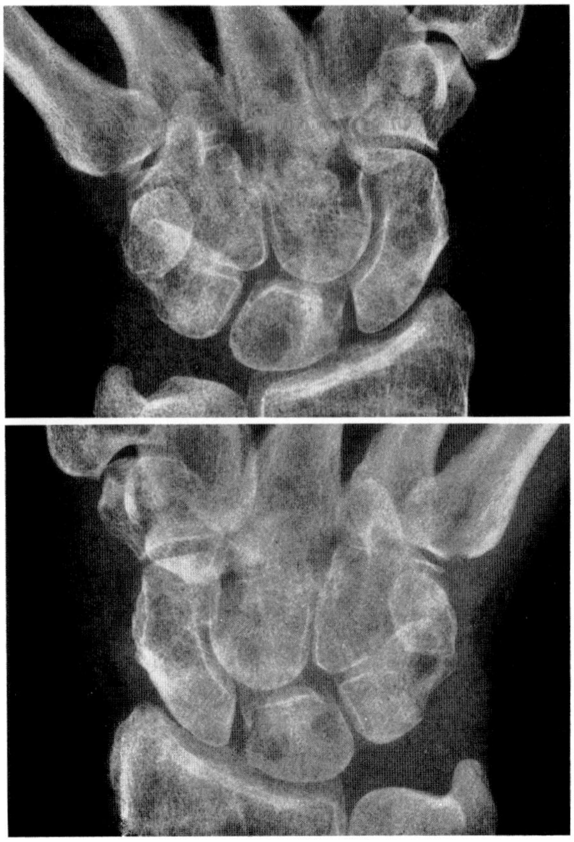

a b

Fig. 9a, b. Possible amyloid arthropathy in a 46-year-old woman. Periarticular osteoporosis of wrists. The radiographic findings are not specific: rheumatoid arthritis, osteoporosis due to disuse, and Sudeck's atrophy are other possible diagnoses

References

1 Nienhuis RLF (1977) Laboratorium onderzoek bij gewrichtsafwijkingen. Laboratory investigations in joint diseases. Merck Sharp and Dohme, Haarlem

2 Carvallo A de, Grandal H (1980) Radiographic progression of rheumatoid arthritis related to some clinical and laboratory parameters. Acta Radiol 21:551–555

3 Martel W (1964) The pattern of rheumatoid arthritis in the hand and wrist. Radiol Clin North Am 2:221–234

4 Marshall TR (1968) Radiographic changes in rheumatoid arthritis in the digits. Radiology 90:121–128

5 Martel W, Hayes JT, Duff IF (1965) The pattern of bone erosion in the hand and wrist in rheumatoid arthritis. Radiology 84:204–214

6 Resnick D, Niwayama (1981) Diagnosis of bone and joint disorders. Saunders, Philadelphia

7 Gold RH, Metzger AL, Mirra JM, Weinberger HJ, Killebrew K (1973) Multicentric reticulohistiocytosis (lipoid dermato-arthritis). An erosive polyarthritis with distinctive clinical, roentgenographic and pathologic features. AJR 124:610–624

8 Freyschmidt J, Wilmowsky H v, Krmpotic L (1978) Multizentrische Retikulohistiozytose als Ursache einer „erosiv-destruktiven Arthropathie". Fortschr Geb Röntgenstr Nuklearmed Ergänzungsband 129:605–610

7.3.5 Rheumatoid Arthritis in Childhood and Adolescence

Rheumatoid arthritis in childhood and adolescence can be divided into the following clinical types [1, 2]:

1. Juvenile rheumatoid arthritis:
   onset before the age of 16 years (mean $7^1/_2$ years)
   polyarthritis, oligoarthritis, or monoarthritis for at least 6 weeks
   frequently iridocyclitis (9%–19%)
2. Still's disease:
   usually affects young children (mean $5^1/_2$ years)
   extra-articular symptoms: mostly arthritis of fingers, carpals, and cervical spine
   extra-articular symptoms: fever, lymphadenopathy, hepatosplenomegaly, high ESR, exanthema (70%), pericarditis, pleuritis, peritonitis, and anemia
   articular symptoms: mostly arthritis of fingers, carpals and cervical spine
3. Juvenile ankylosing spondylitis:
   frequently iridocyclitis
   oligoarthritis (hips, sacroiliac joints, cervical spine)
   mostly HLA-B27 positive
4. Rheumatoid arthritis of the adult type mostly occurs from the age of 16 years. Patients can be sero-positive.

Radiographic Findings [3, 4]

Hand
Periarticular soft tissue swelling
Osteoporosis
Periostitis
Joint space narrowing
Cysts and erosions
Accelerated skeletal maturation
Decreased growth
Bony ankylosis of the wrist

Other Sites
Foot abnormalities
Arthritis of major joints (especially: knee 86%, hip 54%, ankle 75%)
Sacroiliitis (especially in juvenile ankylosing spondylitis)
Ankylosis of apophyseal joints in cervical spine (especially in juvenile ankylosing spondylitis)
Atlantoaxial dislocation

Differential Diagnosis

Carpal fusion: pyogenic arthritis (Sect. 7.3.2)
  adult rheumatoid arthritis (Sect. 7.3.4)
  tuberculous arthritis (Sect. 7.3.9)
  after surgery
  other disorders (Sect. 2.2.7)
Bony ankylosis of cervical spine:
  congenital
  ankylosing spondylitis
  Reiter's syndrome (Sect. 7.3.7)
  psoriatic arthritis (Sect. 7.3.6)
  fibrodysplasia ossificans progressiva (Sect. 7.1.3)

References

1 Stoeber E (1978) Juvenile rheumatoid arthritis and Still's syndrome (in Dutch). Folia Rheumatologica 1–20, Ciba Geigy
2 Ansell BM (1978) Chronic arthritis in childhood. Ann Rheum Dis 37:107–112
3 Ansell BM, Kent PA (1977) Radiological changes in juvenile chronic polyarthritis. Skeletal Radiol 1:129–144
4 Martel W, Holt JF, Cassidy JT (1962) Roentgenologic manifestations of juvenile rheumatoid arthritis. AJR 88:400–423

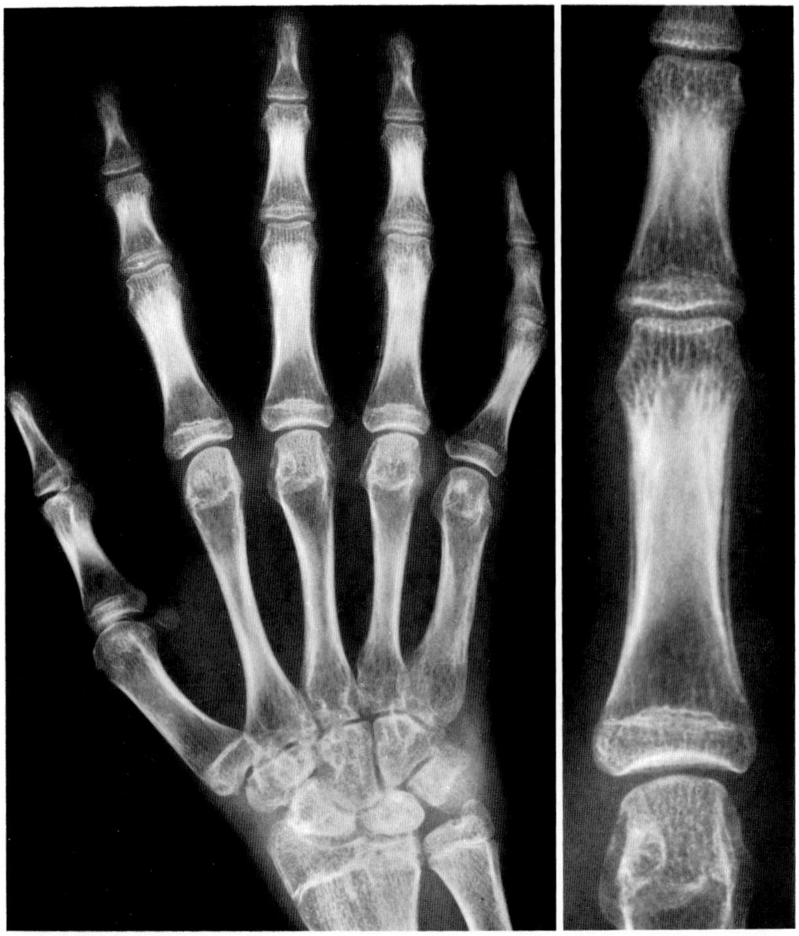

a b

Fig. 1 a, b. Juvenile rheumatoid arthritis in a 13-year-old girl. **a** Left hand: Soft tissue swelling, periarticular osteoporosis, periosteal bone formation, arthritis of wrist with deformation of carpals. **b** Detail: Periosteal bone formation

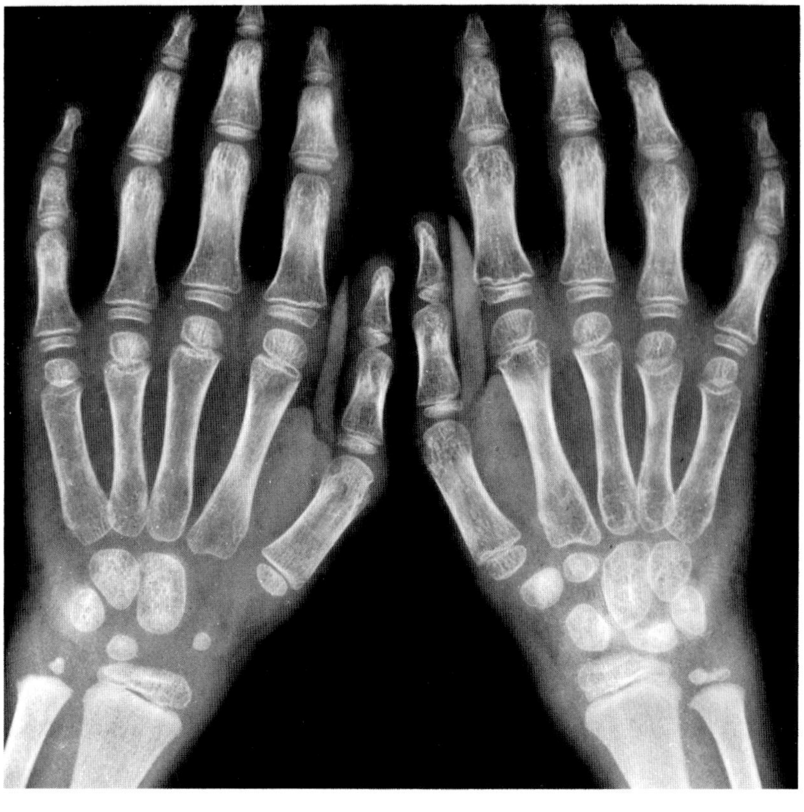

Fig. 2. Juvenile rheumatoid arthritis in a 7-year-old boy. Unilateral accelerated skeletal maturation in the carpal area

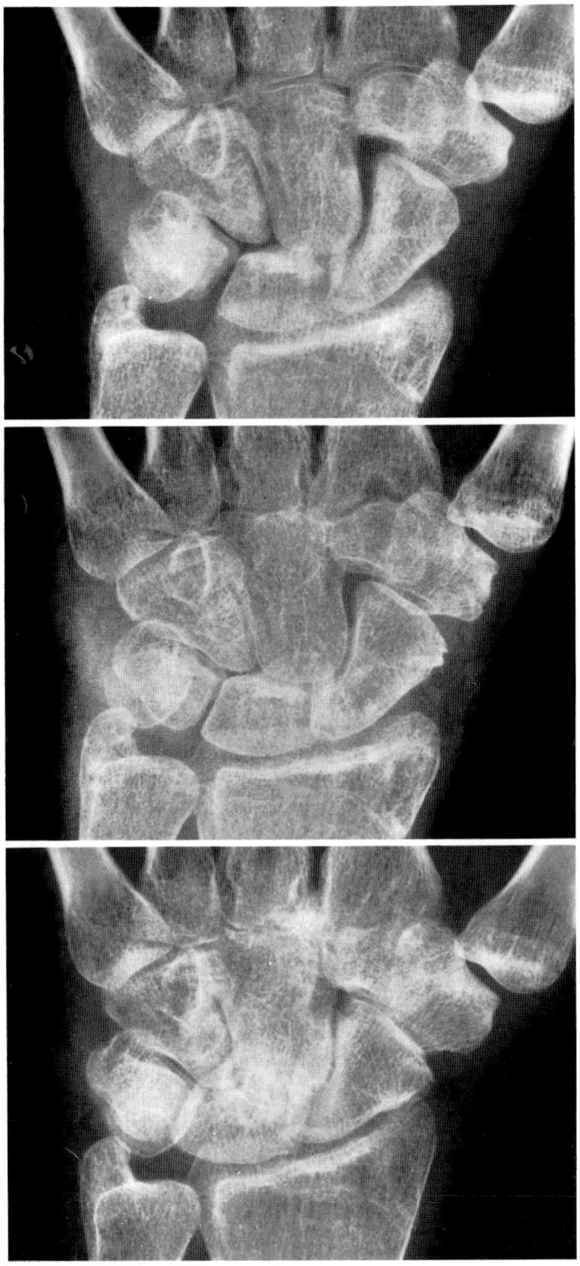

a

b

c

Fig. 3a–c. Bilateral rheumatoid arthritis with systemic extra-articular symptoms (fever, lymphadenopathy, pericarditis) in a 17-year-old girl. **a** Some periarticular osteoporosis. **b** After 2 months: Significant osteoporosis and joint space narrowing (especially carpometacarpal). **c** After 3 years: Carpometacarpal fusion, severe destruction of intercarpal joint spaces

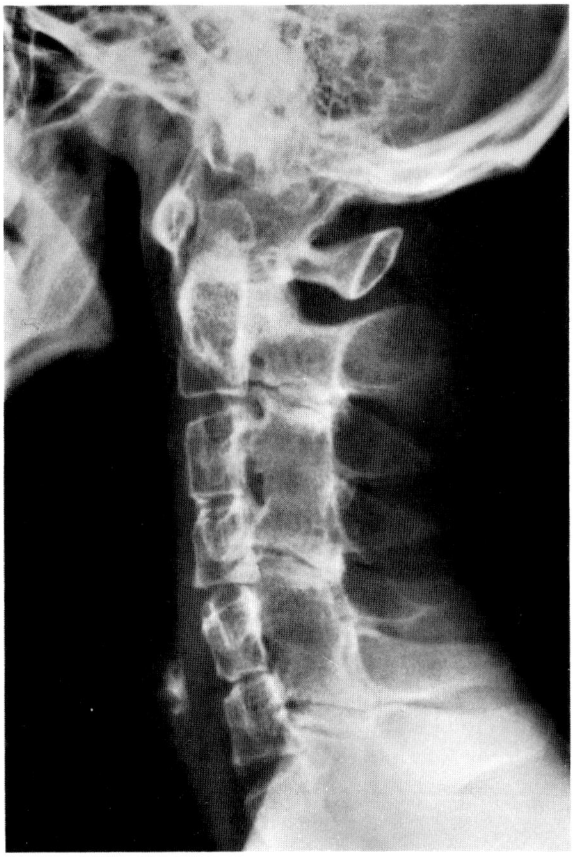

Fig. 4. Juvenile rheumatoid arthritis (since the age of 3) in a 19-year-old woman. Hypoplasia of vertebral bodies, arthritis of apophyseal joints, ankylosis of several vertebral arches, narrowed intervertebral spaces

a 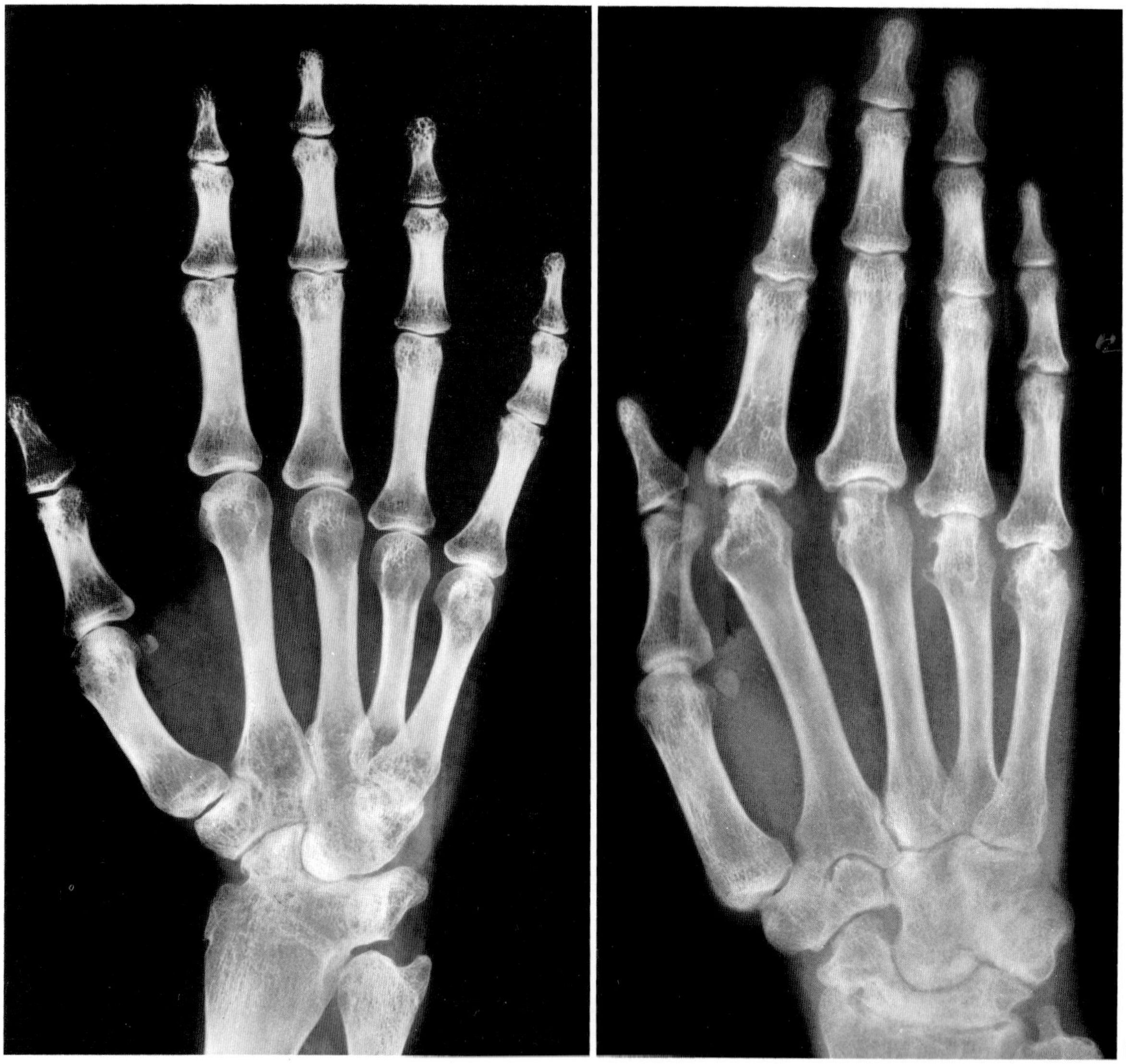 b

Fig. 5. a Juvenile rheumatoid arthritis in a 20-year-old woman: Carpometacarpal and radiocarpal ankylosis. **b** Adult rheumatoid arthritis in a 21-year-old man: Severe destruction of radiocarpal and metacarpophalangeal joints, multiple small cysts, erosions, joint space narrowing

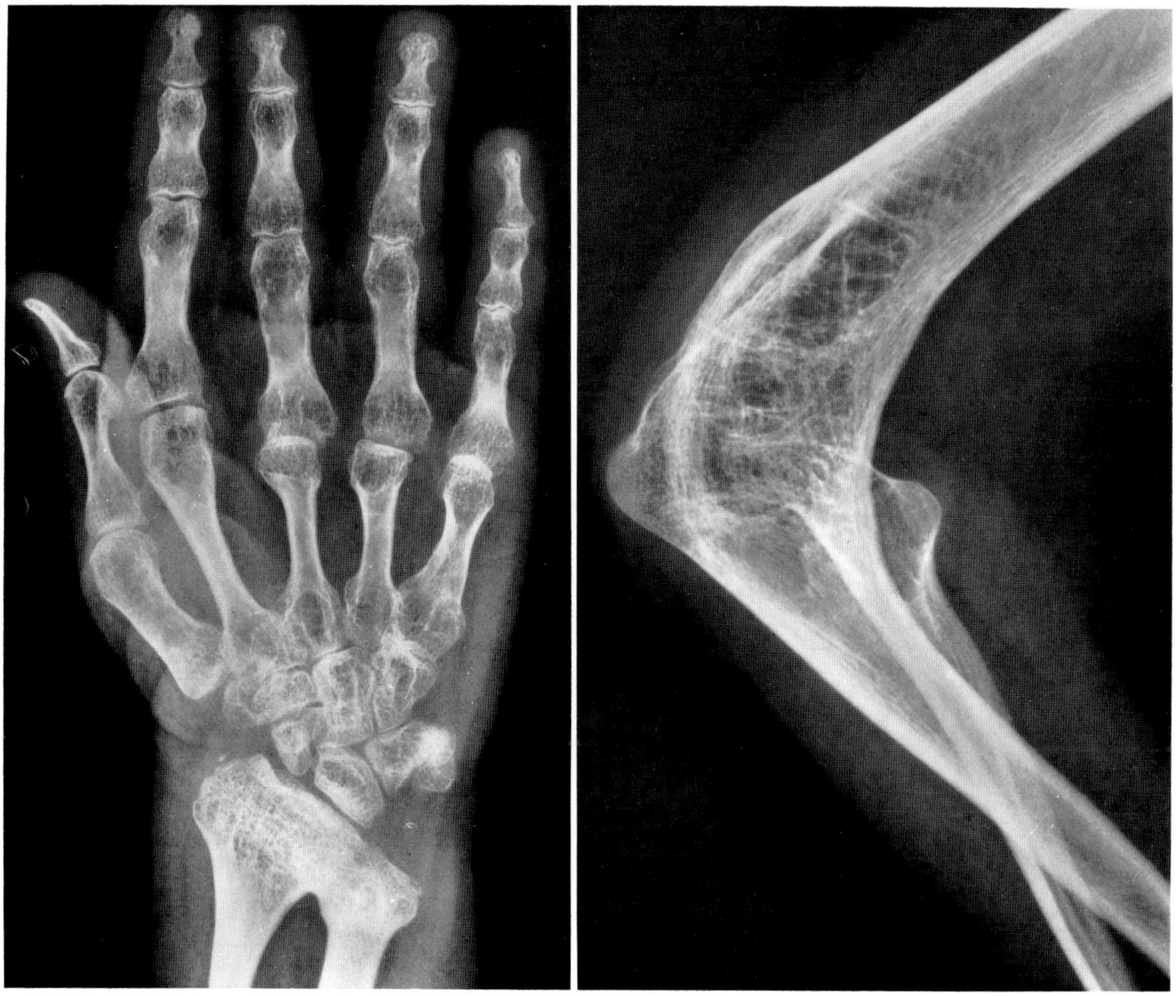

a b

Fig. 6a, b. Juvenile rheumatoid arthritis in a 31-year-old woman who between 7 and 20 years of age was treated for severe manifestations of this disease. **a** Left hand: Deformation and hypoplasia of hand bones, radioulnar ankylosis. **b** Left elbow: Ankylosis

7.3.6 Psoriatic Arthritis

The skin changes of psoriasis are present in about 1% of the general population. In nearly 7% of psoriasis sufferers, polyarthritis is found, and in 25%–60% of this group the HLA-B27 antigen is positive. Other etiologic factors mentioned in the literature are heredity, trauma, infection, and capillary and neurotrophic abnormalities.

Histology

Joints: synovitis with raised levels of lymphocytes and plasma cells, edema, and deposits of fibrin
Entheses: inflammation at the attachments of tendons and ligaments
Synchondroses: inflammation (discovertebral junctions, symphysis pubis, manubriosternal joint)
The interphalangeal joints, tufts, sacroiliac joints, and spine are frequently affected, the wrists, elbows, shoulders, knees, ankles, and hips less frequently.

Radiographic Findings [1–4]

Hand
Soft tissue swelling
Osteoporosis in acute stages
Joint space narrowing or widening
Marginal erosions
Proliferation of bone (mouse ears)
Periostitis
Tuft resorption
Osteosclerosis in later stages (ivory phalanx)
Intra-articular ankylosis
(Sub)luxation
Arthritis mutilans (cup and pencil deformity)

Other Sites
Foot: abnormalities similar to those in hand
Spine: large syndesmophytes
Sacroiliac joints: arthritis
Entheses: erosions
bone apposition
Synchondroses: irregular contours
osteosclerosis
Major joints: arthritis

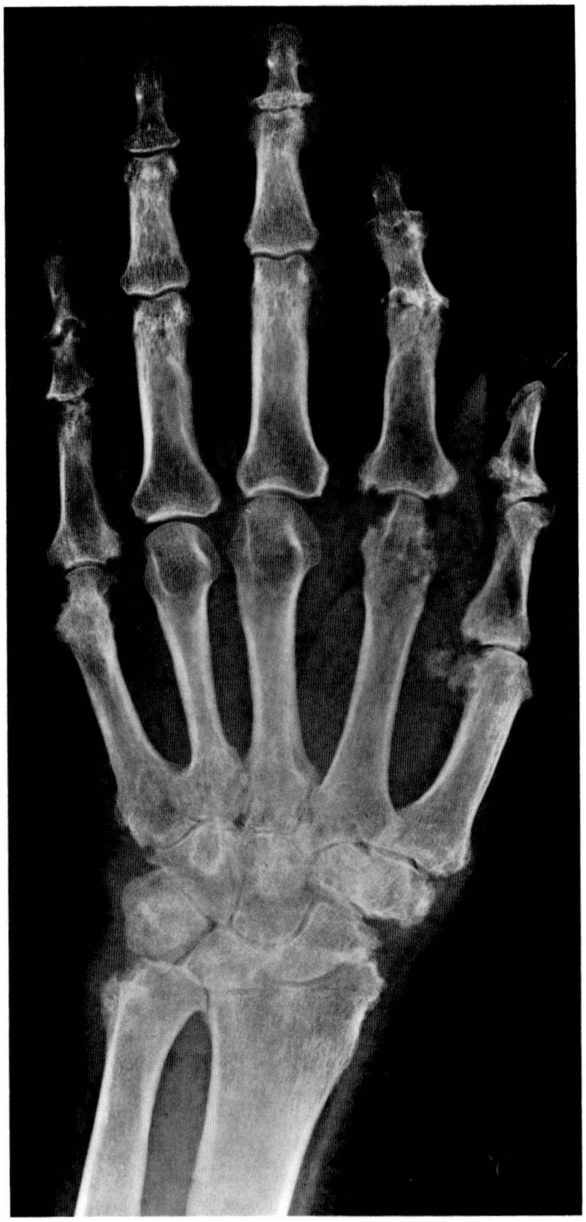

Fig. 1. Psoriatic arthritis. Characteristic features

Differential Diagnosis

Pyogenic arthritis (Sect. 7.3.2)
Rheumatoid arthritis (Sect. 7.3.4)
Juvenile rheumatoid arthritis (Sect. 7.3.5)
Reiter's syndrome (Sect. 7.3.7)
Gout (Sect. 7.3.8)
Osteoarthrosis (Sect. 7.3.13)
Thermal injuries (Sect. 7.6.2)
Scleroderma (Sect. 7.6.3)

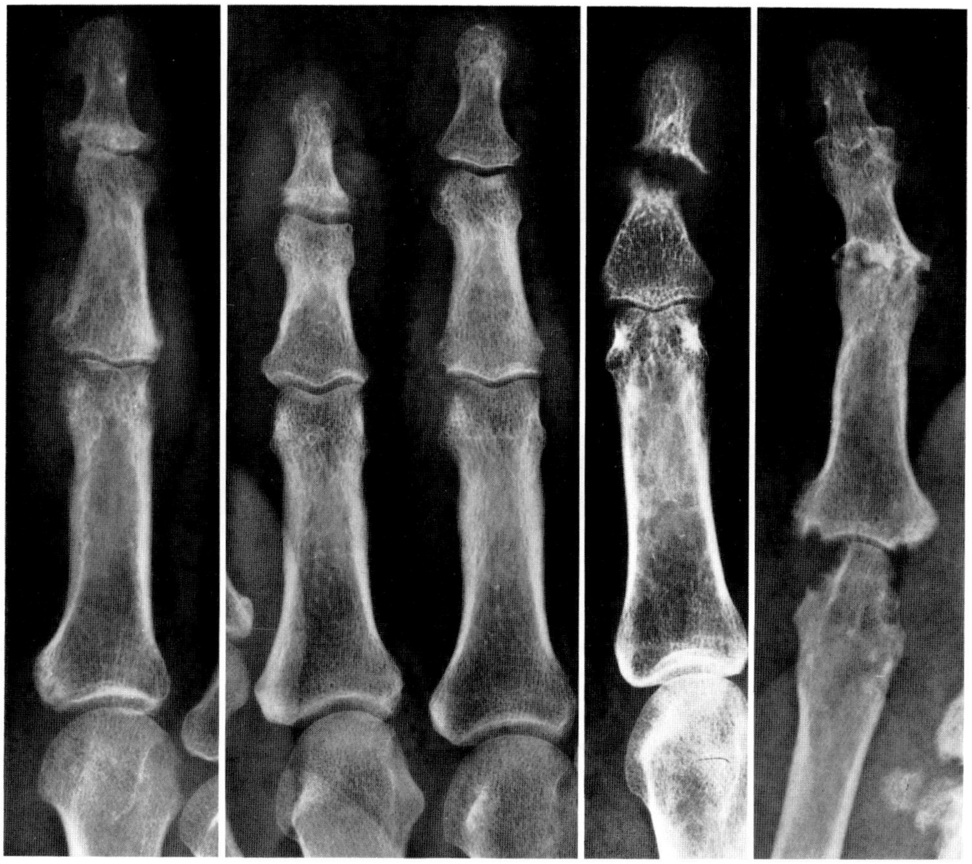

a b c d

Fig. 2a–d. Psoriatic arthritis of fingers. **a, b** Soft tissue swelling, erosions. **c** Arthritis mutilans of distal interphalangeal joint. **d** Proliferation of bone, ankylosis, sclerosis

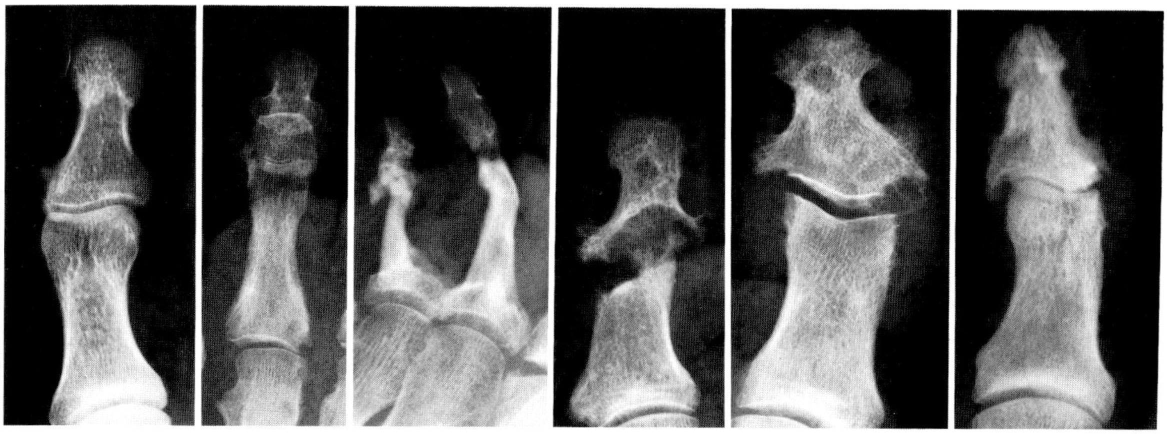

a b c d e f

Fig. 3a–f. Psoriatic arthritis of toes. **a** Slight erosion of distal phalanx. **b** Arthritis of metatarsal joint, periostitis. **c** Sclerosis, ankylosis. **d** Arthritis mutilans. **e, f** Tuft resorption, proliferation of bone, sclerosis

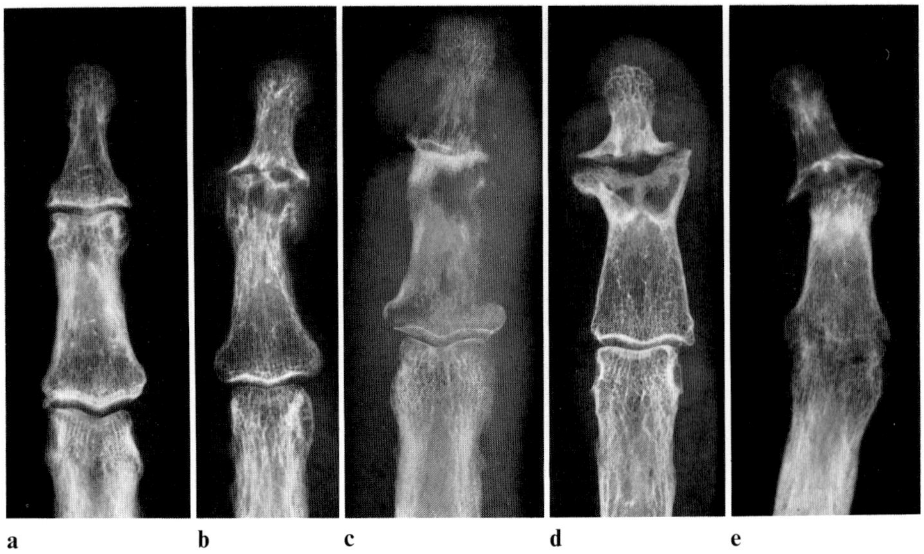

Fig. 4a–e. Some other conditions involving destruction of distal interphalangeal joints. **a, b** Osteoarthrosis. **c** Pyogenic arthritis. **d** Gout. **e** Rheumatoid arthritis

References

1 Resnick D, Niwayama G (1981) Diagnosis of bone and joint disorders. Saunders, Philadelphia
2 Meaney TF, Hays RA (1957) Roentgen manifestations of psoriatic arthritis. Radiology 68:403–407
3 Martel W, Stuck KJ, Dworin AM, Hylland RG (1980) Erosive osteoarthritis and psoriatic arthritis. A radiologic comparison in the hand, wrist and foot. AJR 134:125–135
4 Avila R, Pugh D, Slocumb CH, Winkelmann RK (1960) Psoriatic arthritis: a roentgenologic study. Radiology 75:691–702

7.3.7 Reiter's Syndrome

Synonym: reactive arthritis

Reiter's syndrome is usually asymmetric in presentation, and usually occurs in the lower extremity (knee, ankle, heel, metatarsophalangeal joints). The sacroiliac joints, entheses, and synchondroses are usually also affected [1, 2].

Radiographic Findings [1, 2]

Hand and Foot

Soft tissue swelling, sausage-like fingers and toes
Relative absence of osteoporosis (except in acute episodes)
Narrowing of joint space
Bony erosions at joint margins
Linear or fluffy periostitis
Ankylosis (uncommon)
Severe joint destruction (uncommon in hand)

Other Sites

Entheses: abnormalities of heels, trochanters, and ischial tuberosity, characterized by erosion and adjacent bone proliferation
SI joints: sacroiliitis
Spine: asymmetric vertebral hyperostosis ("parasyndesmophytes")
paravertebral soft tissue calcification
Synchondroses: abnormalities of symphysis pubis and manubriosternal joint

Differential Diagnosis

Chondrocalcinosis (Sect. 6.2.6)
Pyogenic arthritis (Sect. 7.3.2)
Rheumatoid arthritis (Sect. 7.3.4)
Psoriatic arthritis (Sect. 7.3.6)
Gout (Sect. 7.3.8)

Fig. 1a–d. Reiter's syndrome. **a** Slight periarticular osteoporosis of proximal interphalangeal joint. **b** Arthritis of proximal interphalangeal joint and periosteal reaction of proximal phalanx. **c** Significant periosteal reaction and soft tissue swelling. **d** Soft tissue swelling at ulnar side of carpals without involvement of carpals ▷

Fig. 2a–g. Reiter's syndrome. **a–c** and **d–f** Progressive abnormalities of two metatarsophalangeal joints. Significant periosteal reaction, increasing bone density, and joint destruction (**e, f**). **g** Great toe: Soft tissue swelling and severe deformity of tuft and interphalangeal joint

a b c d

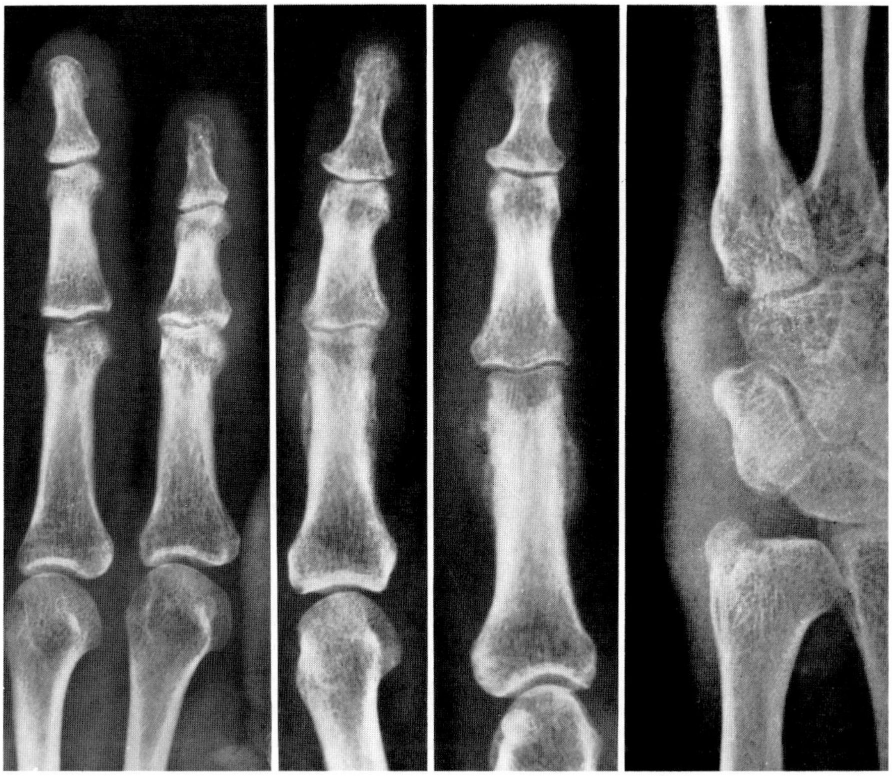

1

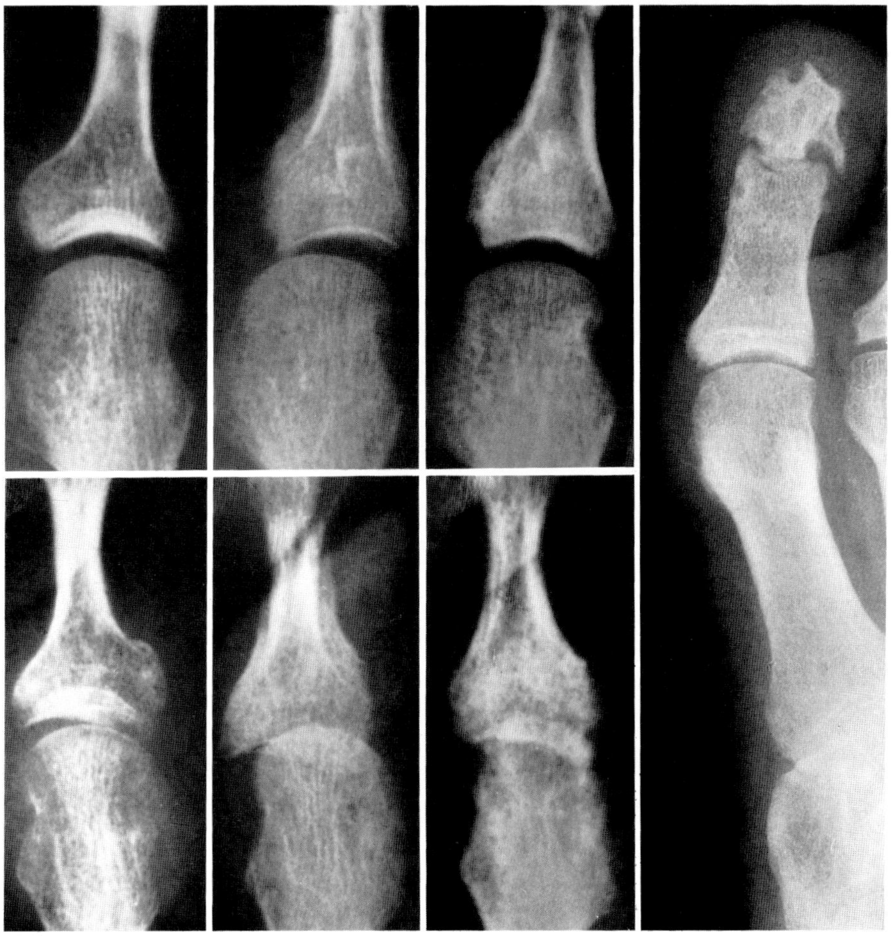

a–c

2

d e f g

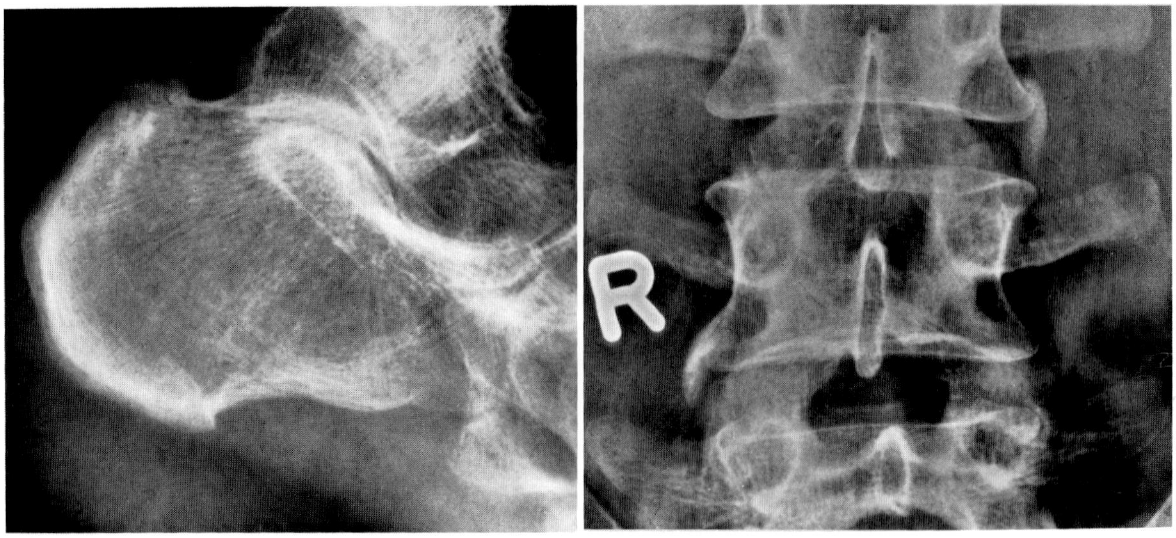

a b

Fig. 3a, b. Reiter's syndrome. **a** Erosions and adjacent bone proliferation of calcaneus, especially at craniodorsal margin. Plantar small exostosis, some sclerosis. **b** Large syndesmophyte (parasyndesmophyte) between L 4 and L 5, paravertebral soft tissue calcification beside L 3–L 4 intervertebral disc

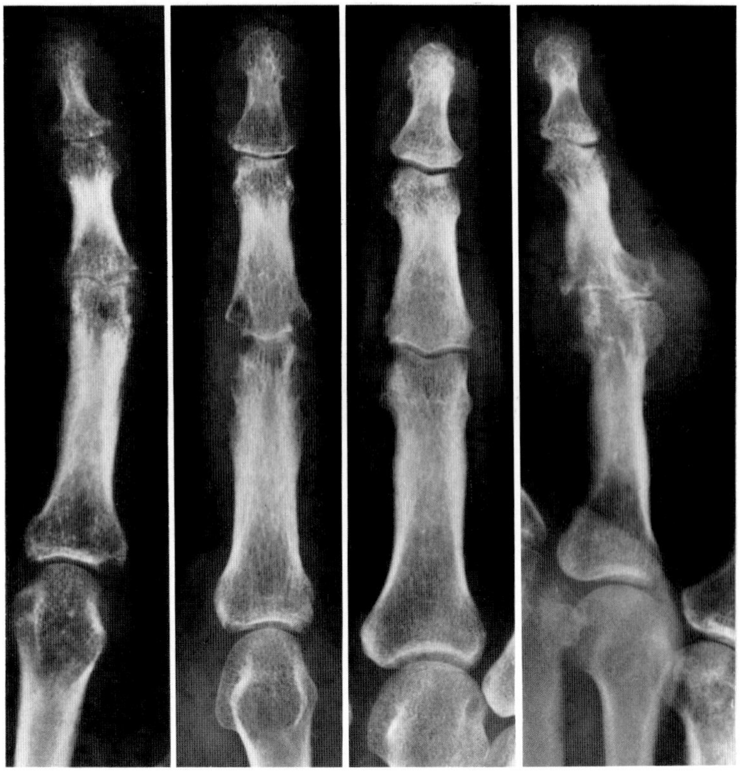

a b c d

Fig. 4a–d. Differential diagnosis. **a** Rheumatoid arthritis. **b** Pyogenic arthritis. **c** Psoriatic arthritis. **d** Gout

References

1 Resnick D, Niwayama G (1981) Diagnosis of bone and joint disorders. Saunders, Philadelphia

2 Martel W, Braunstein EM, Borlaza G, Good AE, Griffin PE (1979) Radiologic features of Reiter disease. Radiology 132:1–10

7.3.8 Gout

Synonym: arthritis urica

Gout is classified as primary or secondary:
Primary gout: hyperuricemia caused by an inborn error of the purine metabolism
Secondary gout: (a) as a complication of other diseases with severe tissue destruction (especially myeloproliferative disorders); (b) induced by drugs (especially diuretics)
Monosodium urate crystals in the synovial membrane cause synovial proliferation with articular cartilage destruction, bony erosions, and joint space narrowing. Crystals in the subchondral bone and the para-articular soft tissue cause tophi within the bone and in the adjacent soft tissue.

Radiographic Findings [1–4]

Hand

Osteoporosis only in acute attacks and immobilization
Tophi (after 10 years in about 60% of patients)
"Punched out" erosions caused by tophi in the articular cartilage, subchondral bone, synovial membrane, and para-articular soft tissue
Soft tissue swelling
Joint space narrowing and/or destruction
Overhanging margins
Amorphous calcifications in tophi
Bone infarction
Periostitis (uncommon)
Coexisting chondrocalcinosis (5–6%)
Bony ankylosis (uncommon)
Secondary osteoarthrosis

Other Sites

Tophaceous deposits and arthritis in feet, heels, ankles, and knees, and less commonly in hips, sacroiliac joints, spine, and shoulders

Differential Diagnosis

Erosive osteoarthrosis (Sect. 7.3.13)
Pyogenic arthritis (Sect. 7.3.2)
Rheumatoid arthritis (Sect. 7.3.4)
Psoriatic arthritis (Sect. 7.3.6)
Hyperlipoproteinemia (Sect. 7.1.5)
Reiter's syndrome (Sect. 7.3.7)
Sarcoidosis (Sect. 7.3.12)
Neuropathic arthropathy (Sect. 7.6.5)
Scleroderma (Sect. 7.6.3)
Systemic lupus erythematosus (Sect. 7.3.14)

References

1 Resnick D, Reinke RT, Taketa RM (1975) Early-onset gouty arthritis. Radiology 114:67–73
2 Bloch C, Hermann G, Yu TF (1980) A radiologic reevaluation of gout: a study of 2000 patients. AJR 134:781–787
3 Resnick D, Niwayama G (1981) Diagnosis of bone and joint disorders. Saunders, Philadelphia
4 Schabel SI, Korn JH, Rittenberg GM, Leman RB (1978) Bone infarction in gout. Skeletal Radiol 3:42–47

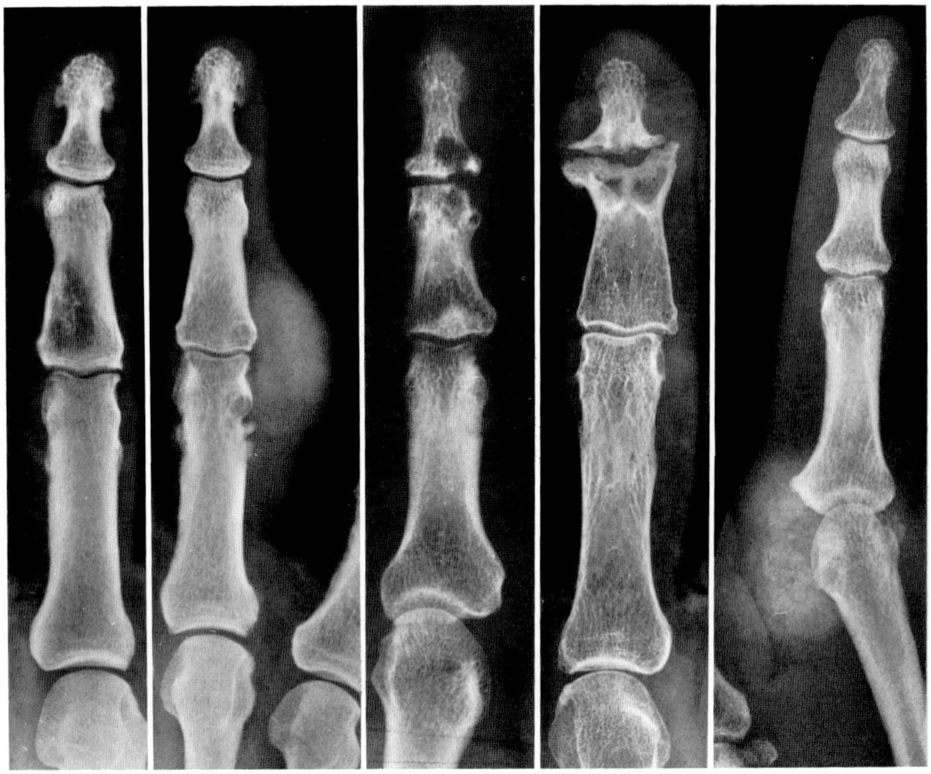

a b c d e

Fig. 1 a–e. Gout. **a** Intraosseous tophus. **b** Bony erosions, soft tissue swelling. Normal bone density. **c** Intraosseous tophi, marginal joint erosions. **d** Destruction of distal interphalangeal joint by large intraosseous tophi, overhanging margins, osteoporosis. **e** Calcifications in large tophus in soft tissue. Normal bone density

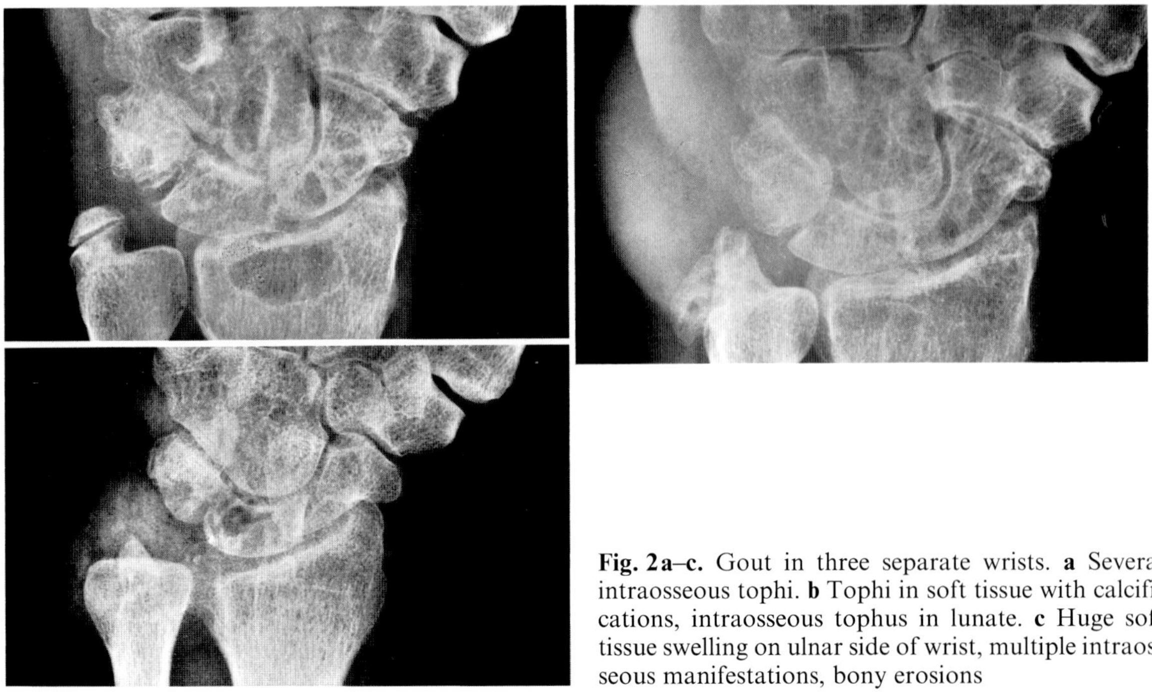

a b c

Fig. 2 a–c. Gout in three separate wrists. **a** Several intraosseous tophi. **b** Tophi in soft tissue with calcifications, intraosseous tophus in lunate. **c** Huge soft tissue swelling on ulnar side of wrist, multiple intraosseous manifestations, bony erosions

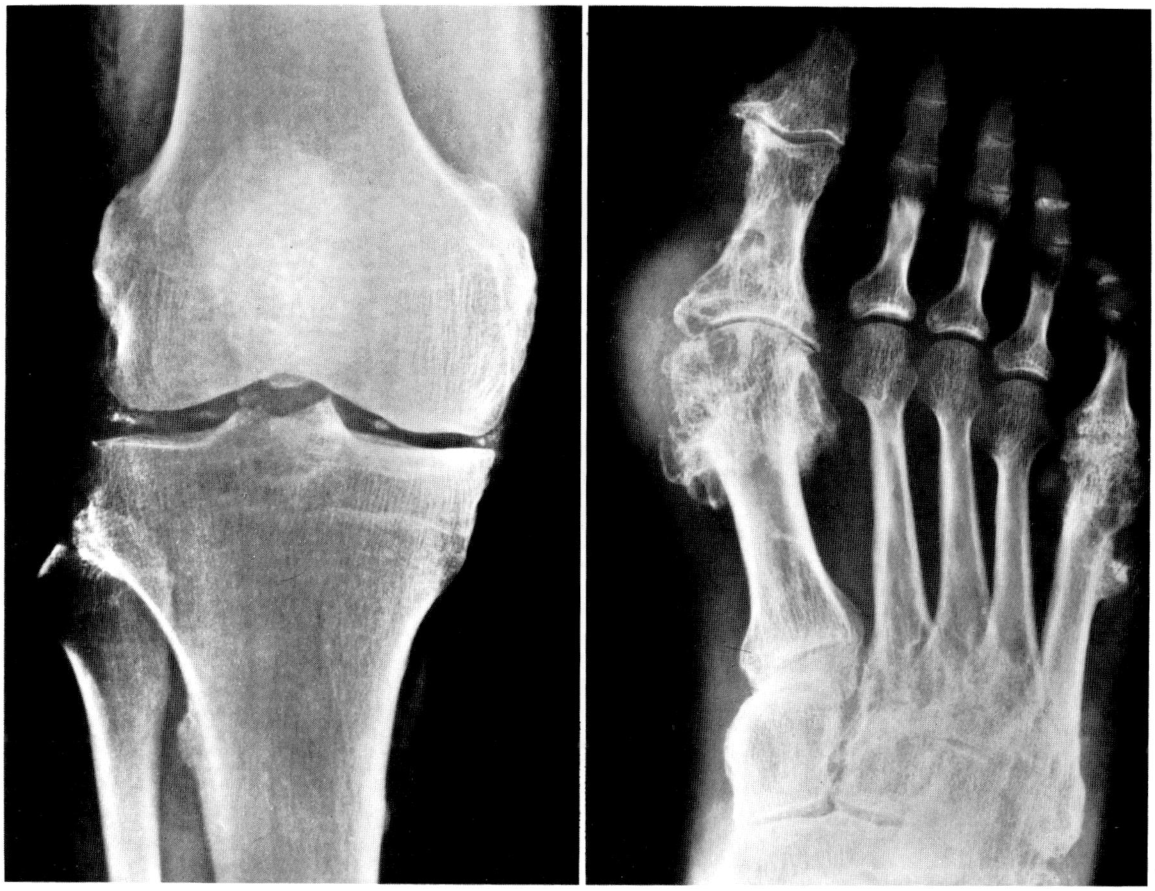

a b

Fig. 3a, b. Gout. **a** Chondrocalcinosis. **b** Multiple affected joints: Large soft tissue swelling at first metacarpal joint, bony erosions, intraosseous tophi. Slight periostitis at proximal phalanx of first toe, thickening of fifth metatarsal

Fig. 4a–k see p. 234

Fig. 4a–k. Differential diagnosis. **a** Hyperlipoproteinemia: Soft tissue swelling, small bony lesions, no demineralization. **b** Pyogenic arthritis and osteomyelitis: Demineralization, osteolysis, soft tissue swelling. **c** Rheumatoid arthritis: Periarticular osteoporosis, joint space narrowing, bony erosions. **d** Reiter's syndrome: Decreased bone density, periostitis at proximal phalanx. **e** Systemic lupus erythematosus with luxation in metacarpal joints. **f** Sarcoidosis: Intraosseous sarcoids in tuft, proximal phalanx, and metacarpal head. **g** Neuropathic joints in syringomyelia: (Sub)luxation in metacarpal joints and in one proximal interphalangeal joint. Increased bone density around latter joint. **h** Severe osteoarthrosis of distal interphalangeal joint with demineralization and joint destruction. **j** Psoriatic arthritis: Mouse ears at metacarpal joint, destruction of interphalangeal joints. **k** Scleroderma: Normal bone density, severe destruction of distal interphalangeal joint

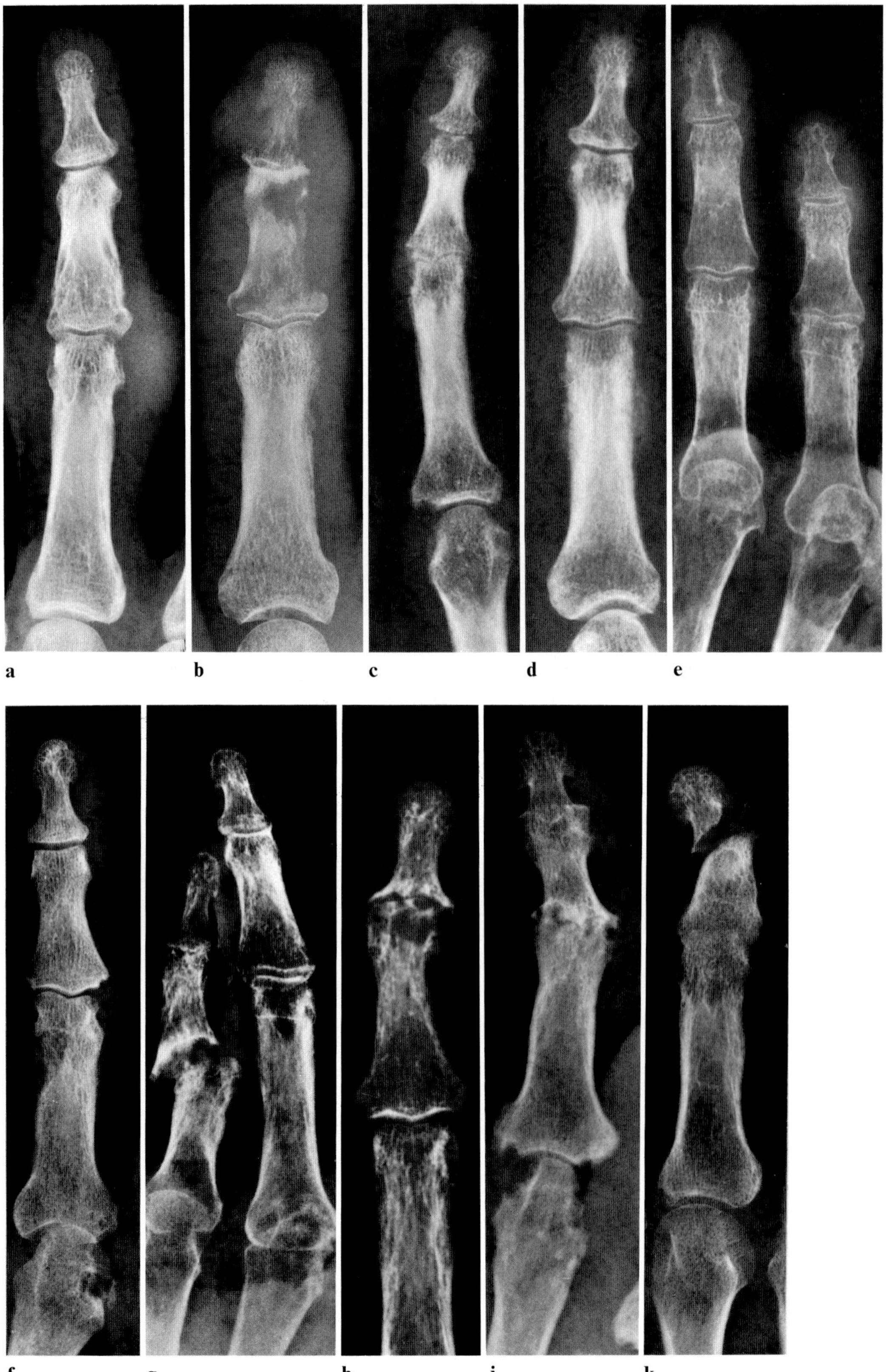

Fig. 4a–k. Legend see p. 233

7.3.9 Tuberculosis

In childhood especially, one of the symptoms of tuberculosis is dactylitis. The infection of a tubular bone can cause spina ventosa. Dactylitis can also occur in adults, but affection of the wrist is more frequent. In these cases demineralization can be the first sign [1, 2].

Radiographic Findings

Hand
Soft tissue swelling
Dactylitis
Periostitis
Spina ventosa
Bone destruction
Pathologic fracture in severe demineralization

Differential Diagnosis

Osteomyelitis (Sect. 7.3.3)
Sarcoidosis (Sect. 7.3.12)
Benign bone tumor (Sect. 7.4.1)
Malignant bone tumor (Sect. 7.4.2)
Fibrous dysplasia (Sect. 7.4.3.1)
Other causes of dactylitis

References

1 Feldman F, Auerbach R, Johnston A (1971) Tuberculous dactylitis in the adult. AJR 112:460–479
2 Cremin BJ, Fischer RM, Levinsohn MW (1970) Multiple bone tuberculosis in the young. Br J Radiol 43:638–645

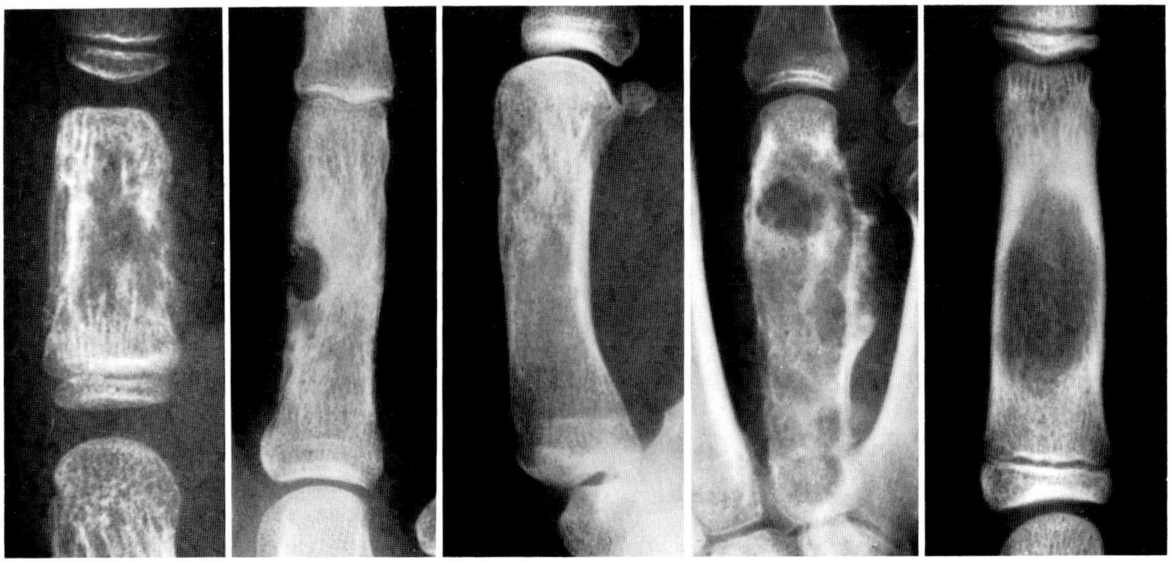

a b c d e

Fig. 1 a–e. Tuberculosis. **a** In a 5-year-old boy: Dactylitis of proximal phalanx, destructive diaphyseal lesion with spina ventosa, periosteal new bone formation. Specific differential diagnosis: Ewing's sarcoma, osteomyelitis, eosinophilic granuloma. **b** In an 18-year-old woman: Dactylitis of proximal phalanx, abnormal bone structure, periosteal reaction, well-circumscribed marginal lytic defect. Specific differential diagnosis: cortical chondroma, pigmented villonodular synovitis. **c** Same patient as **b**: Periosteal new bone formation, abnormal bone structure in first metacarpal, spotty bone density. Specific differential diagnosis: fibrous dysplasia. **d** In an adult male: Tuberculous affection of fourth metacarpal, significant spina ventosa with central lytic defect. Specific differential diagnosis: enchondroma, chondrosarcoma, fibrosarcoma. **e** Some widening of shaft, lytic defect surrounded by zone of sclerosis. Specific differential diagnosis: osteoblastoma

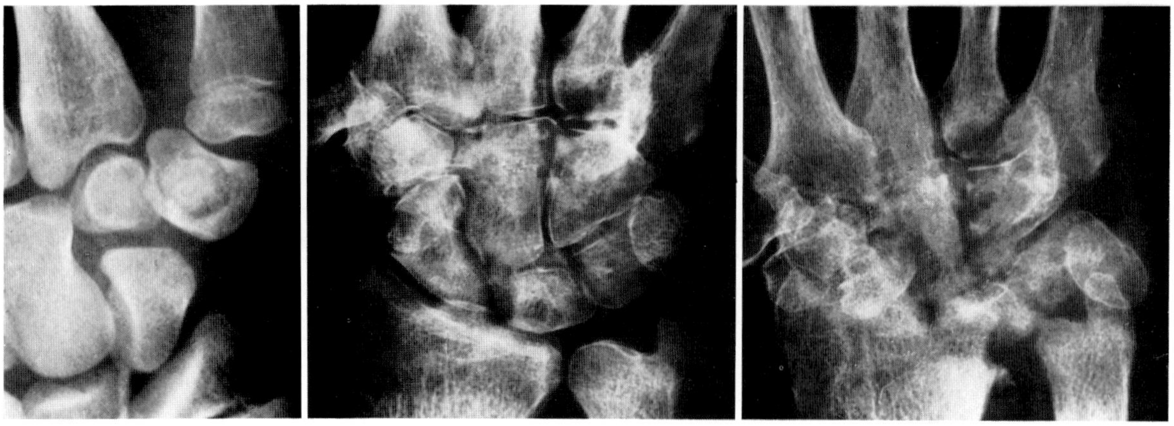

a b c

Fig. 2a–c. Tuberculosis of wrist. **a** Affection of trapezium: Well-defined lesion with reactive new bone formation. Specific differential diagnosis: osteoid osteoma. **b** In an adult: Significant demineralization. **c** Same patient as **b**: Severe destruction of carpals and several joint spaces, demineralization, radiocarpal fusion. Specific differential diagnosis: rheumatoid arthritis, pyogenic arthritis, juvenile rheumatoid arthritis

7.3.10 Leprosy

Synonym: Hansen's disease

In leprosy the abnormalities are caused by *Mycobacterium leprae* and are found mainly in the cooler areas of the body. The nasal mucous membrane, the skin, and the peripheral nerves of the extremities are the favored locations. The small nerves of the skin are particularly affected, and the blood vessels are also commonly involved. In the hand, the radial, medial, and ulnar nerves are characteristically affected, leading to a clawhand deformity. The concentric atrophy of the tubular bones ("licked lollipop" deformity) is probably also due to nerve involvement. Direct affection of the skeleton in leprosy is rather infrequent and may be caused by hematogenous spread of infection. In most cases, bone involvement is secondary to infection of the adjacent soft tissues.

Radiographic Findings [1–4]

Hand

The involvement of the skeleton in leprosy may be specific or nonspecific. The radiographic features in these two types of involvement are different: *Specific bone lesions* (bone affection by the bacilli; 3%–15% of patients):

Soft tissue swelling
Demineralization
Well-defined cyst-like intraosseous lesions in epiphyseal and metaphyseal regions, particularly of phalanges
Enlargement of nutrient foramina of phalanges by granulomas
Severe osseous destruction
Periostitis
Osteosclerosis
Deviation of fingers
Leprous arthritis
Pathologic fractures

Nonspecific bone lesions (neuropathic lesions with or without trauma and infection; 20%–70% patients):

Acro-osteolysis
Osteomyelitis (periostitis, bone destruction, sequestration, septic arthritis)
Fractures
"Licked lollipop" deformity
Fingerless hand
Clawhand
Osteoporosis (hyperemia and disuse)
Nerve calcification (rare)

Other Sites

Foot
Nasal bones

Differential-Diagnosis

Specific bone lesions:
- tuberculosis (Sect. 7.3.9)
- sarcoidosis (Sect. 7.3.12)

Nonspecific bone lesions:
- psoriatic arthritis (Sect. 7.3.6)
- thermal injuries (Sect. 7.6.2)
- scleroderma (Sect. 7.6.3)
- syringomyelia (Sect. 7.6.5)
- congenital insensitivity to pain
- diabetes (uncommon in hand)

References

1 Enna CD, Jacobson RB, Rausch RO (1971) Bone changes in leprosy: a correlation of clinical and radiographic features. Radiology 100:295–299
2 Murray RO, Jacobson HG (1977) The radiology of skeletal disorders. Churchill Livingstone, Edinburgh
3 Resnick D, Niwayama G (1981) Diagnosis of bone and joint disorders. Saunders, Philadelphia
4 Faget GH, Mayoral A (1944) Bone changes in leprosy: a clinical and roentgenological study of 505 cases. Radiology 42:1–13

a 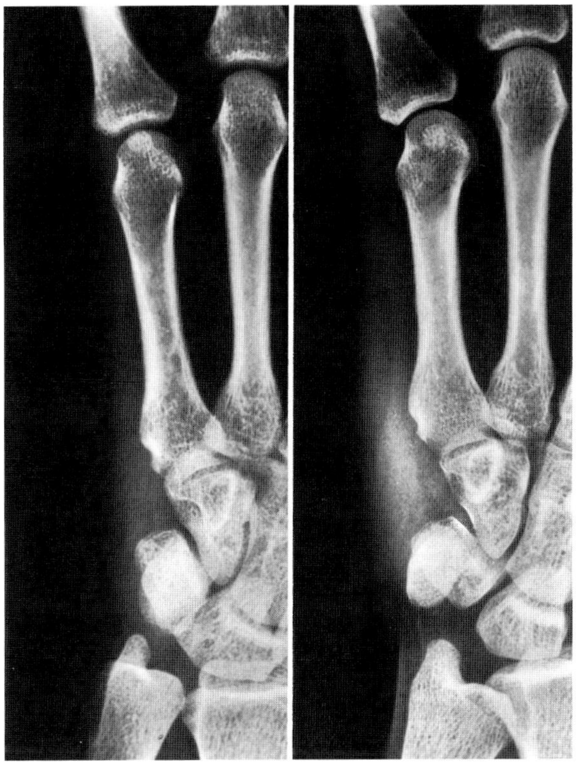 b

Fig. 1a, b. Leprosy in both hands in a 24-year-old woman. Paralysis of ulnar nerve of left hand (**a**), diminution in volume of soft tissues adjacent to fifth metacarpal and wrist. Hand bones not affected

a 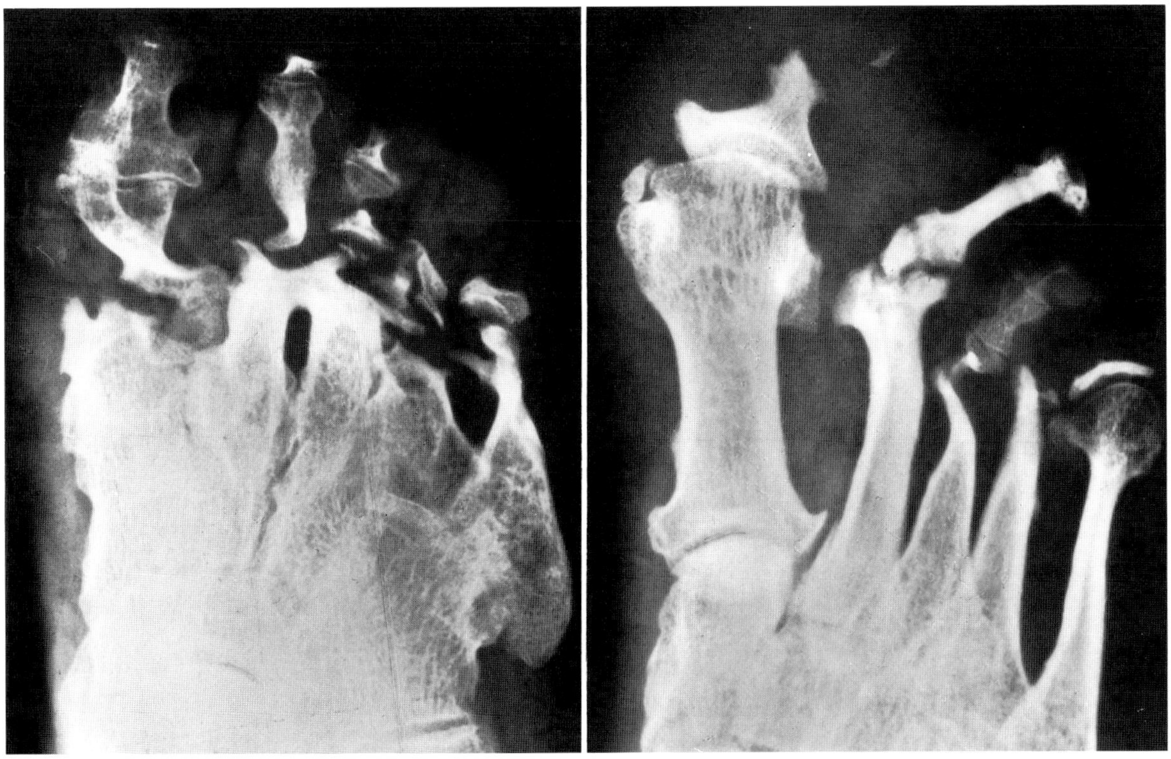 b

Fig. 2a, b. Leprosy in a 44-year-old man. Severe destruction of tubular bones, soft tissue swelling, particularly of right foot (**b**). "Licked lollipop" deformities, acro-osteolysis, increased bone density

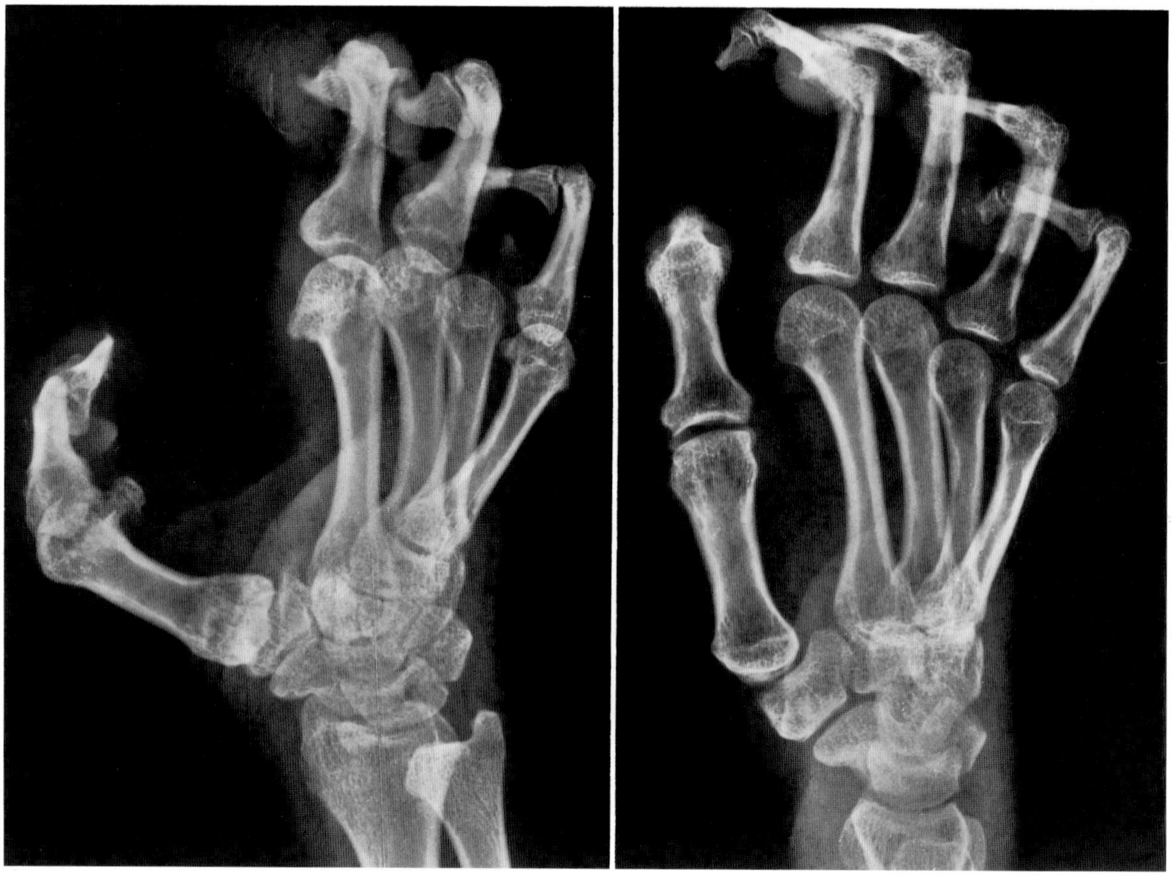

a b

Fig. 3a, b. Leprosy in a 54-year-old man. Paralysis of ulnar and medial nerves, clawhands, concentric atrophy of terminal and middle phalanges of fingers. Previous surgery on right hand with amputation of fourth digit (**a**) and marked thickening of second digit

7.3.11 Yaws

Synonym: frambesia

Yaws is a tropical infection caused by *Treponema pertenue*. Especially in children, bone involvement occurs in the second and third stages of the disease. The tubular bones, skull, pelvis, and facial bones may all be affected.

Radiographic Findings [1–4]

Hand
Dactylitis and bone destruction
Expansion of tubular bones
Sclerosis
Periosteal bone apposition
Usually spared distal phalanges and carpals
Shortening of fingers (telescoping) by severe destruction

Other Sites
Toes
Skull (nose and maxillary bones)
Long tubular bones
Pelvis

Differential Diagnosis

Syphilis (Sect. 7.3.1)
Tuberculosis (Sect. 7.3.9)

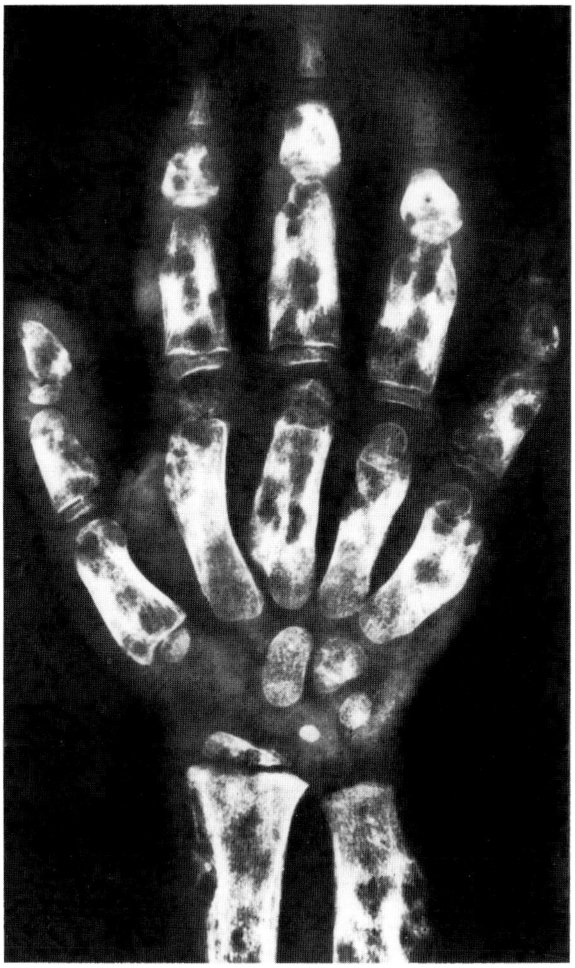

Fig. 1. Yaws in a 6-year-old boy. Severe affection of all tubular bones. Distal phalanges and carpals not involved, except distal phalanx of thumb. Enormous periosteal bone formation. Radius and ulna present identical radiographic findings

References

1 Goldman CH, Smith SJ (1943) X-ray appearance of bone in yaws. Br J Radiol 16:234–238
2 Riseborough AW, Joske RA, Vaughan BF (1961) Hand deformities due to yaws in Western Australian aborigines. Clin Radiol 12:109–112
3 Cockshott WP (1963) Dactylitis and growth disorders. Br J Radiol 36:19–26
4 Jones BS (1972) Doigt en lorgnette and concentric bone atrophy associated with healed yaws osteitis. Report of two cases. J Bone Joint Surg [Br] 54:341–345

7.3.12 Sarcoidosis

Synonym: Besnier-Boeck-Schaumann syndrome

Sarcoidosis is a chronic granulomatous disease of unknown etiology. Involvement of bones is encountered in 1%–36% of all cases (average 5%) [1, 2]. In the hand, the distal and middle phalanges are mostly affected, with soft tissue thickening around the affected bones. Polyarthritis in sarcoidosis does not usually cause significant radiographically visible joint lesions except in cases involving extensive destruction of subchondral bone. About 25% of sarcoidosis sufferers have hypercalcemia, probably caused by generation of $1{,}25(OH)_2D_3$ by the sarcoids themselves [3].

Radiographic Findings [4, 5]

Hand

Involvement especially of distal and middle phalanges
Small or larger well-defined translucent defects with or without sclerotic borders (Jüngling's cysts)
Acro-osteolysis, especially in distal phalanges but also in other phalanges
Honeycomb or lacework pattern of bone destruction
Osteosclerosis
Arthritis
Joint destruction
Uncommon: subperiosteal bone resorption
periostitis and marginal scalloping of bone
soft tissue masses with or without calcifications
chondrocalcinosis by hypercalcemia

Other Sites

Long tubular bones: cystic lesions
Foot: abnormalities similar to those in hand
Skull: well-defined calvarial defects
severe involvement of nasal bone and jaws
Spine: lytic lesions in vertebral bodies

Differential Diagnosis

Arthritis: pseudogout (Sect. 6.2.6)
rheumatoid arthritis (Sect. 7.3.4)
psoriatic arthritis (Sect. 7.3.6)
gout (Sect. 7.3.8)
Osteomyelitis: pyogenic arthritis (Sect. 7.3.2)
tuberculosis (Sect. 7.3.9)
leprosy (Sect. 7.3.10)
Tumors: enchondromatosis (Sect. 7.4.1.3)
primary malignant tumors (Sect. 7.4.2)
myeloma (Sect. 7.4.2.3)
metastatic lesions (Sect. 7.4.2.5)
hemangiomas [6]
Miscellaneous:
basal cell nevus syndrome (Sect. 2.1.2)
renal osteodystrophy (Sect. 6.2.4)
Paget's disease (Sect. 6.2.9)
tuberous sclerosis (Sect. 7.1.2)
hyperlipoproteinemia (Sect. 7.1.5)
fibrous dysplasia (Sect. 7.4.3.1)
fluorosis (Sect. 7.5.1)
mastocytosis (Sect. 7.6.7)

References

1 James DG, Neville E, Carstairs LS (1976) Bone and joint sarcoidosis. Semin Arthritis Rheum 6:53–81
2 Uehlinger E, Wurm K (1976) Skelettsarkoidose. Literaturübersicht und Fallbericht. Fortschr Geb Röntgenstr Nuklearmed Ergänzungsband 125:111–122
3 Barbour GL, Coburn JW, Slatopolsky E, Norman AW, Horst RL (1981) Hypercalcemia in an anephric patient with sarcoidosis: evidence for extrarenal generation of 1,25-dihydroxyvitamin D. N Engl J Med 305:440–443
4 Bonakdarpour A, Levy W, Augerter E (1971) Osteosclerotic changes in sarcoidosis. AJR 113:646–649
5 Fitzgerald P, Meenan FOC (1958) Sarcoidosis of the hands. J Bone Joint Surg [Br] 40:256–261
6 Graham DY, Gonzales J, Kothari SM (1978) Diffuse skeletal angiomatosis. Skeletal Radiol 2:131–135

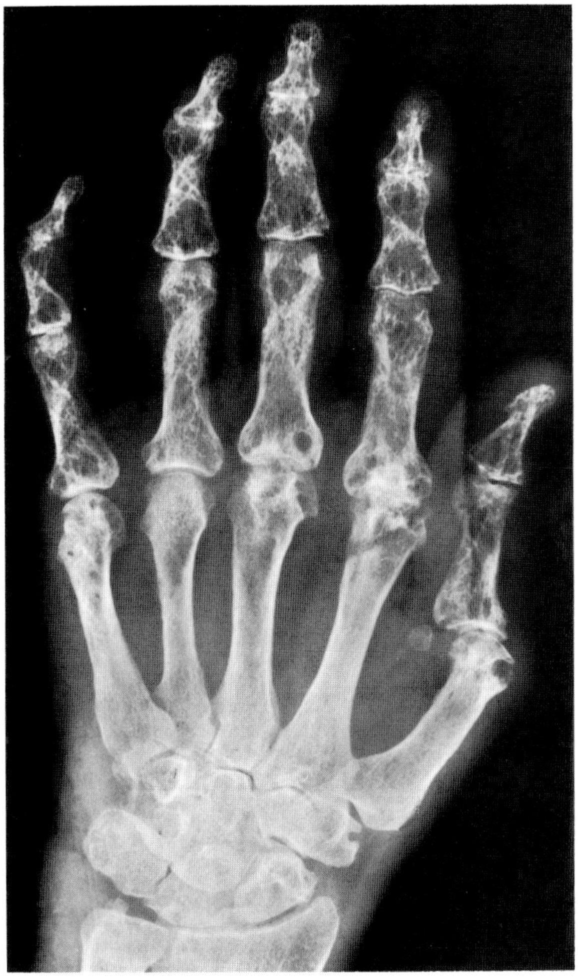

Fig. 1. Sarcoidosis in a 72-year-old woman. Significant lacework destruction of bone structure and destructive polyarthritis

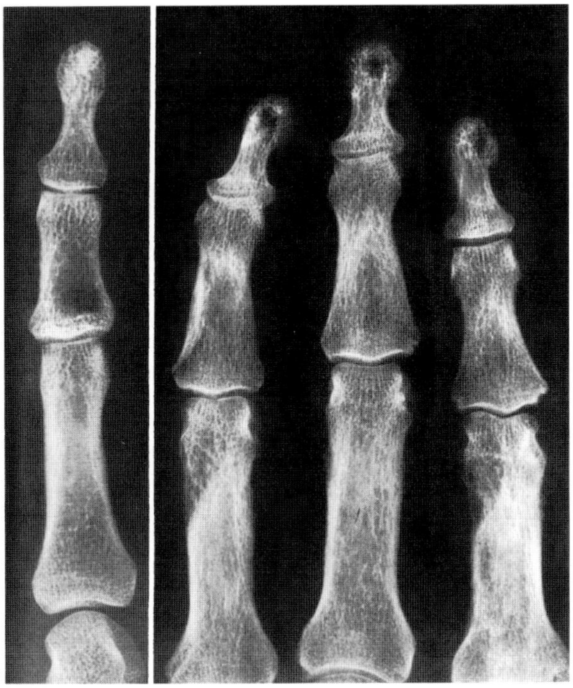

a b

Fig. 2a, b. Sarcoidosis. a In a 27-year-old man: Solitary radiolucent defect in fifth finger. b In a 65-year-old woman: Several osteolytic defects in both tufts and proximal phalanges of second to fourth fingers

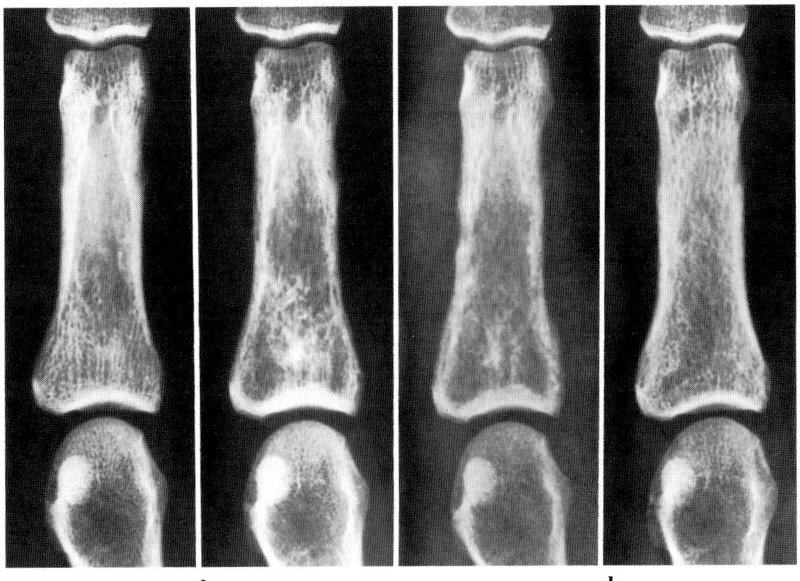

a b c d

Fig. 3a–d. Sarcoidosis in a 48-year-old woman. a 1975: Some endosteal sclerosis of proximal phalanx. b 1978: Soft tissue swelling, permeative osteolytic lesion associated with slight periosteal new bone formation. c 1979: Soft tissue swelling, some increase in periosteal bone formation, scalloped cortical margin. d 1983: Bone abnormalities healed, slight endosteal sclerosis

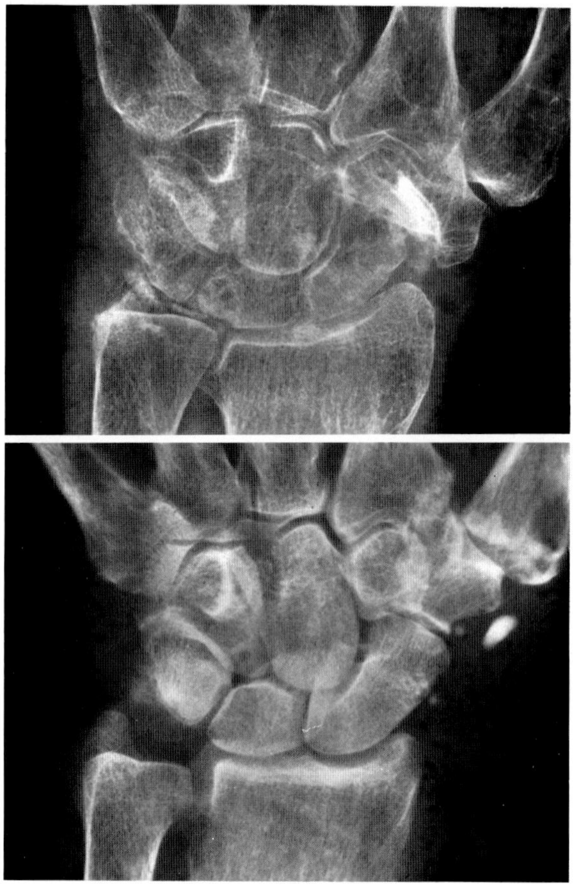

a

b

Fig. 4a, b. Sarcoidosis and hypercalcemia. **a** In a 76-year-old woman: Significant chondrocalcinosis, demineralization of wrist bones, osteoarthrosis. Differential diagnosis: pseudogout. **b** In a 67-year-old woman: Several lytic bone defects, especially in base of fifth metacarpal, soft tissue calcifications

7.3.13 Osteoarthrosis

Synonyms: degenerative joint disease, arthrosis deformans

Osteoarthrosis is subdivided into primary and secondary types: *Primary* osteoarthrosis: particularly common in postmenopausal women. The distal and proximal interphalangeal joints are usually affected. The first carpometacarpal joint and the trapezioscaphoid joint are less frequently abnormal. Heberden's nodes are found in the distal interphalangeal joints and Bouchard's nodes in the proximal interphalangeal joints.
Secondary osteoarthrosis: cartilage destruction due to previous trauma, arthritis, avascular necrosis, or chondrocalcinosis (pseudogout), hemochromatosis, hyperparathyroidism, Wilson's disease, ochronosis)

Radiographic Findings [1, 2]

Asymmetric joint space narrowing
Subchondral sclerosis
Pseudocysts
Osteophytes
Normal bone density
Demineralization in older patients and in postmenopausal women
Small ossicles in joint capsule
Subluxation
Joint destruction ("seagull appearance")
Ankylosis (occasionally)

Differential Diagnosis

Rheumatoid arthritis (Sect. 7.3.4)
Psoriatic arthritis (Sect. 7.3.6)
Gout (Sect. 7.3.8)
Hyperlipoproteinemia (Sect. 7.1.5)
Neuropathic arthropathy (Sect. 7.6.5)
Chondrocalcinosis (Sect. 6.2.6)
Primary biliary cirrhosis

References

1 Martel W, Snarr JW, Horn JR (1973) The metacarpophalangeal joints in interphalangeal osteoarthritis. Radiology 108:1–7
2 Stechen RM (1955) Heberden's nodes. A clinical description of osteoarthritis of the finger joints. Ann Rheum Dis 14:1–10

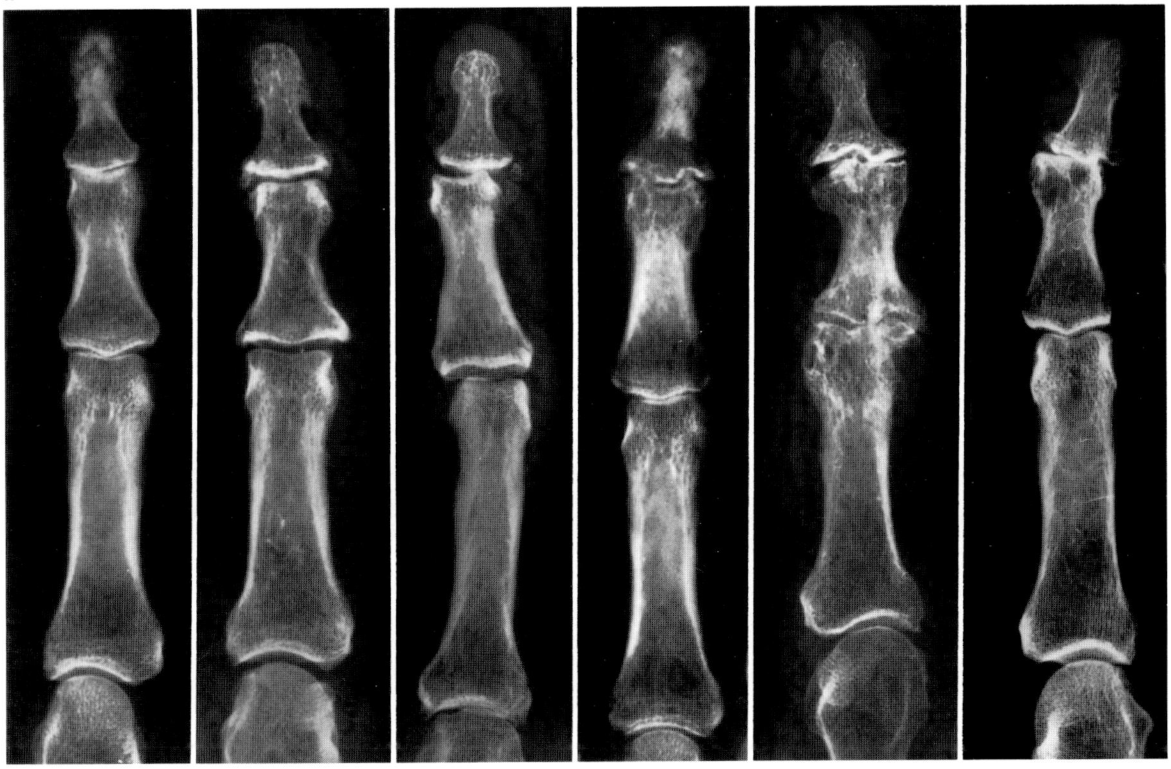

Fig. 1a–f. Osteoarthrosis. **a** Joint space narrowing in distal interphalangeal joint. **b** Osteoarthrosis in both distal and proximal interphalangeal joints: Small osteophytes, subchondral sclerosis. **c** Asymmetric narrowing of joint space and subluxation in distal interphalangeal joint, small paraarticular ossicles. **d** Destruction of distal interphalangeal joint with small pseudocysts, seagull appearance. **e** Destruction of distal and proximal interphalangeal joints by erosive osteoarthrosis: Asymmetric joint space narrowing, pseudocysts, sclerosis, osteophytes. **f** Asymmetric narrowing of distal interphalangeal joint space with sclerosis, cysts, and small exophytes

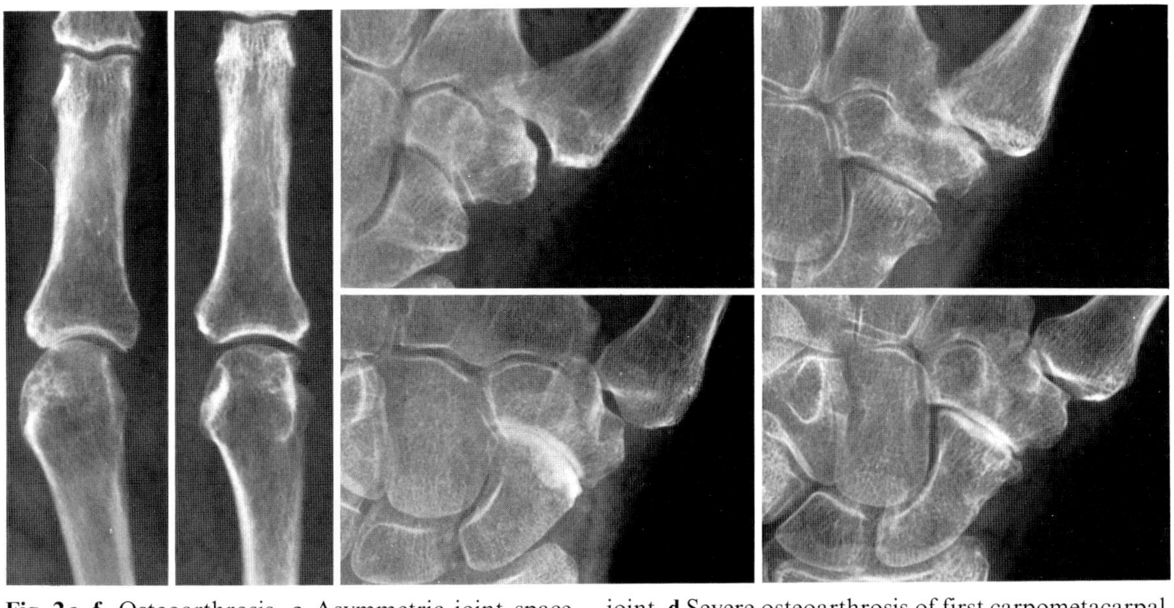

Fig. 2a–f. Osteoarthrosis. **a** Asymmetric joint space narrowing, pseudocysts, and sclerosis of second metacarpophalangeal joint. **b** Principally small osteophytes and slight sclerosis of third metacarpophalangeal joint. **c** Osteoarthrosis of first carpometacarpal joint. **d** Severe osteoarthrosis of first carpometacarpal joint, early osteoarthrosis of trapezioscaphoid joint. **e, f** Intercarpal osteoarthrosis in trapezioscaphoid joint: Joint space narrowing, sclerosis, only small osteophytes

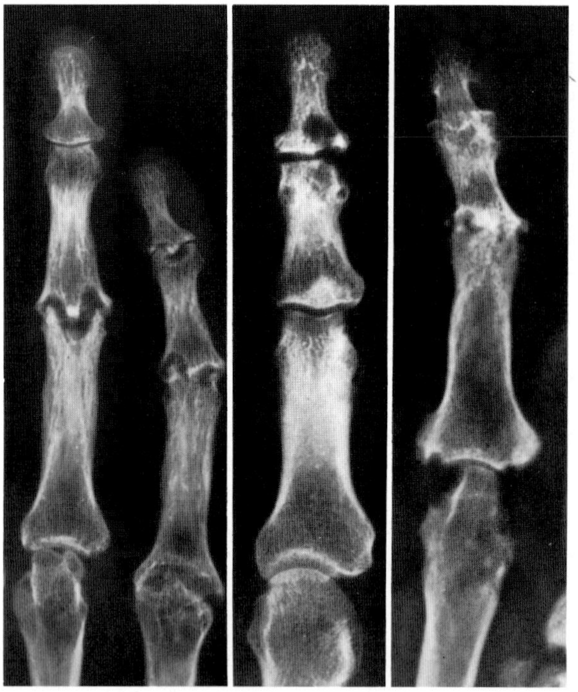

a b c

Fig. 3a–c. Differential diagnosis. **a** Rheumatoid arthritis: Typical seagull appearance, destruction of metacarpophalangeal joints. **b** Gout: Marginal erosions, small tophus in the distal phalanx. **c** Psoriatic arthritis affecting distal interphalangeal, proximal interphalangeal, and metacarpophalangeal joints: Marginal erosions, joint space destruction, mouse ears, ankylosis of distal interphalangeal joint

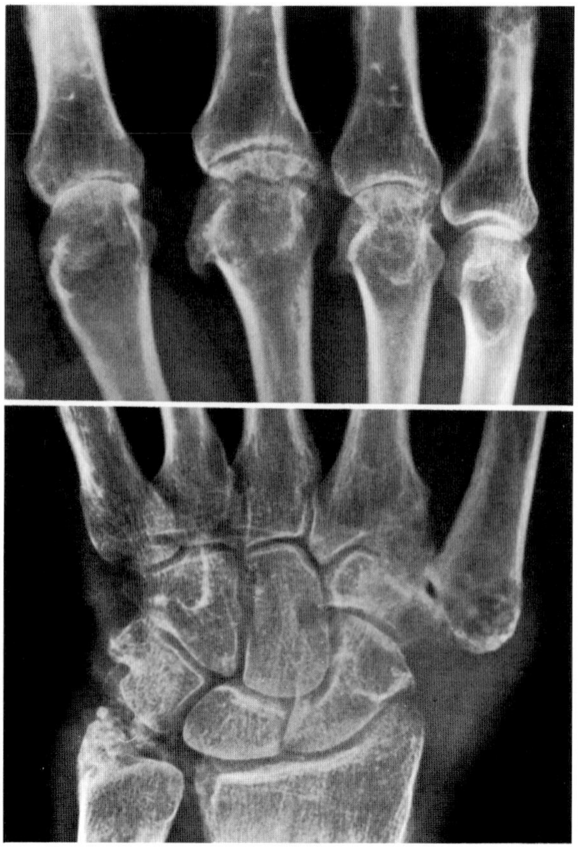

a

b

Fig. 4a, b. Degenerative changes in hemochromatosis and chondrocalcinosis. **a** Hemochromatosis: In this disorder especially the second and third metacarpophalangeal joints are frequently affected. **b** Chondrocalcinosis: Calcifications in carpoulnar joint, severe destruction of first carpometacarpal joint with cysts on both sides of joint space. Clinical examination: arthritis. Aspiration: calcium pyrophosphate crystals

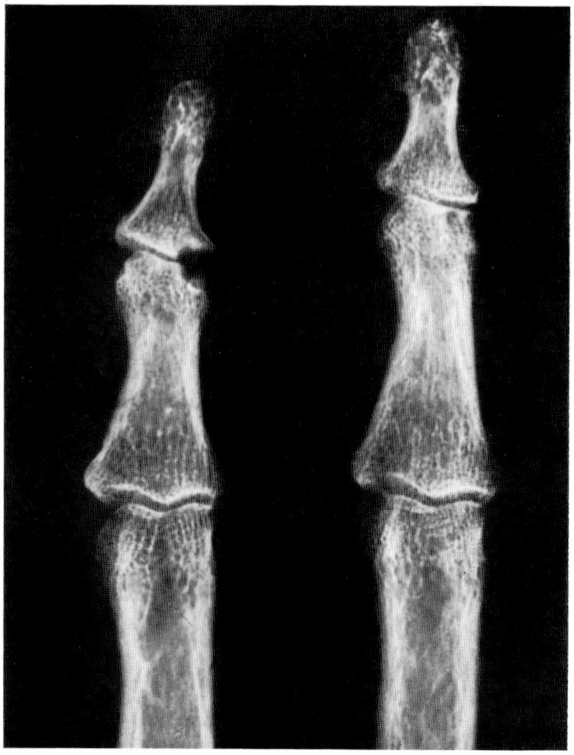

Fig. 5. Primary biliary cirrhosis in a 62-year-old woman: The erosions on both sides of the distal interphalangeal joint space are probably caused by primary biliary cirrhosis. These abnormalities are unusual in osteoarthrosis

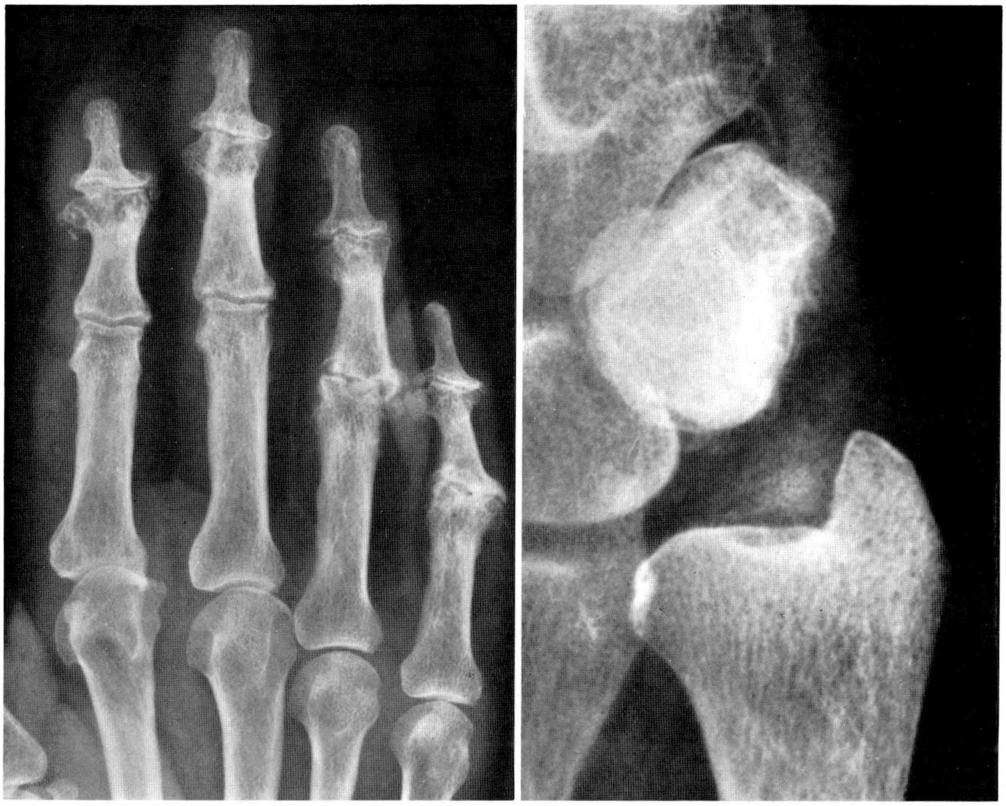

a b

Fig. 6a, b. Osteoarthrosis and chondrocalcinosis in a 64-year-old woman. Severe osteoarthrotic changes of interphalangeal joints. The wrist presented chondrocalcinosis, so the osteoarthrotic abnormalities are possibly influenced by calcium pyrophosphate crystals within these joints

7.3.14 Systemic Lupus Erythematosus

Systemic lupus erythematosus is an autosomal immune disease presenting with signs of inflammation in a variety of organs. A dysregulation of the immune system seems to be the initiating factor. A disturbance of the action of the T cells is said to be an important causal moment, and is followed by hyperactivity of the B cells. In this way many autoimmune antibodies are formed. Many organs are affected [1, 2]:

Skin: exanthema, alopecia, vasculitis, Raynaud's phenomenon (20%)
Joints: arthritis (90%)
Eyes: conjunctivitis, amblyopia
Lungs, pleura: pleuritis, bronchopneumonia, vasculitis
Heart: myocarditis, pericarditis, endocarditis, vasculitis of coronary arteries
Central nervous system: hemiplegia, ataxia and peripheral neuropathy
Kidneys: nephritis
Blood: anemia (70%–80%)
Gastrointestinal tract: peritonitis, pancreatitis, intestinal arteritis

Most of the victims are women aged 20–40 years. Arthralgia is one of the leading clinical symptoms in 75%–90% of cases. The articular findings are usually bilateral and symmetric.

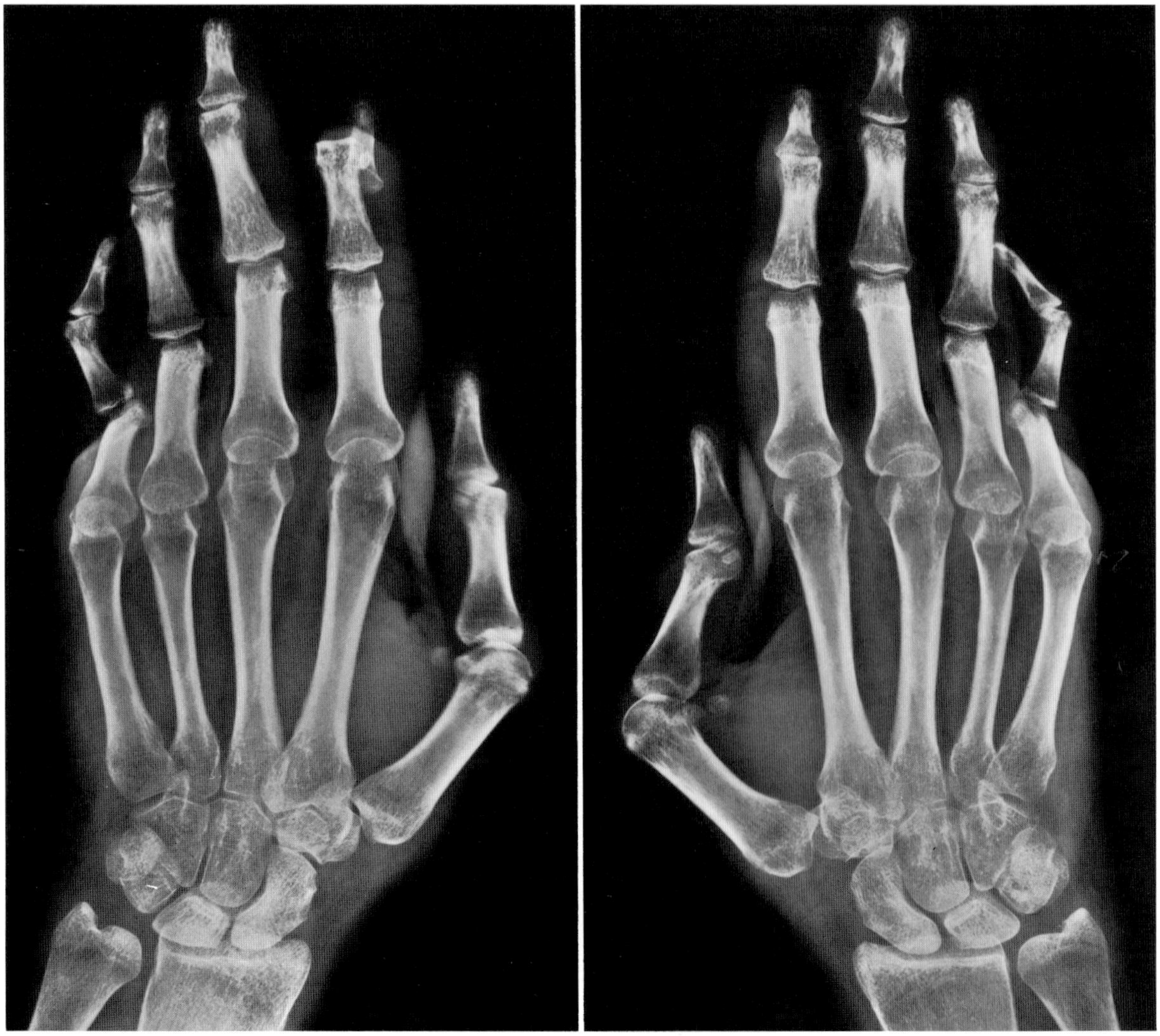

a b

Fig. 1 a, b. Systemic lupus erythematosus in a 27-year-old woman. Both hands: Periarticular demineralization and subluxation of metacarpophalangeal joints. Luxation of distal interphalangeal joint of left second finger (**a**) and hyperextension of several proximal interphalangeal joints

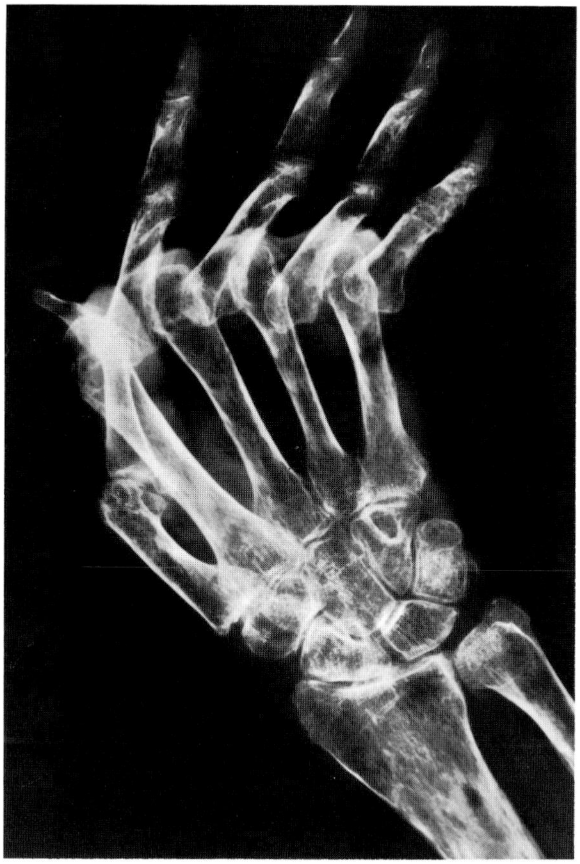

Fig. 2. Rheumatoid arthritis and lupus erythematosus in a 64-year-old woman. Luxation of metacarpophalangeal joints associated with severe osteoporosis and erosive changes at joint margins. Ulnar deviation of second to fifth fingers, hyperextension of interphalangeal joint of thumb and proximal interphalangeal joints of other fingers

Laboratory Findings

See: Adult Rheumatoid Arthritis (Sect. 7.3.4)

Radiographic Findings [1–5]

Hand

Soft tissue swelling
Periarticular demineralization
Joint spaces intact
No erosions
Interphalangeal joints: distal, flexion
  proximal, hyperextension
  thumb joint, hyperextension
Metacarpophalangeal joints: reversible ulnar subluxation
Reversible ulnar subluxation of fingers
Occasionally: soft tissue atrophy in later stages
  joint space narrowing
  avascular necrosis of metacarpal heads
  periarticular calcifications
  tuft resorption

Other Sites

Foot: abnormalities similar to those in hand
Various organs: a variety of abnormalities

Differential Diagnosis

Rheumatoid arthritis (Sect. 7.3.4)
Scleroderma (Sect. 7.6.3)
Chondrocalcinosis (Sect. 6.2.6)

References

1 Weissman BN, Rappoport AS, Leland Sosman J, Schur PH (1978) Radiographic findings in the hands in patients with systemic lupus erythematodes. Radiology 126:313–317
2 Resnick D, Niwayama G (1981) Diagnosis of bone and joint disorders. Saunders, Philadelphia
3 Bleifeld CJ, Inglis AE (1974) The hand in systemic lupus erythematodes. J Bone Joint Surg [Am] 56:1207–1215
4 Russell AS, Percy JS, Rigal WM, Wilson GL (1974) Deforming arthropathy in systemic lupus erythematodes. Ann Rheum Dis 33:204–209
5 Noonan CD, Odone DT, Engleman EP, Splitter SD (1963) Roentgenographic manifestations of joint disease in systemic lupus erythematodes. Radiology 80:837–843

7.4 Bone Tumors

7.4.1 Benign Tumors [1–3]

7.4.1.1 Osteoblastoma

Age

70% younger than 20 years (55% between 10 and 20 years)

Site

Hand	*4.5%*		
Vertebrae	28%	Tarsus	10%
Femur	12%	Sacrum	7%
Tibia	12%	Skull	4%

In vertebrae: neural arch, transverse process, and spinal process
In long tubular bones: metaphysis and diaphysis

Radiographic Findings

The radiographic findings vary widely depending on the location of the tumor. In the long tubular bones the tumor is usually a radiolucent and well-defined lesion surrounded by sclerosis varying from slight to very extensive. Periosteal new bone formation is often marked.

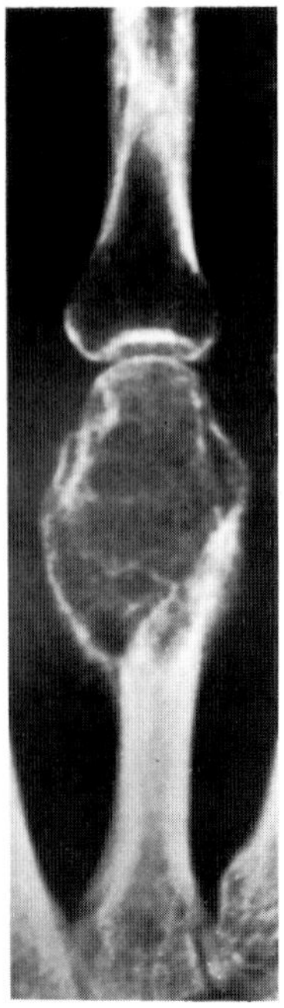

Fig. 1. Osteoblastoma in a 26-year-old woman. Expanding lesion in metaphysis. Periosteal reaction, within the tumor faint trabeculation. Joint space intact. Specific differential diagnosis: aneurysmal bone cyst, giant cell tumor, enchondroma, chondrosarcoma

Differential Diagnosis

Osteoid osteoma (Sect. 7.4.1.2)
Osteomyelitis (Sect. 7.3.3)
Eosinophilic granuloma
Enchondroma (Sect. 7.4.1.3)
Chondromyxoid fibroma (Sect. 7.4.1.4)
Fibrous dysplasia (Sect. 7.4.3.1)
Osteosarcoma

7.4.1.2 Osteoid Osteoma

Age

85% between 5 and 25 years

Site

Hand	*10%*	Vertebrae	19%
Femur	25%	Tarsus	6%
Tibia	22%	Humerus	5%

In vertebrae: neural arch
In long tubular bones: metaphysis and diaphysis

Radiographic Findings

The round or oval-shaped radiolucency (nidus) is up to 1.5 cm in diameter and is often surrounded by a (thin) sclerotic margin facing the normal bone. Calcification in the nidus is commonly seen. In young individuals the periosteal new bone formation may be of the laminar or onion-skin types. Usually the periosteal new bone formation is very extensive, especially if the tumor is located at the end of a bone.

Differential Diagnosis

Osteoblastoma (Sect. 7.4.1.1)
Sclerosing osteomyelitis
Fibrous dysplasia (Sect. 7.4.3.1)

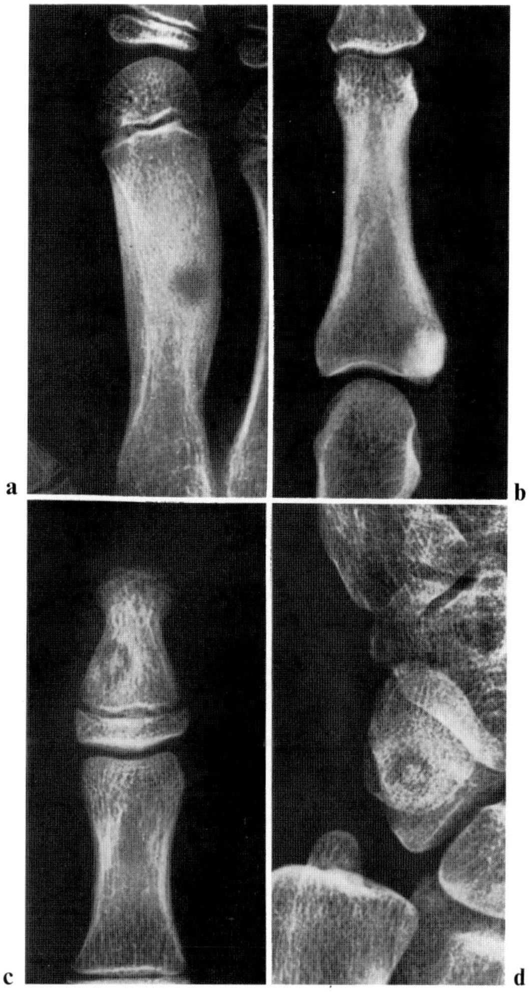

Fig. 1a–d. Four osteoid osteomas. **a** In a 10-year-old girl: Thickening of second metacarpal due to periosteal bone apposition, small central radiolucency. **b** In a 22-year-old woman: Small sclerotic area in proximal phalanx without a central radiolucency. Sharp border. Specific differential diagnosis: bone island. **c** In a 13-year-old girl: Characteristic lesion in distal phalanx. Small nidus surrounded by some sclerosis, calcification within nidus. **d** In a 26-year-old woman: Osteoid osteoma in triquetrum. Tiny calcification in small nidus

7.4.1.3 Chondroma [4]

Enchondroma (Solitary Chondroma)

Age

Majority discovered before 40 years

Site

Hand	40%
Ribs	10%
Femur	9%
Humerus	6%
Scapula	4%

In long tubular bones: metaphysis, epiphysis, and diaphysis

Radiographic Findings

A typical enchondroma appears as a round or lobulated radiolucency demarcated by a thin sclerotic shell. Particularly the eccentrically located enchondroma causes bulging of the cortex. The radiolucent center of the tumor may present trabeculation and spots of calcification and ossification.

Differential Diagnosis

Epidermoid cyst (Sect. 7.4.3.2)
Chondromyxoid fibroma (Sect. 7.4.1.4)
Osteoblastoma (Sect. 7.4.1.1)
Chondroblastoma
Giant cell tumor (Sect. 7.4.1.6)
Aneurysmal bone cyst (Sect. 7.4.1.7)
Solitary bone cyst
Fibrous dysplasia (Sect. 7.4.3.1)
Chondrosarcoma (Sect. 7.4.2.1)

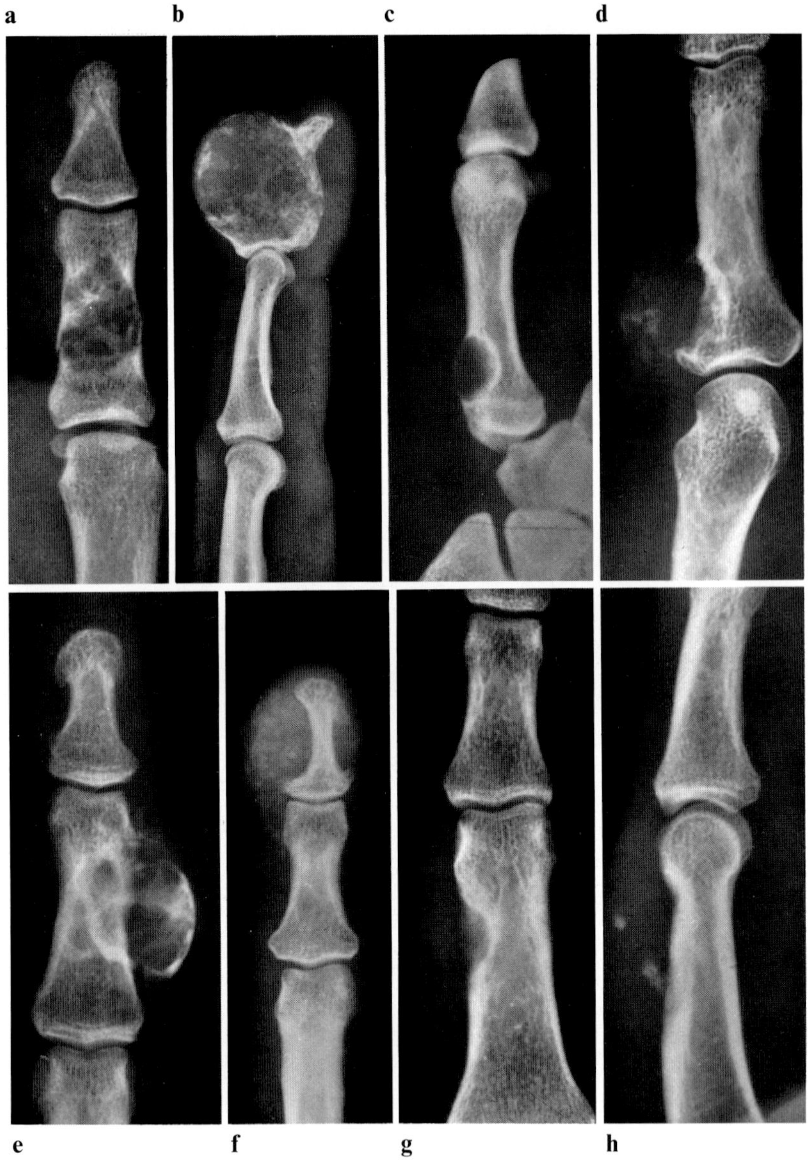

Fig. 1 a–h. Chondromas. **a** In a 14-year-old girl: Enchondroma of thumb with fracture. **b** In a 38-year-old woman: Huge expansive enchondroma of distal phalanx. Multiple calcifications in cartilaginous tissue. Specific differential diagnosis: giant cell tumor, osteoblastoma. **c** In a 30-year-old man: Small cortical chondroma. Well-defined margin, thinned but otherwise intact cortex. **d** In a 44-year-old woman: Cortical chondroma. Extraosseous calcifications in cartilaginous tissue. Well-defined intraosseous defect with some sclerosis. The small spur suggests the cortical origin of the tumor. **e** In a 47-year-old man: Cortical chondroma, partly extraosseous. Fluffy calcifications in the tumor. Specific differential diagnosis: osteochondroma. **f** In a 41-year-old woman: Juxtacortical chondroma with calcifications. Shaft narrowing due to extraosseous erosion. Specific differential diagnosis: chondrosarcoma (uncommon). **g, h** In a 32-year-old man: Cortical chondroma. Well-defined bone erosion and some soft tissue swelling (**g**). Slight irregularity of cortex and several distinct calcifications in adjacent soft tissue (**h**). Specific differential diagnosis: osteochondroma of tendon sheath, synovial sarcoma, chondrosarcoma (uncommon)

Enchondromatosis (Multiple Chondromas)

Synonym: Ollier's disease

The combination of enchondromatosis and multiple cutaneous or visceral hemangiomas is called Maffucci's syndrome.

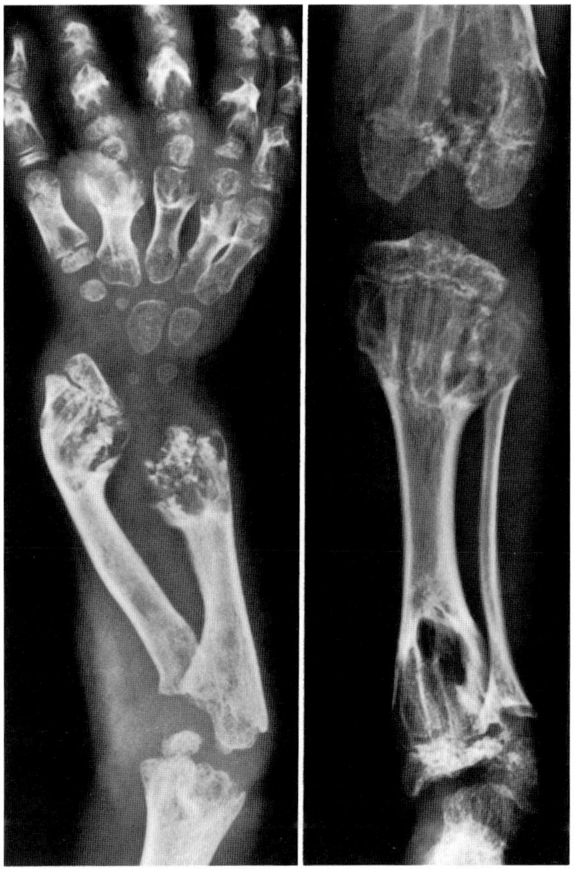

Fig. 1. Unilateral enchondromatosis in a 5-year-old girl

Fig. 2. a Enchondromatosis in a 14-year-old boy: Only the ulnar digits are affected. **b** Maffucci's syndrome in a 17-year-old girl: Large chondromatous masses with deformation of tubular bones, phlebolith in fourth finger. The patient had recently had an operation for an ovarian tumor

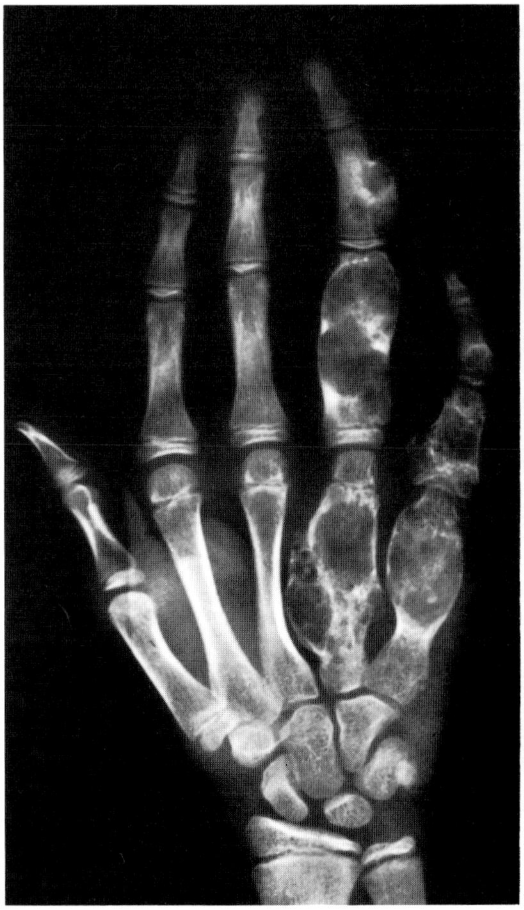

2a

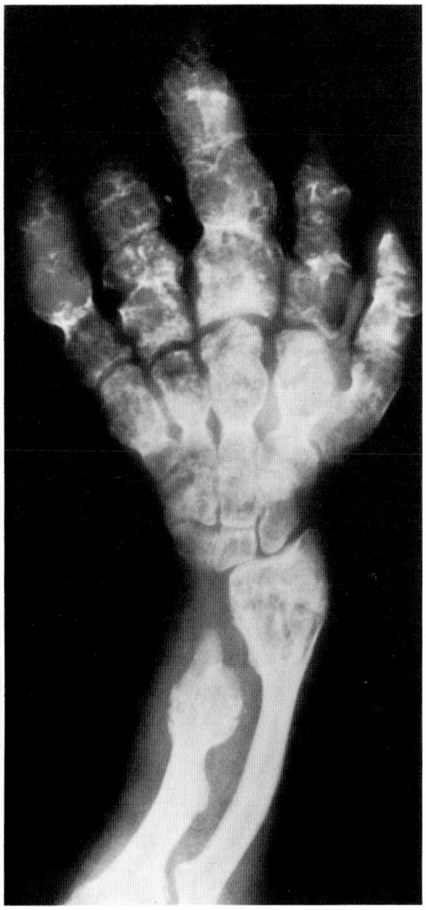

b

7.4.1.4 Chondromyxoid Fibroma

Age

60% between 10–25 years

Site

Hand	3.2%	Fibula	7%
Tibia	38%	Pelvis	7%
Femur	17%	Foot	6%

In long tubular bones: metaphysis

Radiographic Findings

A chondromyxoid fibroma is usually seen as a well-defined, oval or lobular, eccentrically located radiolucency. The borderline with the normal bone structure is often formed by a distinct thin sclerotic zone. Trabeculation in the tumor accentuates the lobulated aspect. If the tumor bulges beyond the bony contours, a large layer of periosteal bone is often present.

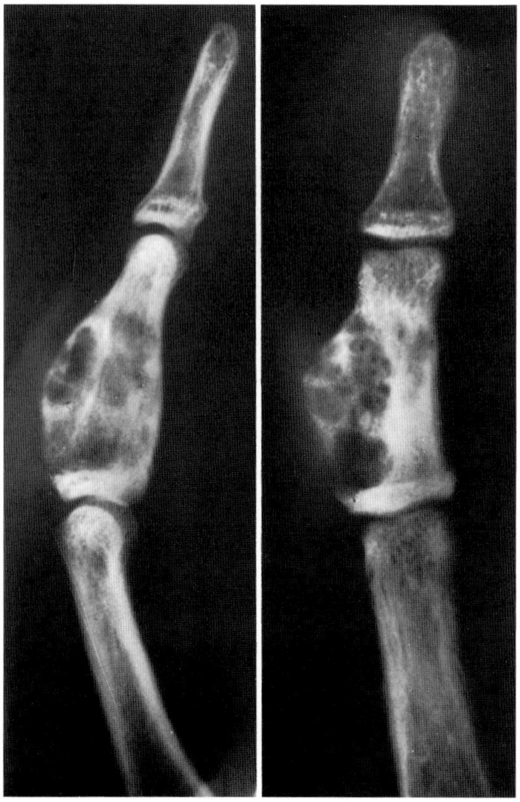

a b

Fig. 1 a, b. Chondromyxoid fibroma in a 19-year-old man: Expansive, lobulated, well-defined, bubbly lesion. Specific differential diagnosis: enchondroma, fibrous dysplasia

Differential Diagnosis

Chondroma or well-differentiated chondrosarcoma (Sects. 7.4.1.3 and 7.4.2.1)
Osteoblastoma (Sect. 7.4.1.1)
Giant cell tumor (Sect. 7.4.1.6)
Chondroblastoma
Solitary bone cyst
Aneurysmal bone cyst (Sect. 7.4.1.7)
Nonosteogenic fibroma
Fibrosarcoma

7.4.1.5 Osteochondroma

Age

Mostly in young individuals (60% before 30 years)

Site

Hand 10%
In long tubular bones: metaphysis
The presence of multiple osteochondromas is also known as osteochondromatosis, multiple osteocartilaginous exostoses, and diaphyseal aclasia [4]. Specific differential diagnosis in multiple osteochondromas: previous irradiation of bone, fibrodysplasia ossificans progressiva, pseudopseudohypoparathyroidism

Radiographic Findings

An osteochondroma is a bony and frequently pedunculated projection of the skeleton. The contour of the lesion may be smooth or irregular. If abundant calcification is present, the connection with the cortex may be difficult to determine. In the hereditary type of osteochondroma, the affected bones may be deformed and curved.

Differential Diagnosis

Myositis ossificans circumscripta (Sect. 7.4.4.1)
Chondrosarcoma (Sect. 7.4.2.1)
Juxtacortical osteosarcoma

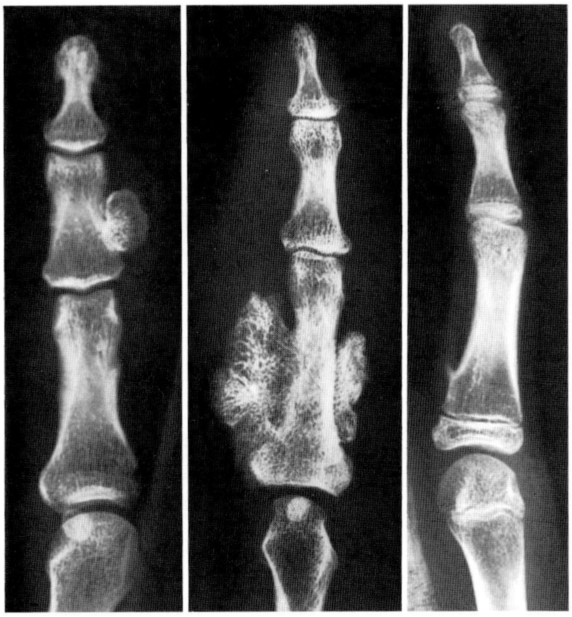

a b c

Fig. 1. a Osteochondroma of middle phalanx in a 34-year-old man: Sharp margin, bony structure in lesion. b Large osteochondroma of proximal phalanx in a 44-year-old woman: Well-defined lesion with bony structure. c Small exostosis in a 15-year-old girl with fibrodysplasia ossificans progressiva

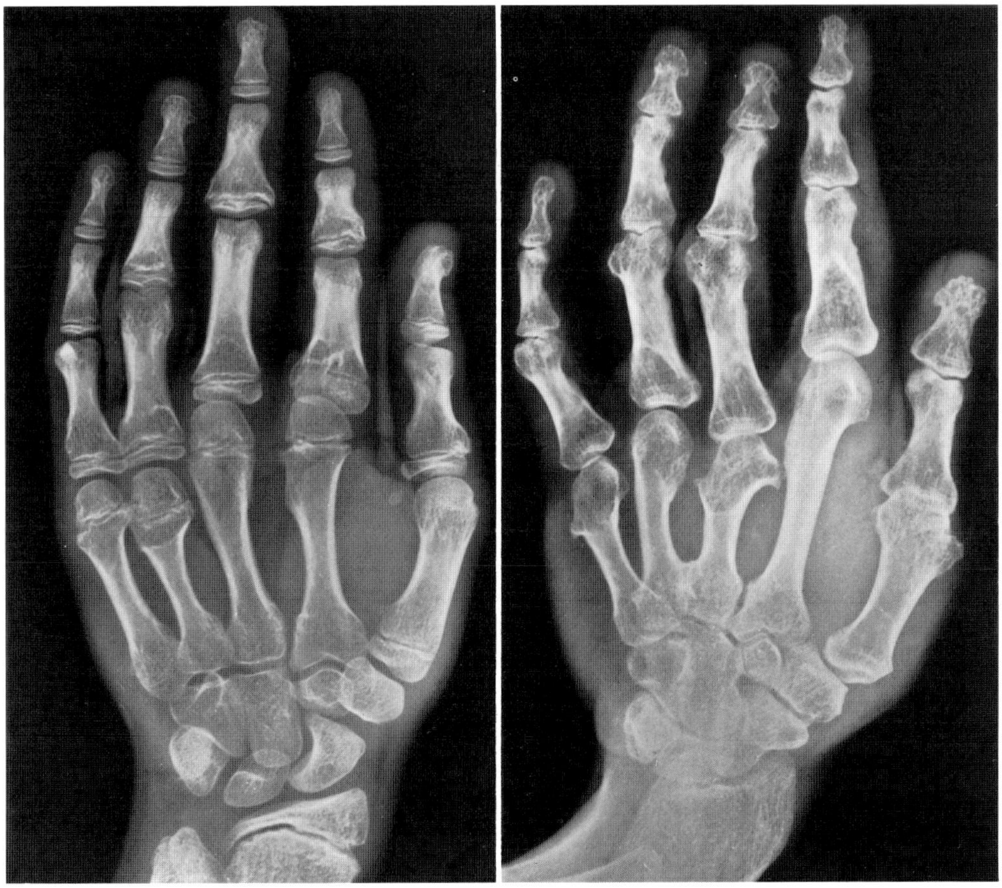

a b

Fig. 2a, b. Multiple osteochondromas. a In a 13-year-old girl: Deformation of multiple metacarpals and phalanges. b In a 58-year-old man: Short third to fifth metacarpals, deviation of fingers, relatively short ulna

7.4.1.6 Giant Cell Tumor

Age

90% older than 20 years
60% between 20 and 40 years

Site

Hand

Grade I and II:	3%
Grade III:	2.8%

Other

Grade I and II:	femur 27%	humerus 7%		
	tibia 17%	vertebrae 4%		
	ulna 10%	fibula 4%		
Grade III:	femur 42%	radius 6%		
	tibia 20%	humerus 6%		
	pelvis 8%			

In long tubular bones: metaepiphysis 95%; metaphysis 5%

Radiographic Findings

The center of the usually eccentrically located and radiolucent giant cell tumor often presents coarse trabeculae. The ballooning and thin cortical bone shell may be entirely intact. The borderline with the normal bone is mostly distinct and slightly sclerotic.

Differential Diagnosis

Aneurysmal bone cyst (Sect. 7.4.1.7)
Chondroma or well-differentiated chondrosarcoma (Sects. 7.4.1.3 and 7.4.2.1)
Chondroblastoma
Chondromyxoid fibroma (Sect. 7.4.1.4)
Fibrous dysplasia (Sect. 7.4.3.1)
Osteoblastoma (Sect. 7.4.1.1)
Fibrosarcoma
Osteolytic osteosarcoma
Multiple myeloma

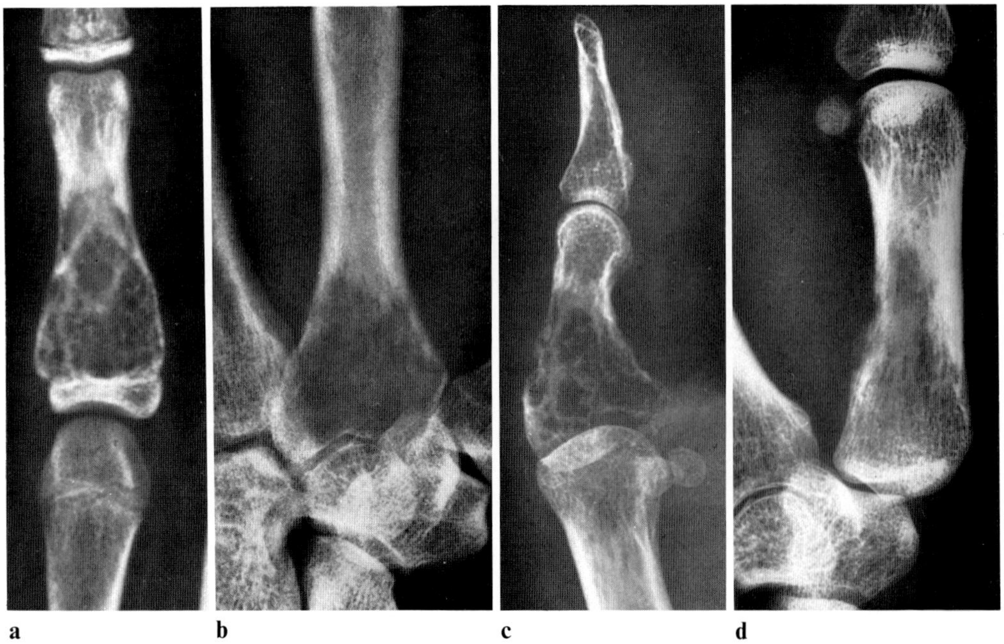

Fig. 1a–d. Giant cell tumors. **a** In a 15-year-old girl: Grade II tumor. Metaphyseal lesion with sharp margin and bubbly, mild expansion. Specific differential diagnosis: aneurysmal bone cyst, chondromyxoid fibroma, osteoblastoma, enchondroma. **b** In a 60-year-old woman: Grade II tumor. Purely lytic tumor in second metacarpal with irregular intraosseous margin, slight expansion. Specific differential diagnosis: fibrosarcoma, osteolytic osteosarcoma, metastatic lesion, myeloma. **c** In a 46-year-old man: Grade III tumor. Marked expansion, some trabeculation, cortex disrupted in some areas. Specific differential diagnosis: fibrosarcoma, metastatic lesion, myeloma. **d** In a 25-year-old woman: Grade III tumor. No expansion, irregular cortical destruction, faint periosteal reaction. Specific differential diagnosis: osteolytic osteosarcoma, metastatic lesion, fibrosarcoma

7.4.1.7 Aneurysmal Bone Cyst [6]

Age

85% younger than 25 years

Site

Hand	4%	Tibia	13%
Vertebrae	20%	Humerus	8%
Femur	14%	Fibula	6%

In long tubular bones: metadiaphysis 40%; diaphysis 30%; metaphysis 20%; metaepiphysis 10%

Radiographic Findings

An aneurysmal bone cyst presents as a central or eccentric, radiolucent lesion bordered by an intact thin layer of periosteal bone formation. The center of the tumor often presents a coarse trabecular structure, and the borderline with normal bone is distinct and usually somewhat sclerotic. Sometimes this bone layer is very thin, so only small Codman's triangles may be seen.

Differential Diagnosis

Giant cell tumor (Sect. 7.4.1.6)
Solitary bone cyst
Chondromyxoid fibroma (Sect. 7.4.1.4)
Fibrous dysplasia (Sect. 7.4.3.1)
Nonossifying fibroma
Chondroblastoma
Osteoblastoma (Sect. 7.4.1.1)
Chondrosarcoma (Sect. 7.4.2.1)
Myeloma (Sect. 7.4.2.3)

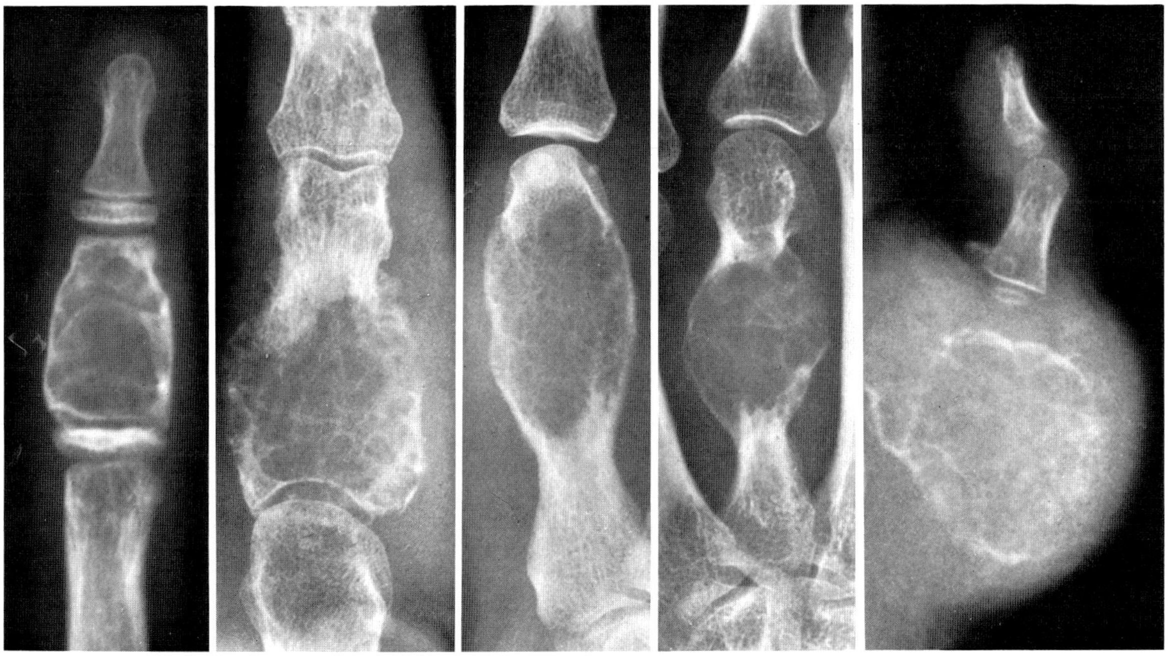

a b c d e

Fig. 1a–e. Aneurysmal bone cysts. **a** In a 10-year-old boy: Well-defined tumor with some coarse trabeculation in middle phalanx. Specific differential diagnosis: fibrous dysplasia, enchondroma, spina ventosa (tuberculosis). **b** In a 57-year-old man: Expansive lesion with cortex disruption and fine trabeculation. Specific differential diagnosis: giant cell tumor, chondroma, metastatic lesion, myeloma. **c** In a 35-year-old woman: Expansive well-circumscribed tumor in fifth metacarpal. Lace-like trabeculations. Specific differential diagnosis: giant cell tumor. **d** In a 24-year-old woman: Diaphyseal tumor, expansive and bubbly with well-defined margins. Specific differential diagnosis: chondroma. **e** In a $2^1/_2$-year-old boy: First metacarpal. Huge tumor with cortex destruction and expansion, sparse trabeculation

7.4.2 Malignant Tumors [1, 3, 7, 8]

7.4.2.1 Chondrosarcoma

Age

No specific predilection

Site

Hand	2% (very rare in phalanges)		
Femur	19%	Tibia	6%
Pelvis	17%	Scapula	6%
Ribs	17%	Vertebrae	5%

In long tubular bones: epiphysis, metaphysis, and diaphysis

Radiographic Findings

The radiographic findings in chondrosarcoma depend on the site of the tumor. A centrally located chondrosarcoma in a long tubular bone may present as a more or less lobular, radiolucent lesion. In the more advanced stages, cortical destruction and some periosteal bone formation may be seen. The center of the tumor contains irregular calcifications (densities) in the tumor tissue. An eccentrically located tumor is usually ill-defined and may mimic an osteochondroma. The adjacent cortex is intact or infiltrated by tumor invasion.

Differential Diagnosis

Chondromyxoid fibroma (Sect. 7.4.1.4)
Chondroblastoma
Bone infarct
Chondroma (Sect. 7.4.1.3)
Osteosarcoma
Fibrosarcoma

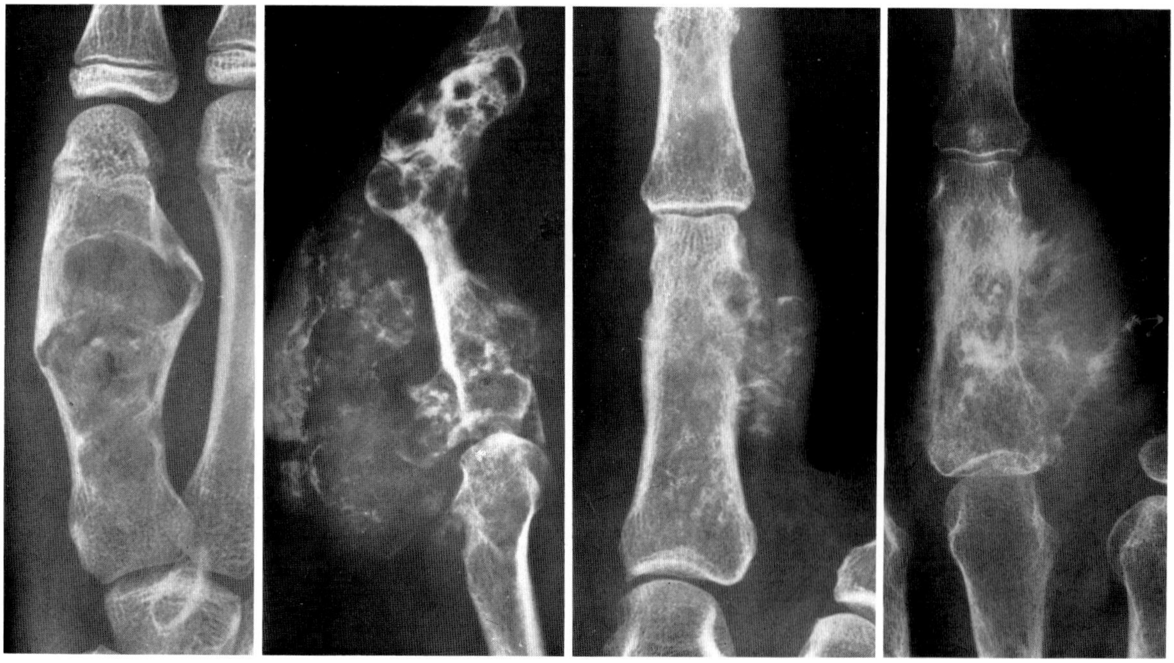

a b c d

Fig. 1 a–d. Chondrosarcomas. **a** In a 16-year-old boy: Grade I, lobular, expansive tumor with shaft distension, very thin cortex, fracture. Radiographically benign appearance! Specific differential diagnosis: benign intraosseous fibrous histiocytoma (see Fig. 2b). **b** In a 57-year-old woman: Multiple enchondromas in fifth finger. Grade I chondrosarcoma in base of proximal phalanx. Calcifications in tumor. **c** In a 63-year-old woman: Grade I tumor. Cortex destruction, periosteal bone apposition, calcifications. **d** In a 76-year-old woman: Grade I tumor. Cortical erosion, periosteal bone apposition, demineralization, calcifications. Specific differential diagnosis: osteosarcoma

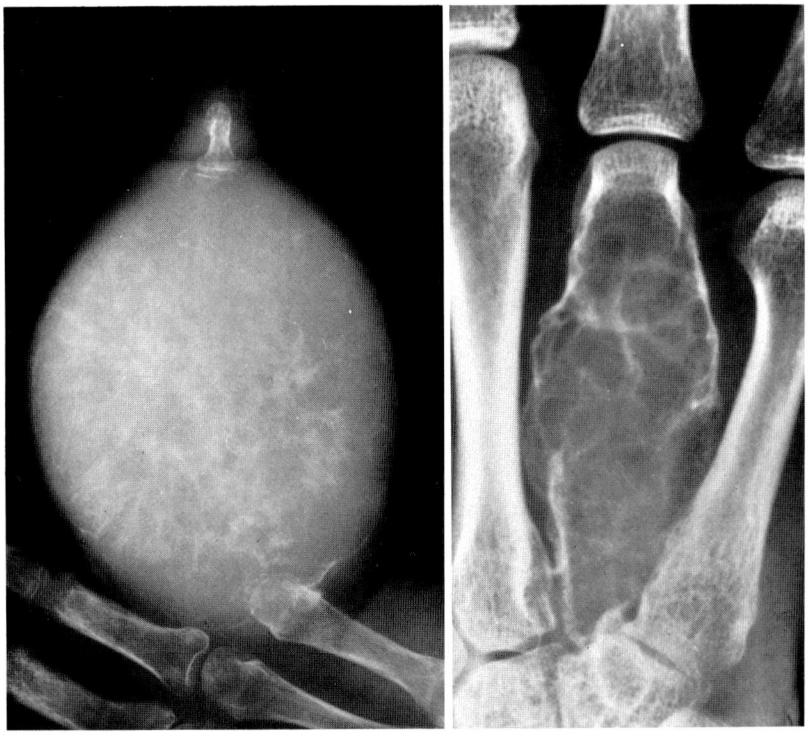

a b

Fig. 2. a Chondrosarcoma in a 66-year-old man. Huge grade I tumor of fifth finger. Tumor growth over a period of 15 years! Proximal and middle phalanges destroyed, multiple calcifications in tumor. Specific differential diagnosis: giant cell tumor, angiosarcoma. **b** Benign intraosseous fibrous histiocytoma (PA diagnosis) in a 19-year-old man. Large bubbly and trabeculated tumor. Specific differential diagnosis: chondroma, giant cell tumor, aneurysmal bone cyst, chondromyxoid fibroma, chondrosarcoma

7.4.2.2 Ewing's Sarcoma

Age

10–30 years (peak incidence 10–20 years)

Site

Hand	0.5%	Tibia	9%
Femur	21%	Humerus	9%
Ribs	17%	Fibula	8%
Pelvis	13%	Scapula	5%

In long tubular bones: diaphysis and metaphysis

Radiographic Findings

The radiographic appearance of Ewing's sarcoma varies considerably. In tubular bones a large part of the shaft may present a permeative type of bone destruction and periosteal bone formation (spiculae or lamellar bone formation). Sometimes bone destruction is minimal and periosteal bone formation predominates. In other cases there is rather circumscribed cortical destruction with periosteal new bone formation and some expansion of bone is present.

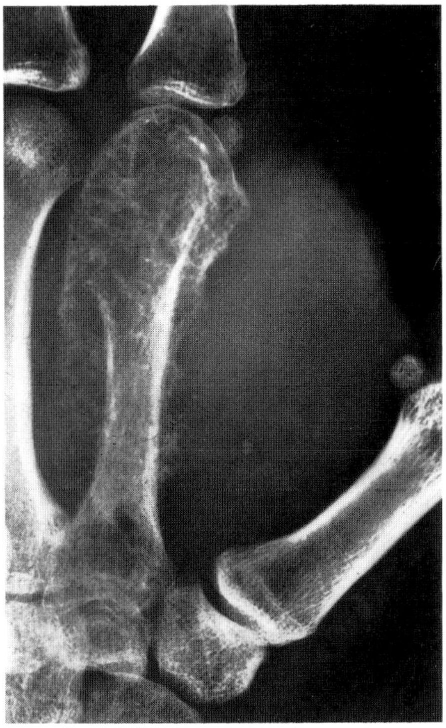

Fig. 1. Ewing's sarcoma of second metacarpal in a 19-year-old man. Large lesion involving both metaphyseal and diaphyseal parts of bone. Permeative destruction in cortical and spongious bone, extensive periosteal new bone formation, large soft tissue mass. Specific differential diagnosis: osteosarcoma

Differential Diagnosis

Eosinophilic granuloma
Osteomyelitis (Sect. 7.3.3)
Osteosarcoma
Lymphoma
Angiosarcoma

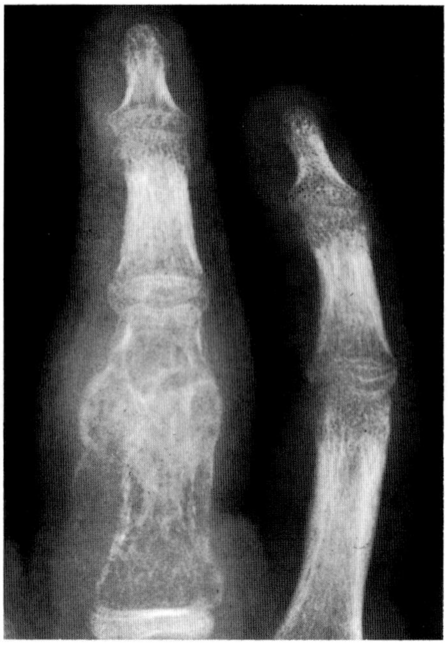

Fig. 2. Hemophilic pseudotumor. Destructive lesion of proximal phalanx with new bone formation. In a hemophilic patient a subperiosteal hemorrhage may cause pressure and erosion of the adjacent cortex. Bony spicules may develop within the organizing hematoma, and new bone formation gives the lesion a malignant aspect. Most of these tumors occur in the femur [8]. Specific differential diagnosis: Ewing's sarcoma, osteoblastoma

7.4.2.3 Myeloma

Age

Vast majority over 50 years

Site

Hand	very rare		
Vertebrae	35%	Ribs	10%
Pelvis	15%	Humerus	7%
Femur	10%	Maxilla	7%

In long tubular bones: metaphysis and diaphysis

Radiographic Findings

Myelomatous lesions in the long tubular bones are usually round or oval-shaped and sometimes surrounded by some osteosclerosis. Periosteal new bone formation near the predominantly osteolytic lesions is infrequently encountered. Myelomas in the marrow cavity lead to destruction of circumscribed areas of the inner cortex. This cortical destruction may sometimes be over a considerable distance.

Differential Diagnosis

Metastatic lesion (Sect. 7.4.2.5)
Aneurysmal bone cyst (Sect. 7.4.1.7)
Chondroma and well-differentiated chondrosarcoma (Sects. 7.4.1.3 and 7.4.2.1)
Giant cell tumor (Sect. 7.4.1.6)

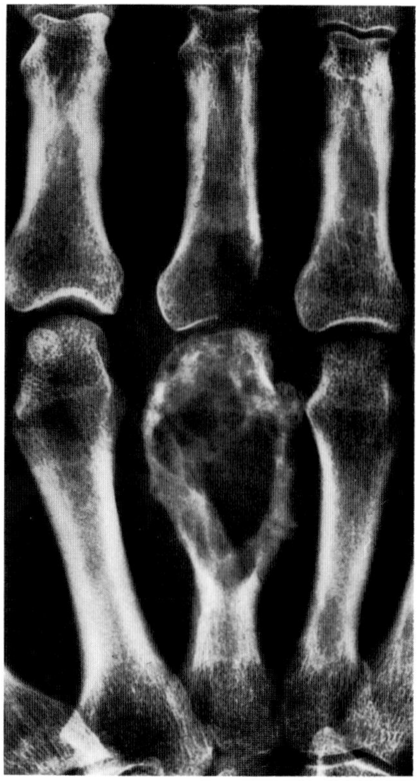

Fig. 1. Myeloma in a 63-year-old man. Destructive lesion in third metacarpal, proximal phalanx also affected. Specific differential diagnosis: pyogenic arthritis, metastatic lesion, pigmented villonodular synovitis

7.4.2.4 *Synovial Sarcoma* [9]

Age

50% between 20 and 40 years

Site

Hand 9%
Thigh 20%
Knee 17%
Foot 12%
Lower leg 10%
In long tubular bones: bone involvement often slight

Radiographic Findings

Synovial sarcoma presents as a soft tissue mass near a joint, containing calcifications in about one third of cases. Involvement of bone, when present, begins with cortical erosion and progresses to invasion of the medulla.

Differential Diagnosis

Soft tissue fibrosarcoma
Rhabdomyosarcoma
Liposarcoma
Soft tissue chondrosarcoma

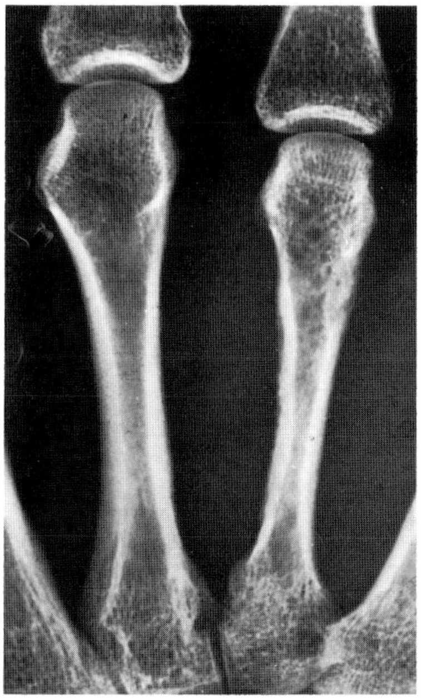

Fig. 1. Synovial sarcoma in a 19-year-old man. Increased density of soft tissue around fourth metacarpal, thinning of metacarpal shaft due to cortical erosion, small lucencies in metacarpal metaphysis. Specific differential diagnosis: soft tissue tumor

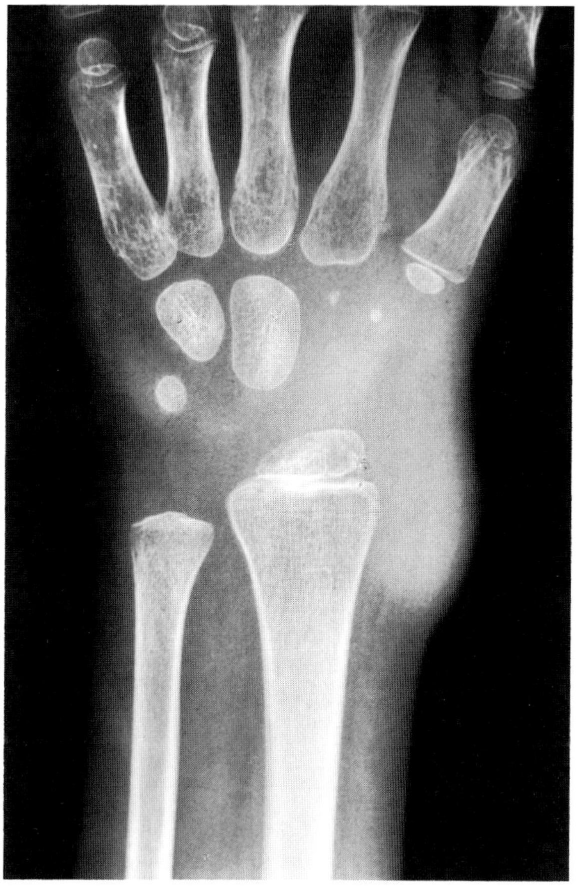

Fig. 2. Rhabdomyosarcoma. Soft tissue swelling, no osseous involvement. Specific differential diagnosis: other soft tissue tumor, soft tissue infection

7.4.2.5 Metastatic Lesions

Age

Vast majority over 50 years

Radiographic Findings

If a solitary osteolytic lesion is present, a metastatic lesion should be considered from the outset.

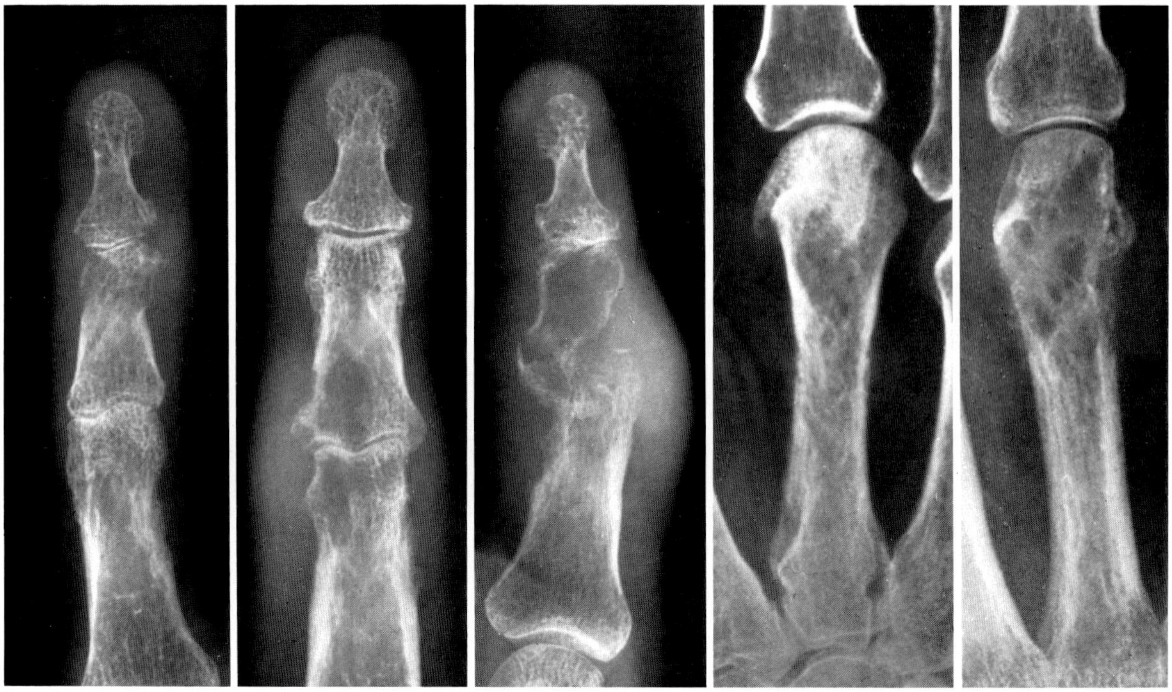

a b c d e

Fig. 1 a–e. Metastatic lesions. **a–c** Multiple metastatic lesions from carcinoma of prostate in a 66-year-old man: Various grades of bone destruction and soft tissue swelling. Specific differential diagnosis: myeloma. **d** Lymphatic leukemia: Infiltrating lesion with cortical erosion. Specific differential diagnosis: lymphoma, osteomyelitis, Ewing's sarcoma. **e** Carcinoma of breast: Significant bone destruction with irregular margins. Specific differential diagnosis: myeloma

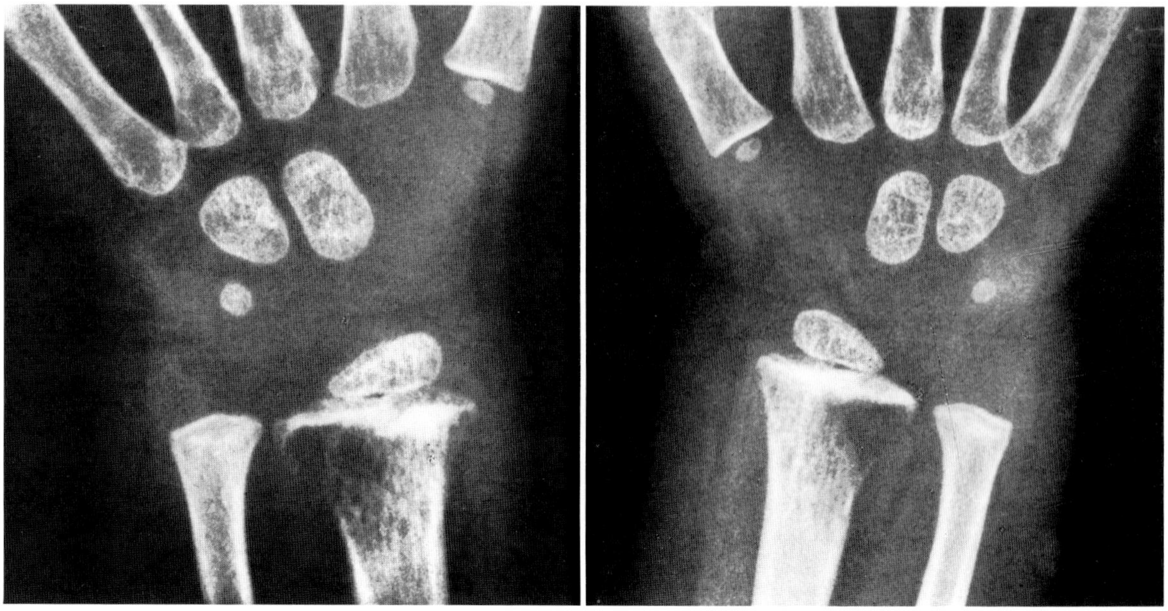

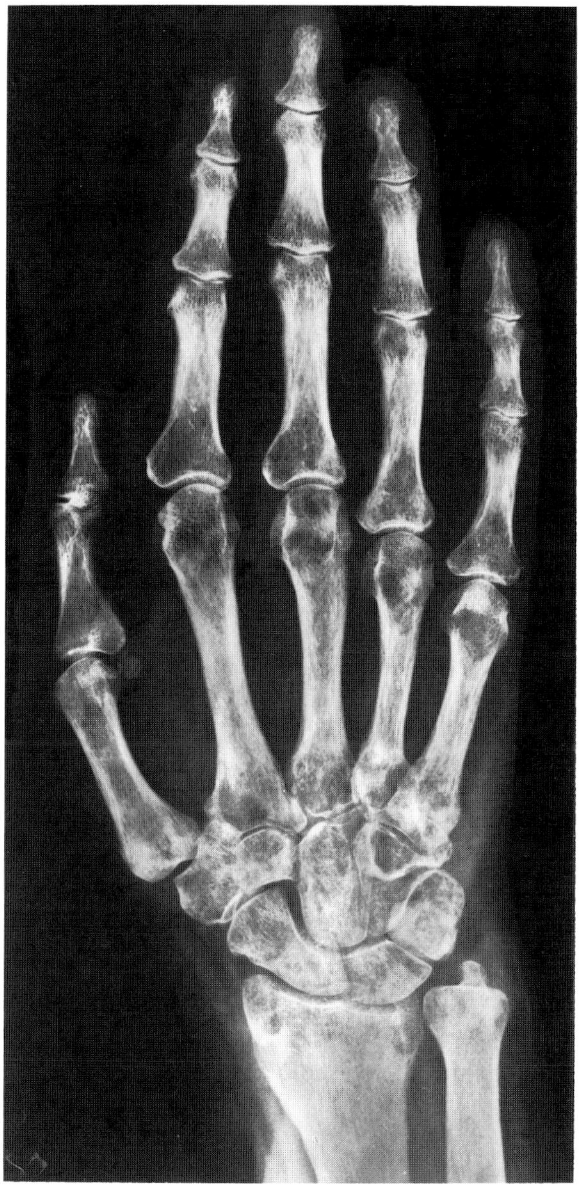

Fig. 2. Metastatic lesions from breast carcinoma

References

1 Netherlands Committee on Bone Tumours (1966) Radiologic atlas of bone tumours, vol 1. Mouton, The Hague
2 Netherlands Committee on Bone Tumours (1973) Radiologic atlas of bone tumours, vol 2. Mouton, The Hague
3 Mulder JD, Poppe H, Von Ronnen JR (1981) Primäre Knochengeschwülste. In: Lehrbuch der Röntgendiagnostik, II/2. Thieme, Stuttgart
4 Takigawa K (1971) Chondroma of the bones of the hand. A review of 110 cases. J Bone Joint Surg [Am] 53:1591–1600
5 Vinstein AL, Franken EA Jr (1971) Hereditary multiple exostoses. AJR 112:405–407
6 Dahlin DC, McLeod RA (1982) Aneurysmal bone cyst and other nonneoplastic conditions. Skeletal Radiol 8:243–250
7 Lodwick GS (1971) Atlas of tumour radiology. The bones and joints. Year Book Medical Publishers, Chicago
8 Ghormley RK, Clegg RS (1948) Bone and joint changes in hemophilia. With a report of cases of so-called hemophilic pseudotumor. J Bone Joint Surg [Am] 30:589–600
9 Wilner D (1982) Radiology of bone tumors and allied disorders. Saunders, Philadelphia
10 Pirschel J, Metzger HOFJ, Wissmann C (1978) Zur Metastasierung maligner Tumoren in die Skelettperipherie. Fortschr Geb Röntgenstr Nuklearmed Ergänzungsband 129:621–626

◁ Fig. 3. Symmetrically distributed metastatic lesions from neuroblastoma in an infant

7.4.3 Benign Nonneoplastic Tumor-Like Bone Lesions

7.4.3.1 Fibrous Dysplasia

Age

Detection in adolescence or adult life: peak incidence 10–20 years

Site

Hand 1%

Ribs	30%	Maxilla	12%	Tibia	10%
Femur	15%	Skull	10%	Pelvis	17%

In long tubular bones: diaphysis, metaphysis

Radiographic Findings

The radiographic findings vary widely. Large amounts of fibrous tissue cause areas of radiolucency, whereas a ground-glass appearance is given by diffuse formation of calcified bone. Bony lesions with extensive osteosclerosis may be encountered, as may multilocular lesions with trabeculation. The borderline with normal bone is usually well-defined, and a zone of sclerosis may be present in that area. Curvature of tubular bones is a well-known finding.

Differential Diagnosis

Nonossifying fibroma
Solitary bone cyst
Paget's disease (Sect. 6.2.9)
Aneurysmal bone cyst (Sect. 7.4.1.7)
Chondroma (Sect. 7.4.1.3)
Hyperparathyroidism (Sect. 6.2.3)
Giant cell tumor (Sect. 7.4.1.6)

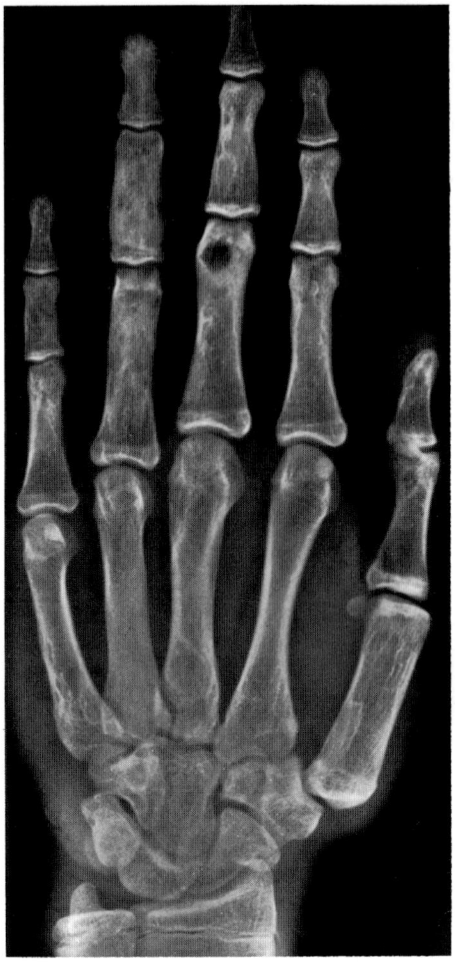

Fig. 1. Polyostotic fibrous dysplasia of hand in a 17-year-old boy. Small radiolucent area in proximal phalanx of middle finger, widening and ground-glass structure of several metacarpals and phalanges

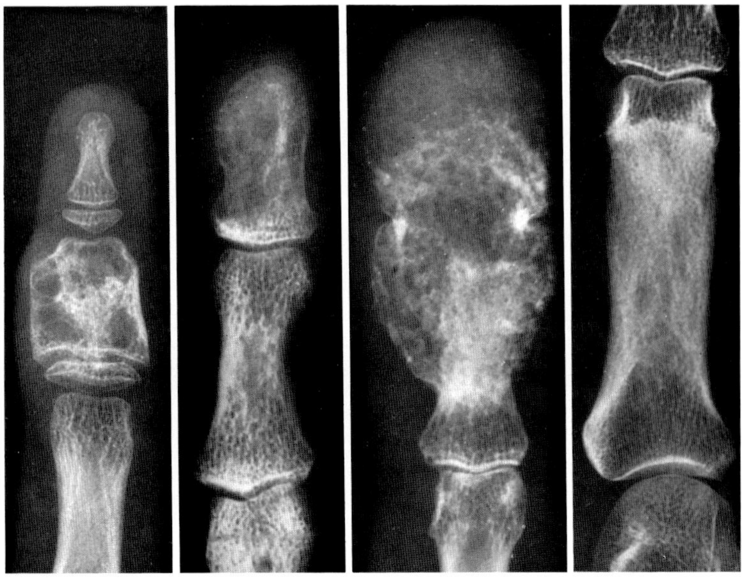

a b c d

Fig. 2a–d. Fibrous dysplasia. **a** In a 6-year-old boy: Widened middle phalanx, fine trabeculation, some formation of bone. Specific differential diagnosis: aneurysmal bone cyst, enchondroma. **b** In a 28-year-old woman: The distal phalanx of the fifth finger is widened: amorphous bone formation. **c** In a 51-year-old man: Severe ballooning of fifth finger with destruction of distal phalanx. Specific differential diagnosis: giant cell tumor, enchondroma, metastatic lesion. **d** In a 60-year-old woman: Sclerosis of diaphysis. Specific differential diagnosis: Paget's disease, osteoid osteoma, sclerosing osteomyelitis. Hodgkin's lymphoma

7.4.3.2 Epidermoid Cyst

An epidermoid cyst is caused by traumatic implantation of epidermoid tissue in bone. Usually the distal phalanges are affected [1, 2].

Differential Diagnosis

Glomus tumor
Giant cell tumor (Sect. 7.4.1.6)
Chondroma (Sect. 7.4.1.3)
Sarcoidosis (Sect. 7.3.12)
Myxoma
Metastatic lesion (Sect. 7.4.2.5)

References

1 Byers P, Mantle J, Ralm R (1966) Epidermal cysts of phalanges. J Bone Joint Surg [Br] 48:577–581
2 Hoessly M, Lagier R (1982) Anatomico-radiological study of intraosseous epidermoid cysts. Fortschr Geb Röntgenstr Nuklearmed Ergänzungsband 137:48–54

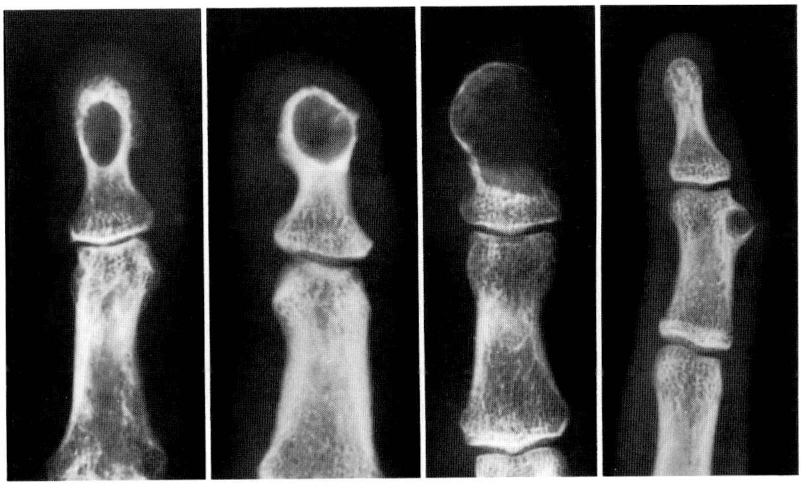

a b c d

Fig. 1a–d. Epidermoid cysts. **a** In a 58-year-old woman: Well-defined lytic lesion with sclerotic margins in distal phalanx. Cortex intact. **b** In a 34-year-old man: Typical lesion. **c** In a 56-year-old man: Large well-defined lesion. Cortex destroyed, no calcifications. Specific differential diagnosis: myxoma, metastatic lesion. **d** In a 14-year-old girl: Small lesion in middle phalanx of fifth finger with overhanging edges (unusual site)

7.4.4 Ossifying Tumor-Like Lesions in the Soft Tissue

7.4.4.1 Myositis Ossificans Circumscripta [1–3, 6]

Myositis ossificans circumscripta is extraosseous cartilage and bone formation after local acute trauma or repeated injuries. The abnormalities occur mostly in the striated muscles.

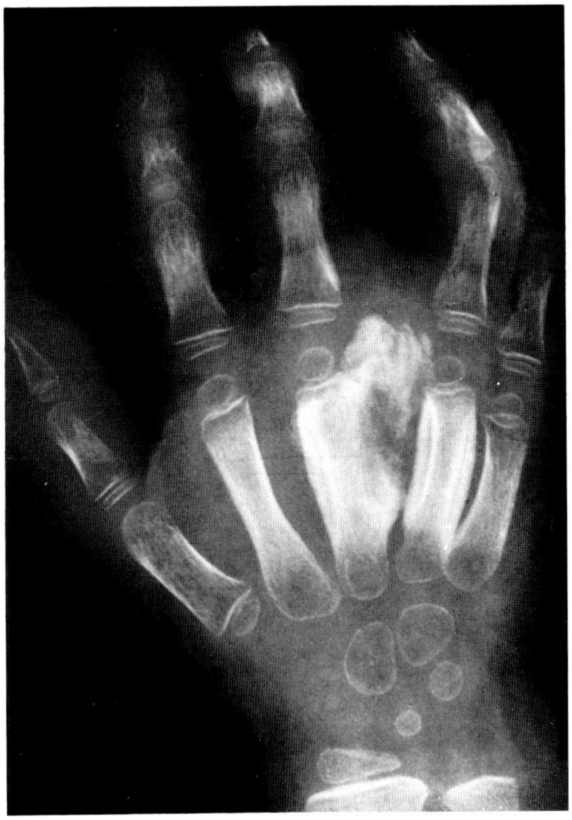

Fig. 1. Myositis ossificans in a 4-year-old girl. Large inhomogeneous dense mass in soft tissue adjacent to third and fourth metacarpals, significant reaction. Specific differential diagnosis: soft tissue inflammation with secondary periostitis

7.4.4.2 Extraosseous Pseudo-osteoblastoma [2, 4–6]

Synonym: pseudomalignant osseous tumor of soft tissue

Extraosseous pseudo-osteoblastomas are well-circumscribed. A definite history of trauma is uncommon, and hematoma formation in the tumor has not been encountered. The tumor is surrounded by a thin layer of mature bone. Spicules of osteoid tissue radiate toward the center, which consists of a large number of spindle cells.

References

1 Ackerman LV (1958) Extraosseous localised non-neoplastic bone and cartilage formation (so called myositis ossificans). Clinical and pathological confusion with malignant neoplasms. J Bone Joint Surg [Am] 40:279–298

2 Netherlands Committee on Bone Tumours (1973) Radiologic atlas of bone tumours, vol 2. Mouton, The Hague

3 Goldman A (1976) Myositis ossificans circumscripta: benign lesion with a malignant differential diagnosis. AJR 126:32–40

4 Jeffreys TE, Stiles PJ (1966) Pseudomalignant osseous tumour of soft tissue. J Bone Joint Surg 48:488–492

5 Chaplin DM, Harrison MHM (1972) Pseudomalignant osseous tumour of soft tissue. J Bone Joint Surg [Br] 54:334–340

6 Wilner D (1982) Radiology of bone and allied disorders. Saunders, Philadelphia

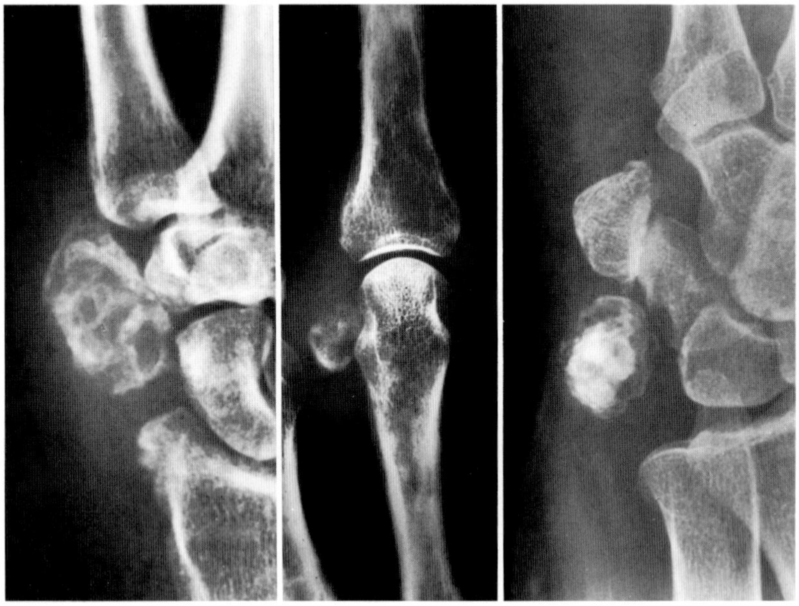

a b c

Fig. 1 a–c. Extraosseous pseudo-osteoblastomas. **a** In a 52-year-old man: Ossifying lesion in soft tissue, periosteal reaction of first metacarpal and distal radius, soft tissue swelling. Specific differential diagnosis: osteochondroma of tendon sheath, chondroma, chondrosarcoma. **b** In a 35-year-old woman: Well-circumscribed ossifying lesion surrounded by a thin bone shell, slight periosteal reaction of second metacarpal and proximal phalanx, soft tissue swelling. Specific differential diagnosis: extraosseous osteochondroma, chondrosarcoma. **c** In a 64-year-old woman: Demarcated ossifying lesion with thin bone shell in soft tissue, degenerative changes in pisiform bone. Specific differential diagnosis: calcification of tendon sheath

7.4.5 Miscellaneous Lesions

7.4.5.1 Fibromatosis

Synonyms: Musculoaponeurotic fibromatosis, periosteal desmoids

Fibromatosis is subdivided as follows [1]:

1. "Adult" fibromatosis
   a) Dupuytren-type fibromatosis
      palmar fibromatosis
      plantar fibromatosis
      Peyronie's disease
   b) Desmoid fibromatosis
      extra-abdominal desmoids
      abdominal desmoids
      intra-abdominal desmoids
      multiple desmoids
      Gardner's syndrome
2. "Juvenile" fibromatosis
   a) Congenital fibrosarcoma-like fibromatosis
   b) Congenital localized or generalized fibromatosis
   c) Juvenile aponeurotic fibromatosis
   d) Fibrous hamartoma of infancy
   e) Recurring digital fibrous tumors of childhood

Fibromatosis may erode and invade adjacent bones. The recurrence rate after surgery is high. Although fibromatosis locally proves to be very aggressive, metastases never occur. Microscopically, the lack of pleomorphism and the low mitotic rate distinguish fibromatosis from fibrosarcoma. Digital fibrous tumors in children differ from the other forms of fibromatosis in being limited to the fingers and toes, having a remarkable tendency to recur, and containing cytoplasm inclusion bodies [2]. Recurring digital fibrous tumors are usually multiple and are either congenital or appear in the first few months of life. A viral causative agent is postulated, usually producing slowly growing tumors, although sometimes more rapid growth takes place. Spontaneous regression of these tumors is normal.

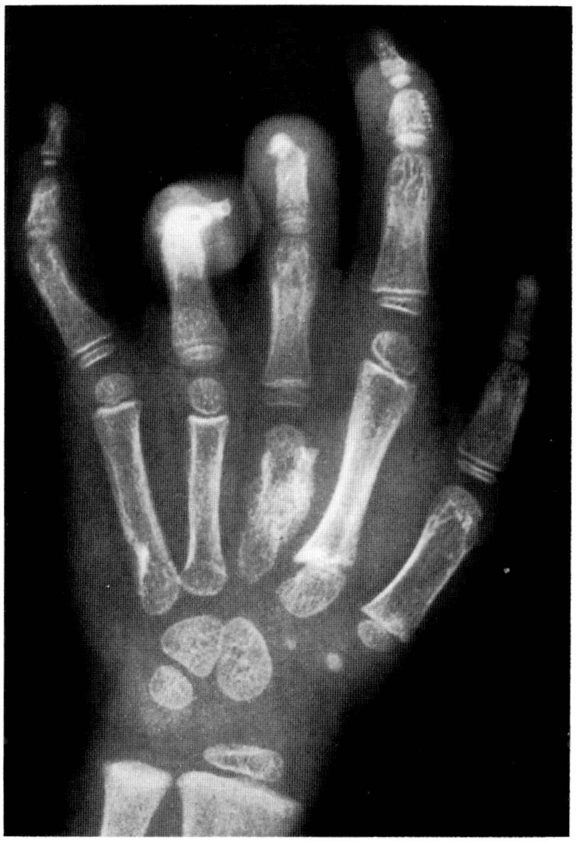

Fig. 1. Recurring digital fibromas in a 3-year-old girl. Erosion of fifth metacarpal and invasion of third metacarpal, deformation of third and fourth digits

Radiographic Findings [1, 3, 4]

The skeleton is not frequently invaded. The affected bones present erosions, intraosseous abnormalities, and/or periosteal new bone formation.

Differential Diagnosis

Soft tissue tumors (benign or malignant)

References

1 Griffiths HJ, Robinson K, Bonfiglio TA (1983) Aggressive fibromatosis. Skeletal Radiol 9:179–184
2 Reye RDK (1965) Recurring digital fibrous tumours of childhood. Arch Pathol 80:228–231
3 Bloem JJ, Vuzevski VD, Huffstadt AJC (1974) Recurring digital fibroma of infancy. J Bone Joint Surg [Br] 56:746–751
4 Bonakdarpour A, Pickering JE, Resnick EJ (1978) Case report 49. Fibromatosis. Skeletal Radiol 2:181–183

7.4.5.2 Bone Metaplasia Due to Mechanical Irritation

In cases of bone metaplasia caused by mechanical irritation the abnormalities develop in the bone tissue and not primarily in the periosteal membrane [1]. The radiographic findings usually include periosteal reaction as well as the bone metaplasia.

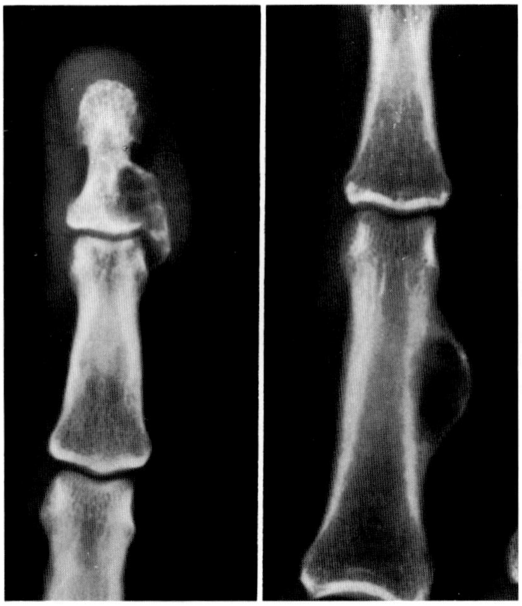

Fig. 1 a, b. Bone metaplasia due to mechanical irritation. **a** In a 53-year-old man: Well-circumscribed expansive lesion of distal phalanx, developed after local trauma. Specific differential diagnosis: chondroma. **b** In a 19-year-old man: Well-defined, juxtacortical, expansive lytic lesion with significant periosteal bone formation. Specific differential diagnosis: cortical chondroma, cortical abscess, calcified hematoma

Reference

1 Netherlands Committee on Bone Tumours (1973) Radiologic atlas of bone tumours, vol 2. Mouton, The Hague

7.4.5.3 Tumors of the Tendon Sheath

Tenosynovial Osteochondromatosis

Tenosynovial osteochondromatosis is a rare and benign condition of the tenosynovial sheath. The intra-articular chondromatosis capsulae is much more common [1].

Differential Diagnosis

Chondroma (Sect. 7.4.1.3)
Extraosseous pseudo-osteoblastoma (Sect. 7.4.4.2)
Other disorders with calcification in the soft tissues (Sect. 6.2.7)

Ossifying Fibroma of the Tendon

This uncommon tumor presents with soft tissue swelling. Tiny ossification centers within the tumor may be encountered.

Reference

1 De Benedetti MJ, Schwinn CP (1979) Tenosynovial chondromatosis of the hand. J Bone Joint Surg [Am] 61:898–903

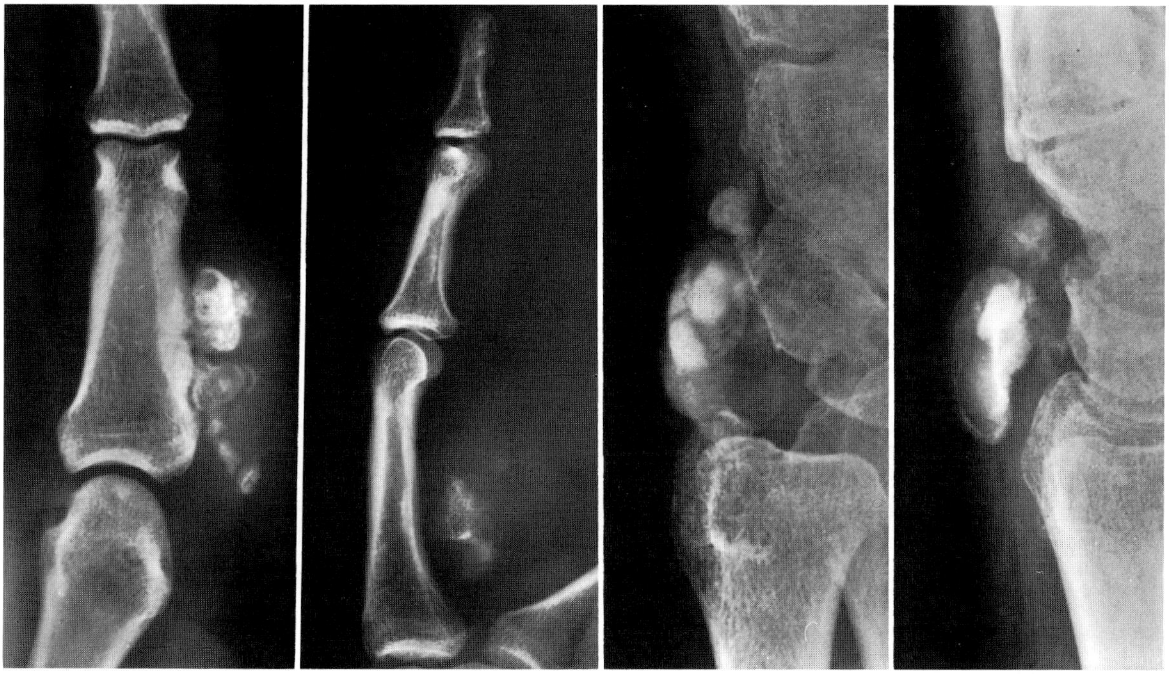

a b c d

Fig. 1 a–d. Tenosynovial osteochondromatosis. **a** In a 31-year-old man: Cartilaginous and osseous structures in tumor, slight cortical thickening. **b** In a woman: Predominantly osseous structures in soft tissue swelling of finger. **c, d** In a 62-year-old man: Several ossifying masses in soft tissue without bone erosions

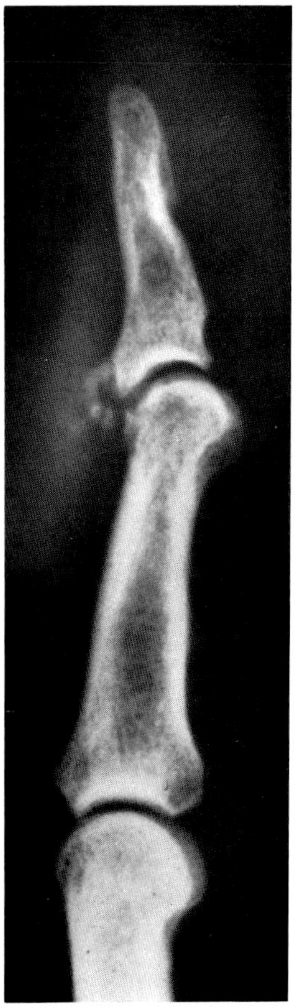

Fig. 2. Ossifying fibroma in a 65-year-old woman. Tiny ossifications in soft tissue dorsal to distal interphalangeal joint. Specific differential diagnosis: parosseous chondroma, other conditions with calcifications in soft tissues

7.4.5.4 Pigmented Villonodular Synovitis

In most cases of pigmented villonodular synovitis only one tendon sheath, bursa, or joint is affected. Proliferation of synovial tissue causes nodules and villi with heavy deposition of hemosiderin.

Tendon Sheath

Depending on the site of the lesion, osseous abnormalities can be present, often in the form of erosions.

Joint

In most cases of intra-articular villonodular synovitis, the bones on both sides of the joint are affected.

a, b 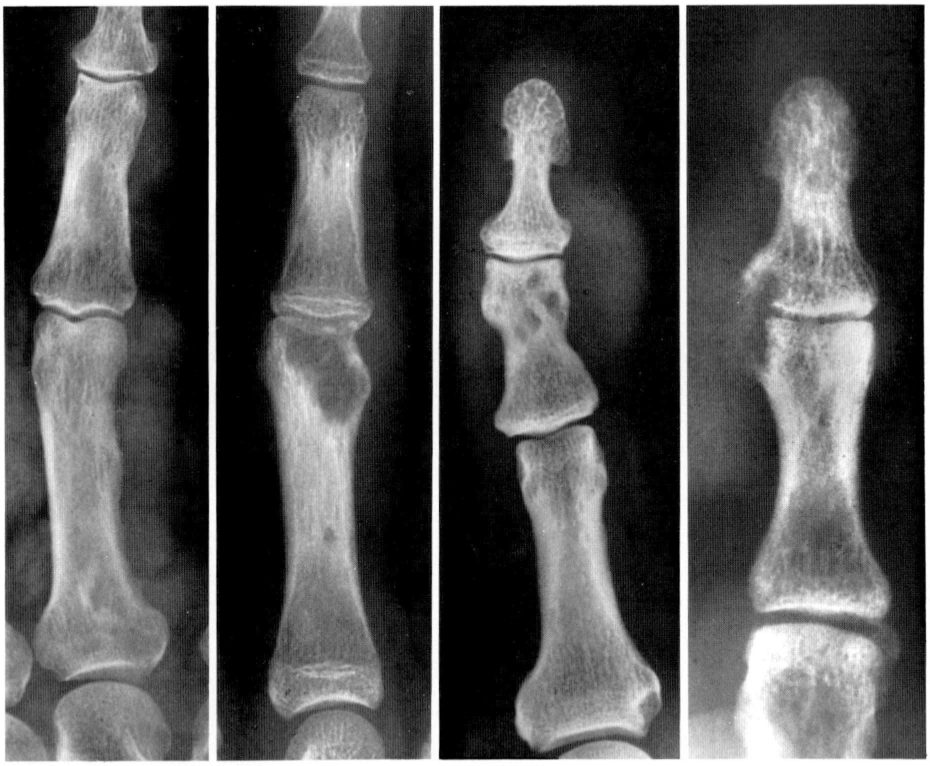 c, d

Fig. 1 a–d. Pigmented villonodular synovitis of tendon sheath. **a** In a 51-year-old woman: Soft tissue swelling and erosion of proximal phalanx. Specific differential diagnosis: other soft tissue lesion with secondary erosion of bone. **b** In a 19-year-old woman: Soft tissue swelling and erosion of proximal phalanx. Specific differential diagnosis: chondroma, giant cell tumor, fibrous dysplasia, sarcoidosis, intraosseous ganglion. **c** In a 41-year-old man: Soft tissue swelling and severe cystic lesions in middle phalanx, distal interphalangeal joint intact. Specific differential diagnosis: sarcoidosis, intraosseous ganglion. **d** In a 49-year-old woman: Eccentric huge soft tissue swelling with bone erosions. Specific differential diagnosis: pyogenic arthritis

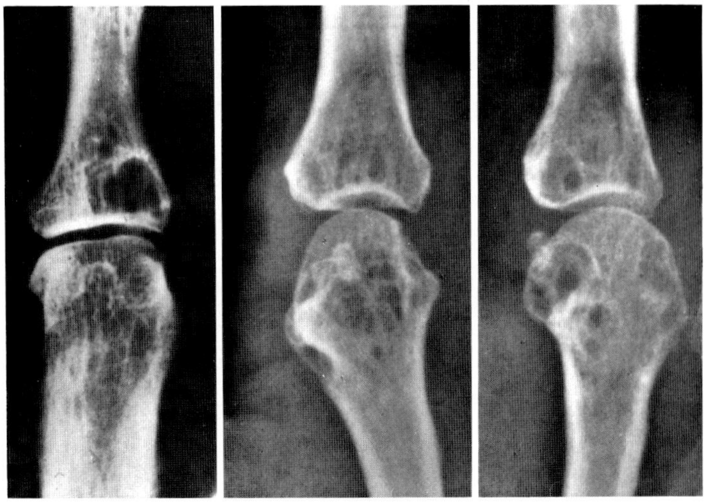

a b c

Fig. 2 a–c. Pigmented villonodular synovitis of joint. **a** In an adult woman: Only this joint affected, cystic lesions on both sides of normal joint space. **b, c** In a 51-year-old woman: Only this joint affected, soft tissue swelling around metacarpophalangeal joint, cystic lesions on both sides of normal joint space

7.5 Chemical Agents

7.5.1 Fluorosis

In small doses, fluorine, in the form of fluoride, prevents dental caries. An excessive intake of fluorine results in dental abnormalities (mottled enamel) and osteosclerosis and osteoporosis of the skeleton. The pathogenesis of the skeletal abnormalities is not entirely clear. As fluorine is an inhibitor of many enzymes, its effect may be to diminish resorption of bone. Raised levels of circulating parathyroid hormone have been found in fluorosis. It is also possible that increased bone formation and resorption are responsible for the radiographic findings [1]. The axial skeleton is particularly affected; the appendicular skeleton presents only relatively mild sclerosis.

Radiographic Findings [1–5]

Hand
Cortical thickening
Osteoporosis and osteosclerosis (especially in carpals)
Coarsening of bony trabeculae
Periosteal new bone formation
Roughening of muscular attachments
Narrowing of marrow spaces

Other Sites
Pelvis: calcification of ligaments (ischial tuberosities, sacrospinous, sacrotuberous, iliac crest)
Spine: calcification of paraspinal ligaments
dense sclerosis
formation of dense osteophytes with encroachment of foramina
thickening of trabecular pattern
kyphosis
Skull: dental abnormalities
Long tubular bones: hyperostosis of ligamentous or muscular attachments
periosteal new bone formation

Differential Diagnosis

Pachydermoperiostosis (Sect. 1.2.8)
Renal osteodystrophy (Sect. 6.2.4)
Paget's disease (Sect. 6.2.9)
Mastocytosis (Sect. 7.6.7)

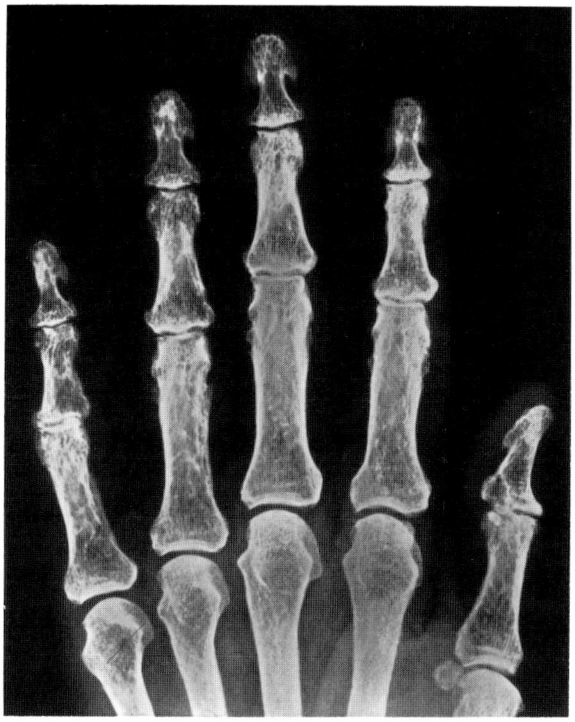

Fig. 1. Fluorosis in a 69-year-old woman. Increased bone density, coarsening of trabeculae, periostitis along radial margin of fifth proximal phalanx, small bony excrescences around interphalangeal joints

Hypertrophic osteoarthropathy (Sect. 7.6.8)
Osteoblastic metastases
Myelofibrosis

References

1 Resnick D, Niwayama G (1981) Diagnosis of bone and joint disorders. Saunders, Philadelphia
2 Morris JW (1965) Skeletal fluorosis among Indians of the American South West. AJR 94:608–615
3 Soriano M, Manchón F (1966) Radiological aspects of a new type of bone fluorosis, periostitis deformans. Radiology 87:1089–1094
4 Teotia M, Teotia SPS, Kunwar KB (1971) Endemic skeletal fluorosis. Arch Dis Child 48:686–691
5 Stevenson CA, Watson RA (1957) Fluoride osteosclerosis. AJR 78:13–18

7.5.2 Lead Poisoning

Only in children does chronic lead poisoning cause skeletal abnormalities detectable on radiographs. The intoxication is usually due to ingestion or inhalation of lead-containing materials. The clinical features of lead poisoning are colic, encephalopathy, peripheral neuritis, and anemia. Lead replaces calcium in the growing metaphyseal areas, inhibiting the action of the osteoclasts but not that of the osteoblasts, and thus stimulating the formation of bony trabeculae containing cores of calciferous and plumbiferous cartilage covered by layers of true bone. Lead accounts for about one-fifth of the density of the lead-containing zone [1, 2]. When lead exposure ceases, the lead lines gradually disappear.

Radiographic Findings [1–4]

Hand

Metaphyseal bands of increased density (lead lines) in radius and ulna
Short tubular bones
Lead lines in carpals
Widening of metaphyses (failure of modeling)

Other Sites

Foot: abnormalities similar to those in hand
Long tubular bones: metaphyseal lead lines
Flat bones: lead lines in iliac crest
Abdomen: lead particles in gastrointestinal tract
Skull: widening of sutures

Differential Diagnosis

Normal, rather dense metaphyses
Bismuth poisoning
Phosphorus poisoning
Healing rickets (Sect. 6.2.1)
Hypervitaminosis D (Sect. 6.2.2)
Cretinism (Sect. 7.2.1)
Osteopetrosis (Sect. 1.2.2)
Leukemia
Scurvy (Sect. 6.2.5)
Hyperparathyroidism (Sect. 6.2.3)

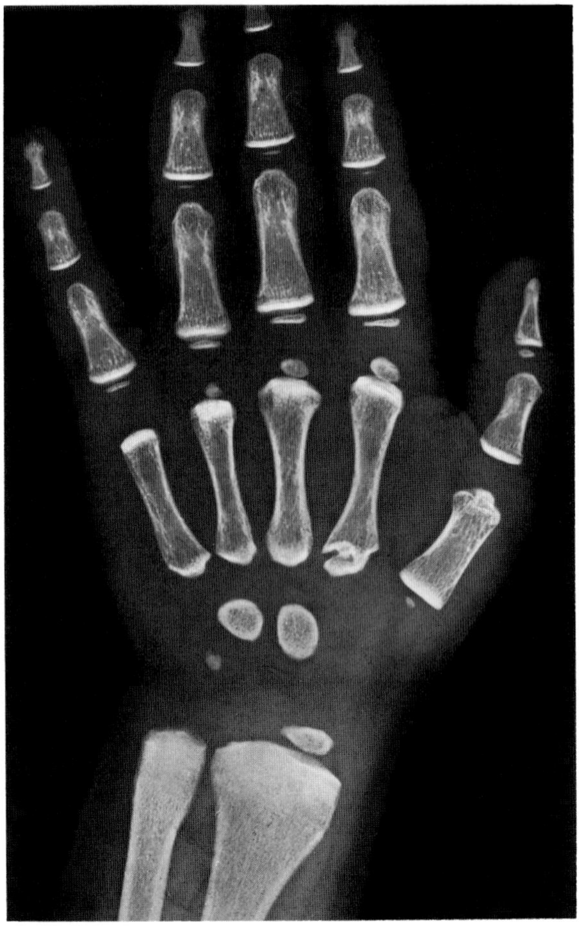

Fig. 1. Lead poisoning in a 3-year-old boy. Widening of very dense metaphyses of radius and ulna, smaller lead lines in metaphyses of short tubular bones, marginal density of carpals

References

1 Leone AJ (1968) On lead lines. AJR 103:165–167
2 Schwörer I, Kaul A, Stolpmann HJ, Hunger J (1983) Bleieinlagerung im Knochen – Röntgenaufnahme als Nachweismethode? Fortschr Geb Röntgenstr Nuklearmed Ergänzungsband 138:84–94
3 Pease CN, Newton GG (1962) Metaphyseal dysplasia due to lead poisoning. Radiology 79:233–240
4 Resnick D, Niwayama G (1981) Diagnosis of bone and joint disorders. Saunders, Philadelphia

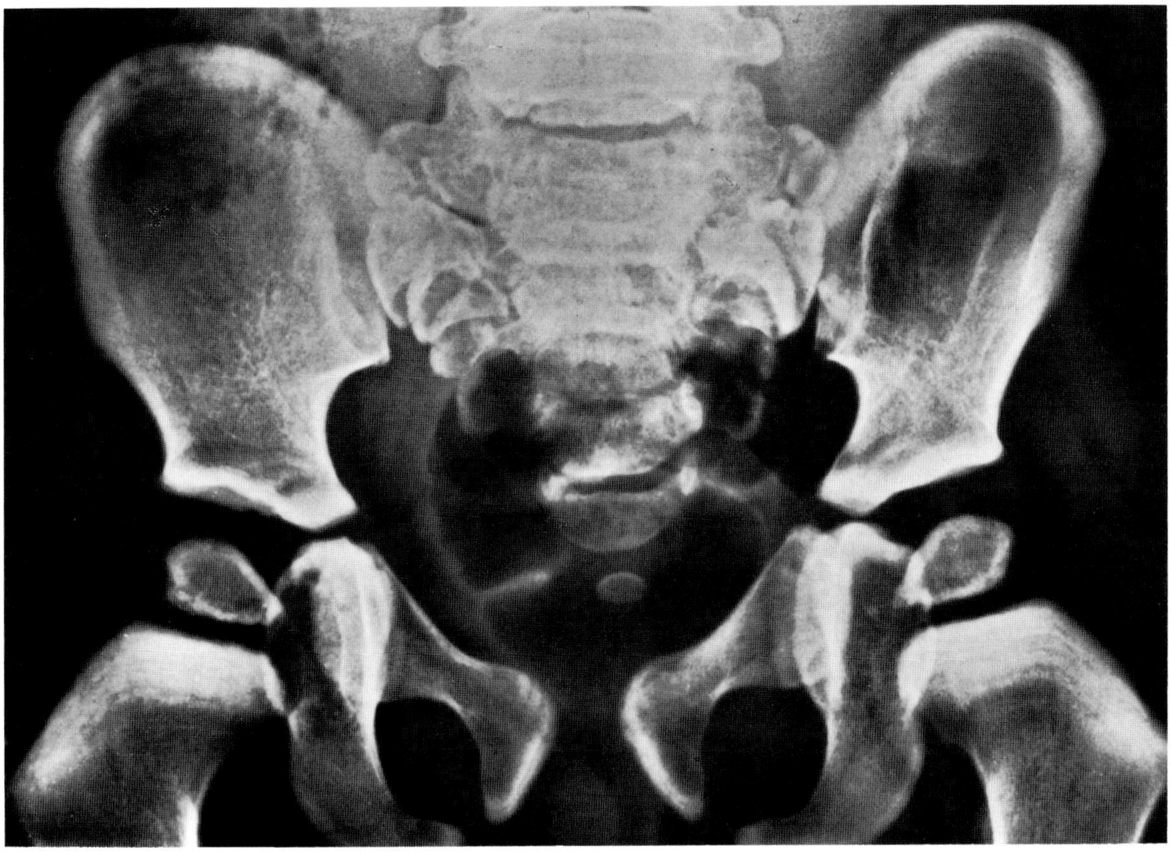

Fig. 2. Same patient as Fig. 1. Lead lines in proximal femoral metaphyses, increased density of iliac crests, acetabula, and margins of sacrum

7.6 Miscellaneous Conditions

7.6.1 Lunatomalacia

Synonyms: aseptic necrosis of lunate, Kienböck's disease

Lunatomalacia is probably of traumatic origin and may develop after acute trauma or as the result of repeated trauma (e.g., from use of pneumatic tools). In many cases a definite history of preceding injury is lacking. A commonly encountered congenital anomaly in patients with aseptic necrosis of the lunate is a relatively short ulna (ulna minus variant). The shortness of the ulna probably puts the lunate under permanent stress [1].

Radiographic Findings [1–4]

Subchondral fracture (seen on tomography)
Increased bone density
Endosteal pseudocysts
Fragmentation
Flattening of lunate
Relatively short ulna (ulna minus variant)
Osteoarthrosis of wrist

References

1 Hulten O (1935) Über die Entstehung und Behandlung der Lunatummalazie (Morbus Kienböck). Acta Chir Scand 75:121–135
2 Gelberman RH, Salamon PB, Jurist JM, Posch JL (1975) Ulnar variance in Kienböck's disease. J Bone Joint Surg [Am] 57:674–678
3 Resnick D, Niwayama G (1981) Diagnosis of bone and joint disorders. Saunders, Philadelphia
4 Pöschl M (1971) Juvenile osteo-chondro-nekrosen. In: Diethelm L (ed) Röntgendiagnostik der Skeleterkrankungen. Springer, Berlin Heidelberg New York (Handbuch der medizinischen Radiologie, vol 5/4)

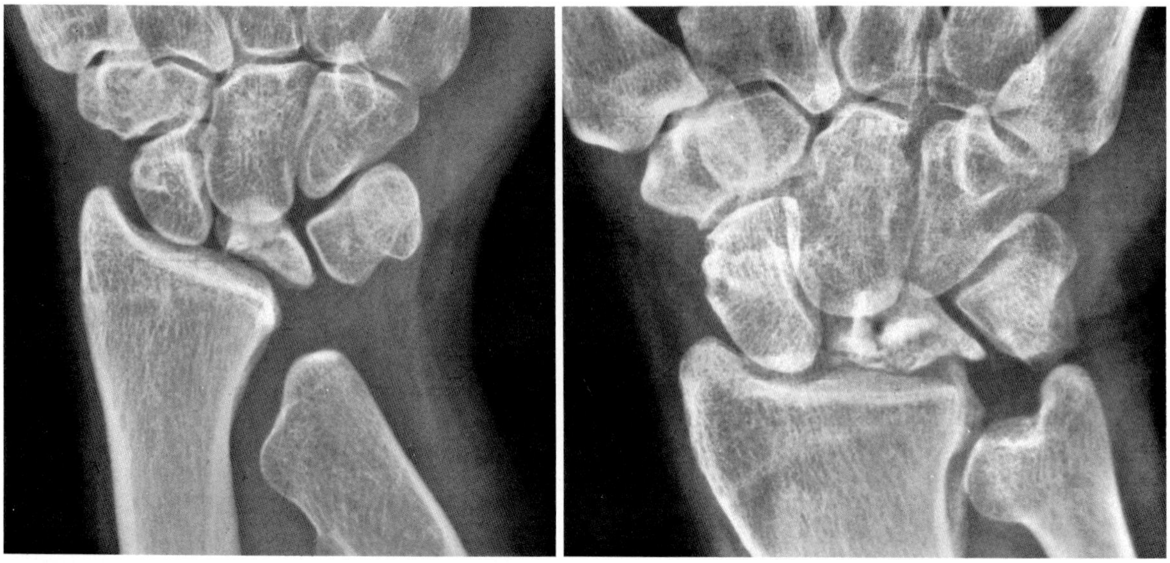

a b

Fig. 1a, b. Lunatomalacia. Congenital shortening of ulna with aseptic necrosis of lunate

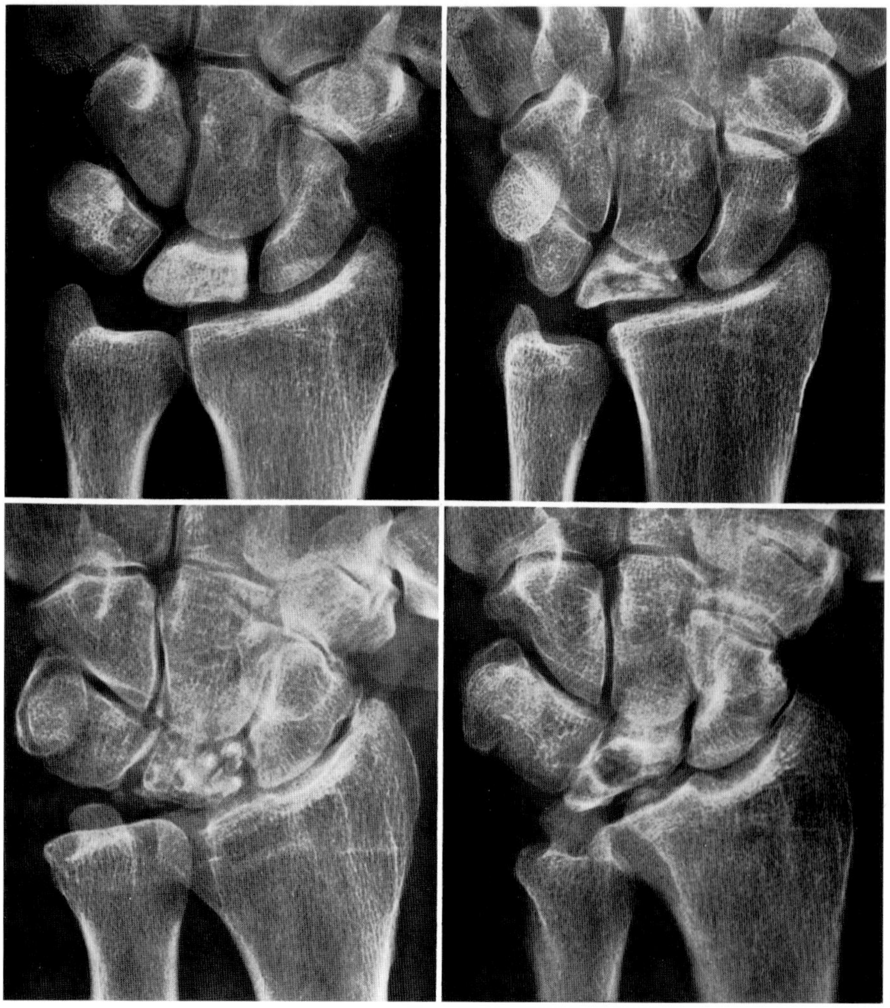

a b c d

Fig. 2a–d. Lunatomalacia in four different patients. **a** Increased bone density, some flattening of lunate. **b** Flattening, pseudocysts, sclerosis. **c** Fragmentation, increased density. **d** Pseudocyst, flattening, increased bone density, osteoarthrosis of wrist

7.6.2 Frostbite

The vascular tree closes in a period of extreme coldness (below −13° C). In the following period of normal temperature vascular occlusion by thrombosis, edema, and cellular aggregation occurs, leading to tissue necrosis and even to autoamputation. The middle and distal phalanges of the fingers and toes are particularly affected. The thumb is usually spared [1]. Milder frostbite may result only in pernio.

Radiographic Findings [1–5]

Hand
Soft tissue swelling
Reduced soft tissue at fingertips
Periostitis
Variable osteoporosis
Acro-osteolysis (especially in tufts)
Juxta-articular pseudocystic lesions
Osteosclerosis
Fragmentation or disappearance of epiphyseal centers
Premature fusion of epiphyses
Joint destruction
Short distal phalanges
Curved fingers
Secondary bone and joint infection

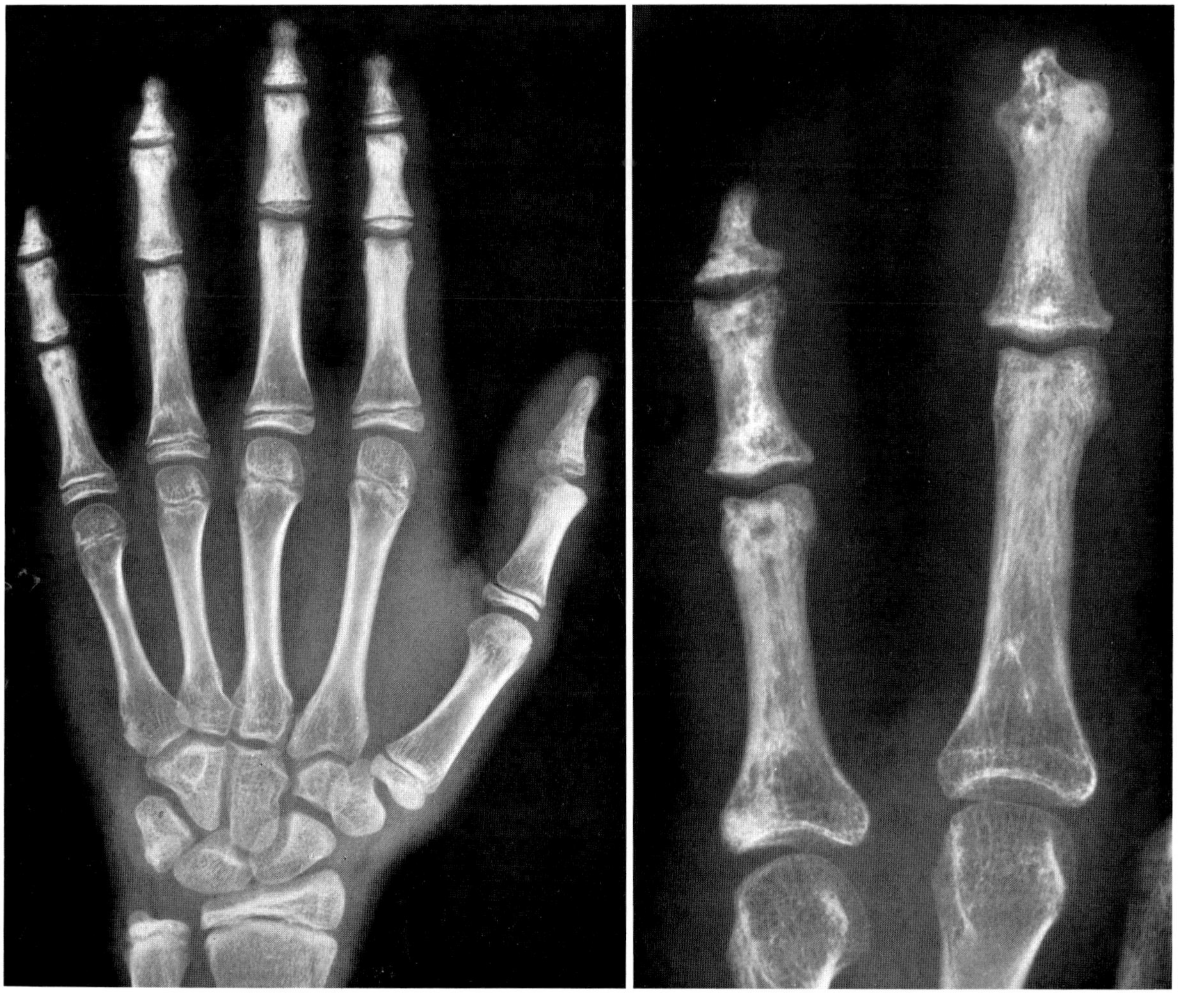

a b

Fig. 1 a, b. Frostbite of right hand in a 17-year-old boy. **a** Osteosclerosis of phalanges and brachydactyly of middle and distal phalanges of second to fifth fingers, premature fusion of several epiphyses and diminution of soft tissues at fourth and fifth fingers. The metacarpals and the thumb are normal. **b** After 3 years, the fourth finger in particular presents progressive deformation at the distal end and intra-articular ankylosis

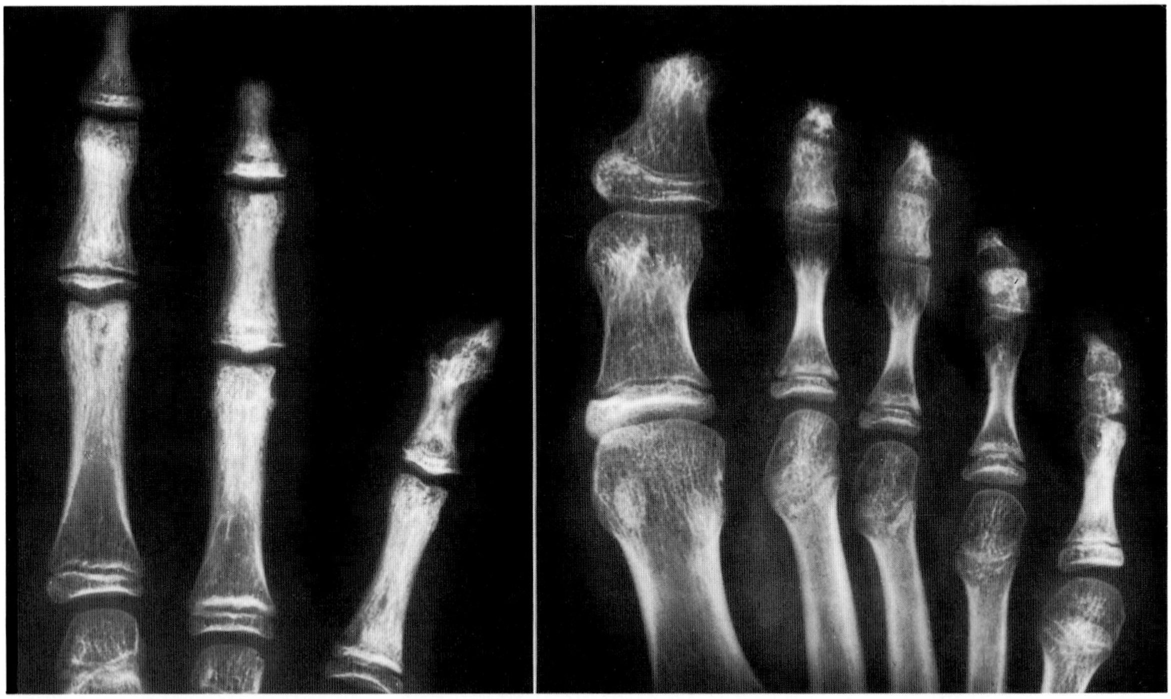

Fig. 2a, b. Same patient as Fig. 1. **a** Left hand: Osteolysis of tuft of fifth finger and destruction of distal joint, premature fusion of almost all epiphyses, brachydactyly, diminution of soft tissues. **b** Left foot: Osteolysis of tufts, brachydactyly

Differential Diagnosis

Thiemann's disease (Sect. 1.1.11)
Other causes of acro-osteolysis (Sect. 3.1)

References

1 Blair JR, Schatzki P, Orr KD (1957) Sequelae to cold injury in one hundred patients. A follow-up study four years after occurrence of cold injury. JAMA 163:1203–1210

2 Tishler J (1972) The soft tissue and bone changes in frostbite injuries. Radiology 102:511–513

3 Selke AC Jr (1969) Destruction of phalangeal epiphyses by frostbite. Radiology 93:859–860

4 Carrera GF, Kozin F, Flaherty L, McCarty DJ (1981) Radiographic changes in the hands following childhood frostbite injury. Skeletal Radiol 6:33–37

5 Blender W (1980) Röntgenologische Veränderungen der Hand nach Erfrierung III. Grades. Fortschr Geb Röntgenstr Nuklearmed Ergänzungsband 133:674–675

7.6.3 Scleroderma

Scleroderma is a generalized, autoimmune connective tissue disorder in which hypergammaglobulinemia, rheumatoid factor, and antinuclear antibodies may be found. The predominantly female patients present involvement of many organs: skin, synovium, gastrointestinal tract, heart, lungs and kidneys. A chronic inflammatory reaction of the collagen fibers leads to their atrophy, and the number of elastic fibers, hairs, and skin glands also decreases. Raynaud's phenomenon is often associated with scleroderma of varying degrees, ranging from skin abnormalities to diffuse skin changes and visceral involvement.
Radiographs of patients with primary Raynaud's phenomenon commonly show soft tissue atrophy. Bone erosions are less common, and no calcifications are found [1]. In the so-called CREST syndrome subcutaneous *c*alcinosis, *R*aynaud's phenomenon, *e*sophageal dysmotility, *s*cleroderma, and *t*elangiectasia occur together.

Radiographic Findings [1–8]

Hand

Soft tissue atrophy (particularly if Raynaud's phenomenon is present)
Osseous destruction (40%–80%): tufts
  carpals
  distal radius/ulna
  Subcutaneous calcifications (10%–20%) of calcium hydroxyapatite
Flexion deformity of fingers
Demineralization
Joint destruction: distal interphalangeal joints
  first carpometacarpal joint
  distal radioulnar joint
  metacarpophalangeal joints
Intra-articular calcifications
Occasional ankylosis

Other Sites

Foot: abnormalities similar to those in hand
Gastrointestinal tract: atony and dilatation (esophagus, jejunum)
Thorax: interstitial fibrosis of lungs
  destruction of ribs and clavicles
  congestive heart disease
  pericarditis
Kidneys: chronic renal failure
Calcifications in tendon sheaths or bursae

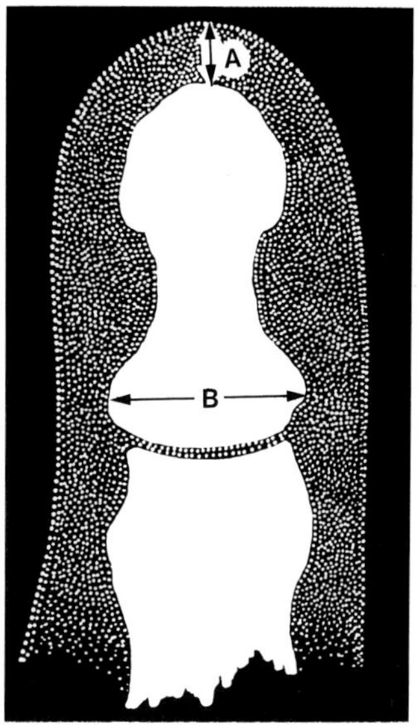

Fig. 1. Soft tissue measurement [1]. Soft tissue atrophy of a fingertip is present if the depth of the pulp (*A*) is less than 20% of the width of the base of the distal phalanx (*B*)

Differential Diagnosis

Bony resorption of phalanges (Sect. 3.1.2)
Periarticular calcifications (Sect. 6.2.7)
Rheumatoid arthritis (Sect. 7.3.4)
Psoriatic arthritis (Sect. 7.3.6)
Osteoarthrosis (Sect. 7.3.13)

References

1 Yune HY, Vix VA, Klatte EC (1971) Early fingertip changes in scleroderma. JAMA 215:113–116
2 Poznanski AK (1984) The hand in radiologic diagnosis. Saunders, Philadelphia
3 Bassett LW, Blocka KLN, Furst DE, Clements J, Gold RH (1981) Skeletal findings in progressive systemic sclerosis (Scleroderma). AJR 136:1121–1126
4 Brandt KD, Krey PB (1977) Chalky joint effusion: result of massive synovial deposition of calcium apatite in progressive systemic sclerosis. Arthritis Rheum 20:792–796
5 Resnick D, Niwayama G (1981) Diagnosis of bone and joint disorders. Saunders, Philadelphia
6 Rabinowitz JG, Twersky J, Guttadauria M (1974) Similar bone manifestations of scleroderma and rheumatoid arthritis. AJR 121:35–44
7 Winter H, Kammerhuber F (1975) Seltene Lokalisation von Knochenveränderungen bei progressiver (diffuser) Sklerodermie. Fortschr Geb Röntgenstr Nuklearmed Ergänzungsband 122:364–366
8 Kauffman GW, Reinbold WD, Hagedorn M (1983) Röntgenmorphologische Befunde bei Sklerodermie. Fortschr Geb Röntgenstr Nuklearmed Ergänzungsband 138:607–613

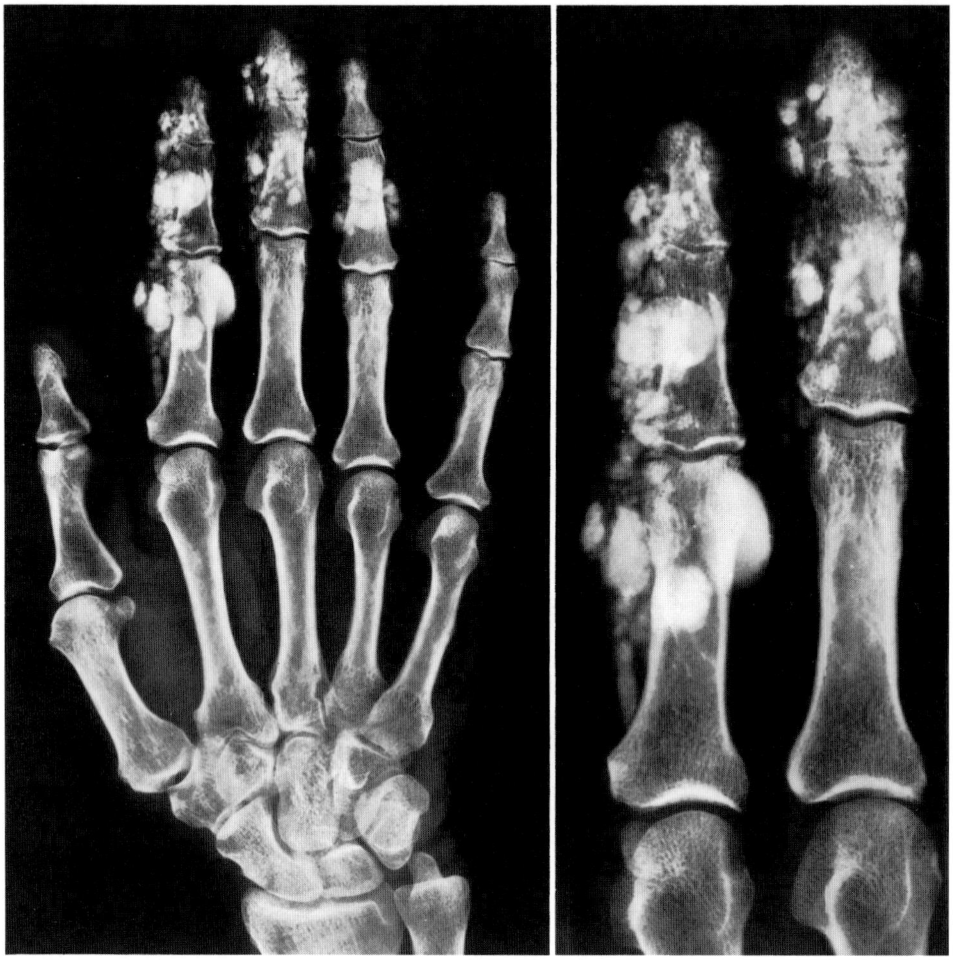

a b

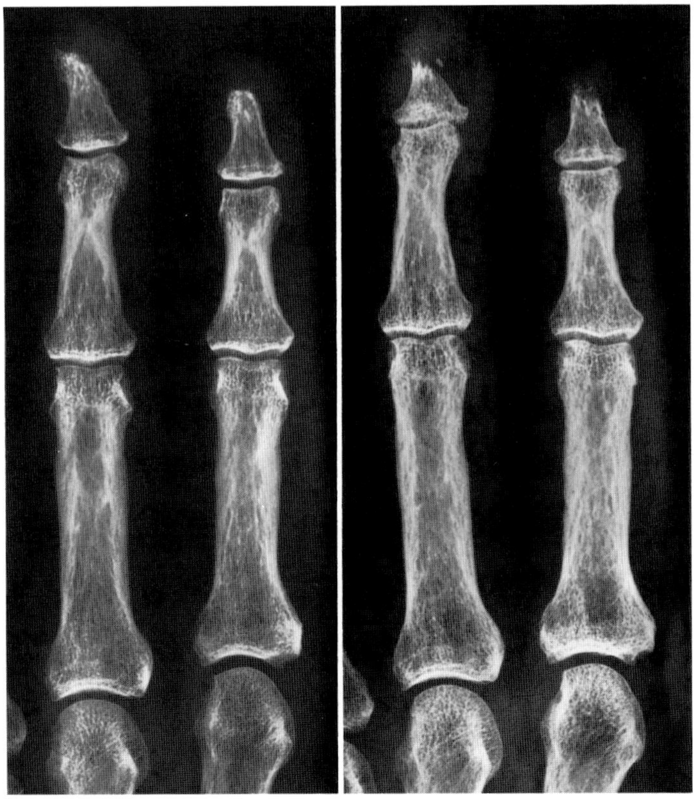

a b

Fig. 2. Scleroderma (CREST syndrome) in a 58-year-old woman. Many deposits of calcium hydroxyapatite in pulp of fingers, some tuftal resorption (detail)

Fig. 3a, b. Scleroderma in a 63-year-old woman. Progressive bone resorption, early calcification of soft tissue (interval between **a** and **b**: $1^{1}/_{2}$ years)

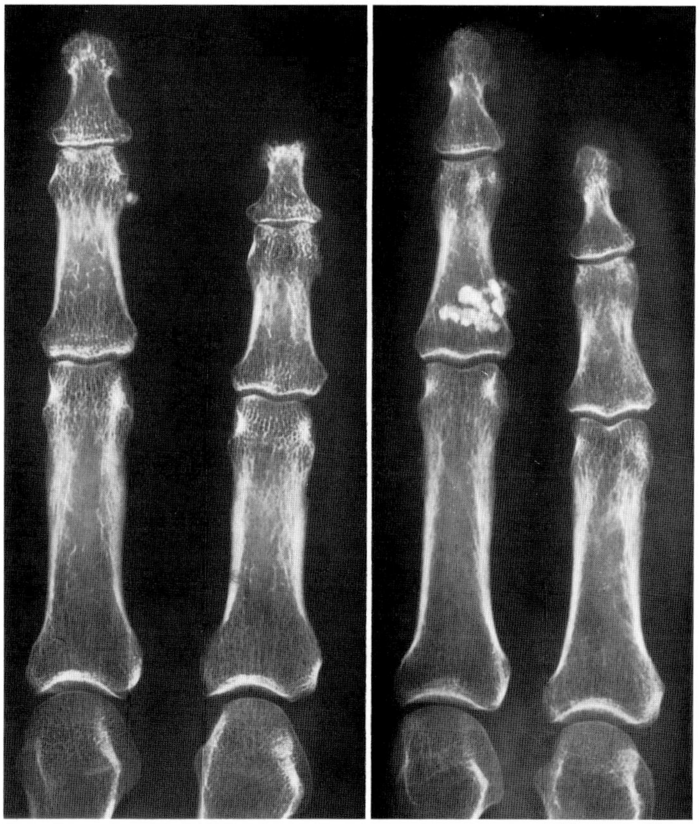

Fig. 4a, b. Scleroderma. a In a 57-year-old man: Predominantly soft tissue atrophy and tuftal erosions, only one small calcification. b In a 72-year-old woman: Calcifications in soft tissue, only minimal tuftal erosions

a b

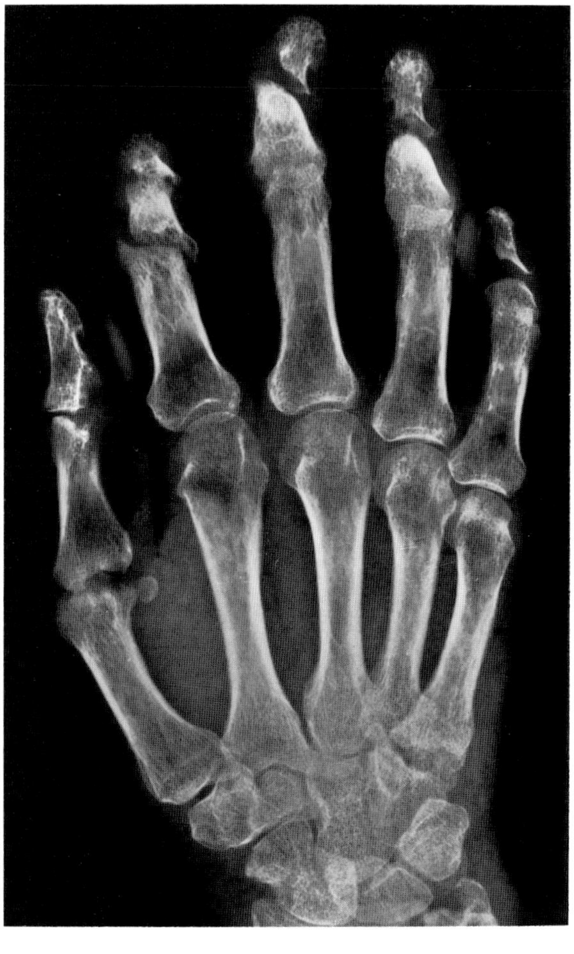

Fig. 5. Scleroderma in a 58-year-old man. Severe involvement of hand and wrist and the proximal end of fifth metacarpal. Erosive arthritis in several joints, destruction of many interphalangeal joints, partial disappearance of phalanges

7.6.4 Metastatic Fat Necrosis

Skeletal lesions caused by metastatic fat necrosis are encountered in patients with acute or subacute pancreatic diseases. An increased circulation of lipase in the blood stream hydrolyzes fat in the lipocytes to glycerol and fatty acids. Microscopically, the surrounding tissue shows an inflammatory reaction with lymphocytic infiltration, giant cells, and obliterating endarteritis. The last-named may lead to medullary ischemia and subsequent bone infarction. Involvement of the periarticular soft tissues and the synovial membrane results in polyarthritis.

Intramedullary foci of metastatic fat necrosis in pancreatic disease are usually present as a metadiaphyseally in the tubular bones of the hands and feet. In children the epiphyses are not affected [1–4].

Radiographic Findings [1–4]

Hand

Soft tissue swelling
Osteolytic lesions in metaphyses and diaphyses
Destruction of cortex
Periosteal new bone formation
Calcification of intramedullary lesions

Differential Diagnosis

Osteomyelitis (Sect. 7.3.3)
Sarcoidosis (Sect. 7.3.12)
Metastatic lesions (Sect. 7.4.2.5)
Sickle cell anemia
Leukemic dactylitis
Histiocytosis

References

1 Schutte HE, Wackwitz JD (1981) Case report 171. Skeletal Radiol 7:147–149
2 Immelman EJ, Bank S, Krige H, Marks IN (1964) Roentgenologic and clinical features of intramedul-

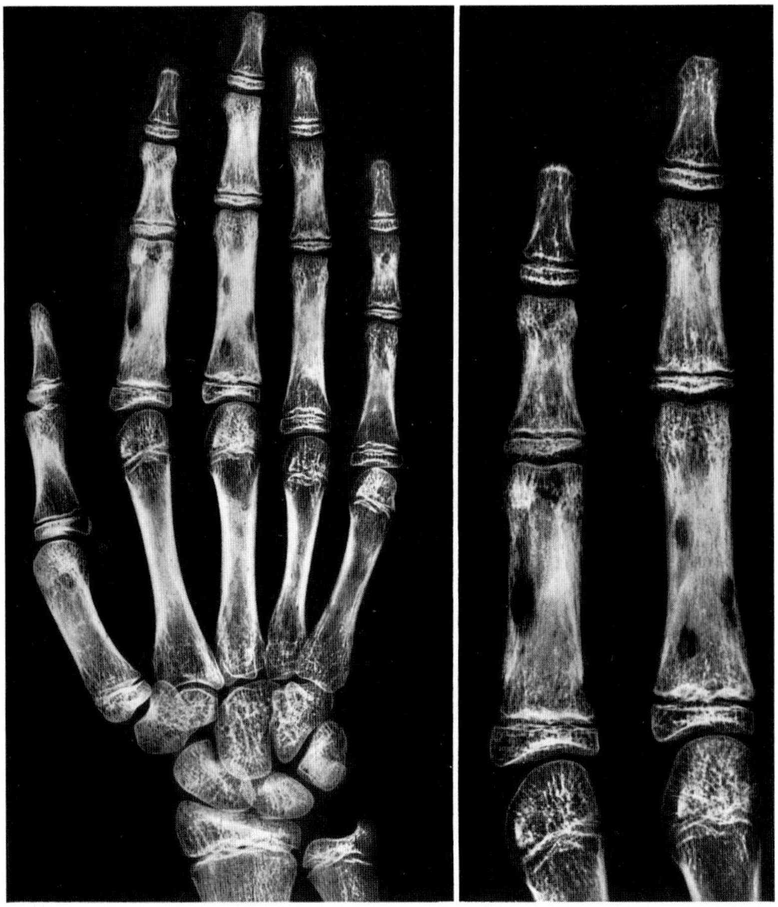

a b

Fig. 1 a, b. Metastatic fat necrosis after traumatic pancreatitis in a 12-year-old girl. Osteolytic lesions in proximal and middle phalanges of second finger with endosteal destruction of phalangeal cortex, osteolytic areas in proximal phalanx of third finger, epiphyses not affected

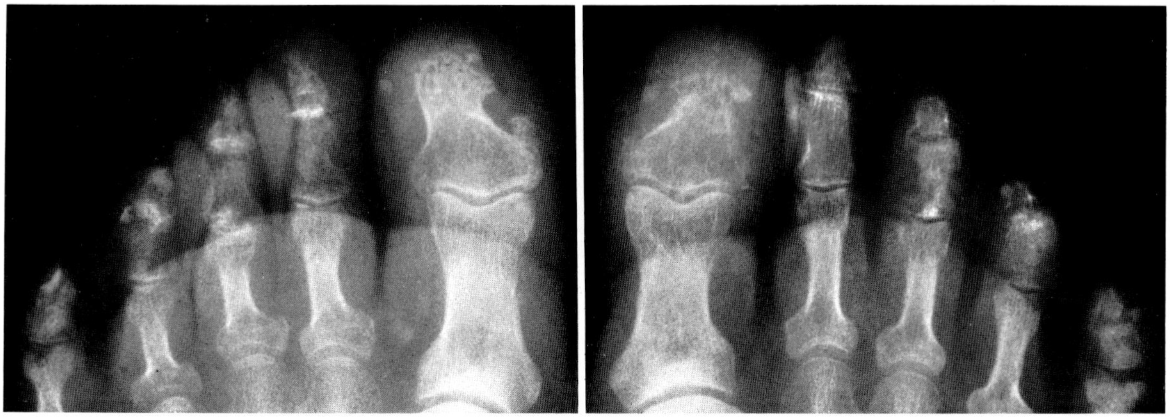

a b

Fig. 2a, b. Metastatic fat necrosis secondary to chronic pancreatitis in a 55-year-old woman. Multiple osteolytic lesions in phalanges of toes, especially in distal phalanx of right big toe (**b**)

lary fat necrosis in bones in acute and chronic pancreatitis. Am J Med 36:96–105

3 Boswell SH, Baylin GJ (1973) Metastatic fat necrosis and lytic bone lesions in patients with painless acute pancreatitis. Radiology 106:85–86

4 Hollingworth P, Isaacs D, Bydder Cr (1979) Recurrent osteolytic lesions and subcutaneous fat necrosis in association with a developmental pancreatic cyst. Arch Dis Child 54:790–792

7.6.5 Neuropathic Arthropathy

Synonym: Charcot's joint

Neuropathic arthropathy may develop in patients with neurological deficits. Common causes are syringomyelia and diabetes, and other less frequent causes are spina bifida, injuries to the brain and nervous system, tabes dorsalis, leprosy, and congenital insensitivity to pain. Neurovascular disregulation and infection are thought to be the most important reasons for the joint features. Misuse and abuse are additional factors.

Whatever the cause, a neurally initiated reflex leads to increased bone blood flow and bone resorption by osteoclasts [1]. Weight-bearing is an important etiologic factor in the development of neuropathic arthropathy. The hands are thus less commonly affected than the major joints, particularly those of the lower extremity.

Radiographic Findings [1–5]

Hand

Soft tissue swelling (joint effusion)
Narrowing of radiocarpal and intercarpal joints
(Sub)luxation
Bone fragments (intra-articular, periarticular)
Cyst formation
Marginal exostoses
Bone resorption (tufts, carpals, bone ends)
Pointed ends of tubular bones
Normal or increased bone density
Ossification of synovial membrane
Osteomyelitis

Differential Diagnosis

Scleroderma (Sect. 7.6.3)
Psoriatic arthritis (Sect. 7.3.6)
Rheumatoid arthritis (Sect. 7.3.4)
Osteoarthrosis (Sect. 7.3.13)
Chondrocalcinosis (Sect. 6.2.6)
Leprosy (Sect. 7.3.10)
Ehlers-Danlos syndrome

References

1 Brower AC, Allman RM (1981) Pathogenesis of the neurotrophic joint: neurotraumatic vs. neurovascular. Radiology 139:349–354

2 Norman A, Robbins H, Milgram JE (1968) The acute neuropathic arthropathy. A rapid severely disorganizing form of arthritis. Radiology 90:1159–1164

3 Resnick D, Niwayama G (1981) Diagnosis of bone and joint disorders. Saunders, Philadelphia

4 Seibert-Daiker FM (1978) Die Osteoarthrosis syringomyelica and ihre Fehldeutungen. Fortschr Geb Röntgenstr Nuklearmed Ergänzungsband 128:79–81

5 Banna M, Foster JB (1972) Roentgenologic features of acrodystrophic neuropathy. AJR 115:186–191

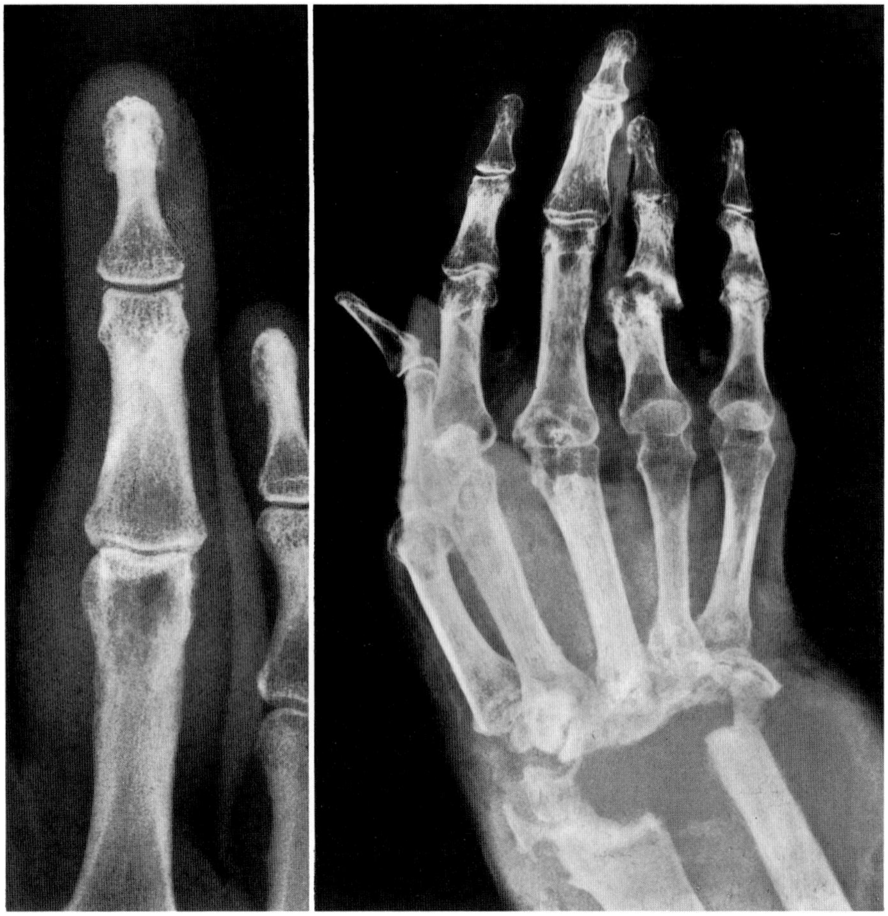

a b

Fig. 1a, b. Neuropathic arthropathy in a 60-year-old patient with syringomyelia. **a** Fourth finger of left hand: Osteolytic area at distal end of proximal phalanx, narrowing of proximal interphalangeal joint space, soft tissue swelling. **b** Left hand 3 years later: Severe neuropathic arthropathy, with disappearance of carpals, soft tissue swelling, involvement of several more distal joints

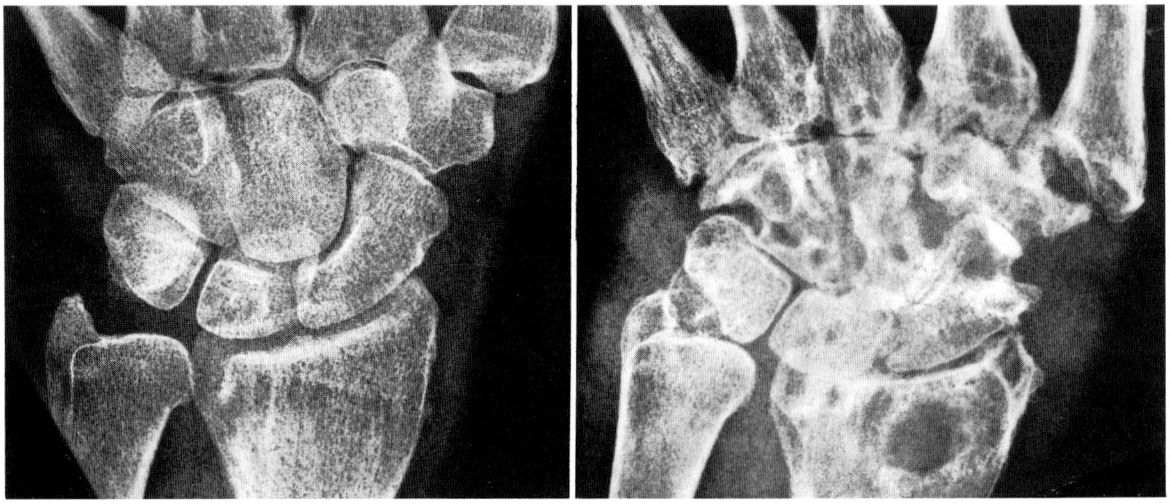

a b

Fig. 2a, b. Same patient as Fig. 1. Right hand. **a** 1972: normal aspect. **b** 1975: severe destruction of intercarpal and carpometacarpal joints

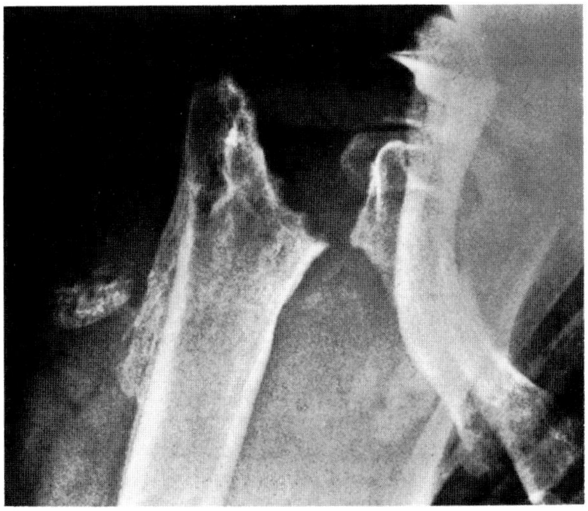

Fig. 3. Same patient. Destructive changes in right shoulder: Periarticular bony fragments, normal bone density, deformation of proximal end of humerus

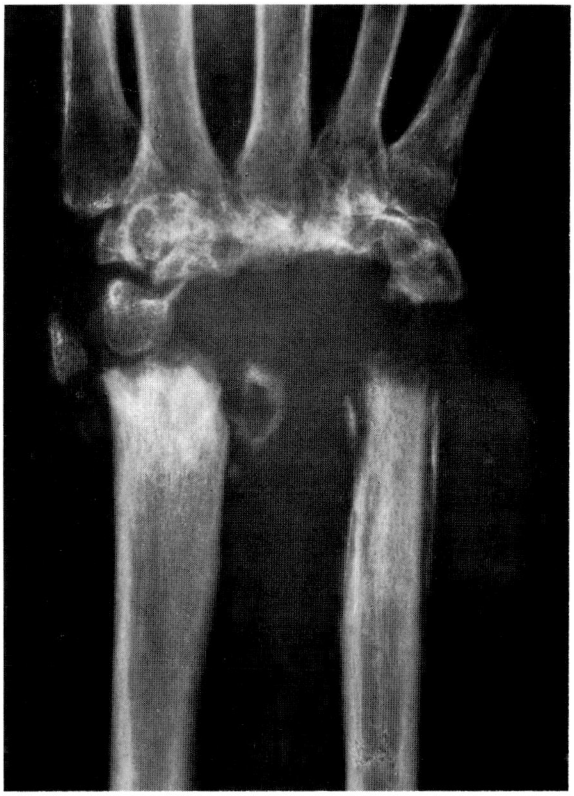

Fig. 4. Same patient 1976. Left hand. Severe destruction of carpals and of distal ends of radius and ulna, ossified masses in soft tissue

7.6.6 Thalassemia

Thalassemia is a hereditary anemia caused by an abnormality in the hemoglobin synthesis leading to erythroid hyperplasia in the bone marrow. There are two forms: The *homozygous* form, thalassemia major (*synonyms*: Cooley's anemia, Mediterranean anemia), is a serious disease involving anemia, hepatosplenomegaly, icterus, facial deformity, growth disturbance, and cardiac enlargement. The *heterozygous* form, thalassemia minor, is a disease usually yielding only mild clinical findings. Skeletal changes are usually detectable before the age of 2 years. Most children with severe thalassemia die before puberty, but modern forms of therapy have resulted in survival of a number of victims into adolescence and even into adult life, by which time the radiographic abnormalities in the peripheral skeleton may have disappeared completely. Severe abnormalities in the skeleton suggest thalassemia major rather then one of the other congenital anemias (congenital hemolytic anemia, sickle cell anemia, hereditary spherocytosis). Acquired anemias may also generate mild skeletal abnormalities.

Radiographic Findings [1–5]

Hand

Coarse trabecular pattern (destruction of some trabeculae and thickening of rest)
Thinning of cortex
Small cortical defects
Medullary widening (biconvex shafts)
Large nutrient foramina
Occasionally: retarded bone maturation
 fractures
 signs of secondary hemochromatosis (repeated transfusions)
 osteomyelitis

Other Sites

Skull: thickening of inner table
 thinning of outer table
 "hair on end" pattern of spiculae deposited by pericranial membrane
 widening of diploic spaces

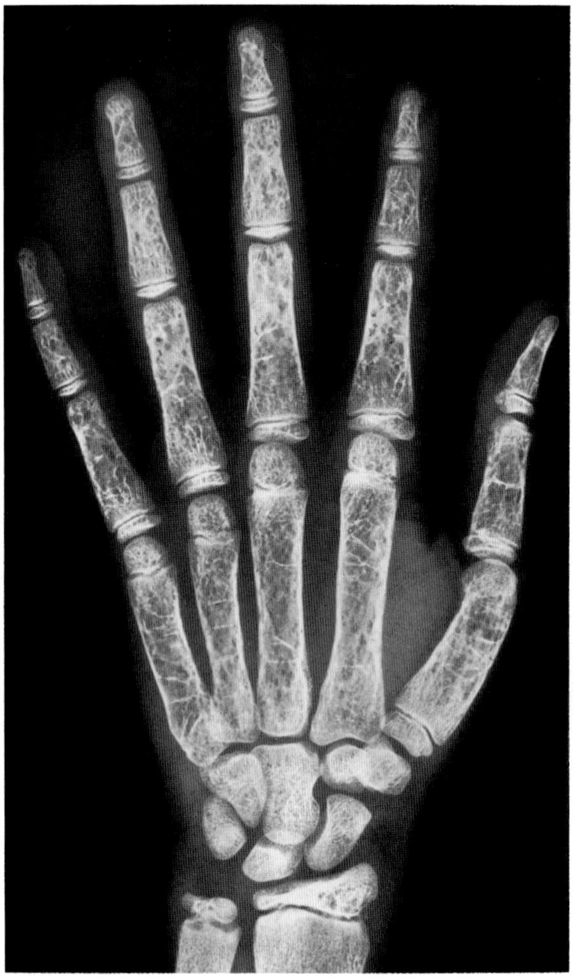

Fig. 1. Thalassemia major in a 15-year-old boy. Widening of tubular bones with cortical thinning, multiple small cortical defects, coarse trabecular pattern. Carpals relatively normal

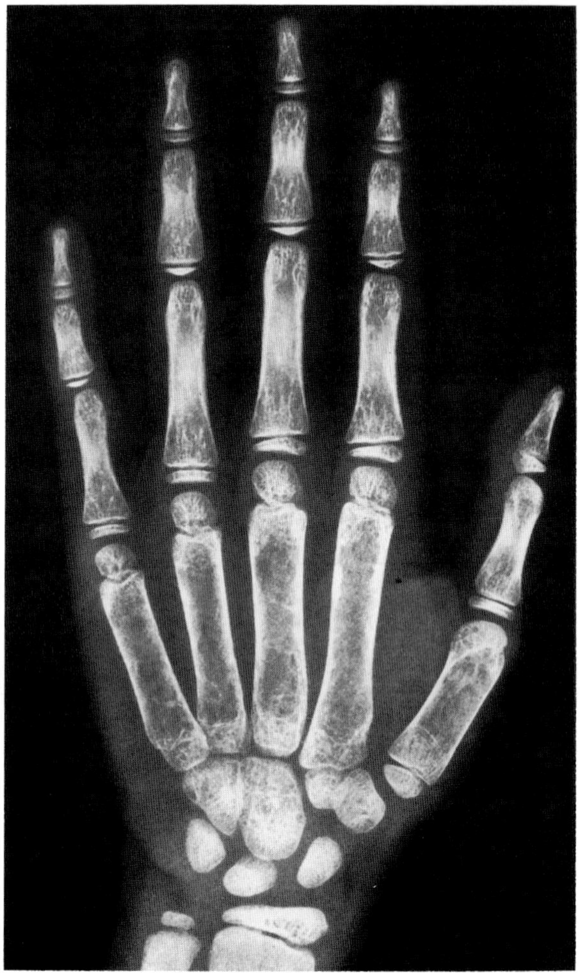

Fig. 2. Congenital hemolytic anemia in a 10-year-old girl. Widening of medullary cavities of metacarpals, cortical thinning, coarse and reticular trabecular pattern. Distal ends of radius and ulna, carpals, and phalanges all relatively normal

bony overgrowth of maxilla (characteristic)
dental abnormalities
malocclusion of jaws
decreased pneumatization of nasal sinuses
hypertelorism

Long tubular bones: bone structure abnormalities similar to those in hand
medullary hyperplasia
flask femora

Spine: reduced number of trabeculae and coarse trabecular pattern
biconcave deformities of vertebral bodies (fish vertebrae)
paravertebral soft tissue mass caused by extramedullary hematopoiesis

Foot: abnormalities corresponding to those in hand

Differential Diagnosis

Congenital hemolytic anemia
Sickle cell anemia
Spherocytosis
Severe acquired anemias

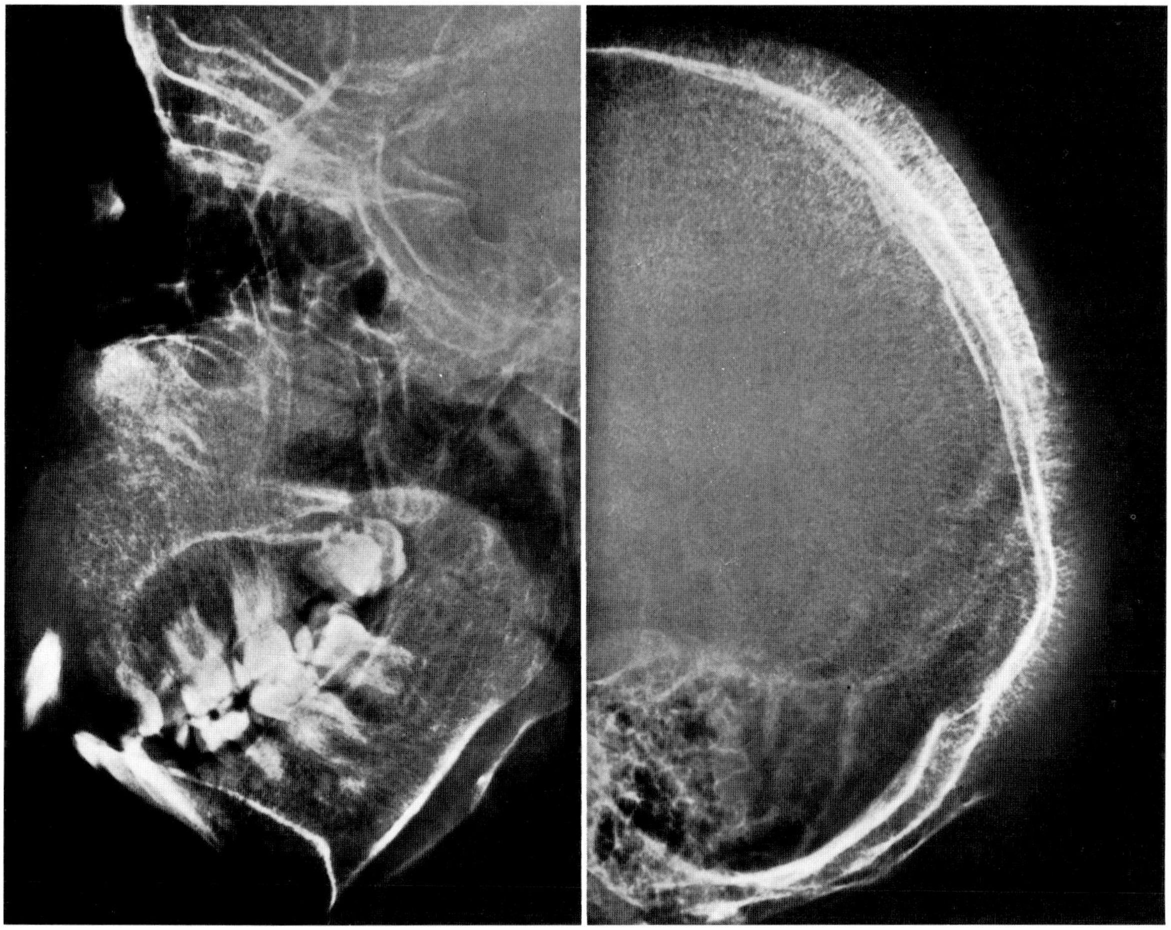

a b

Fig. 3 a, b. Same patient as Fig. 1. **a** Severe bony overgrowth of maxilla, absence of pneumatization of paranasal sinuses, dental abnormalities in maxilla. **b** "Hair on end pattern": spiculae deposited by pericranial membrane

References

1 Middlemiss JH, Raper AB (1966) Skeletal changes in the haemoglobinopathies. J Bone Joint Surg [Br] 48:693–701
2 Caffey J (1957) Cooley's anemia: a review of the roentgenographic findings in the skeleton. Hickey Lecture 1957. AJR 78:381–391
3 Moseley JE (1963) Bone changes in hematologic disorders (roentgen aspects). Grune and Stratton, New York
4 Resnick D, Niwayama G (1981) Diagnosis of bone and joint disorders. Saunders, Philadelphia
5 Currarino G, Erlandson ME (1964) Premature fusion of epiphyses in Cooley's anemia. Radiology 83:656–664

7.6.7 Systemic Mastocytosis

Synonym: urticaria pigmentosa

Mastocytosis is a rare chronic disease characterized by tissue mast cell infiltration of the reticuloendothelial system and the skin. A variety of organs may be involved. On the basis of the clinical features, five types of mastocytosis have been described. In systemic mastocytosis (about 10% of cases) the skin symptoms usually start in adulthood. In decreasing order of frequency the skeleton, liver, spleen, and gastrointestinal tract are also involved. Fifty-six percent of systemic mastocytosis sufferers present diffuse and 6% localized skeletal involvement. The skeletal lesions are due to mast cell proliferation in the bone marrow. Osteoporosis and osteosclerosis are usually present in a mixed pattern. The axial skeleton is particularly affected. Leukemia has been associated with the diffuse skeletal type of generalized mastocytosis [1, 2].

Radiographic Findings [2–7]

Hand

The changes in the hand are usually only minor.
Osteoporosis
Thickened and woven trabeculae
Osteosclerosis and narrowing of marrow space

Other Sites

Depending on the degree of skeletal involvement, localized or diffuse skeletal abnormalities (lytic or sclerotic) are found.
Long tubular bones: osteoporosis
lytic lesions surrounded by a zone of sclerosis
osteosclerosis
osteonecrosis
Skull, pelvis, spine: osteoporosis
lytic lesions surrounded by a zone of sclerosis
osteosclerosis (focal or diffuse)

Differential Diagnosis [2]

Osteoporosis: hyperparathyroidism (Sect. 6.2.3)
osteomalacia (Sect. 6.2.1)
multiple myeloma
Diffuse osteosclerosis: lymphoma
myelofibrosis
osteoblastic metastasis
fluorosis (Sect. 7.5.1)
oxalosis (Sect. 6.2.8)
renal osteodystrophy (Sect. 6.2.4)
Focal osteosclerosis: tuberous sclerosis (Sect. 7.1.2)
osteoblastic metastasis
Cystic lesions: sickle cell anemia
Gaucher's disease
multiple myeloma

References

1 Sagher F, Even Paz Z (1967) Mastocytosis and the mast cell. Karger, Basel
2 Resnick D, Niwayama G (1981) Diagnosis of bone and joint disorders. Saunders, Philadelphia
3 Jensen WN, Lasser EC (1958) Urticaria pigmentosa associated with widespread sclerosis of the spongiosa of bone. Radiology 71:826–832
4 Poppel MH, Gruber WF, Silber R, Holder AD, Christman RO (1959) The roentgen manifestations of urticaria pigmentosa (mastocytosis). AJR 82:239–249
5 Barer M, Peterson LFA, Dahlin DC, Winkelmann RK, Stewart JR (1968) Mastocytosis with osseous lesions resembling metastatic malignant lesions in bone. J Bone Joint Surg [Am] 50:142–152
6 Lucaya J, Perez-Candela J, Aso C, Calvo J (1979) Mastocytosis with skeletal and gastro-intestinal involvement in infancy. Radiology 131:363–366
7 Rohner HG, Bartl R, Koischwitz D, Rodermund OE (1982) Haut- und Knochenbefunde bei der Mastozytose. Radiologe 22:545–552

Fig. 3a, b. Systemic mastocytosis in a 46-year-old ▷ man. **a** 1964: Two small lytic areas in skull. **b** 1980: Enlargement of lytic lesions and progressive skull thickening

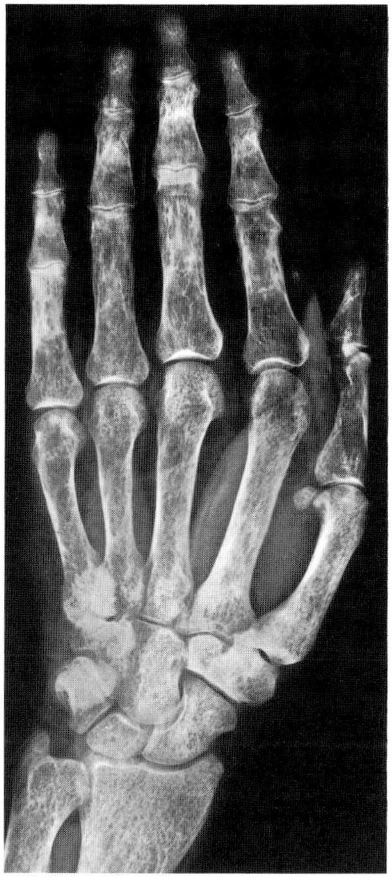

a

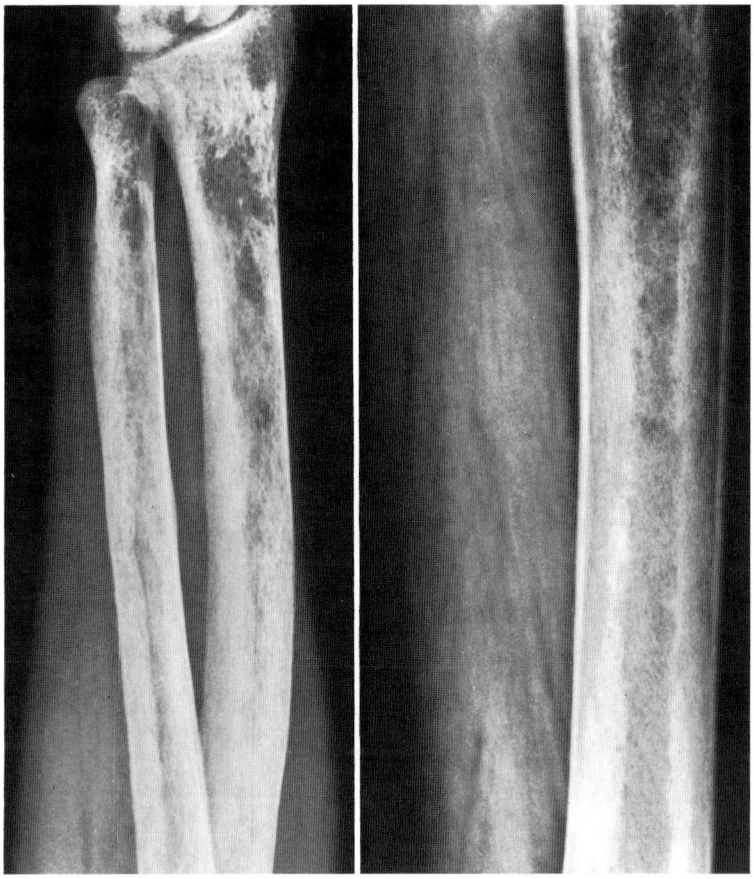

b

Fig. 1. Systemic mastocytosis in a 55-year-old man. Osteoporosis and cortical thinning of phalanges, rather dense metacarpals with a woven trabecular pattern, dense carpals, sclerosis of distal radius and ulna

Fig. 2a, b. Same patient as Fig. 1. **a** Forearm: Narrow medullary cavity, osteosclerosis. Some periosteal bone apposition seems to be present. **b** Cortical thickening of femur, narrow medullary cavity, some periosteal bone apposition

a

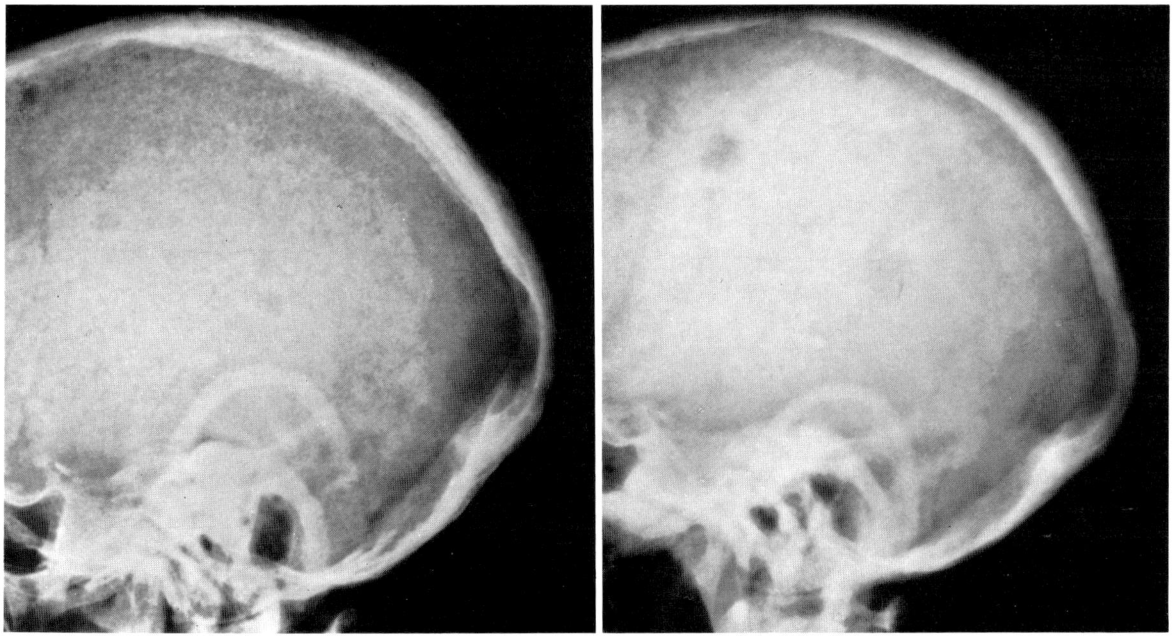

b

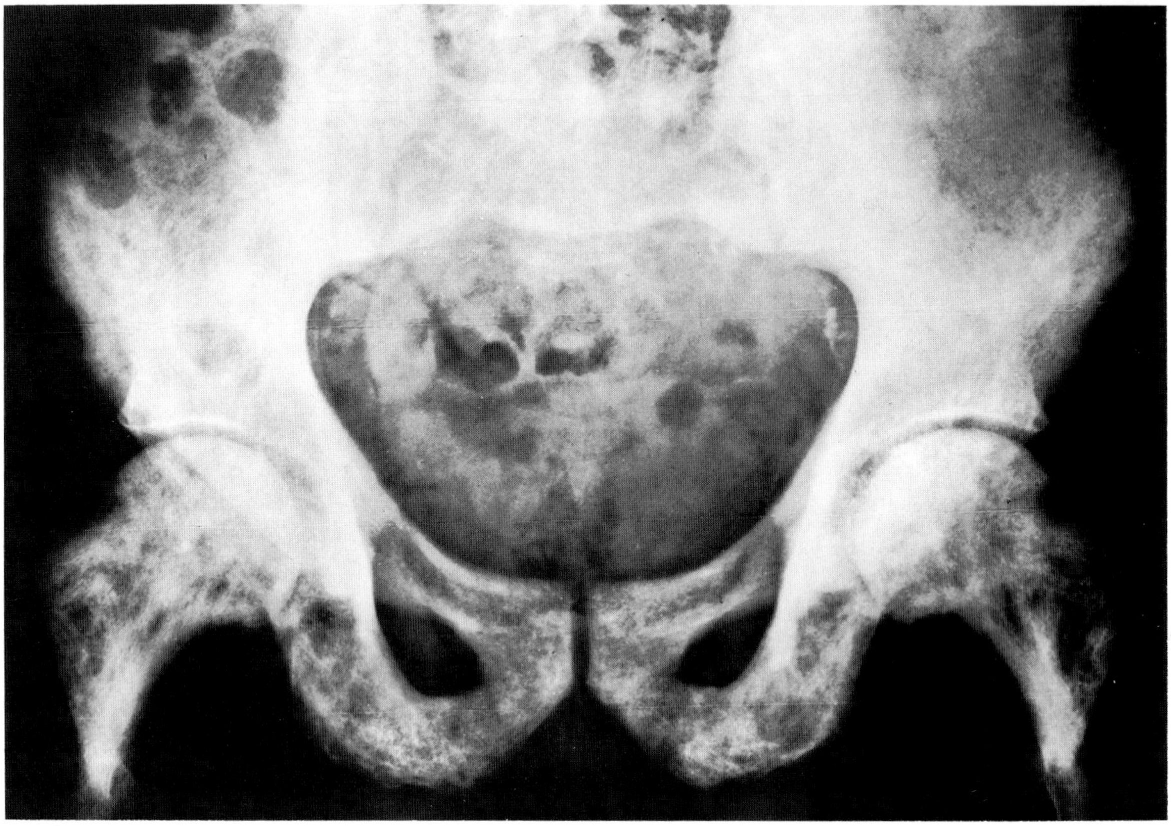

Fig. 4. Same patient as Fig. 3. Mixed osteosclerotic and osteolytic lesions in pelvis, vertebral bodies, and proximal ends of femora

7.6.8 Periosteal New Bone Formation

Periosteal new bone formation along the tubular bones of the hand may be found in a large number of conditions [1, 2].

1. Trauma:
   thermal burns
   healing fracture
   periosteal hematoma
   battered child
2. Osteomyelitis:
   pyogenic arthritis (Sect. 7.3.2)
   tuberculosis (Sect. 7.3.9)
   leprosy (Sect. 7.3.10)
   yaws (Sect. 7.3.11)
   syphilis (Sect. 7.3.1)
   mycetoma
3. Hypertrophic osteoarthropathy [3]
   Thoracic causes: carcinoma of lung
   mesothelioma
   lymphoma
   pulmonary abscess
   bronchiectasis
   pulmonary emphysema
   pulmonary metastases
   cyanotic congenital heart diseases
   pulmonary arteriovenous fistula
   tumor of ribs
   Extrathoracic causes: ulcerative colitis [4]
   dysentery
   lymphoma
   Whipple's disease
   biliary cirrhosis (Sect. 7.3.13)
   cystic fibrosis
   thyroid acropachy [5]
   Takayasu disease
4. Pachydermoperiostosis (Sect. 1.2.8)
5. Rheumatoid arthritis (Sect. 7.3.4)
6. Juvenile rheumatoid arthritis (Sect. 7.3.5)
7. Psoriatic arthritis (Sect. 7.3.6)
8. Reiter's syndrome (Sect. 7.3.7)
9. Sarcoidosis (Sect. 7.3.12)

10. Bone tumors:
    benign (Sect. 7.4.1)
    malignant (Sect. 7.4.2)
        primary
        secondary
    tumor-like conditions (Sect. 7.4.3)
11. Rickets (Sect. 6.2.1)
12. Scurvy (Sect. 6.2.5)
13. Multifocal recurrent periostitis [2]
14. Metastatic fat necrosis (Sect. 7.6.4)
15. Hemophilia
16. Leukemia
17. Sickle cell anemia (Sect. 7.3.3)
18. Fluorosis (Sect. 7.5.1)
19. Hypervitaminosis D (Sect. 6.2.2)
20. Hypervitaminosis A
21. Melorheostosis (Sect. 1.2.6)
22. Tuberous sclerosis (Sect. 7.1.2)
23. Periarteritis nodosa [1]

References

1 Resnick D, Niwayama G (1981) Diagnosis of bone and joint disorders. Saunders, Philadelphia
2 Kozlowski K, Anderson R, Tink A (1981) Multifocal recurrent periostitis. Fortschr Geb Röntgenstr Nuklearmed Ergänzungsband 5:597–602
3 Hammersten JF, O'Leary J (1957) The features and significance of hypertrophic osteoarthropathy. Arch Intern Med 99:431–433
4 Arlart I, Bargon G (1981) Periostale Knochenneubildung bei Colitis ulcerosa im jugendlichen Alter. Fortschr Geb Röntgenstr Nuklearmed Ergänzungsband 135:577–582
5 Scanlon GT, Clemett AR (1964) Thyroid acropachy. Radiology 83:1039–1042

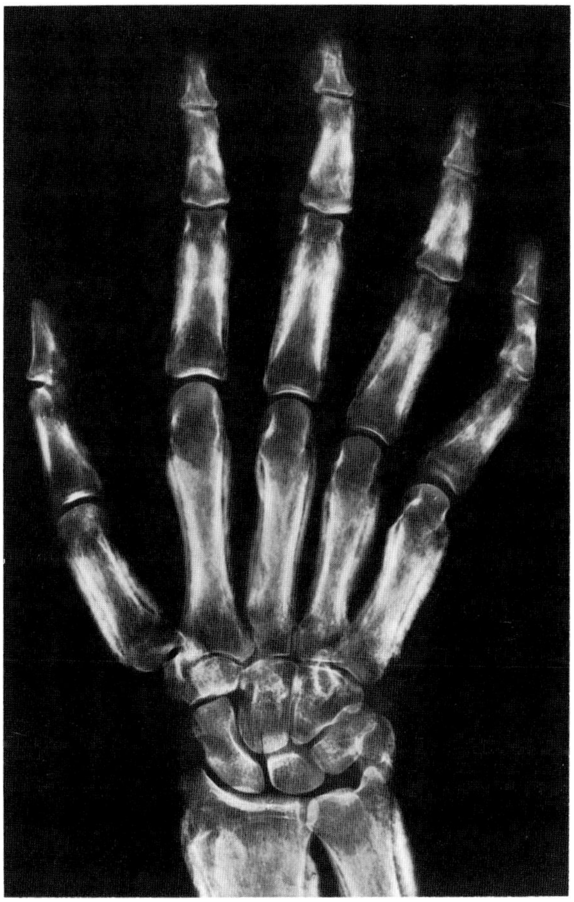

Fig. 1. Hypertrophic osteoarthropathy in a patient with pulmonary carcinoma. Huge periosteal new bone formation along tubular bones of hand and wrist

Figs. 2 and 3 see page 288

Fig. 2a, b. Hypertrophic osteoarthropathy in two patients with pulmonary carcinoma

Fig. 3a–c. Periosteal new bone formation. **a** In vitamin D deficiency rickets. **b, c** Periosteal reaction in a 13-year-old girl with juvenile rheumatoid arthritis

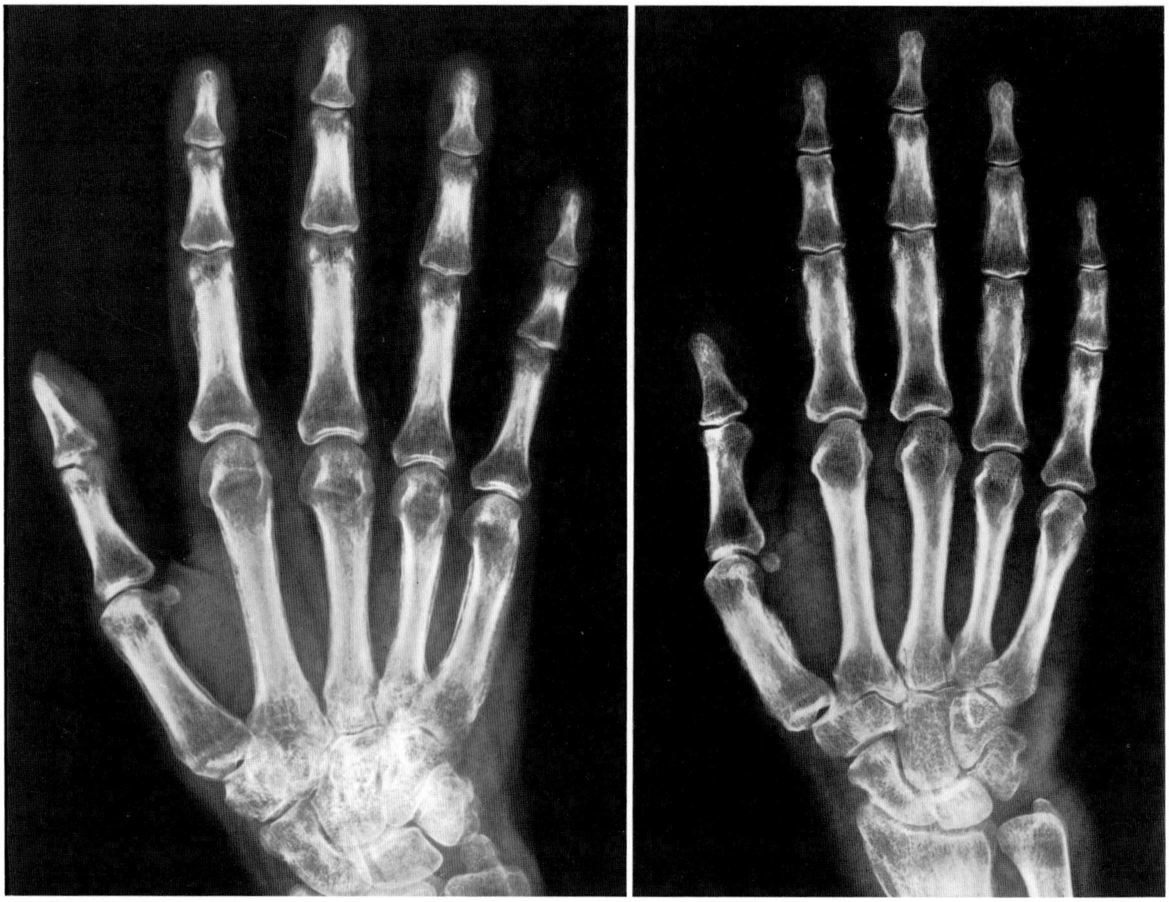

a b

Fig 2a, b. Legend see page 287

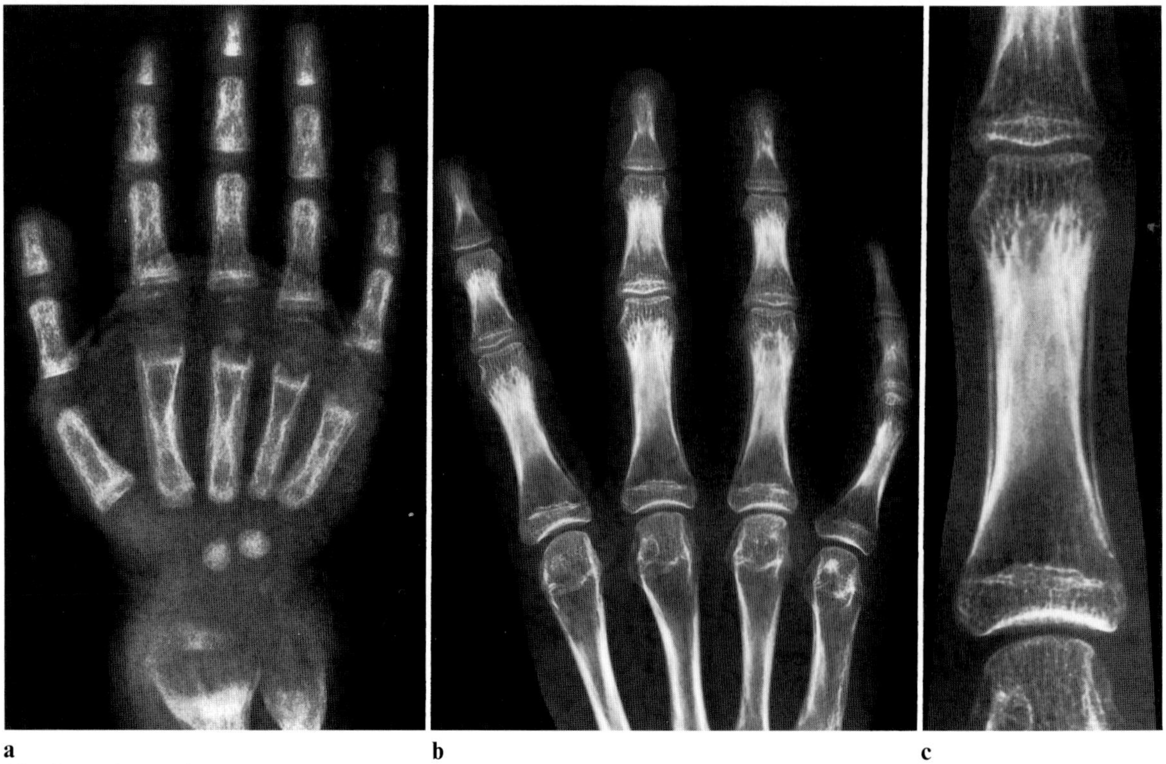

a b c

Fig. 3a–c. Legend see page 287

Fig. 4a–c. Hypertrophic osteoarthropathy in a 46-year-old woman with biliary cirrhosis and osteomalacia (details of second finger and fifth metacarpal)

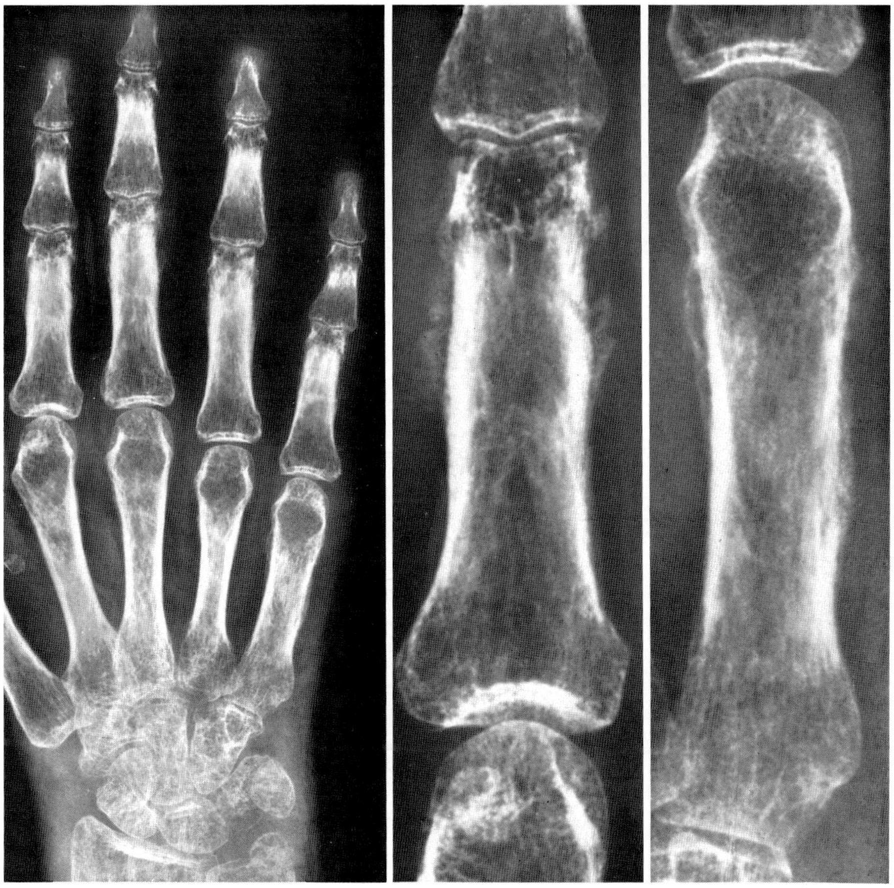

a b c

Fig. 5a, b. Periosteal new bone formation. **a** Psoriatic arthritis. **b** Reiter's syndrome

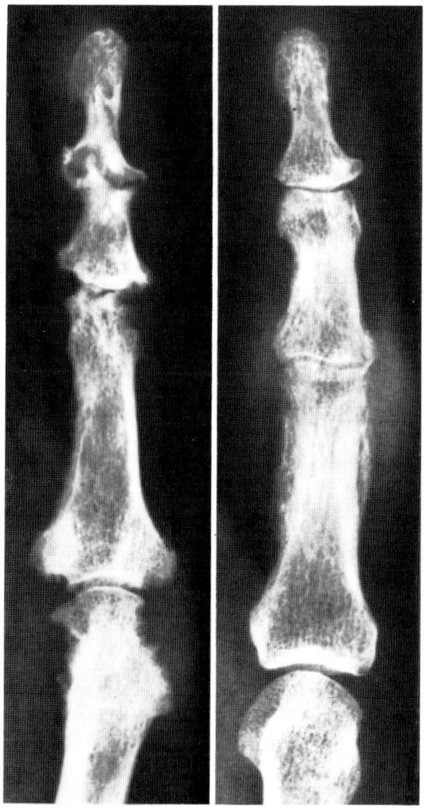

5a b

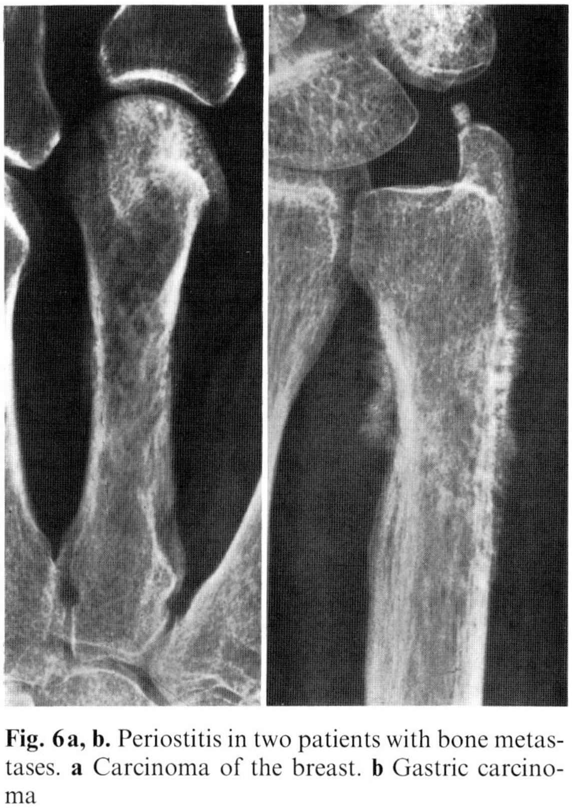

a b

Fig. 6a, b. Periostitis in two patients with bone metastases. **a** Carcinoma of the breast. **b** Gastric carcinoma

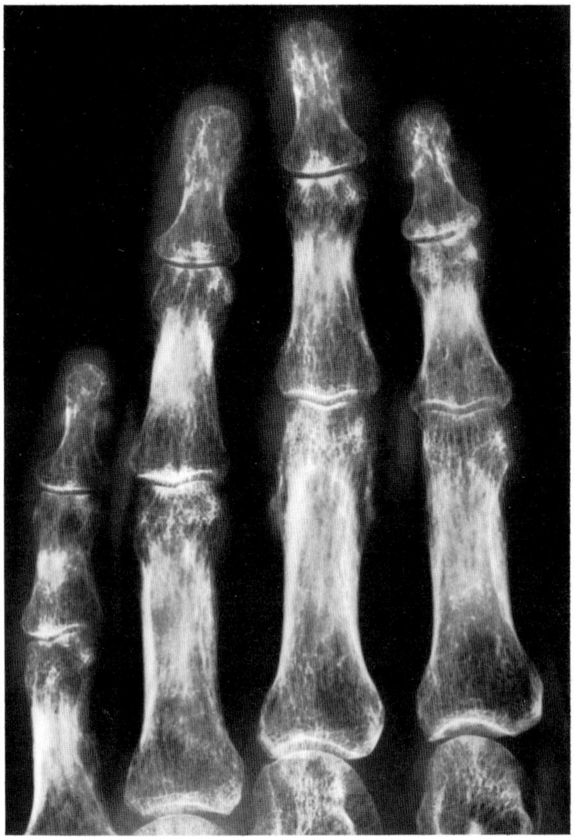

Fig. 7. Periosteal reaction in a 53-year-old patient with hairy cell leukemia

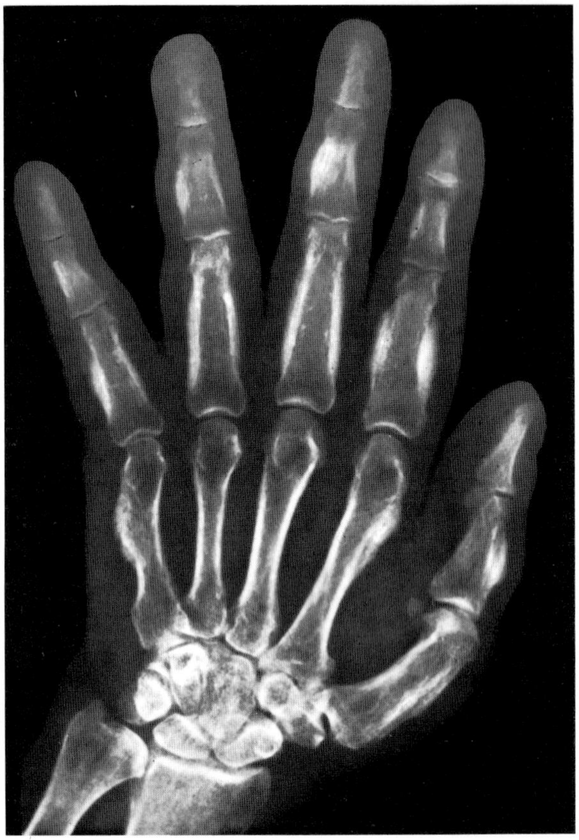

Fig. 8. Thyroid acropachy in an adult patient. Soft tissue swelling and extensive periosteal new bone formation around most phalanges and metacarpals. Periosteal bone formation may be encountered in thyrotoxic patients and in euthyroid and hypothyroid patients who previously suffered from thyrotoxicosis

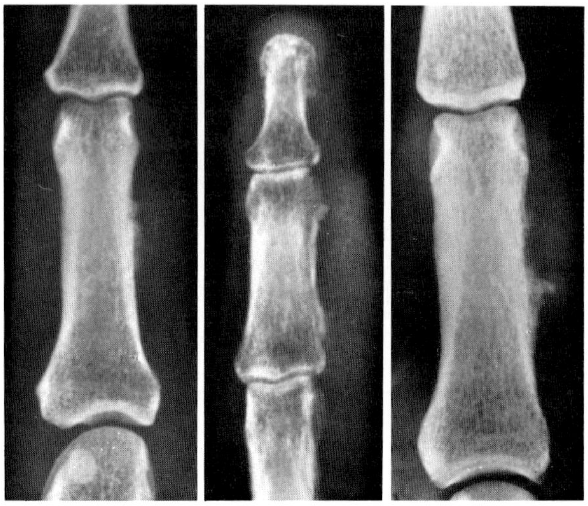

a **b** **c**

Fig. 9a–c. Reactive periosteal new bone formation. **a** In a 41-year-old woman: Slight periosteal ossification, probably post-traumatic. **b** In a 32-year-old woman: Soft tissue swelling with tiny calcifications, probably post-traumatic. Formation of a periosteal bone layer. **c** In a 40-year-old man: Periosteal fibroma with soft tissue swelling and ossification

Subject Index